International Handbook of
Human Response to Trauma

The Plenum Series on Stress and Coping

Series Editor:
Donald Meichenbaum, *University of Waterloo, Waterloo, Ontario, Canada*

Current Volumes in the Series:

BEYOND TRAUMA
Cultural and Societal Dynamics
Edited by Rolf J. Kleber, Charles R. Figley, and Berthold P. R. Gersons

COMMUTING STRESS
Causes, Effects, and Methods of Coping
Meni Koslowsky, Avraham N. Kluger, and Mordechai Reich

COPING WITH CHRONIC STRESS
Edited by Benjamin H. Gottlieb

ETHNICITY, IMMIGRATION, AND PSYCHOPATHOLOGY
Edited by Ihsan Al-Issa and Michael Tousignant

HANDBOOK OF SOCIAL SUPPORT AND THE FAMILY
Edited by Gregory R. Pierce, Barabara R. Sarason, and Irwin G. Sarason

INTERNATIONAL HANDBOOK OF HUMAN RESPONSE TO TRAUMA
Edited by Arieh Y. Shalev, Rachel Yehuda, and Alexander C. McFarlane

INTERNATIONAL HANDBOOK OF MULTIGENERATIONAL LEGACIES OF TRAUMA
Edited by Yael Danieli

PSYCHOTRAUMATOLOGY
Key Papers and Core Concepts in Post-Traumatic Stress
Edited by George S. Everly, Jr. and Jeffrey M. Lating

STRESS, CULTURE, AND COMMUNITY
The Psychology and Philosophy of Stress
Stevan E. Hobfoll

TRAUMATIC STRESS
From Theory to Practice
Edited by John R. Freedy and Stevan E. Hobfoll

International Handbook of Human Response to Trauma

Edited by

Arieh Y. Shalev
Hadassah University Hospital
Jerusalem, Israel

Rachel Yehuda
Mount Sinai School of Medicine
Bronx, New York

and

Alexander C. McFarlane
Queen Elizabeth Hospital
Woodville, South Australia, Australia

Kluwer Academic / Plenum Publishers
New York, Boston, Dordrecht, London, Moscow

ISBN 0-306-46095-5

©2000 Kluwer Academic / Plenum Publishers
233 Spring Street, New York, N.Y. 10013

10 9 8 7 6 5 4 3 2 1

A C.I.P. record for this book is available from the Library of Congress.

To Mrs. Vered Shalev,
a true healer of the soul, whose initiative it was to create this book

Contributors

Libby Tata Arcel, International Rehabilitation Council for Torture Victims, DK-1014, Copenhagen K, Denmark; and Institute of Psychology, University of Copenhagen, DK-2300, Copenhagen S, Denmark

Amit Anand, Department of Psychiatry, VA Medical Center, Yale University School of Medicine, West Haven, Connecticut 06516

Alexandra Argenti-Pillen, Department of Anthropology, University College London, London, WC1E 6BT, England

Dan Bar-On, Department of Behavioral Sciences, Ben Gurion University of the Negev, 84105, Beersheva, Israel

Dora Black, Traumatic Stress Clinic, London, W1P 1LB, England

Sandra L. Bloom, Alliance for Creative Development, P.C., Quakertown, Pennsylvania, 18951-4146

Stanley Bone, Columbia Center for Psychoanalytic Training and Research, New York Psychiatric Institute, New York, New York 10032

Omer Bonne, Center for Traumatic Stress, Department of Psychiatry, Hadassah University Hospital, Jerusalem, 91120, Israel

J. Douglas Bremner, Department of Psychiatry, VA Medical Center, Yale University School of Medicine, West Haven, Connecticut, 06516

Danny Brom, AMCHA, The National Israeli Center for Psychosocial Support of Survivors of the Holocaust and the Second Generation, Jerusalem 93385, Israel

Laura S. Brown, Seattle, WA 98105-4801

Ingrid V. E. Carlier, Department of Psychiatry, Academic Medical Center, University of Amsterdam, Amsterdam, 1101 BC, The Netherlands

Dennis S. Charney, Department of Psychiatry, VA Medical Center, Yale University School of Medicine, West Haven, Connecticut 06516

Carole B. Corcoran, Department of Psychology, Mary Washington College, Fredericksburg, Virginia 22401

D. Cyril D'Souza, Department of Psychiatry, VA Medical Center, Yale University School of Medicine, West Haven, Connecticut 06516

Nancy Dubrow, Taylor Institute, Chicago, Illinois 60622

Edna B. Foa, University of Pennsylvania Health System, Center for the Treatment and Study of Anxiety, Philadelphia, Pennsylvania 19104

Lisa M. Fisher, National Center for Posttraumatic Stress Disorder, Boston Veterans Affairs Medical Center, Boston, Massachusetts 02130

Sara Freedman, Center for Traumatic Stress, Department of Psychiatry, Hadassah University Hospital, Jerusalem, 91120, Israel

Matthew J. Friedman, Veterans Affairs National Center for Post-Traumatic Stress Disorder, White River Junction, Vermont 05009

Merle Friedman, Psych-Action, Sandton, 2046, South Africa

Lisa A. Goodman, Department of Psychology, University of Maryland, College Park, Maryland, 20742

Bonnie L. Green, Department of Psychiatry, Georgetown University, Washington DC, 20007

Stevan E. Hobfoll, Department of Psychology, Kent State University, Kent, Ohio 44242

B. Hudnall Stamm, Institute of Rural Health Studies, Idaho State University, Pocatello, Idaho 83209-8174

Moshe Kotler, Mental Health Center, Faculty of Health Sciences, Ben Gurion University of the Negev, Beersheva, 84015, Israel

Karen E. Krinsley, National Center for Posttraumatic Stress Disorder, Boston Veterans Affairs Medical Center, Boston, Massachusetts 02130

John H. Krystal, Department of Psychiatry, VA Medical Center, Yale University School of Medicine, West Haven, Connecticut 06516

Harold Kudler, Durham Veterans Affairs Medical Center, Durham, North Carolina 27705

Shmuel Lahad, The Community Stress Prevention Center, Tel Hai Academic College, Kiryat Shmona, 11012, Israel

Israel Liberzon, Department of Psychiatry, University of Michigan, Ann Arbor VAMC, Ann Arbor, Michigan, 48105

Randall D. Marshall, Anxiety Disorders Clinic, New York State Psychiatric Institute, New York, New York 10032

Alexander C. McFarlane, Department of Psychiatry, The Queen Elizabeth Hospital, University of Adelaide, Woodville, South Australia 5011, Australia

Elizabeth A. Meadows, Department of Psychology, Central Michigan University, Mt. Pleasant, Michigan 48859

Thomas Alan Mellman, Dartmouth Hitchcock Medical Center, Department of Psychiatry, Lebanon, New Hampshire 03756-0001

Jeannine Monnier, National Crime Victims Research and Treatment Center, Medical University of South Carolina, Charleston, South Carolina 29425

Elana Newman, University of Tulsa, Tulsa Oklahoma, 74104

Martin Newman, St. George's Hospital, London, SW17 0RE, England

Barbara L. Niles, National Center for Posttraumatic Stress Disorder, Boston Veterans Affairs Medical Center, Boston, Massachusetts 02130

Shulamit Niv, The Community Stress Prevention Center, Tel Hai Academic College, Kiryat Shmona, 11012, Israel

Gwenneth Lilian Roberts, Department of Psychiatry, University of Queensland Child and Youth Mental Health Service, Fortitude Valley, Queensland 4006, Australia

Sue Robinson, Institute of Psychiatry, London and Heathlands Mental Health Trust, London, W6 7HH, England

Yehuda Shachem, The Community Stress Prevention Center, Tel Hai Academic College, Kiryat Shmona, 11012, Israel

Arieh Y. Shalev, Center for Traumatic Stress, Department of Psychiatry, Hadassah University Hospital, Jerusalem, 91120, Israel

Derrick Silove, Psychiatry Research and Teaching Unit, Liverpool Hospital, Liverpool, NSW 2170, Australia

Steven M. Southwick, Department of Psychiatry, VA Medical Center, Yale University School of Medicine, West Haven, Connecticut 06516

Zachary Steel, Psychiatry Research and Teaching Unit, Liverpool Hospital, Liverpool, NSW 2170, Australia

Stephan F. Taylor, Department of Psychiatry, University of Michigan, Ann Arbor VAMC, Ann Arbor, Michigan 48105

Onno Van der Hart, Department of Clinical Psychology, Utrecht University, Utrecht, The Netherlands; and Cato-Polm Institute, Zeist, The Netherlands

Eliezer Witztum, Mental Health Center, Faculty of Health Sciences, Ben Gurion University of the Negev, Beersheva, 84105, Israel

Rachel Yehuda, Mount Sinai School of Medicine, Posttraumatic Stress Disorder Program, Bronx Veterans Affairs Medical Center, Bronx, New York 10468

Allan Young, Department of Social Studies of Medicine, McGill University, Montreal, Quebec, H3C 1Y6, Canada

Sahika Yüksel, Istanbul-Psychosocial Trauma Programs, Department of Psychiatry, University of Istanbul, Topkapi, Istanbul, Turkey

Preface

In 1996, representatives from 27 different countries met in Jerusalem to share ideas about traumatic stress and its impact. For many, this represented the first dialogue that they had ever had with a mental health professional from another country. Many of the attendees had themselves been exposed to either personal trauma or traumatizing stories involving their patients, and represented countries that were embroiled in conflicts with each other. Listening to one another became possible because of the humbling humanity of each participant, and the accuracy and objectivity of the data presented. Understanding human traumatization had thus become a common denominator, binding together all attendees. This book tries to capture the spirit of the Jerusalem World Conference on Traumatic Stress, bringing forward the diversities and commonalties of its constructive discourse.

In trying to structure the various themes that arose, it was all too obvious that paradigms of different ways of conceiving of traumatic stress should be addressed first. In fact, the very idea that psychological trauma can result in mental health symptoms that should be treated has not yet gained universal acceptability. Even within medicine and mental health, competing approaches about the impact of trauma and the origins of symptoms abound. Part I discusses how the current paradigm of traumatic stress disorder developed within the historical, social, and process contexts. It also grapples with some of the difficulties that are presented by this paradigm from anthropologic, ethical, and scientific perspectives.

In reflecting on the vulnerability of the current traumatic stress paradigm as reflected by both of the official classification of diseases (i.e., the *Diagnostic and Statistical Manual of Mental Disorders—Fourth Edition* and the *International Classification of Diseases—Tenth Edition*), we realized that the paradigm of traumatic stress implies certain truths that may also not be shared by other cultures. We felt that the issue of cultural diversity in understanding ways to evaluate trauma and the responses to it must follow from a discussion of intellectual and historical origins of the current paradigm. Part II discusses the issue of how traumatic stress is perceived in different cultures.

One of the striking themes of the conference was the commonality of the experience of victimization of women and children worldwide. Although the specific expression of this type of victimization may depend on social and cultural variables, it was impressive that such experiences were ubiquitous. Part III examines how different societies experience and treat the effects of victimization in women and children.

In order to establish the fact of ubiquitous traumatization and its effects, the careful recording and assessment of the facts are essential. On the other hand, much of the currently available literature cannot be currently apprehended and evaluated without understanding the strengths and limitations of systematic descriptions. Part IV therefore focuses on the question of how stable knowledge about trauma and its effects can be generated, recorded, and be made accessible to all.

Among the most salient commonality is the neurobiological template that underlies and determines the human response to stress. While the length of this section does not do justice to the many biological findings that have been accrued in the last decade, it is included within this volume to underscore the potential utility and the enormous relevance of neuroscientific research to questions regarding how human beings may be similar but also dissimilar in their responses to stress. Certainly neurobiology has the potential of adding an important perspective on the expression of the traumatic stress response across gender, society, and culture. Part V provides an accessible review of four major areas in the neurobiology of human responses to trauma.

Discussions about the effect of traumatic stress on individuals and society are incomplete when they do not lead to constructive solutions for alleviating suffering. Part VI consists of a review of three major treatment approaches for Post-Traumatic Stress Disorder (PTSD) as well as for the acutely traumatized individual. Although there is currently no "gold standard" for treating trauma survivors, the six chapters presented provide the clinician with a range of therapeutic tools in order to optimize their treatment of such patients. In view of the effects of trauma on society and culture, treating trauma requires more than attention to the individual and must extend to healing societies of the forces that give rise to, and perpetuate individual and group victimization. The final section (Part VII) of this volume brings forward the courageous efforts among mental health professionals to extend insights gained from the traumatic stress paradigm to heal the larger community.

Work such as this is never done without substantial help from others. In the case of this volume, both organizations and individuals have been supportive and instrumental. We first wish to acknowledge the role of the International Society for Traumatic Stress Studies in sponsoring and supporting the 1996 World Conference, at a time when Jerusalem had been the site of repeated terrorist attacks and uncertainty prevailed. Particular thanks are due to the Society's board of directors and to its successive presidents—Matt Friedman, Terry Keane, and Sandy Bloom—for authorizing the publication of the Society's pamphlet "Childhood Trauma Remembered" (see Appendix) and the unpublished History of the Society (see Chapter 3). Special thanks are due to members of the Center for Traumatic Stress at Hadassah University Hospital, Jerusalem—Sara Freedman and Rivka Tuval-Mashiach—for continuously communicating with authors from five continents and for patiently knitting disparate messages, addresses, and unreadable computer files into one unit. Thanks are also due to Emily Collins of the Queen Elizabeth Hospital (South Adelaide) and to members of the PTSD Research Program at the Bronx VA Hospital for editorial help. Finally, Plenum Press (later Kluwer Academic / Plenum Publishers), and particularly Eliot Werner and Anne Meagher, must be congratulated for having brought this series of disparate discourses, often conceived in languages other than English, into one coherent and well-organized volume.

Contents

I

Human Response to Trauma:
An Evolving Paradigm

The development of a body of knowledge in a particular discipline is a complex process. People become familiar with ideas and often simply repackage them in these days of mass communication. Yet, knowledge accumulates with time, ending by challenging theories and assumptions on which such knowledge was originally sought. Such movements, however, can hardly be captured by reading the specifics of each published article, each piece of the puzzle. Books such as this one offer time for reflection and for drawing the larger picture. Moreover, a complete picture of one's own field cannot be obtained by the sole observations of insiders—hence the need to invite and accommodate outsider critique.

In this section, we begin by reminding the reader that any paradigm has limitations. That there are psychological responses as a direct consequence of trauma exposure represents a current paradigm, but one that may be subject to modification and revision. Indeed, in recent years, this paradigm has needed to expand to accommodate ideas coming from different fields of knowledge that challenge the linear relationship between trauma and response. The longevity of the field depends on its ability to accommodate the diversity of approaches while maintaining the centrality of the impact of human traumatization. Harold Kudler warns us about the danger of simplistic paradigms, and simplistically discarding previous views as irrelevant or outdated. He points to analogies in our understanding of medical diseases in which single-etiology theories have long since been challenged. The dilemma raised by complex, multifactorial etiologies is highlighted in discussions of treatment of trauma survivors. Simplistic paradigms carry the risk of repeatedly implementing partial and ineffective solutions to complex realities. It is indeed necessary to remember that the theories and paradigms presented later in this volume are to be seen in the context of working hypotheses rather than absolute conclusions.

One of the ways to judge current ideas is by viewing them from the lens of the past. Assessing the novelty of new ideas requires an understanding of old ones. However, historical knowledge may also be fraught with posthoc inaccuracies and subjective distortions of project current ideologies. Moreover, past documents may be easily misread in the absence of knowledge about their context. Alexander McFarlane's venture into history provides us with a sophisticated analysis stressing the importance of historical context and demonstrating how history can be conveniently reinterpreted to suit current ideologies. McFarlane demonstrates that debates such as those currently ongoing in the field have been previously held one hundred years ago. At the same time, these demonstrations invite the reader to consider information that may not have made it either into the archives of history or current renditions of it. Such reflection on the life and death of ideas and practices is a prelude for considering the more current history of the field of traumatic stress.

Real history is about things that happen to real people in real time. From a consideration of intellectual history of the field, Sandra Bloom, past president of the International Society for Traumatic Stress Studies, takes us on an inspiring journey into the history of the movement and the events that ultimately led to the official recognition of the consequences of psychological trauma in mainstream mental health. Post-traumatic stress disorder evolved as a concept because many different individuals were able to link their personal experiences of victimization and observations of the effects of victimization on others, to the ongoing political milieu. The impetus for the concept of PTSD was not intellectual, but entirely humanitarian. Yet what has sustained the concept and what ultimately creates a paradigm is the ability to articulate to weave the underlying humanitarian principles with concrete political and social advocacy, in an intellectual framework. Because this "history" is being presented and evaluated by those who can still remember the cultural context of these events, it offers to the reader of this volume a description that is less affected by posthoc interpretation. Yet, paradoxically, it underscores the necessity of understanding events in their cultural and historical context.

An outsider can offer a more critical view, also essential in negotiating the boundaries of current beliefs. Allan Young, an anthropologist and historian by training, reflects on the history of the traumatic stress paradigm, without the constraints associated with being part of the development of the movement. Coming from a largely ethical and historical perspective, Young exposes several inconsistencies that arise when viewing the response to trauma as an advocate or consumer. His very salient argument is an integral part of this volume because nothing solidifies a paradigm more than testing its limits, and its impact on other existing world views. One of the important goals that still need to be achieved by the field of traumatic stress is the integration of the traumatic stress model and the achievement of a greater acceptability.

1

The Limiting Effects of Paradigms on the Concept of Traumatic Stress[1]

HAROLD KUDLER

> *Paradigm: [French.* paradigme, *ad. Latin.* Paradigma*] Pattern, Example, [Greek]: to exhibit beside, show side by side.*
>
> —Oxford Dictionary of the English Language

Paradigms provide a world view. They organize observations, theories, and facts about a given subject into a cohesive working model. Paradigms can shift but not so easily or so often. A momentous discovery is not, in itself, a paradigm shift. When Fleming realized that a certain kind of mold could inhibit bacterial growth, he made an important *discovery.* The subsequent technical development of penicillin and other highly effective antibiotics led to a stunning and permanent change in the role of the doctor. When the practice of medicine was transformed from caring for dying patients in their homes into prescribing life-saving pills in the office, that was a *paradigm* shift.

Paradigms make our surroundings more familiar. They also create the context in which we work toward greater understanding and efficacy. Piaget's concepts of assimilation and accommodation correspond to the cyclic process of paradigmatic development, as seen in growing children. So long as new experiences fit neatly within an existing paradigm, we need only *assimilate* the data into a progressively richer, more stable framework. When a phenomenon cannot be integrated into an existing paradigm, it is the paradigm that must *accommodate.* Changing paradigms make our surroundings less familiar. Such change is often resisted, even when it opens new vistas and creates important opportunities. The resistance can be intransigent, even bitter.

---

[1]Earlier versions of this paper were presented at the Second World Conference of the International Society for Traumatic Stress Studies, June 1996, Jerusalem, Israel, and, in slightly revised form at the Twelfth Annual Meeting of the International Society for Traumatic Stress Studies, November 1996, San Francisco, U.S.A.

HAROLD KUDLER • Durham Veterans Affairs Medical Center, Durham, North Carolina 27705.

International Handbook of Human Response to Trauma, edited by Shalev, Yehuda, and McFarlane. Kluwer Academic / Plenum Publishers, New York, 2000.

"Young Turks" and the "Old Guard" expend excessive energy in contests that often have more to do with the dynamics of power and prestige than the advancement of knowledge. At the bottom of this debate is a contest of world views and a struggle over how, when, or even if those views will change.

Because paradigms create a particular way of seeing the world, they also limit what can be seen and interfere with new ways of seeing. It is sometimes dangerous to assimilate when you should accommodate. On the other hand, a world without paradigms would be a world without stable and familiar contexts. Finally, paradigms may exist in culture, as well as in science, without being explicitly acknowledged by those whose world views and activities they shape.

The concept of psychological trauma has a very long history dating back at least to Homer, but, like most human knowledge, it has developed in paradigmatic cycles. Interest in psychological trauma has been energized and focused by the definition of a clinical post-traumatic stress disorder (PTSD). Among other changes, the International Society for Traumatic Stress Studies (ISTSS) was essentially called into being by the *Diagnostic and Statistical Manual of Mental Disorders* (American Psychiatric Association, 1980) that delineated this mental disorder. Hence, the recognition of PTSD (as well as the initial resistance to this entity) can be seen as reflecting a paradigmatic shift. Now, studies that followed the definition of PTSD have reached a point where it is necessary to consider the effects, positive and negative, of the current paradigm of our understanding of psychological trauma and our ability to treat survivors with PTSD.

The Paradigm of Psychological Trauma

The acceptance of PTSD over the last two decades involved the acceptance of a new paradigm which arose from the recognition that survivors of traumatic events endure specific and painful effects and the realization that this suffering had been largely ignored. In summary, *people deserve to be believed when they speak of traumatic experiences and their painful sequelae.*

Prior to the 1980s, it was unlikely that a clinician would inquire about a history of trauma or connect current problems to past traumatic experiences. When I attended medical school in the late 1970s, there was no mention of post-traumatic psychopathology in the curriculum. As a psychiatry resident in the early 1980s, I was taught that there was a "Vietnam-related stress syndrome" (Figley, 1978) and that some women developed a "rape-trauma syndrome" (Burgess & Holstrom, 1974). Still other survivors developed "stress response syndromes" (Horowitz, 1974). By the time I entered practice in the mid-1980s, it had been suggested that all of these different entities might reflect the same pathological process. The new conceptualization of a post-traumatic stress disorder held that these patients had responded in a similar manner to a variety of traumatic stressors. They were consistent in clinical presentation and course across different populations. Similar treatments might be efficacious across the full spectrum of traumatized patients. These considerations have widened the scope of trauma studies from an early focus on Holocaust survivors and Vietnam veterans to include survivors of domestic violence, rape, and incest.

The broad acceptance of the concept of psychological trauma and its derivative clinical concept, PTSD, spurred research on psychological trauma and increased our ability to help survivors. It has also had its pitfalls. Although the understanding that traumatized people suffer because of their experiences and have a basic right to be believed has undoubtedly improved our recognition of post-traumatic disorders, it has also led us into the murky realm of the false memory syndrome and to psychiatrist John Mack's (Mack, 1992) insistence that we accept reports of abduction by aliens in flying saucers at face value.

Even the term "post-traumatic stress" indicates a degree of confusion in our understanding of this concept. What is the relationship between trauma and stress? Are they simply on a continuum where trauma is a more severe form of simple stress? Does one bend (stress) until one breaks (trauma)? Recent studies indicate that the biology of post-traumatic disorders is qualitatively different from the biology of stress (Yehuda, 1996; Yehuda & McFarlane, 1995). Should we be speaking of "post-traumatic disorders" instead of post-traumatic stress disorder? The question strikes to the heart of our current paradigmatic confusion. If it is true that brain structures are altered in survivors (Bremner *et al.*, 1995), is it still relevant to discuss the psychological meaning of traumatic events? If it is eventually demonstrated that a tendency toward PTSD is predicted by preexisting genetic or physiological markers, does that mean that PTSD is a matter of biological predestination? Is it possible for researchers and clinicians to keep from being split into different camps that reflect their respective disciplines and traditions? Finally, how are we to keep critical human issues in focus as we shift between views of what trauma is?

Trauma studies are unique and particularly difficult because working with survivors of trauma exposes clinicians and researchers to events that are so powerful that many people have never acknowledged that such things could happen or dared to consider what it would be like to actually experience such events. Listeners can either assimilate the survivor's story into their own precepts of what kind of world this is and what people are capable of or accommodate their world views to fit the new information. Assimilation may draw on listeners' compassion, force them to distort what they have heard, or distance themselves from the survivors. Accommodation may produce a more mature and balanced appreciation of reality, generate a sense of danger, or cast the listener into despair. Few other human activities demand this kind of confrontation with reality. Trauma is a break in the continuity of normal experience and in one's previous mode of adaptation. Working with trauma survivors is, by definition, a profound challenge to our view of the world and our place in it.

The current state of trauma theory is very much like the state of medical theory before the rise of germ theory. It may be easier to appreciate the implications of paradigmatic thinking about psychological trauma if we begin by considering a more familiar example from medical history, the development of germ theory.

Germ Theory as a Paradigm in Medicine

Before germ theory, there were several competing schools of medicine. Some of these, such as homeopathy and osteopathy, continue to survive as "alternative forms" to the discipline that is now called "medicine." But, in the mid-nineteenth century, none of the competing schools could claim supremacy because there was no clear understanding of what actually causes disease. Germ theory provided that paradigm. The understanding that microscopic creatures in the environment could enter the human body and cause disease (an idea that was by no means widely accepted until well into the last century) informed the work of Lister, Pasteur, Semmelwiess, and Koch. Each of these men struggled against powerful resistance from the presiding scientific authorities of their day.

Germ theory provided a remarkably powerful and resilient concept of what medicine is and does. On the other hand, even germ theory has its limitations. "One germ, one disease, one antibiotic" remains an apt paradigm when dealing with pneumococcal pneumonia in an otherwise healthy host, but there are many disorders, including the autoimmune disorders, mental retardation, and the problems of aging that cannot be approached from this paradigm. Over the last twenty years, the challenge of a previously unrecognized disorder, acquired immune deficiency syndrome (AIDS), has led to a reevaluation of germ theory and of the medical practices that derive from it.

AIDS: A Challenge to the Germ Theory Paradigm

In AIDS, a virus interacts with the biological, psychological, and social conditions of its host to produce a unique combination of clinical problems in each sufferer. These can involve a variety of infectious agents and degenerative processes. There is one germ, but there is no single disease entity nor is there, as yet, any definitive antibiotic. For what seemed like a very long time, we could not even find a germ. The existence of a deadly and rampant disease for which there was no known germ was a powerful challenge to medicine and its practitioners. For a time, special AIDS wards were being built. Doctors were gloving up before virtually any contact with AIDS patients. There were even physicians who refused to have any physical contact with AIDS patients. The public was terrified by AIDS. Those identified with the disorder were stigmatized, even cast out. Children who were simply HIV-positive were expelled from school, and infected workers were rooted out and driven from their jobs.

Why did the medical establishment and society as a whole respond as they did to this particular disease? There are many infectious diseases that are more contagious, more deadly, and much more common, yet AIDS is perceived as the most threatening medical problem of our time. Perhaps this is because AIDS does not follow the prevailing medical paradigm: it (originally) did not have an identifiable germ; there was no defined disease process; and antibiotics were powerless against it. Thus AIDS has more power to bewilder, frustrate, and even terrify modern physicians and the society to which they minister.

The recognition of AIDS as outside the traditional germ paradigm challenged medicine to reach beyond that paradigm. New research into immune systems, prompted by the emergence of AIDS, has stimulated new ways of understanding disease processes and new ways of improving health. The challenge of AIDS has also helped medical practitioners move beyond the "antiseptic" quality of germ-based medical practice and replace it with a more modest, more humanistic stance focused on maintaining health and standing by suffering patients. Doctors are returning to the broader aim of alleviating human suffering instead of merely hunting microbes.

As this example demonstrates, when existing paradigms are threatened, there is considerable confusion and trepidation. Old ways of seeing are challenged, and although change becomes possible, many resist that change. It is essential that science and society muster the will and the flexibility to shift between paradigms. It is also true that society suffers when a medical paradigm is so powerful that it draws attention away from the appreciation of the patient as a person.

Relevance for Studies of Trauma

As yet, there is no central organizing idea about what psychological trauma is. Many researchers seem to be rushing toward reductionistic solutions along biological, psychological, or social lines. It seems that premature closure is sometimes better than no closure at all. There has been a corresponding explosion in the variety of therapies proposed. Despite claims to the contrary, there is still no well established, generally efficacious treatment for PTSD. Paradoxically, we hear a good deal about specialized therapies that are not based on a theoretical understanding of the consequences of trauma, but instead gain much enthusiasm among clinicians due to the promise of rapid cure. Some of these treatments have been called "power therapies." This is a particularly unfortunate term because real clinical power (efficacy) derives, in large part, from a clear conceptual framework, from the strength of our paradigm.

In our rush toward reductionism and miracle treatments, there is danger that the field of traumatic stress will move away from the basic humanism that initiated the study of psychological trauma in the first place, particularly, of the pioneering efforts of Krystal (1968), Lifton (1967), Shatan (1973), Haley (1974), and others who were drawn to this field by their appreciation of immense human tragedies. If we continue to simply search for the traumatic "germ" (be it neurotransmitter, gene, brain process, or idea) that "causes" PTSD so that we can develop the "antibiotic" against it and "cure" the illness, we run the danger of forgetting that medicine, is already moving beyond the germ model toward a multidimensional, holistic appreciation of disease and of health. It would be ironic if trauma workers jumped to a paradigm that is already being abandoned by our medical colleagues.

An Attempt at Resolution

One way to achieve resolution may be to borrow the psychoanalytic metaphor and put PTSD and its conceptual development on the couch. Psychoanalysis pays attention to process as well as content. It demands that the analyst remain a participant-observer centered on the patient's world view. Analysts must be sensitive to their own responses but refrain from imposing their personal views on patients. This stance is designed to invoke a dialogue of discovery and integration that sorts wish from fact and misperception from reality. Psychoanalysis can be described as a process by which perspectives on reality can be tested, expanded, and, when necessary, cast aside. Psychoanalysis, in effect, is a method for testing paradigms.

Sorting Paradigms of Psychological Trauma: A Brief Historical Analysis

An "analysis" of the history of the concept of traumatic stress over the last 150 years reveals that Da Costa, Weir Mitchell, Charcot, Janet, Breuer, Freud, Mott, and our other predecessors in this field each struggled with the same clinical problems that we face today. Each stumbled upon what we now call PTSD and developed a specific paradigm that reflected their training, clinical experience, and personal world view. Each of these paradigms (irritable heart, exhaustion, hysteria, dissociation, hypnoid states, neurosis, and shell shock) advanced the field of traumatic stress but also distorted future observations and impeded progress along new lines of conceptualization.

As Kobrin (1996) has elucidated, Da Costa and Weir Mitchell were not only contemporaries but actually worked in the same hospital, maintained a close friendship, and even became related by marriage. Despite all they had in common, when these two men confronted the problems of American Civil War veterans, they could understand those problems only in terms of their respective specialties: Weir Mitchell, a neurologist, understood these problems as exhaustion of the nervous system whereas Da Costa, a cardiologist, described "irritable [soldier's] heart syndrome."

Jean Martin Charcot was one of greatest neurologists of his time. He believed that problems of the mind had their origin in problems of the brain. Charcot's theory of hysteria legitimized the scientific study of mental illness but limited it to study of the brain and spinal cord. Although Charcot recognized that hysteria often developed in the wake of a psychological trauma, he assumed that this experiential shock merely triggered a neurological process already latent in a *degenerate* brain. Limited by his paradigm, Charcot failed to consider the psyche as an issue either in the post-traumatic state or in the hypnotic trances that he employed to study the effects of trauma. In fact, Charcot dismissed the concept of suggestion out of hand and participated in long and very public scientific "wars" with Bernheim and Leibault, who ran a rival program at Nancy that championed the concept that hysteria and hypnosis both derived from the power of suggestion. Charcot's famous demonstrations of hysteria (such as the one that Freud attended during his traveling internship to Charcot's Salpêtrière) largely derived from the hypnotic suggestions given to subjects by Charcot's assistant, Babinski. Once the medical community realized the role that suggestion played in Charcot's "neurological" demonstrations, his views were overthrown and relegated to obscurity.

Charcot's essentially neurological views were undermined by the growing realization that psychological forces were involved in the expression of post-traumatic pathology. Had he not been so invested in his own biological paradigm, he might have been less naive in his reliance on hypnosis and more receptive to the scientific study of the psychological issues expressed by his patients.

Joseph Breuer's clinical experience convinced him that traumatic experiences could be pathogenic in and of themselves, even in people who had perfectly normal brains. He and his junior colleague, Sigmund Freud, published their paradigm-shifting *Studies on Hysteria* in 1895. Ironically, this work also contained the seeds of the next paradigm shift. Although both authors agreed that hysteria resulted when traumatic experiences were stored as pathological memories [thus the famous dictum "Hysterics suffer mostly from reminiscences" (Breuer & Freud, 1895, p. 7)], Breuer believed that the traumatic memories were pathogenic only because they had jumped the usual mental track, became misplaced, and, therefore, were inaccessible to further processing. In Breuer's view, this was the reason that hysterical patients were unable to deal with and resolve the implications of traumatic experiences. Freud, however, believed that traumatic memories were pathogenic because they had been actively repressed by forces in the mind. Freud's understanding of hysteria as a dynamic defense against the conscious expression of overwhelming and hence unwanted memories became the cornerstone of psychoanalysis. Although Breuer was willing to accept Freud's notion of repression as the possible cause of some cases of hysteria, he could not accept Freud's concept of psychological defense as a general principle or the discipline of psychoanalysis that evolved from it. The *Studies in Hysteria* were the culmination of a long relationship between two clinician/researchers who shared many views and jointly enunciated the idea that psychological trauma could, by itself, produce mental illness. Their differing paradigms about how traumatic memories produced hysteria split their paths as scientists and as friends.

Avoiding the Pit: The Flexibility to Shift Paradigms

How do we avoid similar pitfalls as we attempt to understand and treat PTSD? Perhaps the problem is not one of finding the *right* paradigm for PTSD because *there is no one right paradigm for PTSD*. By definition, PTSD begins with an external event that is psychologically perceived and transduced into psychological, biological, and social manifestations. These derive both from the external event and from premorbid characteristics of the survivor. No single etiologic factor or germ can suffice as the explanation for all post-traumatic disorders. No single treatment modality can correct all post-traumatic states. What is called for is the ability to flexibly shift between paradigms. Just as a microscopist has the freedom to switch lenses, we should be able to shift our focus as our needs demand. Then we can talk about PTSD at every level. In particular, we are less likely to lose sight of the fact that PTSD affects the individual on every level.

A flexible perspective on paradigms and PTSD frees us from obsessive concerns about single etiologic agents or about biological, psychological, and/or social flaws that allow the pathogen in. Instead, we can ask: *What* existed prior to the trauma, what has been damaged, *and in what ways?* This perspective focuses attention on a complex biological–psychological–social system. This system is as much shaped by early life experience as it is by genetics and subsequent development. It is as delicately modulated by personal and social meanings as it is by the firing of its locus coeruleus and the expression of its genes. We would have to be blind to see anything less complex at work.

References

American Psychiatric Association (1980). *Diagnostic and statistical manual of mental disorders*, 3rd ed. Washington, DC: American Psychiatric Press.

Bremner, J. D., Randall, P. K., Scott, T. M., Bronen, R. A., Seibyl, J. P., Southwick, S. M., Delaney, R. C., McCarthy, G., Charney, D. S., & Innis, R. B. (1995). MRI-based measurement of hippocampal volume in patients with combat-related posttraumatic stress disorder. *American Journal of Psychiatry, 152*, 973–981.

Breuer, J. & Freud, S. (1895). *Studies on hysteria*. Translated by Strachey, J. (1955). London: Hogarth Press.

Burgess, A. W., & Holstrom, L.L. (1974) Rape trauma syndrome. *American Journal of Psychiatry, 131*, 981–986.

Figley, C. R. (1978). Psychosocial adjustment among Vietnam veterans: An overview of the research. In C. R. Figley (Ed.), *Stress disorders among Vietnam veterans: Theory, research and treatment* (pp. 57–70). New York: Brunner/Mazel.

Haley, S. (1974). When the patient reports atrocities: Specific treatment considerations of the Vietnam veteran. *Archives of General Psychiatry, 30*, 191–196.

Horowitz, M. J. (1974). Stress response syndromes: Character style and dynamic psychotherapy. *Archives of General Psychiatry, 31*, 768–781.

Kobrin, N. H. (1996, June). Paradigmatic partners in trauma: J. M. Da Costa & S. Weir Mitchell. Presented at the *Second World Conference of the International Society for Traumatic Stress Studies*. Jerusalem, Israel.

Krystal, H. (1968). *Massive psychic trauma*. New York: International Universities Press.

Lifton, R. J.(1967). *Death in life: Survivors of Hiroshima*. New York: Random House.

Mack, J. E. (1992). Commentary. In *Unusual personal experiences: An analysis of the data from three national surveys* (pp. 7–8). Las Vegas: Bigelow Holding.

Shatan, C. F. (1973). The grief of soldiers: Vietnam combat veterans' self-help movement. *American Journal of Orthopsychiatry, 43*, 640–653.

Yehuda, R. (1996). PTSD: Not the biology of stress. Presented at the *Second World Conference of the International Society for Traumatic Stress Studies.* Jerusalem, Israel.

Yehuda, R., & McFarlane, A. C. (1995). Conflict between current knowledge about posttraumatic stress disorder and its original conceptual basis. *American Journal of Psychiatry, 152*, 1705–1713.

2

On the Social Denial of Trauma and the Problem of Knowing the Past

ALEXANDER C. McFARLANE

> *"The beginning of World War II, while Europe and Asia Minor were still reeling from the effects of World War I, indicates the fragility of the capacity of nations and cultures to learn from the past."*

This catastrophic conflict occurred only 21 years after the war that was supposed to end all wars. It is as though the evocation of John of Salisbury in 1159 that "Who is more contemptible than he who scorns knowledge of himself?" might as well never have been uttered. How is it that our ability to hold on to the past is so fragile when there seems to be some agreement that history can teach worthwhile lessons, if only a willingness to doubt, learn and contemplate existence? Psychiatry and psychology are disciplines that supposedly understand the value of history in understanding human behavior. Taking a history is one of the basic skills of a clinician. Whether clinicians like it or not, they are students of the discipline. However history is a bewildering affair, and the value of historical scholarship is easy to ignore, as Auden has indicated. It is a discipline in its own right with a methodology and tradition. The trouble is that even if we value history, establishing and understanding the past is never straightforward and always involves interpretation. As Salman Rushdie, the novelist who is haunted by condemnation to death by Iranian clerics has said:

> History is always an ambiguous affair. Facts are hard to establish, and capable of being given many meanings. Reality is built on our own prejudices, gullibility, and ignorance, as well as on knowledge and analysis. (Salman Rushdie, " 'Errata': Unreliable Narration," *Midnight's Children* (1981, pp. 99–100))

Therefore, although history has much to teach us, it can also be selectively quoted and used anecdotally to justify interpretations by giving them some enduring lineage and

ALEXANDER C. McFARLANE • Department of Psychiatry, The Queen Elizabeth Hospital, University of Adelaide, Woodville, South Australia 5011, Australia.

International Handbook of Human Response to Trauma, edited by Shalev, Yehuda, and McFarlane. Kluwer Academic / Plenum Publishers, New York, 2000.

validity. When used with care and thoughtfulness, its most valuable contribution is to provide an insight into patterns or processes that cannot be clearly discerned in the present.

This chapter aims to identify some of the lessons from the past which may be relevant to the field of traumatic stress in the present. The first point is to emphasize the durability of this field of inquiry and how it has played a central role in the development of many of the most influential ideas in psychiatry in the twentieth century. It is sometimes argued in legal settings that PTSD is a concept that can be discredited because of its brief history and the arbitrary nature of its definitions that have changed with the revisions of the Diagnostic and Statistical Manuals of the American Psychiatric Association. To address this question, the complex ebbs and flows in the evolution of the concept of traumatic neurosis will be discussed.

Another characteristic of this field has been a remarkable propensity for periods of intense interest and periods where the lessons of the past are dramatically forgotten. Kardiner and Spiegel, two eminent U.S. military psychiatrists, highlighted this phenomenon in 1947, a concern which remains equally valid today.

> The subject of neurotic disturbances consequent upon war has, in the past 25 years, been submitted to a good deal of capriciousness in public interest and psychiatric whims. The public does not sustain its interest, which was very great after World War I, and neither does psychiatry. Hence these conditions are not subject to continuous study ... but only to periodic efforts which cannot be characterised as very diligent.... Though not true in psychiatry generally, it is a deplorable fact that each investigator who undertakes to study these conditions considers it his sacred obligation to start from scratch and work at the problem as if no one had ever done anything with it before. (Kardiner and Spiegel, 1947; p. 1)

One of the challenges is to understand why this discontinuity about the effects of trauma exists in the collective memory of medicine and psychiatry. Perhaps a perspective that can illuminate this issue is the effect that the collective trauma of the world wars has had on the medical profession this century, as this may explain something of the difficulty investigators have had holding onto the subject. There is a tendency for both individuals and societies to try and avoid or even develop amnesia for the fear, suffering, and helplessness that these experiences bring. On the other hand, individuals are often intensely preoccupied by intrusive and distressing traumatic memories of experiences long gone. The extent to which these patterns of reaction characterize individuals' responses to trauma and also that of legal and psychiatric knowledge about trauma will be discussed.

Historic inevitability tends to create symbols and icons who stand above the crowd. Then these individuals are seen to be the originators of trends and ideas when in fact they may have done little more than clarify and be spokespeople for the collective investigation of the time. It is always important to wonder about the apparently minor characters and to look to some of the other events that may have framed interest at the time that knowledge has blossomed.

The Origins of History

History is a fragile form of investigation because it depends upon interpretation and there is not absolute methodology or theorem as in scientific proof. It involves looking to trends and patterns in the past and to the way these relate to the progressive steps in time. One would presume that there is a recurrence of these patterns in the subsequent epochs. Historical knowledge is particularly vulnerable at times when it confronts a society with a future that is incompatible with some powerful ethos. This means that history always has the potential to slip back in time to the world of myth from where it originated. History developed alongside medicine and philosophy in ancient Greece in an age when it was beginning to be understood that the world was not simply at the mercy of the gods and superstition.

In approximately 600 BC a new way of thinking emerged in Greece when people began to look beyond religion for answers to all of their questions. Reason became a challenge to myth. "The myth is a story about the Gods which sets out to explain why life is as it is" (Gaarder, 1996; p. 18). These supernatural explanations were handed down from generation to generation in the form of religious rituals. The challenge of philosophy was to use experience and reason. Natural processes supplanted supernatural explanations. Thus, philosophy was the school that gave birth to scientific reason and the value of primary observation and secondary theory.

In essence, it was believed that there were natural explanations for the processes of nature. Equally, there was the challenge to look back on the past and to find reasons for the course of history. The use of logic implied that it was possible to determine why a country lost a war, other than to look to the vengeance the gods. Equally, the beginning of Greek medicine involved moving away from the idea that sickness was a consequence of the displeasure of the gods. Medical science involved an attempt to find reasoned explanations in nature for the existence of sickness, health, and the fall of governments.

However, as time has passed, it is important to realize that science, philosophy, medicine, and history can also be transmuted into myth. The language of these disciplines can be used to hide belief; myths can come to supplant reason. Although the sophistication of knowledge has progressed, particularly when people feel threatened and uncertain, ideals and rationalizations can come to supplant fact. Investigation and doubt can be replaced by narrative. It is always important to be watchful about the misrepresentation of the past and the dominance of perspectives. This debate has been at times vengefully played out in the post modernist movement. In the field of trauma, it is critical to be watchful when history becomes myth or narrative is claimed to be history.

Traumatic Neurosis in the Nineteenth Century

In medicolegal settings, the apparent brevity of the concept of post-traumatic stress disorder is used to challenge its validity. Is this really the case? One of the central and novel ideas embraced in DSM-III (American Psychiatric Association, 1980) was the notion that a range of traumatic experiences led to one psychopathological syndrome. This implied that there was a single psychopathological end-point independent of whether the traumatic event was a rape, combat, a motor vehicle accident, or witnessing some horrendous death. Essentially, the diagnostic criteria of PTSD described this psychopathological syndrome. At the time, this appeared to be a novel idea.

In 1995, I visited the library at the Saltpetriere Hospital in Paris with Bessel van der Kolk. This was a pilgrimage to the halls where Charcot conducted his famous lectures that were attended by many of the great neurologists and psychiatrists of the late nineteenth century. I took one book off the shelf, titled *Annual of the Universal Medical Sciences—a yearly report of the progress of the general sanitary sciences throughout the world.* This was edited by Charles E. Sugois (1890) and seventy associate editors. Volume III had one topic on psychiatry titled "Traumatic Neurosis." This article by Seguin was written in a style similar to *Current Opinions in Psychiatry*. It was an attempt to summarize and criticize knowledge in the field at that time. The opening paragraph began,

> The detestable terms, "railway spine" and "railway brain," are still employed by a number of authors, but apparently more with the object of clearly indicating the general classification of the cases they report than with the idea of proper scientific designations. It would do much towards finally setting the status of the topic if those terms (railway spine, railway brain, compensation neurosis) as well as the words "concussion" and "hysteria" were dropped. (E. C. Seguin, Traumatic neuroses, 1890; p. N1)

Essentially the idea was advocated that these terms should be grouped under the term "traumatic neuroses." Table 1 lists the conferences where the subject was discussed in the previous summer, and the author concludes "Evidently the subject is now receiving the attention its importance warrants in all civilised countries" (Seguin, 1890; p. N1).

The article summarized many of the debates of the time about the relative role of physical as opposed to psychic shock. One of the debates was about the relative importance of malingering, and several clinicians protested against Oppenheimer's idea that simulation was rare. Oppenheimer's advice was that in obscure cases a positive diagnosis should be made only after observing a patient in a hospital. In relation to the other symptoms, Seguin (1890; p. N3) also noted that "It is somewhat strange that the very important symptom, amnesia, partial or total, as a result of shock, has received no attention in the numerous papers of the last three years." Thus, there was acceptance in the 1890s that repressed memories occurred.

The debate about etiology focused on the relative importance of psychic shock as opposed to vascular changes. Meynert (1890) was particularly interested in the arteria choroidea, which provides circulation to the hippocampus among other structures, including the internal capsule. A debate existed about whether many of the hysterical symptoms observed were a consequence of the effect of impaired circulation involving the internal capsule and hippocampus rather than of a cortical origin, as argued by Charcot (1890; p. N5). There is surprisingly little reference to the theories that we more commonly associate with that time about the role of suggestibility and dissociative states.

In discussing the treatment and prognosis, a vast divergence of views "… exists between writers as to the prognosis of traumatic neuroses" (Seguin, 1890; p. N6). Galvanism and the use of the faradic brush vigorously in anesthetic parts appeared to be an important component of treatment. Wichman (1890; p. N7) advocated that this "… should not be done by the patient or a lay assistant but by a skilled physician." Arsenic and carbolic acid injections were also suggested. Kronthal (1890; p. N7) implied that hypnotic suggestion provided useful improvement. Seguin (1890), the author, argued that bromides, opiates, and stimulants are injurious if used in a routine way. There was

TABLE 1. Conferences Where Trauma Was a Major Theme in 1890

- Congress of German Surgeons
- Association of Southwestern German Neurologists and Alienists
- International Medicolegal Congress
- American Medical Association
- Missouri State Medical Association

a remarkable ring to the dichotomies of debate between the organic and the psychological and the views about prognosis in these accounts. What is striking is the way in which these ideas were subsequently lost and how it took ninety years for the recommendation about a single entity, traumatic neurosis or post-traumatic stress disorder to be accepted.

The field of endeavor was not embraced by the few names that tend to be quoted regularly now as the prominent clinicians of that time. This was a thriving field that was embraced by many clinicians from quite varying backgrounds.

The Social Impetus in the Nineteenth Century

One of the interesting questions is the extent to which the social and political forces of the time played a role in this burgeoning interest. The importance of the Vietnam War and the notion that the soldiers of that conflict could be victims of the U.S. government's social policy played an important role in rethinking the psychopathological consequences of combat. The feminist movement and the general atmosphere of political protest of the 1970s equally advocated a sound rationale for moving from individual vulnerability to the perpetration of violence and the gross denial of the rights of women as a powerful political force for recognizing post-traumatic stress disorder. Thus, the late 1970s was a period when society was ready to begin contemplating the broader social responsibility for the effects of violence and war and to recognize the rights of women.

Charcot and his colleagues have been criticized for their apparent exploitation of their female patients and for the male domination of these intellectual and academic circles. So what were the forces and the immediate social antecedents that preceded this blossoming of knowledge and interest in the 1880s in Paris? Parisian society had entered a period of relative stability after a century of European conflict. Apart from the Napoleonic Wars, there were major conflicts such as the Crimean War in which the French and the Austro–Hungarian Empire were actively involved. The immediacy of war was brought to Paris in the Semaine Sanglante (bloody week) in 1870. In this week, the third republic defeated the republic of the commune. There were 25,000 Parisians massacred, and 5,000 were deported to New Caledonia. This was prompted by a release of 60,000 prisoners by the Germans from the Franco-Prussian War. The size and atrocity of the events of this week would have meant that the sensations and reality of death and trauma would have been known to most Parisians. In the aftermath, the fervor for political freedom and democracy continued.

One of the particularly important domains was the role of women in democracy. The First International Congress of the Rights of Women was held in Paris in 1879. Jules Ferry, a founding father of the third republic, stated "Women must belong to science or they will belong to the church" (p. 17). This was an argument for removing many of the superstitious beliefs about women's behavior and maladies and the importance of medicine for investigating them. In fact, one of Charcot's acts of scholarship was to investigate the role of hysteria in the miracles of the Middle Ages. In 1881 with P. Richter he published *Les demoniaques dans l'art*. Charcot's interest in hysteria was partly driven by his political interest in human rights.

The social forces that drove this interest were not confined to the European continent. The United States had emerged from the Civil War, which was the first conflict where soldiers suffered the awful carnage of the increasingly destructive mechanization of armaments. This was also a war based on the rights and political freedoms of individuals, particularly slaves.

Medicine throughout the world was associated with the emergence of liberal political ideals. For example, South-Australian-born Sir Edward Stirling originally proposed that his native state become the first place in the world to have universal suffrage and gave the vote to women in 1888. Stirling was a medical graduate of Trinity College in Cambridge, where his contemporaries included A. J. Balfour, who became the Prime Minister of Britain, and Frances Darwin, Charles Darwin's son. Subsequently, he became a lecturer in physiology and then was responsible for the statute that founded the Medical Faculty at the University of Adelaide, where he was the first Dean. He was also the first President of the State's Children's Protection Society. While employed by the University, he was elected to Parliament where in an 1885 address to Parliament he proposed that women should be given the vote. He argued,

> It would be another creditable stage in the record of South Australia of yet another measure based upon equity and justice .... should serve as a precedent for the law makers of other countries whom (they) were usually accustomed to imitate rather than to instruct. (Stirling, 1885; p. 331)

Thus, even in the far-flung corners of the British Empire, medical graduates, surgeons by training, were preoccupied by the issues of the rights of women and children. This was not an isolated preoccupation in the sophisticated environs of Paris, where women were the idle curiosity of medical voyeurs.

Thus, there are some striking similarities between the political and social movements of the latter decades of the nineteenth century and those of the twentieth centuries that seemed to have mirrored the political and social environment in which psychological trauma became an acceptable issue for investigation and discourse.

Another factor that may have influenced the embracing of these social and political roles by medical practitioners was the impact of anesthesia on medical practice. In the brutal times of preanesthesia, surgeons had to defend and protect themselves from knowing and feeling the suffering of their patients. The unbridled screams and glazed terror of the patient during and after amputation are well documented in the *Annals of Military Medicine*. Many patients refused surgery because of the lasting effect that this had on the minds of those who physically survived. As with other advances in medical care such as adequate asepsis, anesthesia meant that doctors could begin to come closer to their patients. Encounters were not blessed with significant probability of death or immutable suffering. Doctors could begin to open their eyes to the traumatization of patients who were involved in accidents, had been the victims of sexual abuse, or were terribly injured in combat.

How medicine withdrew from this age of enlightenment is an intriguing question. It seems that two factors were involved. The first was the burgeoning dominance of psychoanalysis and the replacement of the acceptance of knowledge about abuse with the myth of the Oedipal conflict. The second was the terrible consequences of the First World War and its numbing and overwhelming effect. This was an experience which again thrust medical practitioners back into a role of allegiance to the state, where there was a need to distance themselves from the awfulness of the carnage they had to repair, to numb their empathy to the suffering of those who were not killed immediately or were left maimed but alive.

The Reversion of History into Myth

The need to use a myth to create an explanation for a patient's psychopathology is similar to the use of parables by Christ to give moral direction. This is not about science, but the use of a story to justify a point of view. This was the way in which the original philosophers, historians and doctors were attempting to lead the world of ancient Greece from this world of narrative. The myth which Freud chose for his explanation was that of an abused child. Oedipus was given by his parents to a shepherd to be murdered. He had to be done away with because his father had raped his wife while drunk. She had then become pregnant with the child he had been warned would bring about his death if his wife ever conceived. Instead, the shepherd hung Oedipus by his Achilles' heels from the branch of a tree to die. The infant was rescued. He survived to unknowingly kill his father, marry his mother, and put out his own eyes when he realized what he had done. This was not a simple story of murderous fantasies because of an infantile sexual attachment to the parent of the opposite sex. It was a myth paradoxically used to explain away the abuse of children and to root psychopathology in infantile impulses and conflicts.

Freud advocated the importance of trauma somewhat later than Janet, Charcot, and those who viewed psychic shock as critical in spinal disorders. Freud's 1896 proposition was that trauma was the central etiological issue in neurotic disorders: "External events determine the pathology of hysteria to an extent far greater than is known and recognised. It is, of course, obvious that in cases of traumatic 'hysteria' what provides the symptoms is the accident." Breuer and Freud (1893–1895/1955) also saw that dissociative mechanisms play a central role in the psychological process in the disorder. "A tendency to dissociation is the basic phenomenon of this neurosis.... Severe trauma can bring about the splitting of a group of ideas even in people who are otherwise unaffected by mechanisms of psychiatrically acquired hysteria. This contrasts to dispositional hysteria where a hypnoid state was thought to pre-exist the onset of symptoms." These ideas about the central role of dissociation show how few new ideas there are in reality. One of the proposals in DSM-IV (American Psychiatric Association, 1994) was that PTSD be categorized as a dissociative disorder, rather than remain in the category of anxiety disorders.

Freud acknowledged the difficulties clinicians had in establishing the link between a traumatic stress patients' symptoms for a number of reasons: "In the great majority of cases, it is not possible to establish the point of origin by simple interrogation of the patient however thoroughly it may be carried out. In part the patient dislikes discussing it. Principally—genuinely unable to recollect it. Often has not suspicion of the causal connection." Freud saw the critical traumatic event responsible for the neurotic symptoms of most of his patients as childhood sexual abuse. Despite the fact that he had probably seen an autopsy of a child killed while being sexually abused and knew of a study by Tardieur of a number of such postmortems, in 1897 he came to reject his views. This appears to have been partly in response to the increasing alienation from his colleagues that these observations caused: "When I began more and more resolutely to put forward the significance of sexuality in the aetiology of the neuroses, (Breuer) was the first to show that reaction of distaste and repudiation which was later to become so familiar to me, but which at that time I had not learnt to recognise as my inevitable fate."

This process of recanting had a dramatic impact on the acceptance and management of sexually abused children for more than a half century. His final renunciation of the role of sexual abuse occurred in his letter to Wilhelm Fliess on September 21, 1897: "I no longer believe in my neurotica (theory of neuroses) ..." There were several reasons. First, "... the absence of complete success" by the treatment of psychoanalysis and secondly "... then the surprise that in all cases the father, not excluding my own, had to be accused of being perverse ... whereas surely such widespread perversion against children was not very probable." This indicates how the powerful pressures of social conformity come to exercise their influence.

Thus, according to Brown (1964): "Freud had to change his mind concerned with these supposed sexual seductions of childhood (as ...) from the accounts of relatives it seemed clear that the patient was either lying or imagining an event which had never happened. At first it seemed to strike a final blow at Freud's theory, but with characteristic tenacity, he began to seek out a new formulation of his beliefs."

Despite the stories told by millions of patients, the psychiatric community continued to accept Freud's assertions. This suggests that clinicians had a great deal of difficulty in acknowledging the existence of trauma. The reasons for this denial are an interesting issue in their own right. The main problem was that many psychiatrists and psychologists assumed that the symptoms of traumatic events were due to the existing personality traits, and this was based on the theoretical assumptions of psychoanalysis. The Oedipus complex was a powerful myth that tainted the capacity of generations of clinicians to observe the natural world and trust their senses and their reason.

To give Freud his due, he indicated the difference between traumatic neurosis and the other forms of anxiety and depression. The tragedy is that these enlightened ideas were not embraced by the profession as a whole. In 1920, in *Beyond the Pleasure Principle*, Freud coined the term "the stimulus barrier" to explain the onset of traumatic neuroses. He arrived at this view after he examined World War I veterans. He believed that traumatic neuroses occurred when excessive stimuli excited the mind. He suggested that individuals were normally able to modulate anxiety, but when this process failed a traumatic neurosis developed. His ideas were partly stimulated by his involvement in an official Austrian inquiry in 1920 which addressed the use of electric shocks as a treatment for battle-induced conditions. Veterans were attempting to sue members of the medical corps. A variety of repressive measures were used against the German soldiers who developed traumatic stress disorders. They were treated with special diets, isolation in dark rooms, prolonged immersion in water, and were given electric shocks in the name of treatment.

Freud developed a notion of repetition compulsion as a characteristic pattern of response after a traumatic event which could not be explained by his normal theory of wish fulfillment. This led him to propose the death instinct in *Beyond the Pleasure Principle*. He clearly indicated in Lecture 24 (1917) that traumatic neuroses were different from anxiety and depressive neuroses. He wrote, "In a disorder which we are even today far from understanding ... traumatic neuroses ... (the ego) will not allow recovery until repetition of these dangers no longer seems possible." Even in 1933, he wrote that "The traumatic neuroses are not in their essence the same thing as the spontaneous neuroses ...; nor have we yet succeeded in bringing them into harmony with other views, and I hope I shall be able at some time to explain to you the reason for this limitation ... the term traumatic refers to an experience that within a short period of time presents the mind with an increase of stimulus too powerful to be dealt with or worked off in the normal way." Unfortunately, many clinicians failed to acknowledge the caveats that Freud used about his own ideas about anxiety neuroses. Freud wrote about the way the phenomenology of the traumatic dreams of traumatic neurosis was in stark contrast to his theory of wish fulfillment in dreams which was applied to the other neuroses.

Although the intellectual dominance of psychoanalysis is one reason why the role of trauma came to be minimized, the role of World War I was another critical factor. The brutalizing effect of the experience of dealing with mass casualties should not be underestimated. The other real dilemma for the army surgeon was the dilemma of where one's loyalties lay.

Medicine and World War I

The role of trauma as a determinant of psychiatric illness blossomed in the age when the rights of the individual were being considered and the prejudice of the state was being challenged. A nation at war has a structure very different from a nation at peace. There is a very different acceptance of the rights of the individual in contrast to the collective needs of the social group. This is a fundamental social dilemma that impacts upon the conceptualization of trauma. Therefore, this is an enormous gulf for ambivalence about trauma in the medical profession in time of war. The power of the common good and its central role in the motivation for war highlights the challenge to the rational conceptualization of trauma in this setting. The trouble is that nations can continue to fight wars because of the myths that are created about bravery and submission. There is a purity in sacrifice. This is a narrative that loses the sensitive contemplation of memory and the continued suffering of those who return. The memory to be venerated in remembrance is the dead soldier. The grief of the widow and the parent is not to be sullied with graphic knowledge of the horror of carnage, the scar with which the returned veteran sleeps in his bed every night. This is a world where the power of myth is what sustains, and it is very hard for medicine and psychiatry to sit outside the circle of this motivating process.

Thus, in World War I there was a constant tension about how medicine should conceive of the victims of trauma. Many experts saw these men as suffering from "moral inferiority"; they were "moral invalids." In this light, these men did not deserve the status of patients but rather warranted dishonorable discharge or court martial. If treatment was to be provided, it was in the form of disciplinary therapy. The ambivalence of the military in the First World War about dealing with soldiers suffering from shell shock is indicated by the fact that some who claimed to suffer this condition faced the firing squad, accused and convicted of cowardice. These issues are conveyed in the following quotation from *Death's Men* by Dennis Winter, a book about World War I based on men's diary accounts. In this incident, the soldier to be executed by his comrades had previously fought with courage.

> A man was shot for cowardice. The volley failed to kill. The officer-in-charge lost his nerve, turned to the assistant provost marshal and said "do your own bloody work, I cannot". We understood that the sequel was that he was arrested.
>
> Officially, this butchery has to be applauded, but I have changed my ideas. There are no two ways. A man either can or cannot stand up to his environment. With some, the limits for breaking is reached sooner. The human frame can only stand so much. Surely, when a man becomes inflicted, it is more a case for the medicals than the APM. How easy for the generals living in luxury, well back in their chateau, to enforce the death penalty

and with the stroke of a pen sign some poor wretch's death warrant. Maybe of some poor, half-witted farm yokel, who once came forward of his own free will without being fetched. It makes one sick." (Evans in Winter, 1978; p. 140)

The Moral View and Disciplinary Therapy

The debate about the relative importance of the physical cause of neurosis and whether its origins are purely emotional continued into the First World War. This is the maintenance of the debate about the role of concussion of the spine versus psychic shock in the case of railway accidents. There was comfort for those who argued for the war in the physical theory of neurosis. If the microhemorrhages caused by the explosion of shells were the cause of shell shock, it meant that the awfulness of battle was not the pathogenic feature. This relieved the commanding officers of a substantial responsibility for the emotional well-being of their troops. Leri (1919; p. 118) argued that only the commotional disorders "deserved the rights and privileges of disease." On the other hand, those of an emotional origin were due to the failure of the will of the patient. He stated: "After a severe emotional shock, accompanied or not by physical commotion or wounds, the brave soldier becomes a coward. He is shorn of his warrior courage. When he hears the guns he is afraid, trembles, and can neither conquer nor hide his confusion." This failure of courage, it was argued, is caused by some inherited trait which made these men unable to survive the anvil of combat. It was this loss of capacity to "... no longer resist victoriously the agony of the battle field" that led these soldiers to be conceptualized as "a moral invalid, one wanting in courage." It was this same view in the inquiry before the War Office Committee that led MacPather (1922; p. 28) to say that he viewed cowardice and shell shock as the same phenomena. "Cowardice I take to mean action under the influence of fear, and the ordinary kind of shell shock to my mind was a chronic and persisting fear."

Disciplinary therapies emerged out of the use of galvanism as a treatment for conversion disorders and neurosis in the late nineteenth century. Yealland (1918) took the view that the job of the therapist was to persuade the patient to overcome his symptoms, to "... resume his official soldierly and manly function." The idea was that the consequences of the symptom had to be painful if the symptom was to be given up (Leed, 1979). The central method of disciplinary therapy was the induction of pain administered by electrical devices. In the context of applying these painful currents, commands and admonitions were shouted at the patient, and this was done in an environment where the soldier was isolated. In France, the treatment was called "maniegreforte" and "teorpillage," whereas the British called this "Queen's Square" or quick-cure methods. In Germany the name "Uberrumpleng" was coined, whereas in Austria it was called the "Kaufmann technique." An alternative treatment developed by Bellin and Vernet in the French Army was to take them to a dugout near the front line and give a subcutaneous injection of ether (Leed, 1979). This was extremely painful.

Extraordinarily graphic accounts of these treatments are given in Yealland's (1918) volume of his treatment of a variety of hysterical disorders in World War I combatants. Barker in the novel *Regeneration* (1992) gives an almost word-for-word account of one of Yealland's treatment sessions. His particularly chilling account was of a 24-year-old private who had been mute for nine months after an extraordinarily high combat exposure. The patient was taken into a room and told that he would not be able to leave until he had spoken normally. The severity of the electric shocks which were applied for three hours were of such sufficient severity that after application for half an hour the spasm of the neck due to the electrodes placed in the region of his throat ceased.

While applying these treatments, Yealland (1918) made a series of admonitions about this man's manliness and his need to restore his respect as a soldier. After this treatment, the soldier was able to speak. The essential issue in these treatments was to challenge the will of the patient so that he could be restored to his public role, rather than being swamped by the needs for his own selfish survival.

The success of these treatments is something that perhaps should give cause for reflection. They were brutal, inhumane, and horrific, but successful in some patients, at least in the short term. The reconstructed social narrative relates completely unacceptable notions in the current time. However, there are some slightly chilling similarities between what occurs during these treatments and what would occur in some exposure-based treatments. The patients are put into a highly aroused state where the incorrect nature of their thoughts is identified. Here, the patients are actively encouraged to adopt alternative narratives. There is a common sense way of looking at their experience, rather than idiosyncratic cognition.

The enduring force of these attitudes to the suffering of the victims of war continued into the Second World War despite the objective evidence to the contrary. This further exemplifies the power of the social narrative and its force in determining the prevailing formulation of the effects of traumatic stress. These continued conceptualizations of the medical profession are provocatively described by Germaine Greer in *Daddy, We Hardly Knew You*, which is based on her reflections about her father's war experience and his traumatic neurosis.

> When [the medical officers] examined men exhibiting severe disturbance they almost invariably found that the root cause in pre-war experience, mostly "domestic". This strengthened them in the belief that the sick men were not first-grade fighting material.... The military proposition, that it is not war which makes men sick, but that sick men can not fight wars, is clearly wrong, but most of the military medical corps believe it.
>
> The experiences that make real men also reveal that many are not real men at all. Real men are a minority even among heroes. Even the flying aces occasionally flew cautiously; the more sorties they had done the more cautiously they flew. They began to realize that they had more in common with the men who fell past them to crash in flames than with the brass who had ordered them to stalk and kill them.
>
> Military mythology, however, has to pretend that real men are the majority; cowards can never be allowed to feel that they might be the normal ones, and the heroes the insane.... The principal cause of anxiety neurosis, according to the military, is fear not stress. (1989; pp. 327–238)

The power of the social structure has an enormous capacity to influence the allegiance of doctors and psychiatrists in the armed services. Is one's responsibility to the individual or the patient? The same conflict exists in medicolegal cases where the defense is often a large insurance company or even the state. The enormous power of the doctor in this setting highlights how personal resolution would require resorting to an organizing social ethos because the personal responsibility, if faced squarely, is enormous. Butler reflected on this issue in considering the role of the military doctor,

> The question whether a soldier should be shot at dawn as a military criminal or discharged as a battle casualty with a wound stripe and a war pension was determined by the opinion of a medical officer as to which type of this clinical overlap the soldier's behaviour should consign him. (Butler, 1943)

This places an enormous burden on the military psychiatrist if the issues are thought about. One of the simplest ways to resolve this dilemma is to adopt a philosophy which makes the patient's disorder of his making rather than due to the conduct or horror of war. To accept the latter creates a real dilemma of alliegance. This was graphically played out in the Vietnam War, when it was difficult to resolve the issue of the whether the war was just. As Colbach (1985; p. 265) reflected,

> Whether the Vietnam conflict fits these criteria [of just a war] or not is really beyond me to say. I did accept it as just a war when I agreed to serve in it.... I then had to accept that my obligation to my individual patient was far superseded by my obligation to the military and, eventually, to my country.

In this context, many myths are resorted to as rationalizations that defy fact and reason. The moral and ethical dilemmas for a scientific discipline which is part of the engagement in war are enormous as indicated by Maier (1970; p. 1039):

> By acting to "conserve the fighting strength" in this war of boundless immorality ... [the military psychiatrist] partakes of the massive complicity that is the mark of guilt in our time.... Whatever else army psychiatry may be, I see neither moral nor scientific justification for the dignity of its definition as clinical psychiatry.

These attitudes continue to be played out in the compensation arena today, although they are not so floridly stated. The etiological theories about PTSD have little more currency than competing myths or narratives of the same social dilemma of responsibility and obligation in these settings. Is it any wonder that this is a disorder that provokes florid social polarities? The repressed memory debate, where fact, reason, and evidence have little value, has a similar quality. It is rather the power of the accusation which often seems to win the day, based on beliefs which people do not want to have challenged.

The Analytic View

In the First World War, opinion on the most effective treatment of traumatic neurosis was divided. On one hand, analysts criticized disciplinary therapists for using approaches that were ultimately destructive to the patient. On the other hand, the analytical view itself attracted criticism for failing to progress past a developmental model in which the core of symptoms in the adult soldier were largely attributed to influences in the period of his early development as a child. Such a model was problematic in that it neglected to take into account the central role of the soldier's war experience in the etiology of his neurosis.

A further dilemma was the prevalence of conversion symptomatology. This was seen as indicative of a conflict or internal drama that captured some particularly traumatic experience of combat. Focusing on conversion symptoms meant that many of the critical symptoms of traumatic neurosis did not become a primary focus of treatment. One psychiatrist, whose theoretical writings at the time seemed to go beyond this dilemma, were those of W. H. Rivers, the psychiatrist who treated Siegfried Sassoon. He saw that repression was the central mechanism of the failure to process the traumatic memory. Equally, he saw that it was the attempts to keep the traumatic event at bay rather than the primary experience at the time of combat which was critical to the emergence of later symptoms (Rivers, 1918).

The dominance of the views about conflict as the core feature in symptomatology, rather than Janet's (1889) idea that conversion symptoms represented the recurrence of traumatic memories in sensory modalities, impeded the development of a coherent view. Out of the psychoanalytic view emerged a greater understanding about the issue of the limited adaptations that could be made to the extremes of trench warfare. This highlighted the importance of the present as having the capacity to disrupt an individual's psychological functioning. The mechanisms used to contain the enormity of the threat became an issue of investigation. Particularly, the issue of immobilization became a matter of concern.

However, one of the dilemmas with which the analytic view did not contend was that many of the soldiers who subsequently became severely symptomatic coped quite effectively at the time of combat. Once they had overcome the first fear, they often adapted a type of callousness which allowed them to continue to function. The psychoanalytic view did at least temporarily address the fact that the uniqueness of combat had begun to dominate the role of predispositions such as the repression of sexuality. However, the importance of this observation rapidly became lost in the emerging view that the desire for compensation and the issue of secondary gain was the force which maintained symptomatology rather than considering that this may have reflected a characteristic of the underlying psychopathological process. With the passage of time, many clinicians came to distance themselves rapidly from their patients. This again raises the issue of the enormity of the carnage on the medical profession and how its ways of thinking were affected by this exposure.

The Inability to Grapple with the Event

One of the dilemmas of war is to understand the awfulness of what happens. As was said of Tolstoy's reports about the siege of Sebastopol, "The hero of this story," he says, "is truth, and truth is not all lovely and not all reconcilable with the military communiques of war correspondents. The truth is that war is not as people describe it. Everything is unreal. Nobody knows what is happening or will happen" (Tolstoy, 1986; p. 38). These are events which challenge the human imagination and most people are unable to conceive of the intensity of the experience or the horror of the senses. The awfulness of these experiences is what traps and for some, disrupts the mind.

Neither the analytic school or disciplinary schools grappled with this conundrum. Very few psychiatrists would have directly seen the nature of combat. Realization of the awfulness of the war and its capacity to scar the mind was not part of the medical or social narrative. This was one dimension of the avoidance of the experience by the medical profession and is similar to the conflicting perspectives of the Greek natural philosophers. In understanding the continuity of nature, should reason or the senses be trusted? The senses of the soldiers told one story; the myths that the medical profession believed to be reason told another. The destructiveness of horror, the dissociation caused by immobilization, and the permanence of traumatic memory were not understood as a consequence.

In contrast, a few clinicians stood out. Rivers describes how many patients were actively discouraged from ever describing or speaking of what they experienced. This is a striking feature of Yealland's case histories. He tells nothing of what the soldiers went through. Ironically, the cases described by Rivers are perhaps some of the most graphic records of the war and were used by Barker as the basis for the characters of *Regeneration*, a war novel with extraordinary depth.

The other dimension of experience in the medical professions was far more direct. The medical corp had to deal with the dying, mutilated, and dead. The collective impact of this experience on generations of the medical profession should not be underestimated. The enormity of the carnage which faced field surgeons threw them back into the brutalizing days of the preanesthetic era. Just imagine being at a forward first aid post at the Battle of the Somme; there were 60,000 casualties or dead on that day. Most accident and emergency departments in the largest cities are thrown into chaos by a disaster with 100 victims. The need for doctors in the military services meant that an era of graduates was drafted and modified immutably by this experience. Many of these men later became leaders in the profession, so that their past had an enduring effect on the practice of medicine for generations.

Even though it is on the other side of the world, Australia became involved. The depth and intrusion of the experience of the First World War is perhaps illustrated by the overwhelming nature of this involvement of the Australian people. For many, the involvement of Australia in the world wars may seem odd, given that none of its territory was fought over. Its losses and the disruption should have been minimal compared with European and Asian countries.

However, although Australians made up only 10% of the Allied forces, they were often recruited as front-line troops and captured 25% of the territory won. Thus, it is not surprising that of the 331,787 who went overseas, there were 60,000 deaths and 113,370 unfit on return (Butler, 1943). The enduring scars were present to be seen but were not well understood, with 7,929 pensions for psychiatric disability and 18% of those with a disability pension also having a psychological disability. In the 1930s, the suicide rate of veterans was three times that of age-matched peers. This legacy is one national example of a general cultural legacy.

To survive this terrible carnage, most doctors had to distance themselves from the suffering of the soldiers and align themselves with their role in the military. The effect was to numb the medical profession, including the psychiatrists, from the experience of individual suffering. This was how the profession coped with this enormous pool of suffering. Shutting off this pool of human suffering allowed some focus on the future, both for doctors and society at large. There was no political or social advocacy for recognizing and understanding traumatized veterans at this time. Everything conspired to allow people to forget and to seek some solace in the glory of victory to lessen the suffering of the bereaved. The profession was part of this cultural amnesia for the suffering and persecution of memory that these soldiers brought home. This need to forget meant that the lessons, which began to be learned and were recognized by Freud, were not grasped by medicine in the face of this onslaught. The myths about courage and bravery were easier to live with than exploring the legacy of suffering that was left. The isolated endeavors of a few clinicians such as Kardiner were the bridge of observation that resurfaced in DSM-III. So much for allies.

Defeated Germany was no less reluctant to own the pain. One of the first books to be banned by the Nazi Party was *All Quiet on the Western Front* (Remarque, 1987), an extraordinary tale of the comradeship and suffering of men and their enduring alienation from those at home. It is this type of record which makes the romanticization of war hard. The truth destroys myths and is dangerous for those who wish to seduce and manipulate. Myth, not history, is the fertile soil for political leaders such as Hitler.

Conclusion

This account of the history of the role of traumatic stress in psychopathology demonstrates how tenuous is the hold on reason and observation. There are powerful social forces that conspire to prejudice observation in this area of knowledge. It is often hard to know what is fact and what is myth, and history can be both. To distinguish the two depends on constant questioning and skepticism. The words of the German Chancellor to the Bundestag in 1985 are reminiscent of the potential cost if this challenge is to be avoided:

> Anyone who closes his eyes to the past is blind to the present. Whoever refuses to remember the inhumanity is prone to the risks of new infection. (von Weizsacker, 1985)

An enduring problem is that the study of history and the taking of a history from a patient is too often practiced like the reading of novels. As Naipaul warns,

> Because we take to novels our own ideas of what we feel they must offer, we find, in unusual or original work only what we expect to find and we reject or miss what we are not looking for. (Naipaul, 1977; p. 25)

It is easy to find the evidence to support the argument we want to prove; the challenge is to hold onto the facts that tell us novel and other truths that we would rather not know. Traumatic experiences are events that burst such awareness that they cannot deny into people's lives. It is not surprising that the enduring lessons about psychological trauma are hard to learn and hang onto.

References

American Psychiatric Association (1980). *Diagnostic and statistical manual of mental disorders (DSM-III)*, 3rd ed. Washington, DC: American Psychiatric Press.

American Psychiatric Association (1994). *Diagnostic and statistical manual of mental disorders (DSM-IV)*, 4th ed. Washington, DC: American Psychiatric Press.

Auden, W. H. (1950). 1st September 1939. In *Collected shorter poems (1930–1944)*. London: Faber.

Barker, P. (1992). *Regeneration*. New York: Dutton.

Breuer, J., & Freud, S. (1955). Studies on hysteria. In Strachey, J. (Ed. and Trans.), *The standard edition of the complete psychological works of Sigmund Freud*, Vol. II. London: Hogarth Press (original work published 1893–1895).

Brown, J. A. C. (1968). *Freud and the post-Freudians*. Harmondsworth: Penguin Books.

Butler, A. G. (1943). *Official history of the Australian army Medical Service 1914–1918. Vol. III: Problems and Services*. Canberra: Australian War Memorial.

Charcot, J. M., & Richter, P. (1881). *Les demoniaques dans l'art*. Paris: Macula, 1984.

Colbach, E. M. (1985). Ethical issues in combat psychiatry. *Military Medicine, 150*, 265.

Ferry, J. In Bidelman, P. K. (1982). *Pariahs stand up! The founding of the liberal feminist movement in France, 1858–1889* (p. 17). Westport, CT: Greenwood Press.

Freud, S. (1933). In J. Strachey (Ed. and Trans.), *The standard edition of the complete psychological works of Sigmund Freud*, (1955, Vol. 7). London: Hogarth Press.

Freud, S. (1955). Beyond the pleasure principle. In J. Strachey (Ed. and Trans.), *The standard edition of the complete psychological works of Sigmund Freud*, (1955, Vol. 18, pp. 3–64). London: Hogarth Press. (Original work published 1920).

Freud, S. (1963). Introductory lectures on psycho-analysis. In J. Strachey (Ed. and Trans.), *The standard edition of the complete psychological works of Sigmund Freud*, (Vol. 16, pp. 241–496). London: Hogarth Press. (Original work published 1917).

Gaarder, J. (1996). *Sophie's world—a novel about the history of philosophy* (p. 18). London: Phoenix.

Greer, G. (1989). *Daddy, we hardly knew you*. London: Viking Penguin.

Janet, P. (1889). *L'automatisme psychologique: essai de psychologie expérimentale sur les formes inférieures de l'activite humaine*. Paris: Félix Alcan.

Kardiner, A., & Spiegel, H. (1947). *War stress and neurotic illness*. New York: Hober.

Kronthal cited in Seguin, E. C. (1890). Traumatic neuroses. In Sugois, C. E. (Ed.), *Annual of the Universal Medical Scientists: A yearly report of the progress of the general sanitary sciences throughout the world*, Vol. III (p. N7). Philadelphia: F. A. Davis.

Leed, E. J. (1979). *No man's land*. London: Cambridge University Press.

Leri, A. (1919). *Shell-shock, commotional and emotional aspects* (p. 118). London: University of London Press.

MacPather, E. (1922). *Report of the War Office Committee of Enquiry into "Shell-shock"* (p. 28). London: Wyman and Sons. In Leed, E. J. (1979). *No man's land: Combat and identity in World War I* (pp. 163–192). London: Cambridge University Press.

Maier, T. (1970). The army psychiatrist—an adjunct to the system of social control (letter). *American Journal of Psychiatry, 126*, 1039.

Meynert cited in Seguin, E. C. (1890). Traumatic neuroses. In Sugois, C. E. (Ed.), *Annual of the Universal Medical Scientists: A yearly report of the progress of the general sanitary sciences throughout the world*, Vol. III (p. N4). Philadelphia: F. A. Davis.

Naipaul, V. S. (1977). *India—a wounded civilisation*. London: Deutsch.

Oppenheimer, H. Cited in Seguin, E. C. (1890). Traumatic neuroses. In Sugois, C. E. (Ed.), *Annual of the Universal Medical Scientists: A yearly report of the progress of the general sanitary sciences throughout the world*, Vol. III (p. N2). Philadelphia: F. A. Davis.

Remarque, E. M. (1987). *All quiet on the western front*. London: Pan Books.

Rivers, W. H. R. (1918). The repression of war experience. *The Lancet*, Feb. 2.

Rushdie, S. (1981). *Midnight's children*. London: Cape.

Seguin, E. C. (1890). Traumatic neuroses. In Sugois, C. E. (Ed.), *Annual of the Universal Medical Scientists: A yearly report of the progress of the general sanitary sciences throughout the world*, Vol. III. Philadelphia: F. A. Davis.

Stirling, E. (1885). Extension of the franchise to unmarried women. Parliamentary Debates, July 22, 1885, 331.

Sugois, C. E. (1890) (Ed.), *Annual of the Universal Medical Scientists: A yearly report of the progress of the general sanitary sciences throughout the world*, Vol. III. Philadelphia: F. A. Davis.

Tolstoy, L. (1986). *The Sebastopol sketches*. Harmondsworth, England: Penguin Books.

von Weizsacker, R. (1985). Cited in Buruma, I. (1995). *Wages of guilt: Memories of war in Germany and Japan* (p. 228). New York: Meridian.

Wichman cited in Seguin, E. C. (1890). Traumatic neuroses. In Sugois, C. E. (Ed.), *Annual of the Universal Medical Scientists: A yearly report of the progress of the general sanitary sciences throughout the world*, Vol. III (p. N7). Philadelphia: F. A. Davis.

Winter, D. (1978). Ed.), *Death's men: Soldiers of the Great War* (p. 140). London: Allen Lane.

Yealland, L. (1918). Hysterical disorders of speech. In Yealland, L., *Hysterical disorders of warfare*. London: Macmillan.

3

Our Hearts and Our Hopes Are Turned to Peace

Origins of the International Society for Traumatic Stress Studies

SANDRA L. BLOOM

"Our hearts and our hopes are turned to peace as we assemble here in the East Room this morning," said President Johnson on the morning of November 19, 1968. "All our efforts are being bent in its pursuit. But in this company we hear again, in our minds, the sound of distant battles." President Johnson was addressing these words to those gathered for the Medal of Honor ceremony in honor of five heroes of the undeclared war in Vietnam. One of those heroes was a young African-American man from Detroit, Sgt. Dwight Johnson. Dwight, or "Skip" to his family and friends, had always been a good kid, an Explorer Scout, and an altar boy, who could only recall losing control of his temper once in his life, when his little brother was being beaten by older boys. But in Vietnam, when the men whose lives he had shared for eleven months were burned to death before his eyes, he suddenly became a savage soldier, killing five to twenty enemy soldiers in the space of half an hour. At one point, he came face to face with a Vietnamese soldier who squeezed the trigger on his weapon aimed point blank at Skip. The gun misfired, and Skip killed him. According to the psychiatrist who saw him several years later, it was this soldier's face that continued to haunt him.

After receiving the Medal of Honor, Skip, who had been unable to get a job as a simple veteran, became a nationally celebrated hero. But his body and mind started to give way. In September of 1970 he was sent to Valley Forge Army Hospital where the psychiatrist there diagnosed him with depression caused by post-Vietnam adjustment problems. "Since coming home from Vietnam the subject has had bad dreams," read the psychiatric report, "He didn't confide in his mother or wife, but entertained a lot of moral judgement as to what had happened at Dakto. Why had he been ordered to switch tanks the night before? Why was he spared and not the others? He experienced guilt about his survival. He wondered if he was sane" (Nordheimer, 1971).

SANDRA L. BLOOM • Alliance for Creative Development, P.C., Quakertown, Pennsylvania 18951-4146.

International Handbook of Human Response to Trauma, edited by Shalev, Yehuda, and McFarlane. Kluwer Academic / Plenum Publishers, New York, 2000.

On April 30, 1971, Dwight Johnson, now married and the father of a little boy, was shot and killed while attempting an armed robbery of a Detroit grocery store. The store owner told the police: "I first hit him with two bullets but he just stood there, with the gun in his hand, and said, 'I'm going to kill you....' I kept pulling the trigger until my gun was empty." In the exchange, Dwight Johnson, an experienced combat soldier, never fired a shot. His mother's words echo down to us, twenty-seven years later, "Sometimes I wonder if Skip tired of this life and needed someone else to pull the trigger" (Nordheimer, 1971).

It is with this dramatic behavioral reenactment of one young, despairing African-American soldier that the curtain opens on the first act of the story of the International Society for Traumatic Stress Studies. The ISTSS is one organizational part of a late twentieth century social movement aimed at raising consciousness about the roots of violence by enacting and reacting to that violence everywhere. The ISTSS was born out of the clashing ideologies that became so well articulated in the 1960s and 1970s. War crimes, war protests, and war babies; child abuse, incest, and women's liberation; burning monks, burning draft cards, and burning crosses; murdered college kids and show trials of accused radicals; kidnappings, terrorism, and bombings; a citizenry betrayed by its government and mass protests in front of the Capitol in Washington—all play a role in the backgrounds of the people who founded the organization and in the evolution of the organization itself.

If I have learned anything from my contact with victims of violence, I have learned that it is vitally important to remember—and honor—the lessons of the past. We have to know where we came from if we are to know who we are now. But it is extremely difficult to write history as history is being made. Because this chapter can serve only as a marker along the way, I have chosen to concentrate my attention on the origins of the Society, before those roots become lost in the darkness that envelops those who move offstage.

There are two fundamental aspects of the growth of this group. First, there are the individuals who provided the action—both the victims and their advocates. One remarkable aspect of the ISTSS history is the extent to which the founding mothers and fathers have had personal experience with trauma (van der Kolk et al., 1996). It may be that it was this close brush with the Angel of Death that has given the growing field such a continuing sense of passion, devotion, and commitment. Whatever the case, there are a multitude of stories begging to be told, severely limited here by time and space. The second aspect of organizational growth is the group-as-a-whole growth that I hope will emerge in the structure of the chapter. The origins cannot be placed at the foot of one powerful individual and did not derive from a clearly thought out, hierarchical, managerial demand. Instead, it has grown organically from the grassroots and has remained multidisciplinary, multinational, and multiopinioned.

War Takes Center Stage

Dr. Chaim Shatan was familiar with the symptoms of war. His father had fought in three—the Russo–Japanese War, the Balkan Wars, and the First World War before moving from Poland to Canada. His father wrote short stories about his war experiences and the son translated them from Yiddish to English. Shatan had gone to medical school during World War II, when physicians still received training in combat-related disorders and had evaluated men suffering from the traumatic neuroses of war (Scott, 1993). A New Yorker, Shatan read the *New York Times* routinely and when he read the story about Dwight Johnson, he felt compelled to respond. Further, as codirector of the postdoctoral psychoanalytic training clinic at New York University (NYU), he could even harbor hope that it would get published. His editorial to the *New York Times* was published in May, 1972 and titled, "Post-Vietnam Syndrome." In his editorial, Shatan described what came to be called post-traumatic stress disorder and told how he had noticed these symptoms in the Vietnam veterans he and his colleagues had been seeing in "group rap" sessions (Shatan, 1972; 1978a). One of these colleagues to whom Shatan referred was Robert Lifton.

Lifton was an ardent antiwar activist who had served in Korea as a military psychiatrist and had already studied and written about the survivors of Hiroshima (Lifton, 1967). Lifton met Sarah Haley through the New York and Boston chapters of the group Vietnam Veterans Against the War (VVAW). Sarah Haley was a social worker at the Boston Veterans Administration Hospital. Unlike most of her colleagues at the time, Haley recognized that many of her patients who had served in Vietnam were being misdiagnosed as paranoid schizophrenics or had character disorders because mental health professionals were failing to recognize the symptoms related to combat. But she knew them. She had grown up with a father who was a veteran of World War II, a special agent for the OSS and an alcoholic. She had heard stories of trauma and wartime atrocities from the time she was a little girl, and she had personally experienced the long-term impact of war on her father's behavior. What other colleagues found unbelievable, she found entirely realistic. When she met a Vietnam veteran who claimed to have been involved in the massacre of a village called My Lai, she believed him. It was through Haley that Lifton met and interviewed that soldier (Scott, 1993).

In January 1970, Lifton testified to a Senate subcommittee about the brutalization of GIs in Vietnam, a brutalization that he believed "made massacres like My Lai inevitable" (Lifton, 1973, p.17). In April 1970, the U.S. invaded Cambodia, and students across the country rose up in protest. Within days, the Ohio National Guard fired into a crowd at Kent State, killing four students and wounding nine others. Chaim Shatan had arranged for Lifton to speak at NYU, but they decided to change the topic to address the Cambodian invasion and the Kent State killings and advertised it widely around New York City. Many people came who were not students, including some Vietnam veterans who were members of the VVAW (Scott, 1993). The rap groups in New York evolved from this meeting and from correspondence and phone calls between Jan Crumb, then president of the VVAW, Al Hubbard, a veteran from New York, and Lifton, beginning in November, 1970 (Lifton, 1973; Shatan, 1998).

East Coast Rap Groups

When the clinicians sat down with Hubbard and several others from VVAW, the vets described the way the members "rapped" with each other about the war, American society, and their own lives. They told the clinicians that it would be helpful if they were able to turn to professionals who could teach them more about the complex psychological processes attendant upon war experience. Lifton suggested they form more regular rap groups with some professional involvement. With the support of the chairman of the psychoanalytic training program at NYU, Shatan circulated more than three hundred memos asking for professional volunteers to join in efforts to provide clinical consultation to the rap groups. He urged his colleagues to help, telling them that "This is an opportunity to apply our professional expertise and anti-war sentiments to help some of those Americans who have suffered most from the war" (Shatan, 1971). He outlined for them three theoretical questions that he believed needed some clinically informed answers: What are the differences between Vietnam veterans and World War II veterans? Can the psychodynamics of war atrocities be clarified and demonstrated to grow organically out of modern combat training? What is happening in the group process experience between veterans and professionals?

The enticements worked. Within five days, his memo had drawn forty volunteers. A panel of professional psychological and psychiatric colleagues in the New York area was formed. Most came from the NYU postdoctoral psychoanalytic program, others from prestigious programs like the W. A. White Institute for Psychoanalysis and the New York Psychoanalytic Institute. These clinicians participated in the groups until at least 1976 (Shatan, 1987). They called themselves "professionals" rather than "therapists" because they "... had a sense of groping toward, or perhaps being caught up in, a new group form. Though far from clear about exactly what that form would be, (we) found ourselves responding to the general atmosphere by stressing informality and avoiding a medical model" (Lifton, 1973, p.77). Through word of mouth, announcements from church pulpits, and some media coverage, veterans began to hear about the rap groups, and the numbers of people attending the groups began to grow. Jack Smith and Arthur Egendorf, both veterans, were early members of the rap groups in New York.

The VA Response and the "Counter-VA"

In 1971, Shatan and Peter Bourne testified at the court martial of a Marine POW who was being charged with desertion, though he clearly suffered from traumatic stress. The papers written by Bourne and published in 1969 and 1971 about war neurosis were ignored. The refusal to see the damage that had been done to these men motivated Shatan even further. The response to Shatan's op-ed article was overwhelming. He heard from more than 1,250 rap groups from around the country, as well as student health and financial aid offices on many campuses and even veterans in prison. Groups had already been meeting informally with psychiatrists in Philadelphia, Atlanta, and Boston (Shatan, 1987). All were functioning outside of the established Veterans Administration (VA) services either because they were past the two-year limit for service-connected disabilities or because they found those employed to administer traditional service geared to World War II veterans, hostile to them and unwilling to meet their needs (Scott, 1993).

At this time there was tremendous hostility toward the returning Vietnam veterans, particularly those who had become disillusioned with the war. And the hostility came from the left and the right sides of the political spectrum. John Kerry (now Senator John Kerry) was a founder of the VVAW and holder of three Purple Hearts, a Bronze Star, and a Silver Star for his service in Vietnam. He reported that a Minnesota American Legion post excluded Vietnam vets because they had lost the war. Meanwhile, there were antiwar activists and pacifists calling the veterans "baby-killers" (Shatan, 1987). Even the military victimized the vets as they were leaving the war through the practice of giving "bad discharge numbers." According to a discreet coding system, numbers were entered on discharge papers that identified veterans who had been seen as "trouble-makers" while in the service, and then these codes were distributed to employers and personnel officers. In the media, especially television, the stigmatization was furthered by the portrayal of Vietnam veterans as dangerous and psychotic freaks, murderers, and rapists (Leventman, 1978). In 1978, Leventman, citing an earlier article of his own said, "Nothing reflects so much of what is wrong with American society as its treatment of Vietnam veterans ... one can only reiterate that the negative legacy of Vietnam lies more in civilian society than in the psyches of veterans" (p. 295).

In response to this discrimination, the veterans and their supporters organized a counter-VA consisting of therapeutic communes, storefront clinics, vet centers, and bars. They organized social and political protests. They conducted street theater with mock pacification operations in New Jersey villages. In December, 1970 another veterans' group, the "Citizens' Commission for Inquiry into U.S. War Crimes in Vietnam," held the first war crime hearings in Washington at the Dupont Circle Hotel. Shatan and Lifton testified there, as well as Congressmen Conyers and Dellums, who made sure that a report was entered in the Congressional Quarterly in 1971 (Shatan, 1998). In January of 1971, the VVAW organized war crime hearings in Detroit called the "Winter Soldier Investigation," sponsored by Jane Fonda, among others. One hundred and fifteen veterans, as well as Robert Lifton, presented testimony about atrocities committed in Vietnam. Fonda and antiwar activist, Mark Lane, filmed the testimony and arranged for distribution. However, the event got very little national media coverage.

In April 1971, the VVAW organized a march on Washington. The military had called the invasion of Cambodia and Laos "Operation Dewey Canyon II," and the VVAW named their action "Operation Dewey Canyon III," designating it as a "... limited incursion into the country of Congress." Their week-long occupation of Washington culminated in a ceremony on the Capitol steps, a "medal turn-in" ceremony. Jack Smith recalls, "I can still hear the dings of those medals, the Bronze Stars and the Silver Stars bouncing off the statue of John Marshall, and the Purple Hearts, behind the barricades" (Scott, 1993, p.23).

The veterans published an anthology of war poems and used the money to help a Quaker rehabilitation center in South Vietnam and to help rebuild Hanoi's foremost hospital, destroyed in the carpet bombing. They founded free clinics in poverty areas and staffed them with former nurses and medics. They offered legal aid and regular visits to vets in prison. Mental health professionals, moving beyond therapy and detachment to advocacy, participated: "We went, with the vets, wherever we could be heard: to conventions, war crimes hearings, churches, Congress, the media, and abroad. We, too, suffered insomnia and had combat nightmares" (Shatan, 1987, p. 8).

West Coast Rap Groups

Meanwhile, out on the West Coast, a schizophrenia expert, Dr. Philip May, was director of psychological services for the Brentwood Veterans Administration Hospital. In 1971, he recognized that Vietnam veterans were not getting the services they needed, so he hired Shad Meshad, a social worker and Vietnam vet himself, to evaluate the situation. Meshad had already started one of the nation's first rap groups in the Los Angeles area and was highly critical of the VA services. He had been a medic in Vietnam, was seriously wounded, and had endured several painful operations in the States. He knew what veterans were contending with from a first-hand perspective (Meshad, 1997; Scott, 1993). So did William Mahedy, who had served as a chaplain in Vietnam and was working as a social worker at Brentwood, "Most Brentwood psychiatrists that I met during this period had not the slightest clue how to deal with Vietnam veterans ... they didn't know how to treat combat-related stress. Nor could they provide any guidance to the kind of total reintegration into society that we knew was necessary" (Mahedy, 1986, p. 56). In response, Meshad created the highly unconventional Vietnam Veteran Resocialization Unit within the Brentwood VA hospital, with the support of the director at Brentwood, and set up storefront clinics where rap groups were held.

The Churches Help the Cause

By 1973, Robert Lifton's book *Home from the War* was published, the first widely read book about the plight of the Vietnam veterans. He and Shatan had made strong and supportive connections with the American Orthopsychiatric Association and several universities. Both were impressed by the growing grassroots movement and believed that it could be strengthened even further. In 1970, the National Council of Churches (NCC) established an office under Reverend Richard Kilmer, an ordained Presbyterian minister, to help those hurt by the war in Vietnam. At first the NCC focused efforts on draft resisters and antiwar protestors. However, in 1973, at the urging of Shatan and Lifton, the NCC began laying plans for the First National Conference on the Emotional Needs of Vietnam-Era Veterans. According to Jack Smith, the veterans had pointed out to Reverend Kilmer that they had an obligation to minister to people who were *in* the war as well as *out* of it.

The churches began to listen. The Missouri Synod of the Lutheran Church put up $80,000 for expenses and agreed to host the meeting at its seminary in St. Louis, appropriately situated right in the middle of the country. Arthur Egendorf developed a list of veterans, psychiatrists, and others who were actively involved in helping Vietnam veterans around the country. According to Shatan, about 130 people attended the conference: "... 60 vets, 30 shrinks, 30 chaplains, and 10 central office people [VA] who came on at the last minute" (Scott, 1993, p. 45). At the conference, Lifton and Shatan spent time with reporters talking about the problems of Vietnam veterans. The conference lasted for three days, April 26–28, 1973, and out of the conference the National Vietnam Veterans Resource project (NVRP) was created with a governing council of 16 people codirected by Chaim Shatan and Jack Smith, with representatives from all three groups—veterans, chaplains, and mental health professionals. The project was to have several functions: to search and gather data on the effects of combat stress and to help coordinate a self-help movement of veterans groups (Shatan, 1987, 1997a).

The Government Responds

There were direct consequences for this kind of advocacy. Beginning in 1970, Shatan came under government surveillance. Returning from a meeting at the Pentagon in June of 1973, he found that his phone had been tapped. After a visit to Washington to offer assistance to American POW's returning from Hanoi, he discovered that someone had tampered with his mail. In July of 1973, Shatan had been contacted by William Kunstler's Center for Constitutional Rights for help in preparing a "post-Vietnam syndrome" defense for the "Gainesville Eight," veterans who had been charged with planning to blow up the 1972 Democratic and Republican conventions. After this, the interference with his mail was stepped up so that if mail came from veterans' organizations, people who worked with Vietnam vets, or Robert Lifton, it was bound to be searched (Scott, 1993). The FBI tried to infiltrate the rap groups by sending in informers posing as veterans seeking help (Lifton, 1978). Shatan found that plans were even afoot to entrap him with blueprints of government munitions plants. A veteran who was suspected of being a part of the security apparatus of the time, sent both blueprints and letters to Shatan, detailing to him how easy it was to get letters out of the Pentagon. Shatan had friends at the Center for Constitutional Rights, and they urged him to get the documents out of his office and lock them in their safe because they were convinced that he was being set up for a raid. His response was to talk longer, louder, and more frequently to bring attention to the readjustment problems of the veterans and to make their cause more publicly visible and therefore less vulnerable to government sabotage (Shatan, 1987, 1998).

The VA Central Office attacked Lifton and Shatan in the press when the two psychiatrists estimated that 20% of men who had served in Vietnam were paying a heavy psychological price, because the VA claimed that only 5% of the men had combat-related psychological symptoms. Both were labeled as being "hung up on the war" and accused of "dishonoring brave men" (Shatan, 1985). Both Shatan and Lifton knew that it was impossible to separate the professional work they were doing with these men from their political activism. As Lifton recalls, "I believe that we always function within this dialectic between ethical involvement and intellectual rigor, and that bringing our advocacy 'out front' and articulating it makes us more, rather than less scientific … From the beginning the therapeutic and political aspects of our work developed simultaneously" (Lifton, 1978, pp. 211 and 212).

Turning the Government Around

It was difficult for Vietnam veterans to get the services they needed from the VA for several reasons, besides the existing, sometimes virulent, prejudice against the men who had fought in Vietnam and were suffering from the delayed effects of combat stress. First, there was no diagnostic code for combat stress in DSM-II. This latest edition of the *Diagnostic and Statistic Manual for Mental Disorders* had been published by the American Psychiatric Association in 1968. As Art Blank, points out, "As the return of troops from Vietnam was reaching a crescendo, the psychiatric profession's official diagnostic guide backed away from stress disorder even further, and the condition vanished into the interstices of "adjustment reaction of adult life" (Blank, 1985, p. 73). But even under DSM-I, there had been no classification for delayed stress reactions. So, if the symptoms presented more than two years after discharge from active duty, the VA did not consider that they were service-related problems. If veterans presented with post-traumatic psychiatric symptoms, they were misdiagnosed as suffering from depression, paranoid schizophrenia, character or behavior disorders (Blank, 1985; Wilson, 1988).

Senator Alan Cranston, a World War II veteran and a member of the Senate's Committee on Veterans Affairs, became convinced that the psychological needs of Vietnam veterans were different from those of older veterans. Starting in 1971, he tried to bring about changes in the VA system by seeking better funding for the Vietnam veterans to obtain drug and alcohol rehabilitation, as well as specialized readjustment counseling services. The bill he proposed passed the Senate in 1973 and 1975, but the House refused to pass it. The House was dominated by World War II veterans, who had an unwillingness to concede that the Vietnam War had produced different problems than had been previously recognized. In addition, the American Legion, as well as the Veterans of Foreign Wars, lobbied against the bill. Taking a more long-term approach, Cranston appointed Max Cleland as a member of his staff to review the VA hospitals. Max Cleland was a Vietnam veteran who had lost an arm and both legs in the war and had testified for Cranston at the Senate Committee on Veterans Affairs in 1971. In his new position, Cleland visited Shad Meshad's storefront operations at Brentwood. Both Cleland and Meshad testified in 1975 before Senator Cranston's Subcommittee on Health and Hospitals, providing clear evidence that the VA hospitals were not meeting the needs of Vietnam veterans (Scott, 1993).

Besides the problems with the psychiatric diagnostic schemas, there was no organized Vietnam veterans' pressure group advocating a change in benefits (Scott, 1993). The work of the National Vietnam Veterans Resource Project (NVRP), created during the First National Conference on the Emotional Needs of Vietnam-Era Veterans, began immediately after the conference. By 1974, the NVRP had catalogued 2,700 diverse veterans' self-help programs, 2,000 of them on college campuses, some out in the community, and others in prisons (Lifton, 1973; Shatan, 1974). Jack Smith sought funding for an empirical study and called it the Vietnam Generation Study because the intention was to study both veterans and draft resisters. He and a colleague obtained funding from the National Council of Churches, the Russell Sage Foundation, and the Edward F. Hazen Foundation to begin a pilot study (Scott, 1993). In 1975, the Senate Committee for Veterans Affairs initiated a bill, approved by Congress, mandating the VA to conduct a study to assess the needs of Vietnam veterans. As a result, the VA provided funds to Arthur Egendorf and the NVRP to complete the Vietnam Generation Study, which eventually culminated in *Legacies of Vietnam* (Egendorf et al., 1977, 1981; Laufer, 1985).

The Mysterious Disappearance of Combat Stress

The first version of the *Diagnostic and Statistical Manual* formulated by the American Psychiatric Association was published in 1952, while American psychiatrists were actively treating veterans of World War II and Korea. "Gross stress reaction" was used to describe the aftereffects of previously healthy persons who began having symptoms related to intolerable stress. DSM-II was published in 1968, at the height of the Tet offensive in Vietnam and "gross stress reaction" was replaced with "(transient) adjustment disorder of adult life." The only mention of combat—as "… fear associated with military combat and manifested by trembling, running, and hiding"—was put in the same category as an "unwanted pregnancy" (Shatan, 1985).

As Chaim Shatan wrote many years later, "The disappearance of stress reactions from DSM-II remains a mystery. Its causes have not been established. I have not been able to find a soul who will say they know how or why it happened … [but] we can say that the diagnostic lacuna in DSM-II had great political value during the Vietnam war … every diagnosis is a potential political act" (1985, pp. 2–3). For Figley, the absence in DSM-II of a diagnostic category specific to combat trauma can be attributed to the lack of American involvement in a war during that period, as WWII and Korean veterans became integrated into the community (Figley, 1978a).

But Blank also believed that the elimination of "gross stress reaction" had been politically motivated, if not consciously, then unconsciously. On looking back, he concurs with Shatan, "These dramatic shifts from DSM-I to DSM-III suggest the hypothesis that—as part of a highly complex social and intellectual phenomenon—irrational influences have deeply affected the recognition and appreciation of accurate guidance by organized psychiatry" (Blank, 1985, p. 74). Wilson has puzzled over this mystery as well, pointing out that after the death of Freud the collective knowledge about psychological trauma seemed to go underground and by the time of DSM-II had all but evaporated. "What makes this so peculiar is that by 1968, the cumulative historical events involving war, civil violence, nuclear warfare, etc., produced more trauma, killing, mass destruction, and death in a limited time frame than at any prior time in recorded history" (Wilson, 1995, p. 15). Even now, Blank predicts that, for similar reasons, there will be a move to exclude PTSD as a diagnostic category when the DSM-V is formulated in the future (Blank, 1997a).

Whatever the reasons—and there probably were many—as early as 1969, John Talbott recommended that the future editors of DSM-III reintroduce the gross stress reaction listing. Talbott, later to become President of the American Psychiatric Association, had served in Vietnam as a psychiatrist. He conducted some of the initial interviews for the Vietnam Generation Study and was stunned by how much of this "post-Vietnam syndrome" he had been failing to diagnose in part because there was no way to make the diagnosis under DSM-II (Scott, 1990, 1993).

Organizational Efforts Expand

Shatan says that he first heard that traumatic war neurosis had disappeared in 1974 as a result of a phone call from an Asbury Park, New Jersey, public defender. A Vietnam veteran had been charged with violence against property and had amnesia regarding his behavior. The public defender entered a plea of not guilty based on traumatic war neurosis and the judge rejected the defense because there was no longer such a diagnosis. Shatan recommended that the public defender contact the DSM-III Task Force headed by Robert Spitzer. He did so and was told that there were no plans to reinsert any form of traumatic war neurosis in the DSM-III. A reporter from the *Village Voice* got this word back to Shatan, and he was shocked. He got together with Lifton to decide what to do. They realized they had to mobilize, and mobilize quickly (Shatan, 1985).

Their response was to form the Vietnam Veterans Working Group (VVWG), supported, in part, by the American Orthopsychiatric Association, the Emergency Ministry of the United Presbyterian Church, and the National Council of Churches, with some assistance from Amitai Etzioni at the Center for Policy Research, Columbia University (Scott, 1993; Shatan, 1997a; Shatan et al., 1977). In 1974, Sarah Haley published her landmark paper, "When the patient reports atrocities," in the *Archives of General Psychiatry*, one of the publications of the American Psychiatric Association (APA), and it was widely read. John Talbott had easy access to the APA. He sponsored meetings at the New York chapter of the APA, inviting Shatan, Haley, Arthur Egendorf, and others to present papers on "Post-Vietnam syndrome." He also helped them get access to Robert Spitzer at the 1975 APA convention. Jack Smith developed a questionnaire as part of his doctoral thesis, "American War Neurosis, 1860–1970," and Shatan sent the questionnaire to 35 members of the VVWG in 1975, many of whom had been working closely with the veterans in rap groups and individual sessions, some as far back as 1970 (Shatan et al., 1977). He asked them to go through their caseload with the questionnaires. Shatan and Lifton, joined by Jack Smith and Sarah Haley, tabulated the results on 724 veterans and arrived at a classification system very close to the one Kardiner had proposed in 1941 (Shatan, 1997b; Shatan et al., 1977; van der Kolk et al., 1994).

Meanwhile, Charles Figley organized panels in 1975 at the American Sociological Association. He met with Chaim Shatan, Robert Lifton, and others while beginning to work on an edited volume. In 1978, this volume would become a landmark book on Vietnam. Figley, a psychologist, had served in Vietnam in 1965 with the Marines and was one of the first Vietnam veterans to return home. He completed graduate studies and participated in Dewey Canyon III. On campus, he met other Vietnam veterans and became aware of the widespread nature of their adjustment problems. After obtaining his degree, he took a position at Purdue University where he founded and directed the Consortium on Veteran Studies and started studying the post-Vietnam effects intensively. He developed a bibliography about combat trauma and began corresponding with other people interested in similar studies (Scott, 1993).

Meanwhile, John Wilson, a conscientious objector during the Vietnam War, began working on the "*Forgotten Warrior*" project. Wilson had completed his Ph.D. in 1973 and performed three years of alternative service in a crisis intervention center. When two close friends returned from Vietnam as radically changed people, a seed was planted in his mind. His first academic position was in Cleveland where a student of his presented a report on some Vietnam veterans he had interviewed on campus. John was intrigued. He sent out letters to the veterans on campus and more than 100 responded. He and the student he was working with, Chris Doyle, recorded narratives of their lives before, during, and after Vietnam. The work became consuming. His department chairman threatened to block his tenure or promotion if he continued this work, but John was undeterred. He set up rap groups at the university and requested funding from various organizations for a study. But only in 1976 was he able, through the assistance of a disabled veteran, to get the Disabled American Veterans to provide the money he needed to complete the study (Scott, 1993). Drawn from over 450 interviews, Wilson and Doyle published a report on "*The Forgotten Warrior Project*" (Wilson & Doyle, 1977).

In 1977, Figley chaired a research symposium at the American Psychological Association conference where he was able to arrange for the presentation of three papers: Egendorf and colleagues' first version of what would ultimately become the *Legacies of Vietnam* study (Egendorf et al., 1977), his own work from the Consortium (Figley & Southerly, 1977), and Wilson and Doyle's *Forgotten Warrior Project* (Wilson & Doyle, 1977). Each separate study supported and extended the other (Figley, 1978b) and provided even more support for the efforts of the VVWG in their attempt to change DSM-III.

The Lost is Found: Post-Traumatic Stress Disorder

Ironically, the decision to alter the DSM-III in relation to homosexuality may have had something to do with subsequent changes in the DSM allowing PTSD to enter the lexicon. The argument over whether homosexuality was a disease entity was so heated and politically loaded that Spitzer decided it should be put to a vote. This indicated that the DSM-II could end up being completely redone, opening up negotiating room for those who wanted to reintroduce stress reactions into the classification schema.

Shatan had known Spitzer since the 1950s when they were both at Columbia. Spitzer invited Shatan to come to Disneyland to present his findings as a result of his work with Vietnam veterans. The irony that this momentous occasion was opened with greetings from Mickey Mouse and Pluto was not lost on the participants. So, in 1975, Shatan, Lifton, Jack Smith, Sarah Haley, and Leonard Neff presented their work opposite a psychologist from Washington University in St. Louis. The position of the Washington University group was that all of the symptoms seen in the Vietnam veterans could be explained by depression as a preexisting condition. Spitzer challenged Shatan, Lifton, Haley, and the others to refute these findings (Shatan, 1998). In the summer of 1975, the VVWG invited Spitzer to lunch at Columbia Presbyterian in New York City. The group filled him in on their activities, and he was willing to appoint a formal committee, the Committee on Reactive Disorders, to proceed with the inquiry. He appointed himself, Dr. Lyman Wynne, and Dr. Nancy Andreasen to be the representatives on the committee with Andreasen as chair. Andreasen had previously worked with burn victims and knew about the long-term psychological and physical suffering that was involved in recovery from severe trauma. Spitzer instructed Andreasen to work with Shatan, Lifton, and Smith. The appointment of Jack Smith, a nonprofessional, was a highly unusual move. But the burden of proof still remained with the VVWG (Scott, 1993).

Convincing Andreasen of the validity of the long-term reactions to overwhelming stress was key to the success of the venture. The Working Group reckoned that persuasion would be easier if they could show the similarities between combat stress and other forms of traumatic experience. So they recruited Harley Shands who had experience working with job-related trauma and Mardi Horowitz who was working on the physiology of stress. They combined this with the research related to concentration camp victims that William Niederland and Henry Krystal had been doing and contacted researchers working with other survivor groups to join in their mission. Sarah Haley pointed out to Andreasen that in reviewing the charts of the Vietnam veterans in the VA hospital, she had discovered that many of the clinicians were treating the patients *as if* there was a diagnosis of traumatic war neurosis available. This practical reality had a particularly strong impact on the discussions (Scott, 1993; Shatan, 1997a). Shatan, Haley, and Smith presented their position paper at the 1977 annual meeting of the American Psychiatric Association, representing the accumulated work of the VVWG and making specific recommendations to the DSM-III Task Force for changes in the categorization system (Figley, 1978a; Shatan et al, 1977).

Early in 1978, Spitzer called the Working Group together to present their findings to the Committee of Reactive Disorders. Lifton, Smith, and Shatan presented their evidence in a meeting with Spitzer, Andreasen, and Wynne. They emphasized a wide circle of war-zone victims and the similarity between them and other victim groups. Later that month, the Committee released its decision, recommending a diagnosis of "post-traumatic stress disorder." The DSM-III was completed and published two years later, having incorporated most of the recommendations made by the VVWG, which were similar to the observations made by Kardiner in the 1940s (Kardiner, 1941; Scott, 1993; Shatan, 1978b). Interestingly, at the same time as the VVWG endeavored to establish criteria for the DMS-III, another group of mental health professionals was working on a diagnostic system for dissociative disorders. There was no communication between them and the PTSD working group, largely because very little academic conversation had yet occurred about the relationship between dissociation and trauma. As a result, a separate classification for the dissociative disorders was also entered into DSM-III, and separate organizations subsequently developed to study these two related fields (van der Kolk et al., 1994).

Vet Centers

In the meantime, President Carter had appointed Max Cleland as Director of the Veterans Administration, and Alan Cranston assumed the chairmanship of the Senate Committee on Veterans Affairs. Cleland called a meeting with Art Blank, Charles Figley, Shad Meshad, John Wilson, William Mahedy, and others to make specific recommendations for a VA readjustment counseling program. Art Blank, a psychiatrist, had been drafted to serve in Vietnam in 1965. When he returned and was appointed to a position at Yale, one of his clinical positions was at the West Haven VA Hospital treating Vietnam vets. As a result of his own experience, he began diagnosing traumatic war neurosis in 1972, long before his colleagues were willing to see the effects of war on returning veterans. He made contact with Sarah Haley after reading her 1974 paper and through her had met Figley and Shatan (Blank, 1998). Once the Vet Centers became a reality, he became the VA's chief psychiatrist of the Veterans Readjustment Services.

As a result of the changed political climate at the same time as the APA was changing the DSM-III, Congress directed the Veterans Administration to create a nationwide system of specialized counseling centers (Vet Centers) for a wide range of readjustment problems in Vietnam veterans, including PTSD (Blank, 1985). The first Vet Center opened in 1979, and by 1990 there were almost 200 around the country (Blank, 1993). The *Legacies of Vietnam* study was published in 1981. In that year, Robert Laufer, the principal investigator for the study, testified before the Senate Committee on Veterans Affairs. Senator Alan Simpson wrote the Senate report summarizing the testimony and in it he said: "It does appear clear from the report that there is a continuing need for the Vet Center program and, as the findings of that study become more widely known, that need may become greater as veterans and their families come to realize that service during the Vietnam-era may have had an impact on an individual's ability later in life to adjust satisfactorily to his or her social environment" (U.S. Senate, 1981, p. 16).

Convergence Creates a Social Movement

Although the Vietnam War provided the "... general tendency to change which is apparent in many spheres during wartime" (Jones, 1953), other converging and significant social forces played a role in bringing the recognition of the effects of trauma into the public consciousness in the United States and around the world. The two most significant events were the Nazi Holocaust and Hiroshima–Nagasaki. Robert Lifton had published an extensive study of Hiroshima victims (1967). The adjustment problems of the Vietnam veterans, the long-lasting problems of Holocaust survivors, and the suffering of Hiroshima victims were subjects few people wanted to address because they were all "politically incorrect survivors of atrocities" (Milgram, 1998).

Holocaust Studies and World War II Survivors

William Niederland (1968) had already devoted twenty-five years to working with concentration camp survivors, noting that the same delay preceded their "survivor syndrome" as was being recognized in the work with Vietnam veterans (Shatan, 1974). Niederland, whom Shatan had known for a long time, and Henry Krystal, who had also studied concentration camp survivors (Krystal, 1968), organized a conference on victimization at Yeshiva University in 1975 and joined the VVWG (Scott, 1993). Shatan, Lifton, and others working with the Vietnam veterans had already made international contacts, as early as 1973, with other professionals working with veterans—in Canada, Switzerland, and Australia, as well as Israel (Shatan, 1974, 1998).

In the early 70s, Shatan traveled to Israel and met with military psychiatrists there (Scott, 1993). In a letter to the director of the American Orthopsychiatric Association in 1978, Shatan reported that a liaison had been established with the National Institute for Research in the Behavioral Sciences of Israel (1978b). There, Dr. Rappaport and an American consultant, Dr. Israel Charny, were working on a project called the "Genocide Early Warning System," hoping to isolate and identify features in a society that prefigure the later development of genocide (1978b). Studies also began to be published and conferences were held in Israel on the effects of war stress, a logical occurrence given the unremitting nature of warfare in the region (Benyakar & Noy, 1975; Milgram, 1978; Moses et al., 1975; Noy, 1978; Sohlberg, 1975; Steiner & Neumann, 1978).

Noach Milgram organized the first of four international conferences on psychological stress and coping in time of war and peace in January 1975 in Tel Aviv, a year after the Yom Kippur War, and the second in June 1978 in Jerusalem. Both were attended by Israeli and U.S. participants (Milgram, 1998). Israel was naturally the home for a large number of Holocaust survivors, yet there was a "conspiracy of silence" in Israel about listening to their stories (Danieli, 1981), similar to the phenomenon Neff had described in reference to the Vietnam veterans with his observation that Vietnam veterans were invisible patients with an invisible (nonexistent) illness (1975). Danieli and Solomon both provided a framework for understanding the gradual transformation of Israeli society toward a willingness to comprehend the magnitude of post-traumatic problems (Danieli, 1981; Solomon, 1995a–d).

Yael Danieli had served in the Israeli Defense Forces before emigrating to the United States, where she founded the Group Project for Holocaust Survivors and their Children. During this period, she had already begun her life work, exploring the intergenerational transmission of victimization, styles of adaptation to victimization, survivor guilt, and the attitudes and difficulties of mental health professionals working with survivors and children of survivors of the Nazi Holocaust (Ochberg, 1988b). She would later go on to establish strong connections with the United Nations and become instrumental in bringing the concepts of traumatic stress to a wider international audience (Danieli et al., 1996). Ellen Frey-Wouters, originally from the Netherlands and a specialist in international law, coauthored with Robert Laufer the third volume of the *Legacies of Vietnam* study while also writing about survivors of the Nazi Holocaust and working on social policy issues around the area of traumatic stress.

Many studies of concentration camp survivors were being conducted in Europe as well, including comprehensive long-term follow-up studies from Denmark, the Netherlands, and Norway (Bastiaans, 1974; Eitinger 1961, 1964; Thygesen et al., 1970). Meanwhile, also in Norway, Askevold studied the effects of prolonged stress on men who had served in the Merchant Marine in World War II (1976). Nazi occupations and the terrorism perpetrated by the Gestapo played a significant role in sensitizing the European community to the long-term consequences of excessive stress (Malt et al., 1996).

Another effect of World War II was the vast movement of refugees. Eitinger began studies of refugees in Norway and of concentration camp survivors (1960). The Vietnam War and the fall of Saigon in 1975 brought a flood of Vietnamese and Cambodian refugees to the United States. As early as 1979, reports were published about the adjustment problems these refugees were having (Lin et al., 1979), opening up a discourse on how Westerners could most effectively intervene and help refugees from the East (Kinzie, 1978).

Independent of the DSM-III process and the effects of war, a number of other significant developments took place during the 1970s. One was Mardi Horowitz' *Stress Response Syndromes* (1976). Building on Selye's earlier work (1956), this began to provide a psychophysiological basis for understanding the body's responses to overwhelming experience and how that response connected to psychological processes. Charles Figley (1978a,b), edited the first significant collaborative book on Vietnam War veterans. In doing so, he introduced a new psychosocial series for Brunner/Mazel that by 1990 would grow to eighteen volumes of literature spanning every victimization category.

Violence Against Women

Crime rates in the United States rose rapidly in the 1960s, and attention was also brought to bear on crime against women and children, probably for the first time in history. The women's movement was instrumental in bringing attention to the incidence of rape and domestic violence that was being perpetrated against women. The first public speak-out on rape was organized by the New York Radical Feminists in 1971, and the first International Tribunal on Crimes Against Women was held in Brussels in 1976 (Herman, 1992). In 1974, Ann Burgess and Linda Holstrom at Boston City Hospital described the "rape trauma syndrome" noting that the terrifying flashbacks and nightmares seen in these women resembled the traumatic neuroses of war. Susan Brownmiller and other feminist writers and thinkers redefined rape as an act of violence directed at maintaining dominance. In doing so, they placed the act of rape squarely in a political framework of power relationships, laying the groundwork for cross-fertilization with colleagues working with other survivor groups (Herman, 1992).

The feminist politicization of violence deepened understanding of the abuse of power within the family, leading to the "discovery" of domestic battering and sexual abuse. As in the cases of delayed combat stress and rape trauma, domestic violence and sexual abuse awareness began at the grassroots, emerging out of feminist consciousness-raising groups. Lenore Walker published her landmark study of victims of domestic violence (1979), and Gelles and Straus released the results of major studies on family violence (Straus, 1977; Gelles & Straus, 1979). Around the same time, Judith Herman and her colleagues in Boston began to document the effects in adult women of having been sexually abused as children (1981). Rape crisis centers and battered women's shelters began to spring up in various communities around the country, outside of the traditional mental health systems.

Violence Against Children

Finkelhor described the increasing professional concern about child abuse during the last several decades as being the "... result of a broad social movement and a historic moral transformation" (1996, p. ix). C. Henry Kempe, pediatrician at the University of Colorado, first described the "battered child syndrome" in 1962 (Kempe et al., 1962; Kempe, 1978). This conceptualization of child abuse brought the medical profession into this social movement with all the authority, prestige, and legitimacy necessary to bring about legislative change. At first, clinicians and researchers like

Green focused on the physical abuse of children (1978a, b). The 1970s saw the establishment of mandatory child abuse reporting laws and a widened system of child protection that was furthered and supported by the growing feminist movement (Finkelhor, 1996). But then Susan Sgroi (1975), David Finkelhor (1979), and others began to document the widespread incidence of the sexual abuse of children and the harm it caused. In 1973, the Children's Division of the American Humane Association testified before a Senate Committee and estimated that 100,000 children were sexually abused each year. Burgess and her colleagues noted in 1978 that "concern for the victims of sexual assault has become a national priority only during the past five years. In that time, both public awareness of and knowledge about sexual assault and its victims have grown immeasurably" (Burgess et al., 1978, p. ix).

As early as 1975, Shatan was studying the effects of other kinds of trauma on children. In 1972, he chaired a round-table discussion at the IV International Psychoanalytic Forum in New York, comparing delayed survivor reactions in two parent groups, Vietnam veterans and concentration camp inmates, having noted significant symptoms of unresolved mourning in young adults who were children of World War II veterans from 1965–1970. He presented a paper at the 1975 meeting of the American Orthopsychiatric Association (1975) looking at the delayed impact of war-making, persecution, and disaster on children. But there was a great deal of professional resistance to recognizing that previously normal and healthy children could be severely damaged by exposure to psychologically traumatizing events. In 1979, Lenore Terr published the first of her series of papers and a book on the children of the Chowchilla, California, kidnapping which introduced a developmental focus on the effects of trauma. Elissa Benedek recalls hearing Terr present her data before a mocking and hostile professional audience which was determined to deny the effects of trauma and disaster on previously healthy children. As she puzzled over this seemingly irrational response on the part of a professional group she knew well, she concluded that "This meeting was but another form or manifestation of a long tradition of denying psychological and psychiatric sequelae in the child victim of trauma. The audience's response of disbelief in the face of carefully collected documentation, might have been so intense because it was difficult for professionals to accept that traumatic events, caused by fellow humans, in the lives of children might color and shape their lives for years to come" (Benedek, 1985, p. 4).

Crime and Disaster

Crime victimization surveys in the United States led to the development of the Law Enforcement Assistance Administration, a federal agency designated to provide victim service programs in the 1970s. While new services were starting, researchers were gathering data about the consequences of victimization to the individual and to the entire society. In 1975, the National Organization of Victim Assistance (NOVA) was founded and other victim-centered groups emerged, such as Mothers Against Drunk Driving and Parents of Murdered Children (Young, 1988). Morton Bard became involved in the crime victim movement in the 1970s when he consulted with law enforcement agencies in New York City and later the National Institute of Justice (Bard & Sangrey, 1979; Bard & Shellow, 1976). Bard and his associate, Dawn Sangrey, published a volume for crime victims in Figley's psychosocial series for Brunner/Mazel in 1979 that was the first text published on the subject. Both Robert Rich and Susan Salasin became involved in developing mental health programs and social policies to meet the needs of victims (Rich, 1981; Salasin, 1981).

The study of disaster survivors played a vital role in the development of the field. On February 26, 1972, a dam burst in Buffalo Creek, West Virginia, destroying houses, a community, and many lives. K. Erikson wrote a book about the survivors of the Buffalo Creek disaster (1976) and other researchers, including Bonnie Green, and later, Jacob Lindy, followed up on the long-term effects of this disaster on the survivors (Gleser et al., 1981; Lifton & Olson, 1976; Titchner & Kapp, 1976).

On March 28, 1979, a sizeable portion of the Unit 2 reactor at Three Mile Island, outside of Harrisburg, Pennsylvania, experienced a meltdown, in the most serious U.S. commercial reactor accident to date. Some gaseous, but inert material was released, and no serious health consequences were expected. The population, however, had to be evacuated and a Task Force was rapidly set up to evaluate the highly publicized effects of this event (Dohrenwend et al., 1981). Other disaster studies began to emerge in the literature throughout this period as well (Boman, 1979; Parker, 1977; Quarantelli & Dynes, 1977), building on a knowledge base that dated back to Lindemann's landmark paper on the Coconut Grove fire (Lindemann, 1944; Leopold & Dillon, 1963). Manuals on helping disaster victims began to be developed and published (Tierney & Baisden, 1979). An Australian clinician, Beverly Raphael, began publishing her work on disasters and bereavement. She and John Wilson in the U.S. made early contacts with each other, thereby establishing a firm connection between traumatic stress research in Australia and the United States (Raphael, 1977; Raphael & Maddison, 1976; Wilson, 1997). This growing body of literature on the psychological effects of disaster indicated that there could be long-term consequences of overwhelming stress in populations generally considered by the public to be free from any culpability in their experienced victimization. The high level of publicity given to disasters helped to increase the general level of consciousness about the consequences of trauma.

Terrorism and Hostages

Through the seventies and early eighties there were a number of hostage-taking incidents and terrorist actions that caught the attention of the public. In 1974, a robber in Stockholm, Sweden, took a bank teller hostage. They fell in love and had sex during a long siege in the bank vault (Ochberg, 1996). In the same year, the granddaughter of William Randolph Hearst and heiress to the Hearst fortune, Patty Hearst, age 19, was kidnapped by a terrorist group, while sitting at home with her boyfriend. Until September of 1975, she was a captive of the group and was physically, sexually, and emotionally tortured. She developed a new persona and a new name, "Tanya," and was caught by the FBI while participating in a bank robbery with the group. In 1976 she was convicted and sentenced to seven years in jail, three of which she served (Hearst, 1981). This odd form of bonding between kidnapper and victim was later recognized in other types of captivity situations and came to be known as the "Stockholm syndrome" (Strenz, 1982).

Frank Ochberg, a psychiatrist whose career decisions had been in part shaped by the assassinations of Martin Luther King and Robert Kennedy, coauthored a book on violence even as a psychiatric resident (Daniels et al., 1970). He went to work for the National Institute of Mental Health and became the NIMH representative when the U.S. Department of Justice commissioned an inquiry into terrorism in 1975. As a result, he began to focus on victims of terrorism and hostage negotiations. He served as

Associate Director for Crisis Management at NIMH in the late 1970s, consulted with the U.S. Secret Service, and trained Air Force personnel in methods of coping with terrorism and sabotage (Ochberg, 1988a). He published an article on terrorism as early as 1978 in a new journal devoted to the study of terrorism and in 1982 he coedited one of the first books on terrorism (Ochberg & Soskis, 1982). In England, a study was published showing that people not seriously harmed in a terrorist bombing were more incapacitated than would have been expected. This post-terrorism phenomenon was termed an "aftermath neurosis" (Sims et al., 1979).

Across the nation and around the world, the growing global communication network was tuning many people in to tragedy everyday. Trauma was in the air and a budding awareness began to emerge that the various forms of traumatic experience might be similar and even interconnected. As early as a 1977 paper, Shatan, Haley, and Smith were already comparing the catastrophic stress of natural and man-made disasters, combat trauma, incarceration, Buffalo Creek, Hiroshima, and internment in the death camps. The time was ripe for a convergence, for people to come together and share their knowledge, experience, and sorrow.

The ISTSS is Born

Between November and December 1983, Charles Figley sent a letter to more than 60 internationally known scholars inviting them to form an organization, tentatively titled the Society for Traumatic Stress Studies:

> I believe that an organization, tentatively titled the Society for Traumatic Stress Studies, would be a useful contribution. Moreover, that the central purpose of this Society would be to sponsor a scholarly publication, tentatively titled, *Trauma and Its Wake: The Journal of the Society for Traumatic Stress Studies*. Such a journal would publish important advancements in the field of traumatic and post-traumatic stress. A distinguished Editorial Board is already in place in connection with the book I am editing, with the same primary title, that will be published next year.... How appropriate is such a society and journal, in particular, and the emergence of a separate field of traumatic or post-traumatic stress in general? (Figley, 1986a)

The response to Figley's letter was positive and enthusiastic. He believed that the formation of such a group was essential if the establishment of a journal to promulgate research findings about traumatic stress was to become a reality. Creating a journal was an expensive proposition that required a subscription base of at least 600 members to get off the ground (Figley, 1998; Meshad, 1997). Figley recognized that he could use the resources of his organization, the Consortium on Veteran Studies, to provide initial support to start the organization, but a much wider constituency was going to be necessary for a journal to be successful. He sent another memorandum the following year to the people he had previously contacted, and finally, after the birth of his daughter and the completion of *Trauma and Its Wake* by Brunner/Mazel in 1985, he contacted a group to join him at a meeting in Washington, D.C.

A breakfast meeting was held in Washington on March 2, 1985 and at this meeting the Society for Traumatic Stress Studies (STSS) was formally established. Those who attended comprised most of the Founding Board and their names are recognizable from the previous history: Ann Burgess, Art Blank, Yael Danieli, Sarah Haley, Bernard Mazel, Frank Ochberg, Robert Rich, Susan Salasin, Chaim Shatan, and Marlene Young.

Charles Figley was selected as President, Ann Burgess as Vice President and Scott Sheely as acting Executive Director. Others were subsequently elected—John Talbott, Robert Lifton, Bonnie Green, Morton Bard, Peter Erlinder, and John Wilson.

It was agreed that the purpose of the Society would be: "to advance knowledge about the immediate and long-term human consequences of extraordinarily stressful events and to promote effective methods of preventing or ameliorating the unwanted consequences." The objectives of the organization were (1) to recognize achievement in knowledge production, (2) to disseminate this knowledge through face-to-face contact with colleagues and (3) to disseminate this knowledge through other knowledge transfer media, especially print media.

It was decided to call the group a Society because the term connotes a small group of like-minded colleagues, and the concept of traumatic stress signifies the area that encompasses the entire process of traumatization, including the initial and long-term reactions and recovery (Figley, 1986a, b).

Observations and Conclusions

We will leave the story here because the work of the International Society for Traumatic Stress Studies is just beginning. In the decade 1973–1983, individual suffering, collective experience, and clinical observation had merged and had begun to develop into a field of study. In the subsequent years, this field would begin to present a significant challenge to the existing psychiatric paradigm. In the introduction to their important volume on the state of the traumatic stress field published in 1993, Wilson and Raphael observed the changes for themselves: "To establish some perspective on the rate of growth of the field, one only has to recognize that a decade ago there were no reference books on traumatic stress syndromes, few standardized psychological measures of the disorder, little knowledge about the biological basis of disorders associated with PTSD, and a limited understanding of effective therapeutic approaches" (Wilson & Raphael, 1993, p. xxi).

Today, books on the various aspects of traumatic stress fill rooms, not bookshelves. Traumatic stress has, indeed, become a true field of study if we use the criteria that Figley articulated a decade ago. "The criteria for a true field of study must include a body of knowledge and standards of practice that are subsumed within 1) a history, 2) professional organizations, 3) publications, 4) theory, 5) measurement, 6) research methodology, 7) intervention technology, 8) actions affecting policy and the judicial system" (Wilson et al., 1988, p. ix).

The development of such a field cannot come about without the simultaneous development of supporting organizations that provide the safety, mutual exchange, and collegiality that stimulates individual creativity, while also encouraging and supporting opportunities for group contributions. The ISTSS has provided the leaders in the field of traumatic stress with that kind of an intellectual "home."

As demonstrated by this history, the organization began as a grassroots, multidisciplinary, activist, war-biased but multi-interest group. For many reasons, some perhaps inevitable, the grassroots nature of the organization diminished over time and as a result, many of the original voices faded from the ongoing life of the group. This shift came about because of a need to professionalize and thereby legitimize the field of traumatic stress, so that the accumulated evidence about the effects of trauma could be recognized by and influence social policy makers, lawyers, judges, legislators, health care administrators, etc.

But as this account has demonstrated, the ISTSS was founded only as a result of the most profound social activism, and that is the existential heart of the organization. As Art Blank has recently pointed out, "There is no trauma field without advocacy" (1997b). Just as the early workers in the field had to be concerned about personal and professional safety, the danger has not really passed. As the results of traumatic experience become more widely known and accepted, the need to deny these results—and their implications—becomes simultaneously more frantic. Perhaps it is only a coincidence that as we gain the knowledge we require to treat, and perhaps even, prevent, post-traumatic stress disorders, funding for mental health services in the United States is minimized or cut off entirely. Perhaps it was only a coincidence that at the height of the TET offensive, the psychiatric establishment dropped "gross stress reactions." But it is logic and experience, not coincidence, that tells us, as Blank has pointed out (1997b), that organizations that stand to lose financially by paying compensation or damages have a vested interest in denying the profound and long-term effects of trauma. Perpetrators of assault and abuse have a highly vested interest in finding protection from exposure and criminal penalties by continuing to "blame the victim" as they have always done. The larger society will continue to deny the magnitude of the problem, not only because of the emotional arousal exposure causes, but also because it is becoming increasingly clear that fixing the problems and actually preventing trauma will cost a great deal.

There is a moral danger inherent in our work, perhaps best thought of as the medicalization and privatization of what is a socially determined problem (Bloom, 1995). If we fail to provide evidence-based treatment for our patients who suffer from the chronic disorders related to exposure to traumatic experiences, we fail as healers. But if we focus our attention exclusively on deciphering the complex brain processes that lead to the symptoms of post-traumatic stress, we may ignore the social context within which the traumatic stress originally occurred. A senior army officer and Vietnam veteran nurse points out, "It's the government and the country at large that suffer from PTSD: anger, guilt, shame, denial, mistrust, and all the rest. We've been saying that for years. It's good politics to blame the victims. Then America avoids the consequences of its own actions and condemns the veterans to pay the price" (Davis, 1994, p. 134). This is the same charge that has been leveled at mental health professionals from the women's movement as well: "Psychiatry and psychology on either side, believing or disbelieving women and children, defuses the issue by medicalizing it. That, in removing it from the political sphere to that of individual pathology, it is an excellent vehicle for problem management rather than for social change" (Armstrong, 1994, p. 183). It is a discourse that pervades those who work in the field of human rights abuses, "In a context of human rights violations, this problem must also be related to the political context. To be on a survivor's mission in Chile was not only a question of one's own survival but also of the survival of democracy and human dignity.... It appeared that therapists were exposed to the same kinds of trauma as their patients.... Their work, which helped the enemies of the regime, was fraught with danger and could bring on traumatization by direct actions from the regime.... The work could, however, also be experienced as healing for therapists because of the commitment to a higher goal, the struggle for prosocial change and human rights" (Agger & Jensen, 1994, pp. 284 and 285). We are mental health professionals, trained to diagnose and treat mental illness.

We are not as well-trained—or even comfortable with—social activism. However, the ISTSS was created as an organization clearly directed at mobilizing the power of scientific knowledge in the service of social change and we forget—or neglect—this heritage at our peril.

Our work is far from over. It has only just begun. Ahead for the organization lie the same challenges that we pose for our traumatized patients. Can we continue to balance conflicting needs without disintegrating into chaos? Can we contain overwhelming affect and manage the anxiety of change and lack of predictability without becoming destructive? Can we ultimately find ways to successfully integrate conflicting desires, needs, points of view, and agendas into a creative, dynamic whole? Can we hold onto our memories of what we have learned, defying the ever-present tendency to deny and forget the effects of trauma? Zahava Solomon urges us to "constitute a professional system that will retain information so that lessons, once learned, shall not be forgotten.... I believe that it is our duty as the International Society for Traumatic Stress Studies to chip away, however slowly, at these denial tendencies, at professional blindness, and at the tendency of the establishment to refuse responsibility for the treatment and rehabilitation of casualties and their families" (Solomon, 1995d, p. 281).

We still have the opportunity to decide if we, as individual clinicians and as part of a larger whole, are ultimately going to become a part of the problem or a part of the solution. As Chaim Shatan summed it up,

> I propose that our next professional assignment is to go beyond the treatment of new trauma populations: the long-range cure of war-related trauma requires prevention of traumatic stress. We traumatologists can continue to provide first aid as "stretcher bearers of the social order," sophisticated, compassionate, with growing scientific knowledge, but picking up the wounded rather than preventing them from being wounded. Or we can try to eliminate the sources of PTSD in the social order, to dismantle the army-and-enemy system, a human invention, an institutionalized manhunt.... Otherwise, PTSD—an outgrowth of war and persecution—will remain with us unchanged—under whatever name from shellshock to K.Z. syndrome, from DSM-III to DSM-X. (Shatan, 1992, p. 20)

Dedication

This chapter is dedicated to all those who have played a critical role in transforming trauma into wisdom, particularly those I have neglected to mention in this brief and, by necessity, incomplete historical summary.

References

Agger, I., & Jensen, S. B. (1994). Determinant factors for countertransference reactions under state terrorism. In J. P. Wilson & J. D. Lindy (Eds.), *Countertransference in the Treatment of PTSD*. New York: Guilford.

Armstrong, L. (1994.) *Rocking the cradle of sexual politics*. Reading, MA: Addison-Wesley.

Askevold, F. (1976). The war sailor syndrome. *Psychotherapy and Psychosomatics, 77*(27), 133–138.

Bard, M., & Sangrey, D. (1979). *The crime victim's book*. New York: Brunner/Mazel.

Bard, M., & Shellow, R. (1976). *Issues in law enforcement: Essays and case studies*. Reston, VA: Reston.

Bastiaans, J. (1974). The KZ-syndrome: A thirty-year study of the effects on victims of Nazi concentration camps. *Revue de Medecine et Chirurgie, 78*, 573–580.

Benedek, E. P. (1985). Children and psychic trauma: A brief review of contemporary thinking. In S. Eth & R. S. Pynoos (Eds.), *Post-traumatic stress disorder in children*. Washington, DC: American Psychiatric Press.

Benyakar, M., & Noy, S. (1975, January). A suggestion for a therapeutic model for posttraumatic war neurosis. Presented at the *First International Conference on Psychological Stress and Adjustment in Time of War and Peace*, Tel-Aviv.

Blank, A. S. (1985). Irrational reactions to post-traumatic stress disorder and Viet Nam veterans. In S. M. Sonnenberg, A. S. Blank, & J. A. Talbott (Eds.), *The trauma of war: Stress and recovery in Viet Nam veterans* (pp. 69–98). Washington, DC: American Psychiatric Press.

Blank, A. S. (1993). Vet Centers: A new paradigm in delivery of services for victims and survivors of traumatic stress. In J. P. Wilson & B. Raphael (Eds.), *International handbook of traumatic stress syndromes* (pp. 915–924). New York: Plenum.

Blank, A. S. (1997a). Personal interview with author, November 2.

Blank, A. S. (1997b). On the central role of advocacy in the traumatic stress field. *Stresspoints, 11*(3), 4.

Blank, A. S. (1998). Personal interview with author, January 15.

Bloom, S. L. (1995). The germ theory of trauma: The impossibility of ethical neutrality. In B.H. Stamm (Ed.), *Secondary traumatic stress: Self-care issues for clinicians, researchers, and educators* (pp. 257–276). Lutherville, MD: Sidran Foundation.

Boman, B. (1979). Behavioral observations on the Granville train disasters and the significance of stress for psychiatry. *Social Science and Medicine, 13*, 463–471.

Bourne, P. G. (1969). *The psychology and physiology of stress.* New York: Academic Press.

Bourne, P. G. (1971). From boot to My Lai. In R. Falk, G. Kolko, & R. Lifton (Eds.), *Crimes of war.* New York: Random House.

Burgess, A. W., & Holstrom, L. (1974). Rape trauma syndrome. *American Journal of Psychiatry, 131*, 981–986.

Burgess, A. W., Groth, A. N., Holmstrom, L. L., & Sgroi, S. M. (1978). *Sexual assault of children and adolescents.* New York: Lexington Books.

Danieli, Y. (1981). Therapists' difficulties in treating survivors of the Nazi Holocaust and their children. Ph.D. Dissertation. New York University, New York.

Danieli, Y., Rodley, N. S., & Weisaeth, L. (Eds.) (1996). *International responses to traumatic stress: Humanitarian, human rights, justice, peace and development contributions, collaborative actions and future initiatives.* Amityville, NY: Baywood.

Daniels, D. N., Gilula, M. F., & Ochberg, F. M. (1970). *Violence and the struggle for existence.* Boston: Little, Brown.

Davis, W. (1994). *Shattered dream: American's search for its soul.* Valley Forge: Trinity Press International.

Dohrenwend, B. P., Dohrenwend, B. S., Warheit, G. J., Bartlett, G. S., Goldsteen, R. L., Goldsteen, K., & Martin, J. L. (1981). Stress in the community: A report to the President's Commission on the Accident at Three Mile Island. *Annals of the New York Academy of Sciences, 365*, 159–174.

Egendorf, A., Kadushin, C., Rothbart, G., Sloan, L., & Fine, M. (1977, August). Urban males of the Vietnam generation, a mental health perspective: preliminary findings of the Vietnam-era project. Presented at the *Annual Meeting of the American Psychological Association*, San Francisco.

Egendorf, A., Kadushin, C., Laufer, R., Rothbart, G., & Sloan, L. (1981). Legacies of Vietnam: Comparative adjustment of veterans and their peers. Washington, DC: U.S. Government Printing Office.

Eitinger, L. (1960). The symptomatology of mental disease among refugees in Norway. *Journal of Mental Science, 106*, 947–966.

Eitinger, L. (1961). Pathology of the concentration camp syndrome. *Archives of General Psychiatry, 5*, 371–379.

Eitinger, L. (1964). *Concentration camp survivors in Norway and Israel.* Oslo: Universitetsforlaget.

Erickson, K. (1976). *Everything in its path: Destruction of community in the Buffalo Creek flood.* New York: Simon and Schuster.

Figley, C. R., & Southerly, W. T. (1977, August). Residue of war: The Vietnam veterans in mainstream America. Presented at the *Annual Meeting of the American Psychological Association*, San Francisco.

Figley, C. R. Introduction. (1978a). In C. R. Figley (Ed.), *Stress disorders among Vietnam veterans: Theory, research and treatment.* New York: Brunner/Mazel.

Figley, C. R. (1978b). Psychosocial adjustment among Vietnam veterans: An overview of the research. In C. R. Figley (Ed.), *Stress disorders among Vietnam veterans: Theory, research and treatment* (pp. 57–70). New York: Brunner/Mazel.

Figley, C. R. (1986a). History. *Stresspoints, 1*(1), 2.

Figley, C. R. (1986b). *Trauma and its wake,* Vol. two: *Traumatic stress theory, research, and integration.* New York: Brunner/Mazel.

Figley, C. R. (1998). Personal communication with author, January 6.

Finkelhor, D. (1979). *Sexually victimized children.* New York: The Free Press.

Finkelhor, D. (1996). Introduction. In J. Briere, L. Berliner, J. A. Bulkley, C. Jenny, & T. Reid (Eds.), *The APSAC handbook on child maltreatment* (pp. ix–xiii). Thousand Oaks, CA: Sage.

Gelles, R. J., & Straus, M. A. (1979). Determinants of violence in the family: Toward a theoretical integration. In W. R. Burr, R. Hill, & F. I. Nye (Eds.), *Contemporary theories about the family*. New York: Free Press.

Gleser, G., Green, B. L., & Winget, C. (1981). *Prolonged psychosocial effects of disaster: A study of Buffalo Creek*. New York: Academic Press.

Green, A. H. (1978a). Psychiatric treatment of abused children. *Journal of the American Academy of Child Psychiatry, 17,* 356–371.

Green, A. H. (1978b). Self-destructive behavior in battered children. *American Journal of Psychiatry, 135,* 579–582.

Haley, S. (1974). When the patient reports atrocities. *Archives of General Psychiatry, 30,* 191–196.

Hearst, P. (1981). *Every secret thing*. New York: Doubleday.

Herman, J. L. (1981). *Father-daughter incest*. Cambridge, MA: Harvard University Press.

Herman, J. L. (1992). *Trauma and recovery*. New York: Basic Books.

Horowitz, M. J. (1976). *Stress response syndromes*. New York: Jason Aronson.

Jones, M. (1953). *The therapeutic community: A new treatment method in psychiatry*. New York: Basic Books.

Kardiner, A. (1941). *The traumatic neuroses of war*. New York: Paul B. Hoeber.

Kempe, C. H., Silverman, F. N., Steele, B. F., Droegemueller, W., & Silver, H. K. (1962). The battered child syndrome. *Journal of the American Medical Association, 181,* 17–24.

Kempe, R. S., & Kempe, C. H. (1978). *Child abuse*. Cambridge, MA: Harvard University Press.

Kinzie, J. D. (1978). Lessons from cross-cultural psychotherapy. *American Journal of Psychotherapy, 32,* 110–120.

Krystal, H. (1968). *Massive psychic trauma*. New York: International Universities Press.

Laufer, R. S. (1985). War trauma and human development: The Viet Nam experience. In S. M. Sonnenberg, A. S. Blank, & J. A. Talbott (Eds.), *The trauma of war: Stress and recovery in Viet Nam veterans* (pp. 31–55). Washington, DC: American Psychiatric Press.

Leopold, R. L., & Dillon, H. (1963). Psychoanatomy of a disaster: A long-term study of posttraumatic neuroses in survivors of a marine explosion. *American Journal of Psychiatry, 119,* 913–921.

Leventman, S. (1978). Epilogue: Social and historical perspectives on the Vietnam veteran. C. R. Figley (Ed.), *Stress disorders among Vietnam veterans: Theory, research and treatment* (pp. 291–295). New York: Brunner/Mazel.

Lifton, R. J. (1967). *Death in life: Survivors of Hiroshima*. New York: Basic Books.

Lifton, R. J. (1973). *Home from the war*. New York: Basic Books.

Lifton, R. J. (1978). Advocacy and corruption in the healing profession. In C. R. Figley (Ed.), *Stress disorders among Vietnam veterans: Theory, research and treatment*. New York: Brunner/Mazel.

Lifton, R. J., & Olson, E. (1976). The human meaning of total disaster: The Buffalo Creek Experience. *Psychiatry, 39,* 1–18.

Lin, K. M., Tozuma, L., & Masuda, M. (1979). Adaptional problems of Vietnamese refugees. *Archives of General Psychology, 36,* 955–961.

Lindemann, E. (1944). Symptomatology and management of acute grief. *American Journal of Psychiatry, 101,* 141–148.

Mahedy, W. (1986). *Out of the night: The spiritual journey of Vietnam vets*. New York: Ballantine.

Malt, U. F., Schnyder, U., & Weisaeth, L. (1996). ICD-10 Mental and behavioral consequences of traumatic stress. In F. L. Mak & C. C. Nadelson (Eds.), *International Review of Psychiatry*, Vol. 2 (pp. 151–176). Washington, DC: American Psychiatric Press.

Meshad, S. (1997). Personal interview with the author, October 28.

Milgram, N. A. (1978). Psychological stress and adjustment in time of war and peace: The Israeli experience as presented in two conferences. *Israel Annals of Psychiatry and Related Disciplines, 16,* 327–338.

Milgram, N. A. (1998). Personal communication with author, January 9.

Moses, R., Bargal, D., & Calev, J. (1975). A rear unit for the treatment of combat reaction in the wake of the Yom Kippur War. *Psychiatry, 39,* 153–162.

Neff, L. (1975, May). Traumatic neurosis. Presented at the *Annual Meeting of the American Psychological Association*, CA.

Niederland, W. G. (1968). Clinical observations on the "survivor syndrome." *International Journal of Psychoanalysis, 49,* 313–315.

Nordheimer, J. (1971, May). From Dakto to Detroit: Death of a troubled hero. *New York Times 12:41,* 395.

Noy, S. (1978). Stress and personality factors in the causation and prognosis of combat reaction. Delivered at the *Second International Conference on Psychological Stress and Adjustment in Time of War and Peace*, Jerusalem.

Ochberg, F. (1978). The victim of terrorism: Psychiatric considerations. *Terrorism, 1*(2), 147–168.

Ochberg, F. (1988a). Post-traumatic therapy and victims of violence. In F. Ochberg (Ed.), *Post-traumatic therapy and victims of violence* (pp. 3–19). New York: Brunner/Mazel.

Ochberg, F. (1988b). The victim of war and atrocity. In F. Ochberg (Ed.), *Post-traumatic therapy and victims of violence* (pp. 225–226). New York: Brunner/Mazel.

Ochberg, F. (1996). A primer on covering victims. *The Neiman Report, L(3)*, 21–26.

Ochberg, F., & Soskis, D. A. (Eds.). (1982). *Victims of terrorism.* Boulder: Westview Press.

Parker, G. (1977). Cyclone Tracy and Darwin evacuees: On the restoration of the species. *British Journal of Psychiatry, 130*, 548–555.

Quarantelli, E. L., & Dynes, R. R.(1977). Response to social crisis and disaster. *Annual Review of Sociology, 3*, 23–49.

Raphael, B. (1977). Bereavement and prevention. *New Doctor, 4*, 41–45.

Raphael, B., & Maddison, D. C. (1976). Care of bereaved adults: Modern trends. In O. W. Hill (Ed.), *Psychosomatic medicine—3* (pp. 491–506). London: Butterworth.

Rich, R. F. (1981). Evaluating mental health services for victims: Perspectives on policies and services in the United States. In S. E. Salasin (Ed.), *Evaluating victim services* (pp. 128–142). Beverly Hills: Sage.

Salasin, S. E. (Ed.) (1981). *Evaluating victim services.* Beverly Hills: Sage.

Scott, W. (1990). PTSD in DSM-III: A case in the politics of diagnosis and disease. *Social Problems, 37*(3), 294–310.

Scott, W. (1993). *The politics of readjustment: Vietnam veterans since the war.* Hawthorne, NY: Aldine de Gruyter.

Selye, H. (1956). *The stress of life.* New York: McGraw-Hill.

Sgroi, S. (1975). Sexual molestation of children: The last frontier in child abuse. *Children Today, 44*, 18–21.

Shatan, C. (1971). Memo: The Vietnam veteran and the psychoanalytic community. February 2.

Shatan, C. (1972, May 6). Post-Vietnam syndrome. *New York Times*, p. 35.

Shatan, C. (1974). Through the membrane of reality: "Impacted grief" and perceptual dissonance in Vietnam combat veterans. *Psychiatric Opinion, 11*(6), 6–15.

Shatan, C. (1975). War babies: Delayed impact of warmaking, persecution, and disaster on children. *American Journal of Orthopsychiatry, 45*, 289.

Shatan, C. (1978a). Stress disorders among Vietnam veterans: The emotional context of combat continues. In C. R. Figley (Ed.), *Stress disorders among Vietnam veterans: Theory, research and treatment* (pp. 43–52). New York: Brunner/Mazel.

Shatan, C. (1978b). Letter to Dr. Marion Langer, Executive Director, American Orthopsychiatric Association, February 16.

Shatan, C. (1985, September). Johnny, we don't want to know you: From DEROS and death camps to the diagnostic battlefield. Presented at the *Founding Meeting of the Society for Traumatic Stress Studies*, Atlanta, GA.

Shatan, C. (1987, October). Johnny, we hardly know you: The grief of soldiers and the Vietnam veterans' self-help movement. Presented at the *Third Annual Meeting of the Society for Traumatic Stress Studies*, Baltimore, MD.

Shatan, C. (1992, June). Enemies, armies, and PTSD: Divided consciousness and war—our next assignment. Presented at the *First World Conference of the ISTSS*, Amsterdam, Netherlands.

Shatan, C. (1997a). Personal interview with the author, October 28.

Shatan, C. (1997b). Personal memo to author, November 19.

Shatan, C. (1998). Personal interview with author, February 24.

Shatan, C., Haley, S., & Smith, J. (1977, May). Johnny comes marching home: The emotional context of combat stress. Concepts for the new Diagnostic and Statistical Manual (DSM-III) of Mental Disorders. Unpublished paper, based on a panel "Can time heal all wounds: Diagnosis and management of post-combat stress, presented at the *Annual Meeting of the American Psychiatric Association*, Toronto.

Sims, A. C. P., White, A. C, & Murphy, T. (1979). Aftermath neurosis: Psychological sequelae of the Birmingham bombings in victims not seriously injured. *Medicine, Science and the Law, 19*, 78–81.

Sohlberg, S. (1975). Battle stress and fatigue during the Yom Kippur War. Presented at the *Mental Health Conference of the Israel Defense Force*, Tel Hashomer.

Solomon, Z. (1995a). From denial to recognition: Attitudes toward Holocaust survivors from World War II to the present. *Journal of Traumatic Stress Studies, 8*(2), 215–228.

Solomon, Z. (1995b). Attitudes of therapists toward Holocaust survivors. *Journal of Traumatic Stress Studies, 8*(2), 229–242.

Solomon, Z. (1995c). Therapeutic response to combat stress reactions: Current attitudes of military physicians. *Journal of Traumatic Stress Studies, 8*(2), 243–246.

Solomon, Z. (1995d). Oscillating between denial and recognition of PTSD: Why are lessons learned and forgotten? *Journal of Traumatic Stress Studies, 8*(2), 271–282.

Steiner, M., & Neumann, M. (1978). Traumatic neurosis and social support in the Yom Kippur War returnees. *Military Medicine, 143*, 866–868.

Straus, M. A. (1977). Sociological perspective on the prevention and treatment of wife-beating. In M. Roy (Ed.), *Battered women: A psychological study of domestic violence.* New York: Van Nostrand Reinhold.

Strenz, T. (1982). The Stockholm syndrome. In F. Ochberg & D. Soskis (Eds.), *Victims of terrorism* (pp. 149–164). Boulder: Westview.

Terr, L. (1979). Children of Chowchilla: A study of psychic trauma. *Psychoanalytic Study of the Child, 34,* 552–623.

Thygesen, P., Hermann, K., & Willanger, R. (1970). Concentration camp survivors in Denmark. Persecution, disease, disability, compensation. A 23 year follow-up. *Danish Medical Bulletin, 17,* 65–108.

Tierney, K. J., & Baisden, B. (1979). Crisis intervention programs for disaster victims: A source-book and manual for smaller communities. Washington, DC: U.S. Government Printing Office.

Titchner, J., & Kapp, F. T. (1976). Family and character change at Buffalo Creek. *American Journal of Psychiatry, 143,* 1443–1446.

United States Senate. (1981, April 27). Veterans' programs extension and improvement act of 1981. Report No. 97-89.

van der Kolk, B. A., Heron, N., & Hostetler, A. (1994). The history of trauma in psychiatry. *Psychiatric Clinics of North America, 17*(3), 583–600.

van der Kolk, B. A., Weisaeth, L., & van der Hart, O. (1996). History of trauma in psychiatry. In B. A. van der Kolk, A. C. McFarlane, & L. Weisaeth (Eds.), *Traumatic stress: The effects of overwhelming experience on mind, body, and society* (pp. 47–74). New York: Guilford.

Walker, L. (1979). *The battered woman.* New York: Harper & Row.

Wilson, J. P. (1988). Understanding the Vietnam veteran. In F. Ochberg (Ed.), *Post-traumatic therapy and victims of violence* (pp. 227–253). New York: Brunner/Mazel.

Wilson, J. P. (1995). The historical evolution of PTSD diagnostic criteria: From Freud to DSM-IV. In G. S. Everly, Jr., & J. M. Lating (Eds.), *Psychotraumatology: Key papers and core concepts in post-traumatic stress* (pp. 9–26). New York: Plenum.

Wilson, J. P. (1997). Personal interview with author, October 22.

Wilson, J., & Doyle, C. (1977). *Identity, ideology and crisis: The Vietnam veteran in transition: A preliminary report on the forgotten warrior project.* Cincinnati: OH: Disabled American Veterans.

Wilson, J. P., Harel, Z., & Kahana, B. (1988). *Human adaptation to extreme stress: From the Holocaust to Vietnam.* New York: Plenum.

Wilson, J. P., & Raphael, B. (1993). *International handbook of traumatic stress syndromes.* New York: Plenum.

Young, M. (1988). The crime victim's movement. In F. Ochberg (Ed.), *Post-traumatic therapy and victims of violence* (pp. 319–329). New York: Brunner/Mazel.

4

An Alternative History of Traumatic Stress

ALLAN YOUNG

The starting point for this chapter is the belief that post-traumatic stress disorder can be usefully viewed as an episode in a history that stretches back more than a century. The chapter is an *alternative* history because it is an effort to describe familiar events and developments in an unfamiliar way. I write as an anthropologist and a historian, and my goal is to excavate some of the assumptions that underpin and guide PTSD research and clinical practice today. I want to make tacit knowledge explicit—more specifically, ideas about memory—and to suggest how it has been shaped by history and culture.

Memory and the Post-Traumatic Syndrome

In most historical accounts, clinical interest in the post-traumatic syndrome begins with John Erichsen's treatise on "railway spine" (Erichsen, 1866). During the following two decades, the syndrome was commonly associated with events, such as railway collisions, producing shock, fright, and physical and emotional perturbation. Symptoms were variable but generally resembled effects associated with neurological injury. What made the new syndrome special was that (1) it occurred without significant external injury and (2) the putative victims often claimed compensation (from railway companies) for the pain, distress, and loss of income said to result from their invisible injuries.

Opinion divided on the question of its pathogenesis. The majority view was that the vigorous jolts and shakes experienced on these occasions were sufficient to damage the nervous system. Pathogenesis could be understood by analogy with well-known neurological mechanisms, especially concussion. Some physicians, notably Herbert Page (1883), suggested that the arousal of powerful emotions, specifically fear, might have similar effects. There was no obvious way to test the nerve-trauma hypothesis except by

ALLAN YOUNG • Department of Social Studies of Medicine, McGill University, Montreal, Quebec, H3G 1Y6, Canada.

International Handbook of Human Response to Trauma, edited by Shalev, Yehuda, and McFarlane. Kluwer Academic / Plenum Publishers, New York, 2000.

the pathoanatomical method, that is, by postmortem examination. It was recognized that whatever interesting findings this mode of inquiry might eventually produce, it was diagnostically worthless for the present. Further, it was understood that the pathological alterations produced by these accidents might be submicroscopic or "nutritional" (pathophysiological) and therefore effectively invisible. Other physicians, including Jean-Martin Charcot (himself a celebrated neurologist), believed that only some cases of these disorders were attributable to nerve damage inflicted directly by the force of the accident. There were certain symptomatically similar cases that originated in a previously undetected mechanism, a kind of post-traumatic memory that was created at the time of the collision. The prevailing assumption was that, under ordinary conditions, memories are deposited in associative networks, within which they are connected to concomitant emotions, sensations, and dispositions, and likewise to other memories. In contrast, the post-traumatic memories were isolated or dissociated. This explained the patients' characteristic inabilities to recall their traumatic events. Exactly how the characteristic symptoms were connected to the dissociated memory was a matter for speculation. Charcot and, at one point, Freud believed that the link might be explained in physical terms, wrapped up in action potentials and energy flows. In time, the connection assumed a more symbolic quality (Charcot, 1889). Thus Breuer and Freud (1955, orig. 1893–1895) traced symptomatic neuralgia to a mental pain whose substance was hidden in amnesic memory. Whether the connection between memory and somatic symptoms was organic or symbolic or a combination of the two, the effect was the same. The symptoms were transformed into "mnemic symbols" that might lead experts back to memories to which patients had no ready access.

It is at this point in the last decades of the nineteenth century that the traumatic memory makes its appearance. Charcot portrayed it as "a coherent group of associated ideas *which install themselves in the mind in the fashion of a parasite,* remain isolated from all the rest, and may be explained outwardly by corresponding motor phenomena" (cited in Janet, 1901, p. 267). It was an unprecedented kind of memory, and it transformed the ways in which physicians thought about post-traumatic syndromes and how the syndromes would be diagnosed and treated in the future. Although no one denied that the symptoms could also be produced by mechanical forces, now there was a second possibly, a syndrome caused by moral perturbation (extreme psychological stress or conflict), rather than cerebral commotion.

During this period, post-traumatic syndromes were associated with amnesias of one kind or another. Almost without exception, patients were described as unable to recall the events that precipitated their illnesses. Many patients were also reported suffering from retrograde amnesia (loss of pretrauma memory) or anterograde amnesia (loss of on-going post-trauma memory). In each of these instances, amnesia defines and confirms the unusual character of traumatic memory. In a monograph on *idées fixes,* Janet argued that patients continue to store memories acquired during the amnesic periods but are unable to *assimilate* them. In this regard, they resemble the traumatic memory that has created this situation—they are disconnected from the network of memories that constitute the individual's personality and sense of self-awareness. "[Post-traumatic] personalities, blocked at a certain point, can no longer grow through the addition [and] assimilation of new elements" (Janet, 1925, p. 138, cited in Roth, 1996, pp. 7–8). During the following decades, the association of traumatic memory with retrograde and anteretrograde amnesias gradually uncoupled, and after World War II it was much less often reported. Nevertheless, the conclusions that Janet and other physicians inferred from these forms of forgetting—traumatic memory constricts and distorts the self by imprisoning it in a timeless present—have endured, and they continue to shape our understanding of the post-traumatic syndrome.

I want to briefly mention one more obvious development that occurred during this formative period. In *Beyond the Pleasure Principle* (1955, orig. 1920), Freud linked traumatic memory to an unconscious compulsion to repeat. Patients were said to relive their etiological events in dreams, in an unconscious effort to anticipate and master the fright that had originally overwhelmed them. Janet's conception of traumatic memory had been essentially static: he described it as an *idée fixe* lodged in the psyche. Freud injected a dynamic aspect by portraying the patient's relationship to his traumatic memory as a series of encounters. Although only a minority of clinicians and researchers today would accept Freud's claims about the function of traumatic dreams, his basic idea that the post-traumatic syndrome is sustained by recurrent encounters with the traumatic memory (reexperiences) and by efforts to manage these encounters (avoidance and numbing) is generally taken for granted.

In a seminal account of post-traumatic syndromes, that combined Janet's and Freud's ideas, Mardi Horowitz (1976, chapters 3, 6, 7) described traumatized patients as people who are striving to metabolize their pathogenic memories through alternating phases of engagement (during which they work at assimilating and accommodating these memories) and withdrawal (an adaptive response to pain generated during the engagement phase). Here, in a nutshell, we have the post-traumatic syndrome that entered the official psychiatric nosology in DSM-III (1980) as post-traumatic stress disorder. In this and subsequent editions, the PTSD classification is defined by four diagnostic criteria: an etiologic event, recurrent encounters with memories of this event, symptomatic avoidance and numbing, and physiological arousal. Remembering is said to occur in the form of intrusive recollections, during dreams, and on occasions when patients feel they are reliving their etiological experiences, for instance, in "flashbacks." The act of remembering is also said to occur on occasions when patients react, either psychologically or somatically, to stimuli that are symbolically linked to their etiologic events.

Today, as in the days of Charcot, Janet, and Freud, memory is regarded as the key to understanding the origins and pathogenesis of the post-traumatic syndrome. A century after its initial discovery, the idea of a traumatic memory seems natural, even obvious. Indeed, one wonders why it took so long for the idea to come to mind and why, once it was proposed, some physicians resisted. Likewise, one wonders why an idea that now seems self-evident to most Westerners did not emerge spontaneously in other cultures and regions of the world. In the following pages, I want to show that these puzzles are not "academic," fit only for historians or anthropologists, but have interesting implications for clinicians and researchers. My thesis is that, although the idea of traumatic memory now seems self-evident, it is historically determined and rooted in culturally specific beliefs concerning the self and self-awareness. To grapple with this argument, one must entertain the possibility that memory is malleable. I mean this in the obvious sense that episodic memory is subject to a variety of "distortions," including retroactive interference—the influence of subsequent events on the way one recollects earlier events. I mean to imply more than this though, namely that generic "memory"— *the assortment of things that experts and other people count as memories or evidence of memories*—is also malleable. And like traumatic memory, it needs to be seen in the context of history and culture.

History, Memory, and Self-Awareness

The association between episodic memory and the self has a long history in the West. St. Augustine wrote about it in his *Confessions* at the end of the fourth century (Pelikan, 1986). He portrayed memory as a retrospective view through which someone might see the life journey that reveals the meaning of the self. Until a person grasps his memory of the past, he knows the self, not in its wholeness, but in fragments, specific to time and place. Through the prism of memory, he discovers patterns and underlying meanings which, in Augustine's case, are consonant with Christian metaphysics. Memory reveals the self to consciousness but does not contribute to producing the self. This is a *modern* notion.

One of its earliest monuments is John Locke's concept of the *forensic self*—an entity identified with the individual's accountability for his intentional behavior (Locke, 1959, chapter 27). Intentionality and selfhood both presume consciousness, and consciousness is manifestly located in the present time. In what sense am I accountable for acts that I committed in long-ago acts of consciousness? What is the medium for the continuity of the forensic self? The answer is episodic memory. It connects moments of consciousness and renders acts in the past morally equivalent to acts in the present. David Hume's account of the self, written a century later, is still more recognizably modern. Like Locke, he discusses the continuity of the self in terms of episodic memory; unlike Locke, the existence of the self is not only forensic but also psychological. Had we no memory, Hume writes, we would have no knowledge of the chains of causes and effects from which we produce our self-awareness and, perhaps, our very self-existence (Biro, 1993).

These were the opinions of exceptional individuals, and one might argue that we can infer nothing from them about the self-awareness of ordinary people, either then or now. This would be a fair criticism if these ideas about self and memory did not pass beyond the circle of philosophers. In fact, however, Hume's ideas were taken up and elaborated by a Frenchman who profoundly influenced the thinking of Janet and Freud.

Théodule Ribot was a world renowned psychologist and a translator of British empiricist philosophy. In his widely read treatise on forgetting and remembering, *The Diseases of Memory*, first published in 1881, we encounter the self (*moi*) as something that is formed, nourished, and renewed by its memory. Ribot describes it as being a protean phenomenon, ceaselessly passing through phases of growth, degeneration, and reproduction. In his account, the self now acquires an economic dimension because self-renewal is possible only because room is continually being made for new memories, new associations, and new self-narratives. And room is available only when old memories are permitted to fade and their ability to evoke the emotions with which they were first associated gradually weakens to the point where these old memories are no more than the memories of memories. In other words, forgetting is both normal and necessary. Ribot writes,

> To live is to acquire and lose; life consists of dissolution as well as assimilation. Forgetfulness is dissolution…. Without the total obliteration of an immense number of states of consciousness, and the momentary repression of many more, recollection would be impossible. Forgetfulness, except in certain cases, is not a disease of memory, but a condition of health and life. (Ribot 1883:61)

The Grammar of Forgetting and Remembering

Ribot's idea of a *self-narrated self,* held together by memories, found a receptive audience. It had a powerful effect on the thinking of Pierre Janet, who was Ribot's successor in the Seat of Psychology at the University of Paris. Marcel Proust had also been Ribot's student and gratefully acknowledged his teacher's influence on his own thinking about time, memory, and self-knowledge. When Sigmund Freud left Vienna for London in 1938, he brought a mere handful of books, included among which was his copy of Ribot's book on the diseases of memory.

Ribot believed that the self-narrated self is universal. He presumed that people naturally crave a sense of unity and wholeness that will incorporate memories of the personal past. Anthropologists and other investigators working in non-Western societies have no difficulty getting people to talk in autobiographical terms. Does this validate Ribot's claim? Before we can attempt an answer, we need to examine his other assumption, that self-narration is not only universally possible but it is also the predominant medium of self-consciousness. At this point, there is no compelling empirically based body of evidence to support this assumption, even if its truth is routinely taken for granted. Whether Ribot's ideas about the self and self-awareness are universal, one fact is undeniable. His notion of a self-narrated self is integral to the ways in which most clinicians and researchers think about traumatic memory and post-traumatic disorders.

It would be hard to exaggerate the importance of this concept of self for shaping psychiatric knowledge of PTSD. The disorder's pathology is said to reside in the fact that certain memories will neither fade nor submit to a process of assimilation. They refuse to make way for new constellations of memories and, because of this, the self loses its capacity for renarrating itself. Disorders of traumatic memory are not self-destructive in the way of Alzheimer's disease and extreme cases of Korsakov's syndrome. The self is distorted, crippled, even fragmented into part-selves, but it is not lost.

The last decades of the nineteenth century constituted the golden age of memory science, during which experts constructed the grammar of forgetting and remembering that is employed today to connect aberrations of memory to deformations of the self. In Ribot's scheme, the normal self occupies a space bounded on one side by *hypermnesia*—a "condition in which past acts, feelings, or ideas are brought vividly to the mind, which in its natural condition [would have] wholly lost the remembrance of these"—and on the other side by *amnesia,* remembering too little rather than too much.

Ribot was less interested in *cryptomnesia,* a condition in which a person remembers something from the past but forgets, or rather misremembers, the source of the memory. Théodore Flournoy (1994, orig. 1899), a Swiss psychologist and contemporary of Ribot, wrote about a spirit medium in this connection. The medium believed that she was a conduit for a group of spirits who had lived in fifteenth-century India. Flournoy was convinced that the information provided by the spirits was obtained from a history of India stored in the Geneva municipal library. Unfortunately, he could not learn the circumstances in which the medium had come across this book, nor could he explain why she easily recalled obscure details in the book but had no memory of their actual source. Freud self-diagnosed an episode of cryptomnesia, in which he confesses to unconsciously plagiarizing a colleague's ideas about bisexuality (Ceci, 1995, pp. 93–94). Cryptomnesia also labels the occasional cases of "factitious" PTSD among war veterans, in which men transform the combat experiences of other men into their own traumatic recollections. The most frequently reported cases of cryptomnesia today involve accusations, often raised during litigation, of traumatic recollections implanted in patients' minds by their therapists in the pursuit of recovered memories of childhood incest.

The final ingredient in the grammar of forgetting and remembering consists of *phylogenetic memories*. In the early 1800s, the evolutionary biologist, Jean-Baptiste Lamarck, described a species of collective memory that was acquired biologically over multiple generations. Phylogenetic memories are a basic part of Freud's *Totem and Taboo* and *Moses and Monotheism*, and they are intrinsic to Jung's concept of racial archetypes. In each case, the memories incorporate huge amounts of information. Previous to these accounts, Herbert Spencer and Charles Darwin had suggested the possibility of a much simpler kind of phylogenetic memory, observed in "instinctual" reactions associated with fear and anger. Spencer argued that such memories had been engraved into the nervous system over the course of evolution. Countless repetitions— evidence of the survival value of the entailed behavior—would eventually produce neural pathways, along which perceptions and impulses could now race, no longer impeded by cognition or deliberation. The phylogenetic memories discussed by Freud and Jung fell victim to the Mendelian revolution. Their sheer complexity required a Lamarckian framework, as Freud himself acknowledged. On the other hand, the sorts of memories described by Spencer, accounting for instinctual fear and the fight or flight response, had no problem passing through this historical membrane and emerged on the other side in pioneering research on the physiology of the autonomic nervous system by George Crile, Walter Cannon, and others (Young, 1996). The subject of phylogenetic memory continued to be discussed well into the present century. For example, it is mentioned in Kurt Goldstein's book on holistic neurology, *The Organism* (1939). During the subsequent decades, however, the term "phylogenetic memory" entirely disappeared from psychiatry, neurology, and physiology. At the same time, the adaptational structure that Darwin and Spencer described a century ago is a building block in our own understanding of the biology of extreme situations and is continuous with current PTSD research on the hypothalamic–pituitary–adrenal axis.

It is useful to know how this evolutionary structure entered scientific discourse on the post-traumatic syndrome. Beginning with Charcot, physicians recognized that, in some cases at least, the engine driving the post-traumatic syndrome might be an episodic memory. Even earlier, at the time of Erichsen's and Page's investigations, physicians had observed an association between the syndrome and experiences of fear. Most of these doctors limited the association to two points: intense fear might occur at the time of a patient's etiological experience, and fear (in the form a generalized fearfulness or anxiety) might also occur as part of the syndrome. Janet went beyond this position to argue that fear might also occur within a syndrome, as a product of the patient's traumatic memory. That is to say, reexperiencing the etiological event would likewise elicit a fear response similar to the one that accompanied the original occasion. Although Janet coupled the traumatic memory to the fear response, he did not connect the response to a discrete physiological mechanism. Interest in discovering this mechanism dates from the First World War, and it is at this point that we can say that the episodic memory responsible for the post-traumatic syndrome intersected with the structure that Darwin and Spencer had characterized as phylogenetic memory, and that Cannon redescribed as an autonomic nervous system response (equally a product of the species' evolutionary history).

A New Science of Memory

The preceding pages describe a grammar of remembering and forgetting that emerged in the closing years of the nineteenth century. It was (and remains) associated with certain presumptions about the nature of the self and self-awareness. It created the possibility of a new of psychiatric enterprise, organized around concealed memories (episodic and phylogenetic), mnemic symptoms, and the codes and procedures that have been developed for deciphering these clues. The symptoms are behavioral (compulsion to repeat and avoidance behavior), somatic (body memory, conversions, neurophysiological alterations, and numbing), and cognitive (dreams, intrusive images and thoughts). They stand in a mnemic relationship to the disorder, that is, they contain information about the traumatic memory and, in the right hands, can be read like a text.

These developments can be seen coinciding with the birth of a new political economy of memory, in which the person who owns the memory in question (the traumatic parasite that it is stored in his brain and body) is not necessarily the same person who possesses the meaning of this memory or, in some cases, knowledge of the memory's very existence.

The Traumatic Neuroses of War

Abram Kardiner's *The Traumatic Neuroses of War* (1941) is cited in most histories of traumatic memory as a source of the DSM-III criteria for PTSD. In contrast to earlier monographs on this subject, Kardiner's book focuses entirely on patients with chronic disorders. (His clinical observations were made between 1922 to 1925; most of the patients were traumatized in 1918.) Kardiner had been briefly Freud's analysand, but the book's orientation is predominately holistic and psychosomatic. According to Kardiner, trauma initiates an abrupt change in the organism's adaptation to the world. The subsequent neurosis is a new adaptation, characterized by a lower level of functioning and a constriction of the ego. Kardiner describes four types of post-traumatic syndromes: somatosensory, autonomic, a type organized around neurotic "defensive ceremonials," and an epileptoid type marked by periods of unconsciousness and twilight and fugue states. Patients are said to share a set of features, that are provided on a checklist: patients are fixated on their traumas, their conceptions of the selves and the outer world are distorted, they experience characteristic dreams, they are is irritable, and they exhibit a tendency to explosive aggressive reactions. The reader is led up and down innumerable paths and byways and fails to obtain a coherent or unitary vision of the phenomenon Kardiner is describing, except for the checklist.

In 1959, Kardiner restated his conception of the traumatic neuroses of war in a more concise and integrated way. In the original account, Freud was mentioned only in passing, as having made "some extremely important observations" relating to traumatic neuroses. In the later version, Kardiner describes *Beyond the Pleasure Principle* as his own starting point: "Here Freud announced a new definition of trauma as a breakthrough of the [brain's] defense against stimuli. This break-through set up a great amount of anxiety identifiable in dreams and [is followed by] an effort on the part of the organism to free itself of this anxiety by constant repetition" (Kardiner, 1959, p. 247). The new account includes the original checklist and likewise divides the post-traumatic

syndromes into the various types, and the post-traumatic symptomatology is now ratio-
nalized by a psychodynamic principle, the repetition compulsion.

Kardiner's contribution to the PTSD classification in DSM-III consists of this
checklist, its subtext (the repetition compulsion, the symptoms are adaptions to the
organism's changed circumstances), and the idea that the disorder includes a physiological component. Its theoretical significance should not be exaggerated, however.
Kardiner connected the disorder's psychological, behavioral, and biological symptoms
within a psychosomatic frame of reference. By the time of DSM-III (1980), psychosomatic theories of this sort, shared with writers, such as Franz Alexander (1950) and
Kurt Goldstein (1939), had lost their appeal within American psychiatry. Now researchers and clinicians were more inclined to connect mind and body within alternative frames of reference—furnished by classic conditioning theory, neurophysiology,
and brain science—that maintained the historic link between trauma and phylogenetic
memory (fight-flight-freeze, etc.).

The Birth of Post-Traumatic Stress Disorder

The PTSD classification was introduced into DSM-III in the face of opposition. A
segment of the psychiatric establishment, closely associated with the manual's editorial
task force and its publicly affirmed neo-Kraepelinian principles, doubted the validity of
the proposed classification. They believed that the PTSD syndrome was not a unitary
phenomenon, and clinical cases were said to represent the co-occurrence of various
combinations of established classifications—most commonly, depression, generalized
anxiety disorder, and panic disorder.

The opponents argued that PTSD presupposes an etiology—Kardiner's subtext—
that is an unscientific relic of an age of psychiatric ignorance. A century ago, traumatic
disorders (including hysterias) were said to mimic neurological disorders. We believe
that many of these cases had real organic origins, but that nineteenth-century physicians did not possess the technical means or knowledge required to diagnose them
correctly. The proposed PTSD classification was seen as an analogous phenomenon.
The difference between the past and the present is that now the underlying disorders
are psychiatric rather than neurological, and psychiatry possesses satisfactory ways of
diagnosing these syndromes. Likewise, a century ago, Charcot argued that traumatic
hysteria is a unitary entity, comparable to multiple sclerosis or Parkinson's disease. To
audiences at Salpetriére Hospital, he demonstrated that episodes of this disorder
(*grande hystérie* or *hystero-épilepsie*) pass through invariable and well-defined stages. Yet
we know now that Charcot's star performers acquired their symptom complexes
through subtle and unintended forms of suggestion in the clinic and by autosuggestion
in the hospital ward, where they were domiciled alongside epileptic patients (Goetz et
al., 1995, chapters 4 to 6). Once PTSD is integrated into diagnostic and therapeutic
practices, similar effects can be expected—spurious or at least premature evidence of
the existence of traumatic memory. This "evidence" will transform the pathognomonic
meaning of the disorder's other features. Intrusive ruminations are a common symptom of major depression. Phobias, such as the irrational fear of crowds, are a common
symptom of anxiety disorders. When either of these symptom is connected, during
diagnosis, to an antecedent trauma, its meaning is radically changed. Ruminations turn
into intrusive "reexperiences," and phobias become "avoidance behavior" adjusted to

the environmental stimuli that trigger reexperiences. Analogous transformations will account for the physiological symptoms—difficulty in concentrating, irritability, explosions of aggressive behavior, emotional numbing—that were to be part of the proposed classification.

The advocacy group for the new diagnosis consisted of Vietnam War veterans and sympathetic psychiatrists, notably Robert Jay Lifton and Chaim Shatan (Scott, 1990; Young, 1995, chapter 3). They claimed that the Vietnam War had produced a high prevalence of post-traumatic disorders. However, these cases were consistently undiagnosed or misdiagnosed as paranoid schizophrenia, endogenous depression, alcohol abuse, and drug addiction, etc. Consequently, these victims remained untreated or inappropriately treated for a serious exogenic psychiatric disorder. The disorder's symptomatology severely restricted the veterans' employability and undermined their social relationships and family lives. The cumulative pain, distress, confusion, stigma, and hopelessness engendered maladaptive social and psychological responses. This created a pathogenic spiral that deepened the patients' chronicity and despair, and exacerbated their dysfunctional behavior. This, in turn, accounted for high rates of parasuicide and self-dosing with drugs and alcohol.

According to its advocates, a PTSD diagnostic classification was a necessary first step to bringing this epidemic under control. It would provide the post-traumatic syndrome with a standard definition and the institutional authority of the American Psychiatric Association. After some hesitation, the DSM-III editorial task force established a committee to draft an entry. From the outset, a majority of its members was convinced of the validity of the classification and its high prevalence among Vietnam War veterans, and they were committed to ending the veterans' victimization by psychiatry and the larger society. Thus they devised a set of diagnostic criteria that extended the conditions of eligibility for treatment and compensation—including cases of delayed onset associated with a wide range of etiologic events, including atrocities (the patient as a perpetrator), and allowed for codiagnoses. The new entry achieved this effect by adopting an essentially *quantitative* stressor criterion that defines traumatic events as overwhelming experiences that can be expected to cause distress in nearly anyone. Defined this way, PTSD dispenses with the idea of a diathesis—a hereditary, congenital, or developmental factor that explains why only some people develop the characteristic syndrome following exposure to a stressful event. (Charcot and Janet had invoked the existence of diatheses to account for post-traumatic disorders. A similar opinion was shared by many army doctors who treated shell shock during World War I.) The DSM-III stressor criterion implied that, if an etiological event occurred in the course of military service, the consequent disorder would have to be *service-connected* because it involved no prior condition. These circumstances, entrenched in DSM-III, established the veteran's entitlement to appropriate medical treatment. If his disorder were also severe enough to interfere with his ability to make a living, then he would be entitled to a disability pension, as long as the service-connected condition persisted.

Officials within the Veterans Administration were initially opposed to the proposed classification. Patients diagnosed with PTSD (following the publication of DSM-III) were previously diagnosed with disorders that were not service-connected, e.g., schizophrenia, panic disorder, and major depression. These diagnoses entailed no responsibilities on the part of the VA for treatment (which many of the veterans received from the VA, nonetheless) or compensation (which the patients did *not* receive). If PTSD were to become part of the official nosology, these arrangements would have to change.

Disability rating boards would have to be greatly expanded, and specialized treatment programs would have to be created. In the end, the VA adjusted to the change with the encouragement and generous support of the Congress.

Is PTSD a Traumatic Neurosis?

The neo-Krapelinian critics claimed that PTSD was a traumatic neurosis with a new name and that, for this reason, it had no legitimate place in a diagnostic system dedicated to positivist principles, DSM-III (Young, 1995, chapter 3). This is a credible argument. In both instances, the characteristic syndromes are said to be products of toxic memories, intrapsychic conflicts, and secondary adaptations (in which some symptoms, e.g., avoidance behavior, emerge as adaptations to other symptoms). The advocates of the PTSD classification generally ignored this historical comparison and its implications. Their argument in favor of PTSD was *intuitive* (the pathogenic power of traumatic events is self-evident, nearly everyone who experiences them is affected) and *moral* (people suffering from the irresistible effects deserve to be recognized), rather than epistemological. And they succeeded.

The neo-Kraepelinians wanted to invalidate PTSD by attacking its underlying mechanism. In adopting this tack, they ignored a second criticism, although one that may not have been obvious at the time. To grasp this possibility, it is necessary to make certain assumptions that were rejected outright by the neo-Kraepelinians. Assume that the pathogenic mechanism underlying PTSD is not an issue. And assume that horrible experiences can produce a syndrome similar to the one that is attributed to PTSD, and it can be satisfactorily distinguished from syndromes produced by other combinations of psychiatric disorders. Having made these assumptions, we come to the question that the neo-Kraepelinians ignored. Is it possible (and practicable) to consistently distinguish cases in which traumatic memory is the *cause* of the patient's syndrome from cases in which memory is simply the *reason* (or explanation) for the patient's condition?

Episodic Memories: Objects or Processes?

The psychology of PTSD is based on memory: etiologic events create pathogenic memories, and these memories, rather than the events, generate the disorder's characteristic symptoms. Ordinary memories are highly malleable. This is the memory expert's opinion. In popular culture, episodic memories are given a different appearance. They are routinely (and naively) compared with artifacts like photographs and videotapes. They are objects around which time flows in a single direction, from the past (an experience) to the present (storage of memory content of the experience) to the future (a progressive loss or degradation of memory content). To the memory expert, this comparison is profoundly misleading because episodic memory is a process, not an object. Within this process, past and present interact and intermingle, producing multiple drafts of experiences and not photographs (Schacter, 1996). This is what makes traumatic memory so odd, that is, different from both the expert's and the lay person's conception of episodic memory. Traumatic memories are pathogenic precisely because they do not change or fade; they are immutable and indigestible. Further, time runs through them in just one direction. Or so it is said.

Questions concerning the malleability of traumatic memory are not new. A century ago, Janet explored the feasibility of altering these memories in the clinic—replacing a memory's pathogenic content with some innocuous content through the medium of hypnosis and suggestion (van der Hart et al., 1993). Janet and certain of his contemporaries understood that memories were sometimes altered unintentionally as a product of the clinician's tacit suggestions and the patient's unconscious desire to satisfy these expectations. Freud rejected Janet's idea of creating therapeutic fictions. According to Freud, it was partly his fear of creating fictions through suggestion that induced him to replace hypnosis and abreactive therapy with a new technique, free association. Freud and contemporary doctors, such as W. H. R. Rivers, recognized that memory alterations could also originate in the patient's own mind in a process called "autosuggestion," in which patients might unconsciously revise their memories in response to unacknowledged psychological needs or drives. In each of these cases (autosuggestion and heterosuggestion) a nontraumatic episodic memory acquires a traumatic or etiologic potency at some point following the onset of the symptoms for which the memory is ostensibly responsible. Time flows in two directions, as it does in the case of ordinary memories (Young, 1995, chapter 2).

In the years following World War I, psychiatric interest in the malleability of traumatic memory declined. In his monograph on war neuroses, Kardiner essentially ignored this subject. (For example, a chapter on forensic issues is focused on disability issues and makes no reference to problems of establishing etiology.) During World War II, American and British military physicians relied on abreactive therapies and consequently had no compelling interest in the constancy of traumatic memory. Nor did psychiatric attitudes change during the conflicts in Korea and Vietnam.

In the 1980s, this situation changed, partly in response to an "epidemic" of recovered memories of traumatic childhood sexual abuse. The most influential research consisted of attempts to produce a "misinformation effect" through heterosuggestion. In a recent review of this work, Elizabeth Loftus writes: "What do we know as a result of hundreds of studies of misinformation, spanning two decades ...? That misinformation can lead people to have false memories that they appear to believe in as much as some of their genuine memories." In some of these experiments, subjects witness an event, through photographs, videotape, or a staged performance. Following this, a researcher talks about the event and casually interjects significant distortions and new details. Then the subjects are asked to describe the event as they witnessed it. Findings indicate that many of the subjects integrate misinformation into their accounts and memories. In a provocative series of experiments conducted with children, Loftus demonstrated that "a simple suggestion from a family member [colluding with Loftus] can create an entire autobiographical memory for an event that would have been mildly traumatic ... [had it actually occurred]." Because it is relatively easy to produce the misinformation effect experimentally, "how much more powerful would be a combination of [clinical] techniques, over the course of years of therapy?" (Loftus et al., 1995, pp. 65 and 66; also Loftus and Ketcham, 1994).

Almost no analogous research was conducted on PTSD per se during this period. This is historically understandable. From the 1970s onward, PTSD researchers struggled to establish and, following publication of DSM-III, to defend the validity of the disorder. Quite naturally, they had no incentive to undertake a research program that would draw attention to the epistemology of traumatic time. On the other hand, factitious memories (cases where patients invent or borrow their etiologic events) are mentioned in the PTSD literature during this period. These memories represented only a technical problem—namely, the need for procedures for identifying fabrications—and they subverted no assumptions about the durability of traumatic memory. For many PTSD researchers, questions about the malleability of traumatic memory were red herrings. Changes in memory content could be explained in terms of the dynamics of PTSD, the patient's tendency to oscillate between periods in which the traumatic content is engaged (remembering, processing) and, when the pain is too intense, disengages from it (suppressing or repressing painful elements). The therapist helped the patient modulate this process and, in this capacity, exerted no direct influence—conscious or unconscious—on the content of the patient's traumatic memory.

Recently, a team of PTSD researchers has inquired into the malleability of traumatic memories (Southwick et al., 1997). Gulf War veterans were asked to complete a list of nineteen questions about their combat experiences. Responses (either yes or no) were collected at one month and then two years after the soldiers' return from the war zone. A yes response implied greater risk for exposure to trauma-level events. The researchers reported significant inconsistencies between the first and second reports. In general, informants described the experiences as entailing greater exposure when they were queried at the later date (+ 2 years) than at the earlier one (+ 1 month):

> There are ... a number of possible explanations for changes from no to yes. First, material that had been forgotten, denied, suppressed, or repressed at 1 month may have become conscious by 2 years. Second, memories may have become exaggerated after exposure to media accounts, after conversations with other traumatized reservists, or after multiple retellings of the same events. Third, it is possible that individuals with intrusive memories, nightmares, and flashbacks gradually recalled traumatic memories as a result of their involuntary reexperiencing of symptoms. Fourth, it may be that individuals who became increasingly symptomatic over time [regardless of actual etiology] unknowingly exaggerated their memory for traumatic events as a way to understand or explain their emerging psychopathology. (Southwick et al., 1997, p. 176)

The authors conclude that we cannot merely assume the "accuracy of recall of traumatic events." There are two ways to interpret the word "recall" in this context. One, it might imply that the traumatic memory is equivalent to whatever content is recalled. Alternatively, it might imply that the content recalled changes over time but that the traumatic memory that underlies these performances remains immutable. If the authors interpret their data in the first way, the findings undermine the uniqueness of traumatic memory and, by extension, the validity of PTSD. It is more likely that they are interpreting their findings in the second way, in which case they are not attacking the validity of PTSD, but rather our ability to diagnose between (1) events/memories that produce the PTSD syndrome and (2) events/memories that become etiologically significant only after the fact (that is, as attributions). In these circumstances, diagnosis would be especially problematic in cases of delayed-onset PTSD, where a lengthy period has elapsed between the etiologic event and the onset of intrusive memories and other symptoms, and in cases of co-occurring psychiatric disorders. Delayed onset is a common feature of chronic combat-related PTSD, and chronic cases of all sources are associated with comorbidity. A recent review of 26 studies of PTSD symptomatology reports that "PTSD rarely appears as a singular disorder at any point in its course." (Exceptions occur with acute PTSD and short-duration traumas in otherwise healthy individuals.) "[The] comorbid disorders are not truly separate from PTSD and, in some cases, may even precede and create vulnerability to PTSD" (Deering et al., 1996, p. 344). Although this finding does not undermine the validity of PTSD (a syndrome is said to possess "a distinct set of core symptoms"), it raises questions about the diagnostic practices employed by PTSD researchers:

> [Future] studies should be prospective, with adequate lengths of follow-up to discern the onset, chronology, and interrelationship between core PTSD symptoms and other symptom clusters. Research specifically designed to compare psychiatric symptoms from different sources of trauma, controlled for gender, age, compensation, and/or treatment seeking, time since trauma, and psychopathology would also help to clarify ways in which PTSD may follow a different course depending on the source of trauma. (Deering et al., 1996, p. 344)

In other words, retrospective accounts are problematic, especially when external factors, such as the hope of compensation, may influence how patients recall and report their memories. What can we conclude about chronic cases involving memories of trauma-level stressors? Findings based on retrospective accounts are dubious; findings based on prospective research can help establish chains of causes and effects and therefore help determine whether the PTSD diagnosis is justified in specific cases. The presumption is that researchers either possess or will eventually develop methods for differentiating between traumatic memories—that is, memories that play a primary causative role in producing and maintaining of the syndrome—and distressful memories whose subjective significance (and ostensible pathognomonic significance) is itself a product of antecedent psychiatric problems. Is the presumption justified? In *The Harmony of Illusions*, I have argued that current diagnostic techniques based on clinical interviews, protocols, and psychometric scales are incapable of making this distinction (Young, 1995, chapters 4 and 5). Nor is it obvious how *these* techniques might be suitably modified or revised. I will return to this point in the conclusions to this chapter.

Clinical Reality or Scientific Truth?

For the moment, assume that I am correct in claiming that we do not possess diagnostic methods that can distinguish between traumatic memories and distressful memories whose subjective significance is a product of antecedent psychiatric problems. Is this necessarily a bad thing? I believe that there are two equally valid answers to this question. For the researcher committed to scientific standards of truth, the inability to make this distinction *is* a bad thing because it is an obstacle to aggregating diagnostically homogeneous samples of subjects and to making valid epidemiological inferences. (Keep in mind that these comments are specific to chronic and delayed-onset cases.) For the clinician whose priority is to reduce distress and impairment, the distinction may be less critical.

A large number of psychotherapies are practiced today. Efforts to compare their relative efficacy have failed to demonstrate significant differences. According to some experts, notably Jerome Frank (1973), psychotherapies are intrinsically nonspecific. Despite doctrinal and practical differences, they do the same thing. Frank's thesis is that every psychiatric case is an amalgam of disorder-specific symptoms and "demoralization." Disorder-specific symptoms are beyond the effective reach of psychotherapies, and they wax and wane according to their own (neurophysiological?) logic. Demoralization is nonspecific, and its effects can be altered by psychotherapy.

Demoralization originates in the patients' self-perceived inability to control their emotions, solve their problems, or manage everyday situations that healthy people handle with ease. It is fueled by the patients' uncertainty about the meaning and seriousness of their conditions and by their feelings of helplessness and vulnerability. According to Frank, psychotherapies work by restoring .the patient's sense of self-efficacy through "myths" and "rituals"—clinical beliefs and practices (incorrectly) believed to affect disorder-specific symptoms.

PTSD's therapeutic potential, its capacity for remoralizing certain patients, can be explained by the disorder's etiology (exogenous rather than endogeneous) and a deeply rooted cultural association between memory and self-awareness, described earlier in this chapter. Take the common case of the Vietnam War veteran whose pre-PTSD psychiatric history includes multiple stigmatizing disorders—alcohol and substance use disorders, paranoid schizophrenia, chronic depression. PTSD wipes his slate clean. Ruminations become reexperiences, chemical dependency becomes self-dosing, etc. Because PTSD is an exogenic disorder and a normal response to abnormal situations (a position recently contested in Yehuda and McFarlane, 1995), onset imputes nothing negative about the patient's moral character or mental constitution (Young, 1995, Chapter 5).

Conclusion

The PTSD diagnosis is not inherently therapeutic. There are circumstances in which the classification contributes to chronicity and disability, especially when the diagnosis establishes the patient's eligibility for compensation and other secondary gain. Nevertheless, diagnosis and treatment function as therapeutic myth and ritual in a significant proportion of cases, as described by Frank. The psychotherapist's ability to distinguish between a traumatic memory and another kind of distressful memory in such cases is not merely problematic, it is also unimportant.

PTSD researchers are in a different position, however, if we are to believe that retrospective diagnosis interferes with their ability to aggregate homogeneous samples of subjects with chronic and chronic delayed-onset PTSD. To grasp the dimensions of this problem, one must understand the role of Vietnam War veterans in PTSD research. As I have indicated, the PTSD classification is a historical legacy of the Vietnam War and its aftermath. (This does not impugn the classification's validity.) The majority of patients diagnosed and treated for PTSD over the last two decades passed through the Veterans Administration (VA) Medical System. The majority of research published about PTSD during this same period has been funded by the VA and conducted by VA researchers on VA patient populations. These patients are distinctive in that they were diagnosed with PTSD many years after the war and after the onset of psychiatric symptoms, and consequently, their clinical profiles are complicated by high levels of comorbidity, chronicity, and disability.

In short, a large segment of scientific literature on PTSD is based on a patient population for which current retrospective diagnostic practices yield ambiguous results. This possibility was anticipated by the neo-Kraepelinian critics of the PTSD classification during the period leading up to the publication of DSM-III. Will prospective techniques based on episodic memory—that is, techniques focused on reexperiences and avoidance behavior—significantly reduce ambiguity (related to memory malleability) in cases of chronic and delayed-onset PTSD? Research into the neurophysiology and neuroanatomy of PTSD promises a path beyond this impasse—a way to delineate chains of syndromal causes and effects without engaging subjects' episodic memories or language.

References

Alexander, F. (1950). *Psychosomatic medicine: Its principles and applications.* New York: W.W. Norton.

Biro, J. (1993). Hume's new science of mind. In D.F. Norton (Ed.), *The Cambridge companion to Hume* (pp. 33–63). Cambridge: Cambridge University Press.

Breuer, J., & Freud, S. (1955). *Studies on hysteria.* New York: Basic Books.

Ceci, S. J. (1995). False beliefs: Some developmental and clinical considerations. In D. L. Schacter (Ed.), *Memory distortion: How minds, brains, and societies reconstruct the past* (pp. 91–125). Cambridge, MA: Harvard University Press.

Charcot, J.-M. (1889). *Clinical lectures on diseases of the nervous system delivered at the infirmary of la Salpetriére.* London: New Sydenham Society.

Deering, C. G., Glover, S. G., Ready, D., Eddleman, H. C., & Alarcon, R. D. (1996). Unique patterns of comorbidity in post-traumatic stress disorder from different sources of trauma. *Comprehensive Psychiatry, 37,* 336–346.

Erichsen, J. E. (1866). *On railway and other injuries of the nervous system.* London: Walton and Maberly.

Flournoy, T. (1994). *From India to the planet Mars: A case of multiple personality with imaginary languages.* Princeton: Princeton University Press.

Frank, J. (1973). *Persuasion and healing.* Baltimore, MD: Johns Hopkins University Press.

Freud, S. (1955). *Beyond the pleasure principle.* London: Hogarth Press.

Goetz, L. G., Bonduelle, M., & Gelfand, T. (1995). *Charcot: Constructing neurology.* New York: Oxford University Press.

Goldstein, K. (1939). *The organism: A holistic approach to biology derived from pathological data in man.* Cincinnati: American Book.

Horowitz, M. (1976). *Stress response syndromes.* New York: Jason Aronson.

Janet, P. (1901). *The mental state of hystericals: A study of mental stigmata and mental accidents.* New York: G. P. Putnam.

Janet, P. (1925). *Neuroses et idées fixes,* 4th ed. Paris: Alcan.

Kardiner, A. (1941). *The traumatic neuroses of war.* Washington, DC: National Research Council.

Kardiner, A. (1959). Traumatic neuroses of war. In S. Arieti (Ed.), *American handbook of psychiatry* (pp. 245–257). New York: Basic Books.

Kardiner, A., & Spiegel, H. (1947). *War stress and neurotic illness.* New York: Paul B. Hoeber.

Locke, J. (1959). *An essay concerning human understanding.* Oxford: Oxford University Press.

Loftus, E. F., & Ketcham, K. (1994). *The myth of repressed memory.* New York: St. Martin's Press.

Loftus, E., Feldman, J., & Dashiell, R. (1995). The reality of illusory memories. In D. Schacter (Ed.), *Memory distortion: How minds, brains, and societies reconstruct the past* (pp. 47–68). Cambridge, MA: Harvard University Press.

Page, H. W. (1883). *Injuries of the spine and spinal cord without apparent mechanical lesion, and nervous shock, in their surgical and medico-legal aspects.* London: J. and A. Churchill.

Pelikan, J. (1986). *The mystery of continuity: Time and history, memory and eternity in the thought of Saint Augustine.* Charlottesville, VA: University Press of Virginia.

Ribot, T. (1883). *Diseases of memory: An essay in positive psychology.* London: Kegan Paul, Trench.

Roth, M. (1996). Hysterical remembering. *MODERNISM/modernity, 3,* 1–30.

Schacter, D. (1996). *Searching for memory: The brain, the mind, and the past.* New York: Basic Books.

Southwick, S. M., Morgan, C. A., Nicolaou, A. L., & Charney, D. S. (1997). Consistency of memory for combat-related traumatic events in veterans of Operation Desert Storm. *American Journal of Psychiatry, 154,* 173–177.

Scott, W. (1990). PTSD in DSM-III: A case in the politics of diagnosis and disease. *Social Problems, 37,* 294–310.

Van der Hart, O., Steele, K., Boon, S., & Brown, P. (1993). The treatment of traumatic memories: Synthesis, realization, and integration. *Dissociation, 6,* 162–180.

Yehuda, R., & McFarlane, A. (1995). Conflict between current knowledge about post-traumatic stress disorder and its original conceptual basis. *American Journal of Psychiatry, 152,* 1705–1713.

Young, A. (1995). *The harmony of illusions: Inventing post-traumatic stress disorder.* Princeton, NJ: Princeton
University Press.

Young, A. (1996). Bodily memory and traumatic memory. In P. Antze & M. Lambek (Eds.), *Tense past: Cultural
essays in trauma and memory* (pp. 89–102). New York: Routledge.

II

Trauma and Culture

In the preceding section we focused attention on the development of the paradigm of psychological trauma. Certainly, the social and political forces that guided the development of this conceptual framework were born out of Western culture. Although several discontinuities within that framework are expressed in Part I, the debate is still within the constraints of a single cultural approach. In Part II we consider the relevance and applicability of the traumatic stress paradigm to other cultures, particularly to those with quite different conceptions of adversity and its aftermath.

B. Hudnall Stamm and Matthew Friedman discuss the relevant variables related to the concept of cultural differences and point out that there is substantial diversity in the way societies view and treat survivors of adversity. Then they identify elements within the construct of PTSD that may be more universal and contrast them to those whose expression may be more influenced by cultural effects. One striking observation has been that the more "biological" symptoms of PTSD—intrusive thoughts and hyper-arousal symptoms—appear more universal than avoidance and dissociative symptoms. Drs. Stamm and Friedman postulate that part of the diversity in the expression of these latter symptoms may be related to differences in the perception of both the traumatic event and the appropriate responses to such events. Indeed, even the assumption that one should or could heal oneself of the psychological effects of traumatic stress may not be universally shared.

An important issue raised by Stamm and Friedman is the permeability of most current cultures to the effects of other cultures. Now that geography no longer defines cultural affiliation, many individuals in current societies are influenced by more than one culture. This makes the study of cultural diversity and its effects even more complex. Indeed, the blending of current cultures and the process of migration have not only produced new hybrid cultures, but have also left many individuals pegged between two traditions and others alienated from any culture or social support. Certainly this raises new questions regarding vulnerability to the effects of trauma in such persons.

Alexandra Argenti-Pillen challenges the inherent supremacy of Western culture in interpreting human tragedy and its aftermath. The idea that traumatic stress exposure causes psychological disruption may not be particularly helpful or validating in cultures that place a premium on fate, determinism, and spiritual influences. Argenti-Pillen argues that there is inherent logic and structure in non-Western cultures, and that concepts of reflecting cosmological or teleological conceptions of why trauma occurs and what its restorative function may be to individuals should not be so easily dismissed as primitive by Westerners. Indeed, Western-born idioms of distress such as the concept of PTSD are similarly attempts to create cohesion and clarity in the fact of chaotic experiences of traumatization. The logical extension of these observations is that not all traumatic stress responses should be "treated" in the medical–psychological sense of treatment.

Indeed, the cultural influences affecting the way trauma survivors are viewed and treated are demonstrated more concretely by Eliezer Witztum and Moshe Kotler who trace the way combat stress reactions have been differentially appraised and treated in an evolving Israeli society. In tracing social and cultural changes that took place between the birth of the nation in 1948—clearly a national highlight in Israeli history—and its later controversial 1982 war, the authors describe parallel evolution in the treatment of traumatized soldiers moving from initial ostracizing denial of war stress reactions, to ignoring, to painful confrontations with human vulnerability.

Complementing Witztum and Kotler's observation, Dan Bar-On's essay addresses a more subtle need of evolving cultures—that of having a visible enemy. It is the case, argues Bar-On, that heroic myths may organize societies and shape their world view, even though at the same time they lead to perpetuation of hostilities, projection of hatred, major human losses, and repeated traumatization. Interestingly, such organizing myths are reluctantly abandoned when opportunities for peace arise. Bar-On suggests that the prospect of losing one's enemy has generated the current identity crises in Israeli society because it serves to shatter the previously rigid ethos born as a reaction to the Holocaust.

5

Cultural Diversity in the Appraisal and Expression of Trauma

B. HUDNALL STAMM AND MATTHEW J. FRIEDMAN

... [and they], went on the assumptions that the Dakotas had nothing, no rules no social organization, no ideals. And so they tried to pour white culture into, as it were, a vacuum. After all, they concluded that the Indians were impossible to change and train. What they should have done first, before daring to start their program, was to study everything possible of Dakota life, and see what made it go, in the old days, and what was still so deeply rooted that it could not be rudely displaced without some hurt ...

Letter from E. C. Deloria to H. E. Beebe, 2 December 1952;
DeMallie, 1990/1988, pp. 237–238

... it is important that the clinician take into account the individual's ethnic and cultural context in the evaluation of each of the DSM-IV axes ...

Appendix I, *Diagnostic and Statistical Manual of Mental Disorders*,
4th ed., p. 843

The challenge that we face, when considering post-traumatic stress disorder (PTSD) from a cross-cultural perspective, is to find an appropriate balance between modern and traditional conceptualizations of traumatic exposure and its consequences. Each perspective has a richness and complexity that must be respected and understood if we hope to provide effective clinical interventions for trauma survivors from traditional backgrounds.

B. HUDNALL STAMM • Institute of Rural Health Studies, Idaho State University, Pocatello, Idaho 83209-8174. **MATTHEW J. FRIEDMAN** • Veterans Affairs National Center for Post-Traumatic Stress Disorder, White River Junction, Vermont 05009.

International Handbook of Human Response to Trauma, edited by Shalev, Yehuda, and McFarlane. Kluwer Academic / Plenum Publishers, New York, 2000.

To state one conclusion at the outset, the important question is not whether PTSD can be detected among trauma survivors from traditional ethnocultural backgrounds. Indeed, PTSD has been found among Southeast Asians, Latin Americans, Middle Easterners, American Indians, and other trauma survivors from non-Western cultures (see below). Rather, the important question is whether PTSD or some other idiom of distress reflects the best conceptualization of the impact of traumatic stress on survivors from certain ethnocultural groups.

Universal, Cultural, and Personal Aspects of Human Existence

There is a rapidly growing literature on ethnocultural aspects of mental disorders in general and PTSD in particular (for overviews, see Danieli et al., 1996; Gaw, 1993; Marsella et al., 1996a; Suzuki et al., 1996; Ponterotto et al., 1996; Chemtob, 1996). However, there is little methodologically sound research on transcultural aspects of traumatic stress (Marsella et al., 1996b). This is unfortunate because such research would help us understand the generalizability of specific empirical observations.

For many clinicians and researchers, one of the most difficult aspects of this problem is defining culture. Herein lies a paradox. To understand a culture, it is necessary to have deep knowledge of it. However, it is that very understanding that prevents one from seeing that which it is *not*. Being embedded in a particular culture means interpreting the world through it. Yet, for many cultures, changes in global economics, communications, technologies, and ideas increasingly encourage appropriation of other cultures to create a blended modern culture (Gellert, 1994; Sampson, 1989; Stamm, in press; Stamm, 1999; Stamm & Stamm, 1999).

These transformations and adaptations of culture from one group to another only intensify the need to attend to culture, even it if does make it more difficult to measure. Marsella et al. (1996b) point out that there are actually three dimensions which need to be considered: (1) universal dimensions, (2) cultural aspects, and (3) personal uniqueness.

Universal Dimensions

Is it even possible to identify universal dimensions of the human experience? Universal elements are those that would be important to any person, regardless of cultural context. To answer this question, the most obvious place to look for universal elements is in human evolutionary biology (Cziko, 1995; Cosmides & Tooby, 1990; Izard, 1992). A number of authors have concluded that all humans are similar with respect to their capacity to experience and express a number of fundamental emotions such as joy, fear, anger, sadness, disgust, shame, and guilt (Averill et al., 1994; Eibl-Eibesfeldt, 1989; Izard, 1994; Scherer, 1994). Others have strongly challenged this proposition. Russell (1994) has questioned the fundamental hypothesis of universality, and Lutz (1988) asserts that emotions are cultural constructs. Matsumoto (1989) has taken an intermediate position and argued that fear is expressed and perceived universally, whereas the expression of other emotions may be modified by cultural influences.

With respect to PTSD, extrapolating from Matsumoto's formulation, we suggest that all humans have the capacity to experience and express fear, helplessness, or horror, when exposed to traumatic stress. In other words, all humans have the capacity to meet the response criterion (A2) of the PTSD diagnosis (APA, 1994), although cultural factors may influence the likelihood that fear will be evoked or expressed by a person from a specific ethnocultural group when exposed to a specific traumatic event.

The question of universal versus culture-specific responses to traumatic events can be considered from a psychobiological perspective. We have argued elsewhere (Friedman et al., 1995), that the capacity to cope with stress is a crucial theme in human evolution. Psychobiological mechanisms characterized as "the fight or flight response," the "general adaptation syndrome," the startle response, fear conditioning, and behavioral sensitization have evolved to promote coping, adaptation, and preservation of the species. To carry this argument one step further, we proposed elsewhere that PTSD intrusion (B criterion) and arousal (D criterion) symptoms may be universal post-traumatic indications of the psychobiological evolutionary process, whereas expressions of avoidant/numbing (C criterion) symptoms may be determined more by cultural than by universal factors (Friedman & Marsella, 1996).

Cultural Aspects

According to Marsella et al. (1996a), culture is the second important dimension of the human experience. There is no universally accepted definition of culture. Marsella (1988) defines it as

> ... shared learned behavior which is transmitted from one generation to another to promote individual and group adjustment and adaptation. Culture is presented externally as artifacts, roles, and institutions, and is represented internally as values, beliefs, attitudes, cognitive styles, epistemologies, and consciousness patterns.
>
> But, individual subscription to these shared values may vary, as does the authority that the culture has in any individual's life. Therefore, knowledge of an individual's degree of ethnocultural identity is important for understanding the influence of culture on his or her perceptions of the world. (p. 10)

Draguns (1994) provides an overview of culture and mental illness and points out that although there is evidence that certain psychiatric disorders such as schizophrenia and depression affect people throughout the world, the range of cultural expressions of such disorders is nearly limitless. Based on a review of the literature, Draguns (1994) maintains that mental illness is a mix of universal and culture-specific factors. This is certainly consistent with the DSM-IV approach (Appendix 1) which recommends that ethnocultural factors be carefully considered in any diagnostic assessment. Such factors include: (1) cultural identity of the individuals, (2) cultural explanations of the individual's illness, (3) cultural factors related to psychosocial environment and levels of functioning, (4) cultural elements of the relationship between the individual and the clinician, and (5) overall cultural assessment for diagnosis and care.

Another way to characterize differences in culture is the individualism–collectivism dichotomy (Keats et al., 1989). People from traditional cultures are often collectivists who perceive the self as part of a larger whole (family, community, or tribe). They are concerned with the effects of their decisions on others, share material and nonmaterial resources, and are willing to accept the opinions and views of others. The Zulu concept of umbutu ("I am because we are") is a good example of collectivism. By comparison, individualists are motivated by their own preferences, needs, and rights, giving priority to personal rather than group goals (Hui & Triandis, 1986; Triandis, 1995). A person's position on the individualism–collectivism spectrum appears to have important implications for assessment and treatment of post-traumatic and other psychiatric syndromes (Rosenthal & Feldman, 1992).

Personal Uniqueness

Idiosyncratic aspects of the person, those that can neither be attributed to universal nor cultural aspects, are what Marsella and colleagues (Marsella et al., 1996a) call personal uniqueness. As previously stated, the influence of ethnocultural factors may vary from one individual to the next, so it is necessary to assess and to understand the importance of cultural heritage on every individual.

Western mental health clinicians generally focus on the patient as an individual. Sometimes, however, the family or small group is a more appropriate unit for treatment (Roland, 1996). Such an approach focuses therapeutic attention on the relationship between the individual and his/her family or small group. In this context it is necessary to understand that the subjective experience of patients may be collectivist rather than individualist, so that the clinician must address a more traditional "we-self" rather than the Western "I-self" for therapy to be relevant, accessible, and successful (Roland, 1996).

Diagnostic Issues

Does PTSD Occur in Trauma Survivors from Traditional Ethnocultural Backgrounds?

Because culture may modify the experience or expression of post-traumatic distress, it is important to identify key differences between trauma survivors from Western-industrialized cultures compared to those from traditional settings. However, regardless of the culture of origin, it must be emphasized that, according to empirical data, most trauma survivors do not experience profound long-lasting pathology or develop a psychiatric disorder as a result of such exposure (Marsella et al., 1996a; Kessler et al., 1995; Yehuda & McFarlane, 1995; Stamm, 1999). If psychopathology does develop, PTSD may not be the best clinical characterization of an individual's post-traumatic distress (Marsella et al., 1996a).

Some have argued that a DSM-IV diagnosis such as PTSD should never be applied in a cross-cultural context. Bracken et al. (1995) contend that the PTSD diagnosis should never be applied to non-Western children or adults. They claim the underlying assumptions of the disorder implicitly endorse a Western ontology and should not be applied to non-Western peoples. Lewis-Fernandez and Kleinman (1995) question not only PTSD but the cross-cultural validity of the entire DSM-IV. In their opinion, the nosology that undergirds the DSM-IV does not reflect the mind–body interaction often observed in non-Western cultures.

It is beyond the scope of this chapter to rehash the arguments for and against the DSM-IV approach. The DSM/ICD is the official taxonomy of psychiatric health care and the frame of reference within which we must address all questions of psychiatric nosology. Therefore, we believe we must review the literature on post-traumatic distress among non-Western people from the DSM/ICD perspective. We will assess the goodness-of-fit of PTSD in contrast to other diagnostic formulations as the best conceptual tool for characterizing post-traumatic distress among non-Western individuals.

There is no question that PTSD can be detected among non-Euro-Americans. The list keeps growing as researchers assess post-traumatic distress among survivors of war, torture, forced migration, sexual assault, natural disasters, and industrial accidents. To be more specific, PTSD has been detected among Southeast Asian refugees (Kinzie, 1993, 1989; Smiths Fawzi et al., 1997); Sri Lankans exposed to civil war (Somasundaram & Sivayokan, 1994); civilian survivors of the war in Afghanistan (Wardak, 1993); cyclone survivors in Fiji and Sri Lanka (Fairley, 1986; Patrick & Patrick, 1981); earthquake survivors in Mexico, Ecuador, Japan, and China (Conyer et al., 1987; Lima et al., 1989; McFarlane & Hua, 1993; Odouia et al., 1993; Kato et al., 1996); volcano survivors in Columbia (Lima et al., 1987) and political torture detainees in South Africa (Simpson, 1993). In addition, PTSD has been detected in American Vietnam veterans from African-American, Hispanic-American, American-Indian, Asian-Pacific Islander, as well as Caucasian backgrounds (Kulka et al., 1990; Beals et al., 1997).

Are There Formulations Better Than PTSD?

Showing that PTSD can be detected among traumatized people from non-Western backgrounds does not tell us anything about the goodness-of-fit of the PTSD diagnosis with the experience and expression of post-traumatic distress among traditional people.

> The received categories of affective, anxiety, dissociative and somatoform disorders are not natural divisions in the world or in the phenomenology of disease, disorder, or illness. Once established, nosological categories tend to become reified and to obscure the variation and overlap between disorders in patients.... (Kirmayer, 1996, p. 154)

Two major components of post-traumatic distress among non-Western people are somatization and dissociation (Kirmayer, 1996; Jenkins, 1991; Hough et al., 1996). Somatization is completely missing from the PTSD diagnostic criteria, dissociation is the focus of only one symptom (DSM-IV A3: psychogenic amnesia), and one can meet the diagnostic criteria for PTSD without any evidence of dissociation.

Dissociation

Dissociative disorder has been observed in Turkish women, most of whom reported a history of childhood sexual abuse. PTSD was not assessed in this study (Sar et al., 1996). Berger and colleagues report that a history of sexual abuse was associated with dissociation among Japanese women 15–20% of whom also exhibited symptoms of post-traumatic stress, multiple personality, and eating disorders (Berger et al., 1994). Two studies investigated PTSD, dissociation, depression, and anxiety among Cambodian refugees. The first study, done after 4–6 years in the United States, detected significant symptoms of PTSD, depression, and dissociation in 80–96% of the refugees (Carlson & Rosser-Hogan, 1991). The second study, done on the same cohort of Cambodian refugees 10 years after resettlement, showed similar rates of distress. Ninety percent of the refugees exhibited marked symptoms of at least two of the following disorders: PTSD, depression, anxiety, or dissociation (Carlson & Rosser-Hogan, 1993). After the Exxon Valdez oil spill, 25% of the native people who lived in the close vicinity met criteria for PTSD, and 29 and 42% exhibited depression and generalized anxiety disorder, respectively, one year after the oil spill (Palinkas et al., 1993).

Somatization

There is a strong clinical belief and growing empirical evidence to support the notion that people from traditional cultures experience somatic distress following extremely stressful events (Kirmayer, 1996; Jenkins, 1991; Hough et al., 1996; Robin et al., 1996). Furthermore, there is evidence that PTSD may also be a risk factor for medical illnesses (Friedman & Schnurr, 1995). Therefore, physical symptoms are often an important component of postexposure distress in traditional cultures. Among Asian and Central American refugees, there is an important association of physical health complaints and psychological symptoms, including post-traumatic distress (Palinkas, 1995). Among those native people who lived in the area of the Exxon Valdez oil spill, regardless of high or low exposure, there was a self-reported decrease in perceived health status and some believed that they had developed a medical illness as a direct result of the spill (Palinkas et al., 1993).

Although illness-oriented medicine may not adequately reflect the wellness orientation of traditional medicine, at least among indigenous peoples in North America, it is generally believed that illness can occur as a result of misfortune (Joe, 1994). Extending this concept, Kirmayer (1996) conceptualizes traumatic stress as a sociopolitical and psychophysiological experience that has an explanation and a narrative theme with cultural and sociopolitical variations.

Depression

Depression is often found comorbid with PTSD (Buchwald, Monson, Dinges, Keane, & Kinzie, 1993; Kessler et al., 1995; Kinzie et al., 1989). This may be so because traumatic stress is frequently associated with significant losses. In fact, one important conceptualization of PTSD is derived from a model of bereavement and impacted grief (Horowitz, 1976). According to Raphael and Martinek (1997), the Lidemann conceptualization of loss may have actually been a conceptualization of traumatic stress. Separating traumatic stress and depression is further complicated by the fact that the depression associated with PTSD may be neurobiologically distinct from the classic melancholia of DSM-IV major depressive disorder (Friedman & Yehuda, 1995). The nature of the relationship among trauma, PTSD, and depression is a fundamental question that transcends cross-cultural considerations. We mention it here for the sake of completeness and suggest that it is one of many important areas for future research.

Complex PTSD

Dissatisfaction with PTSD as the only official DSM-IV post-traumatic diagnostic formulation is not restricted to cross-cultural psychologists/psychiatrists and medical anthropologists. Researchers and clinicians who work with survivors of prolonged trauma (such as childhood sexual abuse or political torture survivors) among Euro-American individuals have also criticized the limitations of the PTSD diagnosis. They have argued that it omits a number of major symptoms seen in such patients and have proposed a new diagnosis, "complex PTSD." As first operationalized by Herman

(1992), complex PTSD includes symptoms such as dissociation, somatization, affect lability, pathological changes in relationships, pathological changes in identity, self-injurious or suicidal behavior, and revictimization. Complex PTSD applies to those who have experienced sustained stressors, frequently as hostages or captives. Thus, the post-traumatic distress of many of the world's traditional peoples, who have experienced profound oppression and loss of freedom (for example, black South African activists), may be better defined by complex PTSD than by other diagnostic formulations.

We are not aware of systematic attempts to diagnose complex PTSD among traumatized people from non-Western backgrounds. Turner (1996) has argued that political refugees and asylum seekers from non-Western cultures seem to exhibit complex PTSD rather than DSM-IV PTSD. One obvious cross-cultural advantage of complex PTSD is that it emphasizes both dissociation and somatization more than DSM-IV PTSD; however, it also includes some symptom categories that may not be applicable to people from traditional backgrounds when captivity is not an important aspect of the traumatic experience. Clearly, rigorous investigations are needed to determine the relative advantages of complex versus DSM/ICD PTSD as a post-traumatic diagnosis for trauma survivors from non-Western cultures. Such research must control for exposure to interpersonal violence (torture, rape, forced captivity, etc.) because many refugees and asylum seekers from non-Western cultures have been subjected to such abusive violence during their difficult flight to safety.

Post-Traumatic Culture-Bound Syndromes

There are idioms of distress specific to particular cultures. Moreover, as groups of traumatized people relocate around the world, there is a "migration" of these culturally specific syndromes. Littlewood (1985) suggests that the appearance of these syndromes outside their country of origin may be less an indication of a culture-bound syndrome and more a reaction to Western-industrialized biomedicine. For example, in one case history, similar symptoms were exhibited across two generations in a mother and daughter; the mother attributed her symptoms to possession by spirits/ancestors, and the daughter attributed her symptoms to depression (Ullrich, 1993).

Culture-bound syndromes may be expressed in the Western host country after migration from the original homeland. Van Boemel & Rozee (1992) reported on psychosomatic blindness (despite normal ophthamalogical examination results) among 150 female Cambodian refugees residing in California who witnessed and survived the atrocities of the Khmer Rouge regime. Van Boemel and Rozee believe that those traumatic experiences precipitated this symptom. In addition to the blindness, 90% of refugees reported severe crying spells daily, feeling isolated, experiencing a number of physical symptoms, being sad, and having nightmares. It is noteworthy that these symptoms, including the visual difficulties, improved during group therapy in which the women discussed their traumatic experiences and provided social support for each other.

A well-documented culturally identified syndrome among Latin Americans is *ataques de nervios* which is a "... culturally sanctioned response to acute stressful experiences ... characterized by shouting uncontrollably, trembling, heart palpitations, a sense of heat in the chest rising to the head, fainting, and seizure-like episodes.... [It] mobilizes the support of the person's social network ... the person regains consciousness rapidly and does not remember the *ataque*" (Guarnaccia, 1993, p. 158). Following a disaster in Puerto Rico, 912 people were interviewed, and 16% reported having experienced *ataques de nervios*. These people were also more likely to have met the DSM criteria for PTSD, depression, and anxiety disorders than those who did not exhibit *ataques de nervios*. Although there appears to be a relationship between *ataques de nervios* and certain depressive and/or anxiety disorders, many diagnostic symptoms associated with the DSM-IV disorders are clearly distinguishable from those that characterize *ataques de nervios*.

Culture-bound idioms of distress must be carefully weighed in any post-traumatic assessment. They must also be rigorously evaluated with respect to specificity. In *ataques de nervios*, as an example, it is unclear whether *ataques* occur only after a stressful/traumatic event or whether they are a more general expression of distress that may occur (as do many affective and anxiety disorders) without a distinct traumatic precipitant.

To our knowledge, the only research in which individuals from different ethnocultural backgrounds were assessed for PTSD in response to the same traumatic event are the series of studies carried out on American Vietnam veterans (Kulka et al., 1990; Beals, 1997). These studies compared premilitary, military and postmilitary risk factors for PTSD among African-American, Hispanic-American, American-Indian, and Caucasian Vietnam veterans. Results indicated that race/ethnicity per se was a very weak predictor of PTSD. Premilitary factors such as exposure to childhood physical abuse or parental alcoholism were much more powerful predictors. The military risk factor of exposure to atrocities in Vietnam and the postmilitary factor of perceived social support were also powerful predictors of PTSD. In other words race/ethnicity was truly a risk factor for exposure to specific events such as physical abuse, parental alcoholism, atrocities in Vietnam, and social support. These events, in themselves, were the most important predictors of the development of PTSD. The current data, therefore, do not suggest that race/ethnicity per se is an indicator of intrinsic vulnerability or resistance to PTSD.

Treatment

Because there is a paucity of published randomized clinical trials of psychotherapy and pharmacotherapy for PTSD patients in general, it is especially difficult to discuss PTSD treatment for non-Euro-Americans (Soloman, in press; Friedman & Jaranson, 1994). Therefore, much of the following discussion draws on current knowledge concerning general psychiatric treatments for people from traditional cultures. In addition, we will cite some valuable writing on specific treatments for traumatized/PTSD patients from traditional cultures (Kinzie, 1989; Friedman & Jaranson, 1994; Marsella et al., 1996a).

Our specific emphasis will be on important considerations concerning the following: traditional healers, ports of entry to treatment, treatment context, pharmacotherapy, and individual as well as group treatment and disclosure.

Traditional Healers

The scientific revolution began in the mid seventeenth century. Therefore it is only during the past 350 years that traditional healers have had to compete with empirically trained Western clinicians. In many non-Western cultures, the traditional healer remains the primary source of treatment during episodes of physical and emotional distress. Neither migration to a new country nor the encroachments of Western medicine into traditional cultures have changed this pattern of treatment-seeking behavior, especially when the sociocultural infrastructure supports the preservation of such traditions. Urban enclaves, such as Chinatown and Little San Juan, specific geographic areas, such as refugee camps, American-Indian reservations, or countries relatively unaffected by Western culture, are places where traditional linguistic, dietary, religious, and healing practices are preserved. For refugees, traditional healing that has been utilized for generations may continue to be favored over Western scientific approaches, even among second or third generation descendants (Kinzie, 1993, 1989; Lee & Lu, 1989). Indeed, one extreme example of the antipathy to Western medicine is Bernier's (1992) report that when a vaccination program was initiated in a refugee camp because of the outbreak of a serious epidemic, one Khmer tribe resisted the procedure and hid from medical authorities. For them, the concept of "contagion" was inconceivable because they believe that spirits rather than microorganisms cause illnesses.

We believe that such treatment-seeking patterns are based on powerful beliefs that should be respected. Educational initiatives on the "superiority" of Western technology and expertise are at minimum disrespectful and most likely fruitless attempts to "convert" traditional people to reject the "old ways." We suggest that partnerships with indigenous healers and the development of multicultural treatment approaches will provide better access to and for clients and will produce better clinical results than have been generally achieved to date (Hulkrantz, 1983; Joe, 1994; South-central Foundation, 1995). One successful example of this model was developed by Hiegel (1984) for Khmer refugees in Thailand, where Western professionals rarely saw patients themselves but rather provided support and consultation to traditional healers.

Ports of Entry

Euro-Americans with PTSD are less likely to seek treatment from mental health practitioners than from primary or specialty medical clinics (Soloman, in press) because PTSD is not only associated with somatic symptoms but is also a risk factor for bona fide medical illness (Friedman & Schnurr, 1995; Williams, 1995). Such concerns deserve even greater consideration with regard to trauma survivors from traditional ethnocultural settings. As noted earlier, such individuals are more likely to express their post-traumatic distress through somatic complaints and to seek treatment for bodily rather than psychological symptoms. This is where collaborative relationships with primary or specialty medical clinicians are important. For example, some Indochinese refugees spontaneously seek out medical but not mental health consultation both in refugee camps and in host countries (Kinzie, 1989) because they view mental illness as the result of an energetic disequilibrium and possession by evil spirits for which the remedy is purification with lustral waters and exorcism (Bernier, 1992). Therefore, medical consultation may be the only opportunity for mental health intervention.

The detection of any history of trauma should be a mandatory part of any medical assessment, especially for people from traditional backgrounds. If the trauma history is positive, a culturally sensitive assessment should be carried out to identify PTSD or some other expression of post-traumatic distress. If feasible, an appropriate clinical intervention should always be instituted when indicated.

Treatment Context

Awareness of cultural expectations about the healing/treatment process is necessary for patient retention and treatment compliance. For example, the age and gender of the clinician may have an important bearing on ultimate success. It may be harder for older persons to respect or accept the expertise of a young mental health professional if they believe that clinical wisdom can emerge only later in life. For example, some clients might refuse to see a young therapist whose age may preclude their qualification for healer status by prevailing cultural standards. From the traditional perspective, a twenty- or thirty-year-old could never acquire the necessary wisdom and spiritual power needed to treat psychic ills (Stamm & Stamm, 1999). Similarly, rigid gender role separation in some cultures may complicate attempts for a female clinician to treat male clientele and vice versa.

Perhaps the most obvious of these barriers is that of not having a shared language. Using translators adds a complicated dimensions to the clinical interchange (Berthold & Baker, 1997; Kinzie, 1989; Southcentral Foundation, 1995). Beyond accurate translation of the actual words, there are a host of potential complications. Using a family member as translator may put several family members at risk of learning information about one another that they would rather keep secret. Children may be asked to speak for their parents, thus causing role reversals and difficulties with familial authority. Sometimes, a translator will refuse to translate messages because of perceived cultural insult to one or the other parties in the interchange. Simple difficulties, such as tone of voice, time factors, whom to address (client or interpreter), and the like, must be worked out in advance of the session (Berthold & Baker, 1997).

There are many barriers to the therapeutic process that may inadvertently be created by lack of knowledge. For example, the question and answer method of obtaining a medical history may not yield useful information when confronted by the more slowly unfolding narrative style of self-expression utilized by many traditional people. Even if the pace is slowed, the question and answer process may seem puzzling to the patient. When asked why she would not answer the clinician's questions, an elderly Alaska Native woman commented: "Why would I tell him anything about me, he just kept asking me questions and never told me anything about himself." Kinzie (1989) described how he unwittingly activated traumatic memories of political detention and torture among Cambodian refugees when a physician in a white coat was present during a psychiatric assessment.

Pharmacotherapy

We have argued previously that there are universal aspects to the fear (helplessness and horror) experienced by all humans exposed to catastrophic stress. We have also proposed that the intrusive and hyperarousal symptoms of PTSD may have a common psychobiological basis and be less affected by cultural influences than the avoidant/ numbing symptoms. This suggests that pharmacotherapy may be a very effective transcultural treatment for PTSD. After all, nonbiological psychotherapeutic approaches must incorporate a multitude of linguistic, behavioral, historical, conceptual, and spiritual factors that may vary widely from one culture to the next. Lacking experimental data, we will speculate on major factors that may affect pharmacotherapy for people from diverse ethnocultural backgrounds.

First, through centuries, if not millennia, of ethnocultural segregation, there are cross-cultural genetic differences with respect to the efficacy and pharmacokinetic properties of different drugs. For example, Line, Poland, Nuccio, and Matsuda (1989) have shown how the same dose of a given drug is metabolized differently by Asian versus Caucasian-Americans who suffer from the same disorder.

Second, there is robust scientific literature on coping and adaptation showing that appraisal is a psychological activity with psychobiological consequences. For example, two people, one of whom appraises a given stimulus as a threat and the other appraises the same stimulus as a challenge, will have distinctly different psychobiological responses to the same stimulus (Blascovich & Tomaka, 1996).

Third, cultural factors affect the symptomatic expression of psychological distress. This means that people with the same level of subjective distress may express it differently and that people who exhibit the same pattern and intensity of symptoms may actually experience different levels of emotional distress. For example, Norwegians and Japanese tend to be much less emotionally demonstrative than Italians and Filipinos, although their subjective distress may be comparable. It follows that when the expressed emotion of Norwegians or Japanese equals that of Italians or Filipinos, the former group may actually be suffering more subjective distress than the latter group.

Therefore, people from different ethnocultural backgrounds who were exposed to the same highly stressful event, exhibit similar symptoms, and are given the same dose of the same drug, may have very different qualitative and quantitative responses. Although the drug received by each individual is the same, it may be acting on different genetically induced pharmacological/metabolic receptivity, different culturally induced threat/challenge appraisal, and/or different culturally mediated expressions of psychological distress. This is obviously a rich area for future research.

Individual Versus Group Treatment and Disclosure

Choice of treatment may be dictated by cultural factors in a variety of ways. As noted earlier, individual treatment for someone whose self-identity is collectivist (I–we) rather than individualist (I–me) may be incomprehensible or at best, ineffective. On the other hand, when the trauma violates a cultural taboo (e.g., rape of an unmarried woman), cultural beliefs and practices may weigh strongly against group approaches. In such cases, the advantages of group treatment (e.g., normalization of responses, mutual support) may be overshadowed by the risks of publicly disclosing private catastrophes that are culturally indigestible. Here, the consequences of the trauma itself are amplified by the possibility of therapeutically induced social stigma, marginalization, and opprobrium. There are no hard and fast rules, however, except that any culturally sensitive treatment plan must pay careful attention to the way the traumatic event is experienced by each individual within his/her specific cultural context. Furthermore, there is much room for exploring these issues systematically because there are always important exceptions to any treatment guidelines. Clinical experience has shown that group therapy with unmarried women who have been raped has been both feasible and effective with Bosnian refugees and rape survivors in the Middle East as long as the therapist is also female and strict confidentiality is maintained. Again, more data is needed, but we must ensure that trauma survivors are not exposed to unnecessary therapeutically induced social risks as different treatment approaches are explored.

In some cases, the treatment of individuals may be best accomplished by treating the community, as well as the individuals within the community. For example, one of the more successful treatments for alcoholism and related traumatic stressors (e.g., increased family and personal violence) among Native North Americans has been the Sobriety Movement. Healing circles (similar to a free-form group therapy) are held for both those with the drinking problem and for the community at large. Often a whole town or village agrees to enter supportive treatment activities for those who are recovering from traumatic stress and related drinking (Dill, 1997). Similarly, community development projects may be powerfully therapeutic for individual and community trauma. In South Africa, the KwaZulu-Natal Programme for Survivors of Violence conducted groups for various members of a community devastated by civil war. The youth groups chose to put on sports fairs, but the mothers asked for gardens. The effect of the gardens was far beyond what the clinicians had expected. While the mothers tended their gardens, they shared their stories of horror. From the stories of pain, they grew the food of their futures (Stamm et al., 1996). A similar successful approach was initiated in Chile in which mothers attended sewing circles during which they processed the traumatic deaths and disappearances of loved ones perpetuated by the government (Agger & Jensen, 1992).

Acculturation and Treatment

We are only beginning to understand which treatments are best and for whom. We have focused on additional concerns that must be addressed when considering treatment for non-Western individuals in exploring post-traumatic distress. Dichotomies such as traditional versus Western-industrialized culture may facilitate the construction of book chapters such as this, but they fall short of portraying the richness of the human experience. There is abundant literature suggesting that ethnocultural identity is a more important predictor of the way an individual will respond to a situation or treatment than genetic, familial, or social factors. It is not enough to know that a specific second-generation immigrant to North America or western Europe (who can trace his or her ancestry back many generations) is genetically 100% West African or Japanese or Brazilian. It is even more important to know his or her cultural identity, genetic pedigree notwithstanding. Broadly, there are four possibilities:

1. traditional people from traditional cultures whose ethnocultural identity remains traditional with respect to customs, beliefs, and behavior;
2. assimilated people from traditional cultures who have rejected their heritage and embraced Western customs, beliefs, and behaviors;
3. bicultural people who are comfortable and fluent in both traditional and Western cultural settings and who can easily match their cultural perspective and behaviors to the demands and expectations of the moment;
4. alienated people from traditional cultures who do not identify themselves in terms of their ethnocultural background but who also have been unable to identify with the beliefs and behaviors of the majority culture in their present home in North America or western Europe.

This chapter has focused primarily on treatment for trauma survivors with a traditional ethnocultural identity. We believe that these are people who may benefit most from (1) culturally sensitive diagnostic assessment; (2) collaborative treatment programs involving traditional healers and Western-trained doctors; (3) treatment settings designed to foster access, comfort, and continuity; (4) pharmacotherapy that respects unique cross-cultural challenges; and (5) psychotherapy that incorporates crucial cultural factors both in format and process. In the case of refugees, it is also important that treatment address stress related to acculturation loss and change in addition to post-traumatic distress per se (Bernier, 1992). Assimilated individuals will benefit from Western approaches that research has shown appropriate for Euro-American clientele. Bicultural trauma survivors benefit from both traditional and Western treatment in the same way that they have been able to enrich their lives from two very different cultural traditions.

It is not at all clear what to say about alienated individuals as a group because there may be many roads to the end state of alienation. Some of these paths could include pretraumatic mental disorders, alcoholism, poverty, and homelessness among poorly functioning individuals, as well as anomie and cultural detachment among highly functioning individuals. Perhaps some subgroup of ethnoculturally alienated individuals may prove an important cohort on which to test some of the hypothesized universal aspects of post-traumatic distress because they may be less influenced by culturally mediated aspects of post-traumatic distress than traditional, assimilated or bicultural individuals. This is another important area for further research.

Conclusions

In addition to the extreme stressors of war, disease, sexual and family violence, another important stressor for traditional cultures is the speed at which they are being required to change as they are confronted by Western culture. Although Western-industrialized culture required centuries to evolve to its current form, traditional cultures must sometimes absorb the impact of Western values, beliefs, and practices in a matter of months or days. Consequently, a traditional culture sometimes becomes overwhelmed by the dominant culture that suddenly engulfs it, resulting in alienation, acculturation stress, and other consequences.

Sensitive and appropriate Western-trained clinicians must consider many issues when conceptualizing the sequelae of traumatic events among traditional people. Understanding the idioms of post-traumatic distress depends on our ability to identify universal aspects of human existence, as well as the patient's ethnocultural identity and fluidity with Western-industrialized culture. It also depends on the willingness of the clinician to understand, respect, and integrate such different beliefs and values into an appropriate treatment.

Until we know more, the fit between Western-industrialized science and traditional culture medicine will be uneven. There is obviously a need for culture-appropriate clinical approaches and carefully designed research. Future progress will depend on our determination to address diagnostic and treatment questions with patience, openness, sensitivity, rigor, and creativity.

References

Agger, I., & Jensen, S. B. (1992). Human rights and post-traumatic stress—the human rights movement as an important factor in prevention and healing of severe trauma following human rights violations. *Psychiatria Fennica, 23,* 35–40.

American Psychiatric Association (1994). *Diagnostic and statistical manual of mental disorders*, 4th ed. Washington, DC: American Psychiatric Press.

Averill, J. R., Ekman, P., Ellsworth, P. C., Frijda, N. H., Lazarus, R., Scherer, K. R., & Davidson, R. J. (1994). How is evidence of universals in antecedents of emotion explained? The nature of emotion: Fundamental questions. In P. Ekman & R. J. Davidson (Eds.), *Series in affective science* (pp. 142–177). New York: Oxford University Press.

Beals, J., Holmes, T., Ashcraft, M., Fairbank, J., Friedman, M., Jones, M., Schlanger, W., Shore, J., & Manson, S. (1997). A comparison of the prevalence of post-traumatic stress disorder across five racially and ethnically distinct samples of Vietnam theater veterans. (Manuscript submitted for publication).

Berger, D., Saito, S., Ono, Y., Tezuka, I., et al. (1994). Dissociation and child abuse histories in an eating disorder cohort in Japan. *Acta Psychiatrica Scandinavica*, *90*, 274–280.

Bernier, D. (1992). The Indochinese refugees: A perspective from various stress theories. In A. S. Ryan (Ed.), *Social work with immigrants and refugees* (pp. 15–30). Hawthorne Press: New York.

Berthold, M., & Baker, R. G. (1997). Working with interpreters: Providing culturally relevant debriefing and consultation. Presentation at the *6th Annual Conference of the International Association of Trauma Counselors*, Charleston, SC.

Blascovich, J., & Tomaka, J. (1996). The biopsychosocial model of arousal regulation. *Advances in Experimental Social Psychology*, *28*, 1–51.

Bracken, P. J., Giller, J. E., & Summerfield, D. (1995). Psychological responses to war and atrocity: The limitations of current concepts. *Social Science and Medicine*, *40*, 1073–1082.

Buchwald, D., Manson, S. M., Dinges, M. G., Keane, E. M., & Kinzie, J. D. (1993). Prevalence of depressive symptoms among established Vietnamese refugees in the United States: Detection in a primary care setting. *Journal of General Internal Medicine*, *8*(2), 76–81.

Carlson, E. B., & Rosser-Hogan, R. (1993). Mental health status of Cambodian refugees ten years after leaving their homes. *American Journal of Orthopsychiatry*, *63*, 223–231.

Carlson, E. B., & Rosser-Hogan, R. (1991). Trauma experiences, post-traumatic stress, dissociation, and depression in Cambodian refugees. *American Journal of Psychiatry*, *148*, 1548–1551.

Chemtob, C. M. (1996). Post-traumatic stress disorder, trauma, and culture. In F. L. Mak and C. C. Nadelson (Eds.), *International review of psychiatry*, *2* (pp. 257–292). Washington, DC: American Psychiatric Press.

Conyer, R. C., Amor, J., Medina-Mara, M. C., & De La Fuentes, J. R. (1987). Prevalence of the post-traumatic stress syndrome among the survivors of a natural disaster. *Salud Publica de Mexico*, *29*(5), 406–411.

Cosmides, L., & Tooby, J. (1990). Beyond intuition and instancy blindness: Toward an evolutionary rigorous cognitive science. *Cognition*, *50*(1–3), 41–77.

Cziko, G. (1995). *Without miracles: Universal selection theory and the second Darwinian revolution*. Cambridge: MIT Press.

Danieli, Y., Rodley, N. S., & Weisaeth, L. (1996). *International responses to traumatic stress: Humanitarian, human rights, justice, peace and development contributions, collaborative actions and future initiatives*. Amityville, NY: Baywood.

Dill, J. S. (1997). *The sobriety discussion/mailing list*. Available online at http://www.dickshovel.com/aho.html.

DeMallie, R. J. (1990/1988). Afterward. In Deliria, E. C. *Waterlily*. Lincoln, NB: Bison Books of University of Nebraska Press.

Draguns, J. G. (1994). Pathological and clinical aspects. In L. Adler & P. G. Uew (Eds.), *Cross-cultural topics in psychology* (pp. 165–177). Westport, CT: Praeger/Greenwood.

Eibl-Eibesfeldt, I. (1989). *Human etiology*. Hawthorne, NY: Aldine de Gruyter.

Fairley, M., Langeluddecke, P., & Tennant, C. C. (1986). Psychological and physical morbidity in the aftermath of a cyclone. *Psychological Medicine*, *16*(3), 671–676.

Friedman, M. J., Charney, D. S., & Deutch, A. Y. (Eds.). (1995). *Neurobiological and clinical consequences of stress: From normal adaptation to post-traumatic stress disorder*. Philadelphia: Lippincott-Raven.

Friedman, M. J., & Jaranson, J. M. (1994). The applicability of the post-traumatic stress disorder concept to refugees. In A. J. Marsella, T. Bornemann, S. Ekblad, & J. Orley (Eds.), *Amidst peril and pain: The mental health and well-being of the world's refugees* (pp. 207–227). Washington, DC: American Psychological Association.

Friedman, M. J., & Marsella, A. J. (1996). Post-traumatic stress disorder: An overview of the concept. In A. J. Marsella, M. J. Friedman, E. T. Gerrity, & R. Scurfield (Eds.), *Ethnocultural aspects of post-traumatic stress disorder: Issues, research, and clinical applications* (pp. 11–32). Washington, DC: American Psychological Association.

Friedman, M. J., & Schnurr, P. P. (1995). The relationship between trauma, post-traumatic stress disorder and physical health. In M. J. Friedman, D. S. Charney, & A. Y. Deutch (Eds.), *Neurobiological and clinical consequences of stress: From normal adaptation to post-traumatic stress disorder* (pp. 507–524). Philadelphia: Lippincott-Raven.

Friedman, M. J., & Yehuda, R. (1995). Post-traumatic stress disorder and comorbidity: Psychobiological approaches to differential diagnosis. In M. J. Friedman, D. S. Charney, & A. Y. Deutch (Eds.), *Neurobiological and clinical consequences of stress: From normal adaptation to post-traumatic stress disorder* (pp. 429–445). Philadelphia: Lippincott-Raven.

Gaw, A. C. (1993). *Culture, ethnicity & mental illness.* Washington, DC: American Psychiatric Press.

Gellert, G. (1994). Global explanation and the credibility problem of alternative medicine. *Advances, 10,* 60–67.

Guarnaccia, P. J. (1993). Ataques de nervios in Puerto Rico: Culture bound syndrome of popular illness? *Medical Anthropology, 15,* 157–170.

Herman, J. L. (1992). Complex PTSD: A syndrome in survivors of prolonged and repeated trauma. *Journal of Traumatic Stress, 5*(3), 377–391.

Hiegel, J. P. (1984). Collaboration with traditional healers: Experience in refugees mental health care. *International Journal of Mental Health, 12*(3), 30–43.

Horowitz, M. (1976). *Stress response syndromes.* New York: Aronson.

Hough, R. L., Canino, G. J., Abueg, F. R., & Gusman, F. D. (1996). PTSD and related stress disorders among Hispanics. In A. J. Marsella, M. J. Friedman, E. T. Gerrity, & R. M. Scurfield (Eds.), *Ethnocultural aspects of post-traumatic stress disorder: Issues, research, and clinical applications* (pp. 301–338). Washington, DC: American Psychological Association.

Hui, C. H., & Triandis, H. C. (1986). Individualism-collectivism: A study of cross-cultural researchers. *Journal of Cross-Cultural Psychology, 17*(2), 225–248.

Izard, C. E. (1992). Basic emotion, relations among emotions, and emotion-cognition relations. *Psychological Review, 99*(3), 561–565.

Izard, C. E. (1994). Innate and universal facial expressions: Evidence from developmental and cross-cultural research. *Psychological Bulletin, 115*(2), 288–299.

Jenkins, J. H. (1991). The state construction of affect: Political ethos and mental health among Salvadoran refugees. *Culture, Medicine and Psychiatry, 15*(2), 139–165.

Joe, J. (1994). Traditional Indian health practices and cultural views. In D. Champagne (Ed.), *Native America portrait of the peoples* (pp. 525–547). Detroit: Visible Ink Press.

Kato, H., Asukai, N., Miyake, Y., Minakawa, K., & Nishiyama, A. (1996). Post-traumatic symptoms among younger and elderly evacuees in the early stages following the 1995 Hanshin-Awaji earthquake in Japan. *Acta Psychiatrica Scandinavica, 93*(6), 477–481.

Keats, D. M., Munro, D., & Mann, L. (1989). Heterogeneity in cross-cultural psychology. Selected papers from the *9th International Conference of the International Association for Cross-Cultural Psychology.* Newcastle, Australia.

Kessler, R. C., Sonnega, A., Bromet, E., Hughes, M., & Nelson, C. (1995). Post-traumatic stress disorder in the national comorbidity survey. *Archives of General Psychiatry, 52,* 1048–1059.

Kinzie, D. (1989). Therapeutic approaches to traumatized Cambodian refugees. *Journal of Traumatic Stress, 2*(1), 75–91.

Kinzie, D. (1993). Post-traumatic effects and their treatment among Southeast Asian refugees. In J. P. Wilson & B. Raphael (Eds.), *International handbook of stress syndromes* (pp. 311–319). New York: Plenum.

Kinzie, J. D., Boehnlein, J. K., Leung, P. K., Moore, L. J., Riley, C., & Smith, D. (1990). The prevalence of post-traumatic stress disorder and its clinical significance among Southeast Asian refugees. *American Journal of Psychiatry, 147,* 913–917.

Kinzie, J. D., & Manson, S. M. (1983). Five-years experience with Indochinese refugee psychiatric patients. *Journal of Operational Psychiatry, 14,* 105–111.

Kinzie, J. D., Sack, W. H., Angell, R., Clarke, G., & Ben, R. (1989). A three-year follow-up of Cambodian young people traumatized as children. *Journal of the American Academy of Child and Adolescent Psychiatry, 28*(4), 501–504.

Kirmayer, L. J. (1996). Confusion of the senses: Implications of ethnocultural variations in somatoform and dissociative disorders for PTSD. In A. J. Marsella, M. J. Friedman, E. T. Gerrity, & R. M. Scurfield (Eds.), *Ethnocultural aspects of post-traumatic stress disorder: Issues, research, and clinical applications* (pp. 131–163). Washington, DC: American Psychological Association.

Kulka, R. A., Schlenger, W. E., Fairbank, J. A., Hough, R. L., Jordan, B. K., Marmar, C. R., & Daniel, S. (1990). *Trauma and the Vietnam war generation: Report of findings from the National Vietnam Veterans Readjustment Study.* New York: Brunner/Mazel.

Lee, E., & Lu, F. (1989). Assessment and treatment of Asian-American survivors of mass violence. *Journal of Traumatic Stress, 2*(1), 93–120.

Lewis-Fernandez, R., & Kleinman, A. (1995). Cultural psychiatry. Theoretical, clinical, and research issues. *Psychiatric Clinics of North America, 18*, 433–448.

Lima, B. R., Chavez, H., Samaniego, N., Pompei, M. S., Pai, S., Santacruz, H., & Lozano, J. (1989). Disaster severity and emotional disturbance: Implications for primary mental health care in developing countries. *Acta Psychiatrica Scandinavica, 79*, 74–82.

Lima, B., Pai, S., Santacruz, H., Lozano, J., & Luna, J. (1987). Screening for the psychological consequences of a major disaster in a developing country: Armero, Colombia. *Acta Psychiatrica Scandinavica, 76*(5), 561–567.

Lin, K. M., Poland, R. E., Nuccio, I., Matsuda, K., Hathuc, N., Su, T. P., & Fu, P. (1989). A longitudinal assessment of haloperidol doses and serum concentrations in Asian and Caucasian schizophrenic patients. *American Journal of Psychiatry, 146*(10), 1307–1311.

Littlewood, R. (1985). Jungle madness: Some observations on expatriate psychopathology. *International Journal of Social Psychiatry, 31*(3), 194–197.

Lutz, C. A. (1988). *Unnatural emotions: Everyday sentiments on a Micronesian atoll & their challenge to Western theory.* Chicago: University of Chicago Press.

Marsella, A. J. (1988). Cross-cultural research on severe mental disorders: Issues and findings. *Acta Psychiatrica Scandinavica Supplementum, 344*, 7–22.

Marsella, A. J., Friedman, M. J., Gerrity, E. T., & Scurfield, R. M. (Eds.) (1996a). *Ethnocultural aspects of post-traumatic stress disorder: Issues, research, and clinical applications* (pp. 105–129). Washington, DC: American Psychological Association.

Marsella, A. J., Friedman, M. J., & Spain, E. H. (1996b). Ethnocultural aspects of PTSD: An overview of issues and research directions. In A. J. Marsella, M. J. Friedman, E. T. Gerrity, & R. M. Scurfield (Eds.), *Ethnocultural aspects of post-traumatic stress disorder: Issues, research, and clinical applications* (pp. 105–129). Washington, DC: American Psychological Association.

Matsumoto, D. (1989). Cultural influences on the perception of emotion. *Journal of Cross-Cultural Psychology, 20*, 92–105.

McFarlane, A. C., & Hua, C. (1993). Study of a major disaster in the People's Republic of China: The Yunnan earthquake. In J. P. Wilson & B. Raphael (Eds.), *International handbook of stress syndromes* (pp. 493–498). New York: Plenum.

Odouia, T., Iwadate, T., & Raphael, B. (1993). Earthquakes and traumatic stress: Early human reactions in Japanese society. In J. P. Wilson & B. Raphael (Eds.), *International handbook of stress syndromes* (pp. 487–498). New York: Plenum.

Palinkas, L. A. (1995). Health under stress: Asian and Central American refugees and those left behind. *Social and Science Medicine, 40*, 1591–1596.

Palinkas, L. A., Downs, M. A., Petterson, J. S., & Russell, J. (1993). Social, cultural, and psychological impacts of the Exxon Valdez oil spill. *Human Organization, 52*, 1–13.

Patrick, V., & Patrick, W. R. (1981). Cyclone 78 in Sri Lanka—The mental health trail. *British Journal of Psychiatry, 138*, 210–216.

Ponterroto, J. G., Casas, J. M., Suzuki, L. A., & Alexander, C. M. (Eds.). (1996). *Handbook of multicultural counseling.* Thousand Oaks, CA: Sage.

Raphael, B., & Martinek, N. (1997). Assessing traumatic bereavement and post-traumatic stress disorder. In J. P. Wilson & T. M. Keane (Eds.), *Assessing psychological trauma and PTSD.* New York: Guilford Press.

Robin, R. W., Chester, B., & Goldman, D. (1996). Cumulative trauma and PTSD in American-Indian communities. In A. J. Marsella, M. J. Friedman, E. T. Gerrity, & R. M. Scurfield (Eds.), *Ethnocultural aspects of post-traumatic stress disorder: Issues, research, and clinical applications* (pp. 239–253). Washington, DC: American Psychological Association.

Roland, A. (1996). How universal is the psychoanalytic self? In R. M. P. Foster, M. Moskowitz, & R. A. Javier (Eds.), *Reaching across boundaries of culture and class* (pp. 71–90).

Rosenthal, D. A., & Feldman, S. S. (1992). The nature and stability of ethnic identity in Chinese youth: Effects of length of residence in two cultural contexts. *Journal of Cross-Cultural Psychology, 23*(2), 214–227.

Russell, J. A. (1994). Is there universal recognition of emotion from facial expressions? A review of the cross-cultural studies. *Psychological Bulletin, 115*, 102–141.

Sampson, E. (1989). The challenge of social change for psychology: Globalization and psychology's theory of the person. *American Psychologist, 44*, 914–921.

Sar, V., Yargic, I., & Tutkun, H. (1996). Structured interview data on 35 cases of dissociative identity disorder in Turkey. *American Journal of Psychiatry, 153*, 1329–1333.

Savin, D., Sack, W. H., Clarke, G. N., & Meas, N. (1996). The Khmer adolescent project: III. A study of trauma from Thailand's Site II refugee camp. *Journal of the American Academy of Child and Adolescent Psychiatry, 35*, 384–391.

Scherer, K. R., & Wallbott, H. G. (1994). Evidence for universality and cultural variation of differential emotion response patterning. *Journal of Personality & Social Psychology, 66*(2), 310–328.

Simpson, M. A. (1993). Traumatic stress and the bruising of the soul: The effects of torture and coercive interrogation. In J. P. Wilson & B. Raphael (Eds.), *International handbook of stress syndromes* (pp. 493–498). New York: Plenum.

Smith Fawzi, M. C., Murphy, E., Pham, T., Lin, L., Poole, C., & Mollica, R. F. (1997). The validity of screening for post-traumatic stress disorder and major depression among Vietnamese former political prisoners. *Acta Psychiatrica Scandinavica, 95*(2), 87–93.

Smith Fawzi, M. C., Pham, T., Lin, L., Nguyen, T. V., Ngo, D., Murphy, E., & Mollica, R. F. (1997). The validity of post-traumatic stress disorder among Vietnamese refugees. *Journal of Traumatic Stress, 10*(1), 101–108.

Soloman, S. (in press). Trauma: Prevalence, impairment and service use. *Journal of Clinical Psychiatry.*

Somasundaram, D. J., & Sivayokan, S. (1994). War trauma in a civilian population. *British Journal of Psychiatry, 165*(4), 524–527.

Stamm, B. H., & Stamm, H. E. (1999). Ethnocultural aspects of trauma and loss in Native North America. In K. Nader, N. Dubrow, & B. H. Stamm (Eds.), *Cultural issues in the treatment of trauma and loss: Honoring differences.* Philadelphia: Brunner/Mazel.

Stamm, B. H. (1999). Creating virtual community: Telehealth and selfcare updated. In B. H. Stamm (Ed.), *Secondary traumatic stress: Self-care issues for clinicians, researchers and educators,* 2nd ed. Lutherville, MD: Sidran Press.

Stamm, B. H. (1999). Empirical perspectives on contextualizing death and trauma. In C. R. Figley (Ed.), *Death-related trauma: Conceptual, theoretical, and treatment foundations.* Philadelphia: Brunner/Mazel.

Stamm, B. H., Higson-Smith, C., Terry, M. J., & Stamm, H. E. (1996). Politically correct or critically correct? Community and culture as context. Symposium at the *12th Annual Conference of the International Society for Traumatic Stress Studies,* San Francisco, CA.

Stamm, H. E. (in press). *People of the Wind River.* Norman, OK: University of Oklahoma Press.

Suzuki, L. A., Meller, P. J., & Ponterotto, J. G. (1996). *Handbook of multicultural assessment.* San Francisco: Jossey-Bass.

Triandis, H. C. (1995). *Individualism and collectivism.* Boulder, CO: Westview Press.

Turner, S. W. (1996). *Beyond PTSD: Complex trauma reactions.* Symposium at the *2nd World Conference of the International Society for Traumatic Stress Studies,* San Francisco, CA.

Ullrich, H. E. (1993). Cultural shaping of illness: A longitudinal perspective on apparent depression. *Journal of Nervous & Mental Disease, 181*(10), 647–649.

Van Boemel, G. B., & Rozee, P. D. (1992). Treatment for psychosomatic blindness among Cambodian refugee women. In E. Cole, O. M. Espin, & E. D. Rothblum (Eds.), *Refugee women and their mental health: Shattered societies, shattered lives* (pp. 239–266). New York: Harrington Park Press.

Wardak, A. W. H. (1993). The psychiatric effects of war stress on Afghanistan society. In J. P. Wilson & B. Raphael (Eds.), *International handbook of stress syndromes* (pp. 349–364). New York: Plenum.

Williams, R. B. (1995). Somatic consequences of stress. In M. J. Friedman, D. S. Charney, & A. Y. Deutch (Eds.), *Neurobiological and clinical consequences of stress: From normal adaptation to post-traumatic stress disorder* (pp. 403–412). Philadelphia: Lippincott-Raven.

Yehuda, R., & McFarlane, A. C. (1995). Conflict between current knowledge about post-traumatic stress disorder and its original conceptual basis. *American Journal of Psychiatry, 152*(12), 1705–1713.

6

The Discourse on Trauma in Non-Western Cultural Contexts

Contributions of an Ethnographic Method

ALEXANDRA ARGENTI-PILLEN

> *Between seventy and a hundred thousand people have disappeared in Sri Lanka, there is a cultural collapse, the normal rituals performed after death cannot be performed.... Now people cannot go through the process of burial and mourning.... This is a big confusion or trauma or something.... Like the Diagnostic and Statistical Manual says; the problem of Post Traumatic Stress Disorder.... Trauma is due to the fact that people cannot forget and cannot say their men are dead. This is that confusion ...*

(counsellor, Sri Lanka, 1996)

Introduction: Culture as a Protective Shield?

A counsellor working in a clinic for torture victims in Sri Lanka speaks of cultural collapse, confusion, and trauma. This interpretation is one among the many ways in which people speak about trauma, the many ways in which the word trauma has taken up a meaning in diverse cultural contexts. What is mentioned first is the experience of cultural collapse, of cultural destabilization. This is a common experience for the large number of people living in war-torn societies, refugee camps, or as political refugees in host countries.

The destruction of war has brought about social disruption and has also severely disabled social processes which we loosely put together under the name "culture." When peace reigns, religious leaders, artists, ritual specialists, or traditional healers play a pivotal role in constructing a shared sense of reality and meaning. People are used to

---

ALEXANDRA ARGENTI-PILLEN • Department of Anthropology, University College London, London, WC1E 6BT, England.

International Handbook of Human Response to Trauma, edited by Shalev, Yehuda, and McFarlane. Kluwer Academic / Plenum Publishers, New York, 2000.

dealing with the minor misfortunes of everyday life and express unhappiness by the tools their culture offers them. But then, when political violence, war, or disaster have destroyed their life-worlds, the struggle for survival becomes a struggle for cultural survival, too. A confusion sets in which might be the beginning of long-term cultural uncertainty. The cultural experts within the community might have passed away, and the rituals which used to maintain the cultural tradition alive cannot be performed. Eventually even the mere knowledge about their culture might slowly become vague or uncertain.

It is at such moments that people come into contact with mainly Euro-American understandings of extreme suffering, such as post-traumatic stress disorder, trauma, and psychological survival. Refugees are referred to trauma clinics, local professionals enroll in training programs run by trauma specialists, and others fill in the trauma questionnaires of epidemiologists. Amidst the general confusion, "trauma" stands out as a master term, a way to communicate extreme suffering to the international community of professional helpers. However, beneath this general label of "traumatized population," survivors struggle to maintain cultural processes, while at the same time trying to grapple with the notion of trauma and the confusion that might go along with the introduction of this new concept coming from another culture: post-traumatic stress disorder (PTSD).

As revealed in Chapter 7, the contemporary concept of PTSD is largely a product of Euro-American history and culture. Nevertheless, epidemiological research shows how traumatic stress can be found among a variety of populations with different cultures and political and religious systems (for example, Hinton et al., 1993; Kroll et al., 1989; Mollica et al., 1987; Westermeyer et al., 1989). But "culture" often remains the unknown factor, a variable difficult to approach with the available research methodologies. Trauma specialists who work in cultures that are relatively unknown to them often wonder whether the local culture is playing a protective role.

This question can be posed concerning the initial traumatization or regarding the long-term effects of traumatic events. Strong religious beliefs that provide survivors with a coherent world view and an interpretation of suffering might be able to reduce the initial impact of extreme events substantially. In the long run, where certain cultural healing practices have survived, they might reduce the risk of chronic psychological disorders and functional impairment. For example, the "therapies" provided by traditional healers such as witch doctors or spirit mediums might be highly effective for the "treatment of illnesses" related to outbreaks of extreme violence. These questions all relate to the role of culture as a protective shield in extreme circumstances, as a sort of cultural immunity, and are typically posed from the perspective of the trauma specialist involved in non-Western cultural contexts (for example, Boehnlein & Kinzie, 1992; Eisenbruch, 1992; Straker, 1994).

To address the issue of trauma and culture, however, I would like to further deconstruct such questions about the "protective value of culture against trauma." "Trauma" is not necessarily a bottom rock, empirical reality against which the myriad of non-Western interpretations of suffering might play a protective role. When anthropologists are being trained in the study of other cultures, they are simultaneously taught to observe their own cultures from a certain distance. From that perspective, PTSD researchers and trauma counselors can be seen as a Euro-American, culturally-specific protective shield against massive disasters. In these ways, our culture protects us and helps us to survive atrocities. It helps people from other cultures, too, as part of humanitarian actions and refugee programs.

In these non-Western contexts, the discourse on trauma becomes one among many ways of dealing with suffering. In much of the world, religious understandings of suffering that belong to what are usually called a world religion (Buddhism, Islam, Christianity, and Hinduism) together with interpretations related to local cosmologies (beliefs in spirits and ancestor worship) exist side by side with Western notions of trauma (Fig. 1). Each of these diverse ways of dealing with suffering often plays a role in the lives of survivors. A complex cultural dynamic develops. Although world religion and local cosmology are known to influence one another, the discourse on trauma has only recently joined the forum of cultural negotiation. This is but a brief and very general situation sketch of this triad, of the wider context in which to contemplate the question of trauma and culture.

But what is the question? As the title of this introduction suggests, is it about the role of culture as a protective shield against "PTSD"? This goes hand in hand with another frequently stated problem: how can trauma specialists "overcome" cultural differences? I propose to work through a more detailed analysis of the context of this problem, the triad of world religion, local cosmology, and trauma discourse to rethink these questions. In the first section, I explore the link between indigenous interpretations of suffering and the organization of society and its moral order. Second, I bring in the cultural factor formed by the discourse on trauma. And in the third section, I look at the cultural processes involved in remembering and forgetting. Gradually, throughout this chapter, the focus of analysis will be shifting and so will the question. Finally, in the conclusion, I contemplate the possible cultural impact of the discourse on trauma in war-torn non-Western societies.

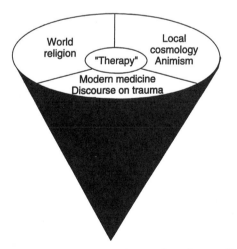

FIGURE 1. The triad of world religion, local cosmology, and modern medicine/trauma discourse; the historical construction of the discourse about "therapy."

Interpretations of Suffering as Indigenous Sociologies: The Locus of Moral Authority

Local Cosmologies, Illness, and Suffering

Before considering the implications of the interaction among world religion, local cosmology, and modern medicine, I will start with a brief characterization of the role of local cosmologies in the experience of suffering and illness. Anthropologists have documented how, in non-Western societies, misfortune and illness are attributed to the intrusion of evil spirits, the magic of sorcerers or witches, the breach of taboos, the loss of one's soul, or the intrusion of an object. These are the five major traditional explanations of illness and suffering that can be found around the world (Last, 1993).

Anthropologists, born and bred in the West, communicate their findings about unfamiliar healing practices by using the vocabulary of a European or North American cultural world (for example, Levi-Strauss, 1963). Hence the frequent use of words like "magic," "the supernatural," "spirit possession," or "the irrational." These words are used to describe "traditional medical systems" and are usually associated by the Western public with the fantastic, a feeling of mystery, the sense of not being "real." Especially when compared to modern medicine, stereotypes about "traditional medicine" proliferate. For some Western observers, "traditional medicine" has become an exotic form of psychotherapy bordering on the religious.

The tendency of anthropologists to make these practices more exotic by using European languages to describe them has been critically reassessed (de Sardan, 1992). For example, many African languages do not have words corresponding to "the supernatural" or "magic," and it has been suggested that practices related to local cosmologies do not have a great deal in common with Western notions of religion, faith, dogma, magic, or the occult. On the contrary, in many cultures, "sorcery," "witchcraft," "ghosts of ancestors," or "spirits" are very ordinary, everyday concepts, a commonsense way of talking about social relationships. For example, wealthy people can be bewitched by envious neighbors (Kapferer, 1983), maltreated spouses may become possessed by vengeful and demanding spirits (Lewis, 1971; Lewis et al., 1991), and the bereaved might engage in a relationship with the ghosts of the deceased (Schieffelin, 1976; Vitebsky, 1993). These notions are frequently used in everyday language in a matter-of-*fact* way (Evans-Pritchard, 1976). Words such as "sorcery" or "spirit" evoke invisible forces. However, it could be argued that such "forces" are no more invisible than our Western notions of "having luck," and our experiences of "transference" or (secure/insecure) "attachment." Such concepts reveal *real* (albeit largely invisible) social forces. Local cosmologies can no longer be merely classified as the irrational and magical worldview of a not yet fully modernized world, a "developing" world, and a Western person's understanding of the situation does generally not benefit by labeling the survivor's experiences of being haunted by evil spirits or disgruntled ancestors with stereotypical words such as "superstition" or "magic."

The Triad of World Religion, Local Cosmology, and Modern Medicine

Alternatively, Western researchers could approach the rituals related to local cosmologies as "therapy," which then could be compared with Western forms of psychotherapy. Then possession by spirits, demons or deities is seen as a "local idiom of distress," or a "local language to talk about traumatic stress." Local healers perform rituals and thereby treat culture-bound syndromes, illnesses particular to their culture. Such practices have been called folk "psychiatries" (see Gaines, 1992 for an overview), or indigenous "psychologies" (Heelas & Lock, 1981)—in other words, traditional forms of psychotherapy. Within this framework of analysis, each culture is described with its own repertoire of emotions (Abu-Lughod & Lutz, 1990; Harré, 1986; Lutz, 1988; Shweder, 1988), its own types of expressions of distress and illnesses (Currer & Stacey, 1986; Helman, 1990), and its own healers and therapies.

Long before the birth of modern psychiatry, traditional healers have dealt with survivors of war, extreme poverty, and disasters. Modern trauma specialists show interest in the ways in which indigenous healers treat traumatized patients. However, attempts to explain non-Western therapeutic strategies with the vocabulary of Western psychology (Obeyesekere, 1981, 1990) remain controversial. Translation of therapies based on the local cosmology into the language of psychology or psychoanalysis (see Devisch & Brodeur, 1996, for a critical discussion) has been described as complicated, imperfect, impossible, or even inappropriate (Cantlie, 1994; Kakar, 1982, 1985).

This way of looking at non-Western healing processes is further complicated by another strategy of doubt so typical and necessary for cross-cultural research. Are spirit possession, sorcery, exorcism of demons, or the undoing of evil spells primarily about psychological illness and therapy as people know them in the West? Anthropologists have pointed out the danger of looking at a variety of non-Western rituals with a gaze borrowed from mental health professionals (de Sardan, 1994; Kapferer, 1988; Littlewood, 1992). A variety of local practices can be described as "therapy" and can be given a significance related to the mental health of the individual patients, but it would not do justice to the complexity of traditional "healing" systems to stop the analysis there. Especially in the context of political violence or excessive social inequalities—chronic crimes against humanity—a wider approach is mandatory.

The previously mentioned triad of world religion, local cosmology, and trauma discourse based on modern medicine needs to be considered. For example, the fact that many local ritual practices in Africa are described as "therapy" could partly be a result of the competition between animist beliefs, world religion, and Western medicine (Last, 1991; Lewis, 1971). Before the spread, first of world religion and then of modern medicine, local cosmologies played a more central role in the social life and politics of non-Western societies. Today, these ritual practices sometimes take up a marginal position and are categorized as "therapy" or "traditional medicine." Traditional ritual specialists increasingly refer to their "therapeutic expertise" to present themselves to outsiders and underplay their religious and political roles.

This could be seen as a strategy for the cultural survival of animist practices in the face of their suppression by purist and dominant world religions. The prestige and "therapeutic" success of Western medicine has formed a role model of sorts that continuing ritual activities of traditional experts in the guise of "therapy" for the chronically ill (de Sardan, 1994). It is important not to take for granted the rhetoric of non-Western healing systems as "psychotherapy" and not to neglect other aspects of the contemporary role of local cosmologies in managing extreme suffering.

"Supernatural" Moral Orders and Traditional Retributive Justice

Sorcery, divination, witchcraft, spirit possession and exorcism are indeed not only a means of expressing personal suffering or a "therapy for the traumatized." Being more than mere "superstition," "magic," "therapy," and "religion," such practices have been described as indigenous sociologies, local ways of looking at society (Kapferer, 1997). For example, they reveal how a community establishes a relationship with its past, how powerlessness and abuse is made public, and how revenge can be carried out. Especially in the context of traumatic events, be it abuse of individuals within the community or the devastation of whole communities, such practices distinguish between Good and Evil, and make possible the re-encounter of some kind of moral authority and accountability. It *does* make a difference whether one is diagnosed as suffering from post-traumatic stress disorder, spirit possession, or an illness caused by the evil eye. These are not necessarily cultural variations on the same theme or diverse "idioms of distress" essentially pointing at the same underlying biological disorder. Indigenous interpretations of suffering simultaneously point at a moral order or disorder, a locus of moral authority that greatly differs across cultures. Through the presentation of suffering and illness in traditional ways and the consultation of ritual specialists, ancestral laws and what Western ethnographers would call a "supernatural" or religious moral order are brought to the fore (Brow, 1988).

For a Western observer familiar with secular forms of moral authority and jurisdiction, these traditional ways of making somebody morally responsible for Evil and suffering within the community seem opaque or even arbitrary. The examples to which Western analysts commonly refer are witch hunts (Allen, 1998; Girard, 1986; Reynolds, 1996; Yamba, 1997) where the people being killed and held accountable are not really morally responsible in the way Euro-American people would understand it. Witchcraft accusations and trails are called a scapegoat mechanism, an unjust way of taking revenge upon somebody to restore health and harmony within the community. When massive misfortune strikes, this interpretation of suffering might exacerbate the cycle of revenge and violence.

At a more general level, this scapegoat mechanism might surface as extreme nationalism and interethnic strife (Kapferer, 1997), when whole groups of people or nations are used as a scapegoat. The media often tend to highlight these extreme examples, while leaving the virtues of these indigenous sociologies and types of moral authority unmentioned. Spirits talking through the voices of the possessed—and the supernatural moral order they present in doing so—have proved a crucial force in conflict resolution at the community level (Brow, 1990). The threat of supernatural sanctions hovers around those abusing their power, and the gaze ("evil eye") of those who do not have the power to speak makes the powermonger sick and miserable. Abused spouses are possessed by vengeful and demanding spirits, and their husbands sometimes are forced to accede to their demands.

These ways of dealing with suffering are thoroughly embedded in a local, indigenous sociology, a local commentary upon power relationships, abuse, and revenge. While illness and well-being are being negotiated with the ritual expert in contact with supernatural beings, subtle adjustments are sometimes effected within the community, as minuscule shifts in the hierarchy of the powerful and the less powerful.

Trauma and its undoing are addressed within what Euro-American people would call "the realm of the supernatural." For example, severely ill patients who undergo a healing ritual might take revenge by casting an evil spell upon their enemy or by performing a sacrifice in which an object or an animal that represents the enemy is ritually killed. This, it is supposed, will bring illness, misfortune, or death upon the enemy, his/her family, or friends (Wirz, 1954). For Western people, this circle is not fully closed, the "cycle of revenge and violence" as we know it within Euro-American culture has been interrupted by ritual means, by relying upon supernatural sanctions for revenge (Kapferer, 1997).

Similar instances sometimes have relevance for the war-torn society at large. In Sri Lanka, a new type of story about ghosts has recently emerged (Perera, 1995). The stories relate how ghosts of the tortured and the disappeared now haunt and make ill members of the security forces known to be war criminals. In Cameroon, soldiers who recently destroyed whole villages, and important sacred places, are said to have gone mad as a result of their acts. Soon after the violence, traditional healers predicted that many more would end up in mental hospitals as they now have to face the vengeance of the angry and implacable gods (Mbunwe, 1997).

This is a form of revenge which equally could be called traditional retributive justice. For people socialized within Western culture, this form of justice seems opaque, not very clear-cut. The distinction between Good and Evil seems to be in the hands of many, spirits, gods, demons, ritual experts, traditional healers, the ancestors, priests, and victims. For people used to a secular form of moral authority and justice, the moral orders involved seem multiple and the resulting state of affairs seems arbitrary.

Traumatic Stress: Our Contemporary Discourse about Suffering and Its Diffusion Across Cultures

A Secular Moral Order and a Flow of Knowledge

Now I want to return to the concept of post-traumatic stress disorder and subject it to a similar type of analysis. I have argued before that the ways in which suffering and illness are presented publicly play an important role in the moral fabric of a community and bring about a recognition of certain sources of morality. If one takes this train of thought further, one can ask the same question about PTSD and try to draw the line between this Euro-American articulation of suffering and a locus of moral authority.

The diagnosis of PTSD places the source of Evil outside the sufferer; it allocates moral responsibility outside the victim. This particular way of dealing with extreme suffering in Euro-American culture might be more ancient than the multiple historical accounts of the development of the notion of traumatic stress during the last two centuries suggest. Helman (1990) argues that "stress" is a secular version of European traditional concepts of witchcraft and sorcery. The bewitched and the possessed were threatened by evil forces coming from outside the self, over which one had very little control and for which one did not feel morally responsible. Today, the locus of moral responsibility for PTSD victims is still shifted away from the self, but the prevailing moral order has become secular. Witches, sorcerers, and priests are no longer involved; the secular institutions of the state and civil society create the moral order.

Being diagnosed as suffering from PTSD entails a particular experience of Good and Evil; it makes people *belong* to a particular moral order. Almost all aspects of our Western moral culture seem self-evident; victims of natural disasters, domestic abuse, or terrorist actions receive recognition or compensation for chronic psychological suffering that might ensue. The State apparatus emits messages about Good and Evil, and its moral authority distinguishes between good and bad citizens, victims, and perpetrators. A crucial and controversial aspect of this secularized moral culture has to do with the values and attitudes people hold vis-à-vis their military apparatus. Generally speaking, citizens tend to recognize the suffering of soldier-victims who fought for the State, and they perceive that the State is morally responsible for their actions as perpetrators. Soldiers might become victims of the enemy, but when history turns its back on them, they might also become victims of an evil State that forced war upon them but has since changed its policy (e.g., the Vietnam War) (Young, 1993).

In this sense post-traumatic stress disorder is more than a set of symptoms; it presupposes a perception of Good and Evil, usually pitting the victim and the State against the evil forces. Just as non-Western interpretations of suffering reveal an indigenous sociology and a culture-specific locus of moral authority, one could argue that the notion of traumatic stress is embedded within a culture-specific moral culture that coalesces around the secular moral authority of the modern State.

Thus, can one state that "PTSD" is a contemporary *discourse* about suffering that Western mental health professionals present to people from other non-Western cultures? Calling the expertise on PTSD a "discourse" (Foucault, 1972) means that Euro-Americans recognize that their current knowledge is greatly determined by their history, organization of society, Euro-American institutions, and moral culture. An analysis of this "discourse on trauma" does not imply a denial of the empirical reality of PTSD. It simply calls attention to the cultural specificity of focusing on this particular empirical reality and to the fact that other cultures that have other non-Western political systems and forms of moral authority have not established the notion of trauma and developed other ways of dealing with extreme suffering throughout their history.

The Western discourse on trauma has entered diverse cultural realities. It has become a "flow of knowledge" (Lyotard, 1979), for example, with a particular pattern of distribution in war-torn societies worldwide. In this global network of communication that channels the flow of knowledge on PTSD, a variety of specialists, organizations, and institutions are active: Trauma researchers, clinicians, the Societies for Traumatic Stress Studies, the United Nations, donor agencies, nongovernmental organizations (NGO), local professionals trained by foreign trauma specialists, rural mental health workers trained by NGOs, or war widows trained to be counselors all take part in this global distribution of knowledge on PTSD.

All are using the word "trauma," which has taken up a slightly (or, in some cases, substantially) different meaning in each context. To a researcher specialized in the neurobiology of PTSD, "trauma" will mean something different than to an official from a donor agency or a rural mental health worker. Such diversity can indeed lead to confusion and to the loss of any specific meaning. But what do mental health professionals achieve if they try to narrow the concept of "trauma" to the meanings given to it in the context of international conferences on PTSD? It would improve the specificity of what trauma means for Western trauma specialists, but at the same time it would make people lose sight of the other participants who currently form a real force within this flow and distribution of knowledge; for example, NGO personnel and rural mental health workers from non-Western cultures.

Thus I will use the notion "trauma discourse" in its broadest sense, as including the discourse of people with very different professional or cultural backgrounds who use the notion "trauma" when referring to extreme suffering. Together these diverse understandings and uses of the word trauma constitute the discourse on trauma, a flow of knowledge on PTSD that simultaneously leads to the diffusion of a secular interpretation of suffering and moral culture.

Questions about the Ideal and the Real

Thus the discourse on trauma forms one instance of the "global cultural traffic" (Appadurai, 1990) that includes a myriad of cultural elements coming from the West, such as fashion, music, mass consumption and party politics. In most cases these Western cultural influences are incorporated in the local culture in a very creative and culture-specific way. They lead to an ever-continuing "cultural work-in-progress" (Hannerz, 1987; Friedman, 1990) in which the foreign and the traditional mutually influence each other. An openness to foreign cultural influences does not necessarily impoverish the local culture. The new is added to the traditions of the past, which continue to fulfill culture-specific roles that the new cultural elements might not provide.

However, in the aftermath of extreme events, the vitality of the local culture cannot be taken for granted, and the trauma discourse is commonly introduced in culturally destabilized communities. In situations where social relationships are disrupted, a shared sense of reality is challenged, and cultural experts and their expertise are not available, people tend to borrow from other available worldviews rapidly to repair their impoverished systems of meaning, morality, and dignity (Nordstrom, 1992). The world-view implicit in humanitarian actions and the discourse on trauma form one such instance on the basis of which people reconstruct a life-world.

In the long run, when traditional healers and religious specialists manage to re-establish their services for the community, traditional and foreign worldviews exist side by side. This is a crucial moment in situations of recurrent "cycles of violence," where people try to reconstruct disabled life-worlds, with the available local and foreign moral discourses, in ways that do *not* reproduce the conditions and discourses that fueled violence and atrocities (Nordstrom, 1992).

Some people have received the diagnosis of PTSD together with Western forms of treatment (e.g., political refugees in Western host countries); others have consulted a ritual specialist and are trying to cope with an evil spirit haunting them, the loss of their soul, or the evil spell of a sorcerer. The latter makes survivors relate to a "supernatural" moral order, whereas the discourse on trauma makes a secular moral culture available. Most often, forms of moral authority based on the supernatural seem arbitrary and opaque to the Western observer.

Arguments about the *reality* of witch hunts or other "irrational" traditional forms of community rehabilitation are close at hand, whereas the more subtle traditional forms of social negotiation and moral authority remain largely outside a Western observer's field of vision. Having the *ideal* of the modern welfare State in mind, traditional Western categories of Good and Evil are used: the goodness of the State versus an evil enemy, the army versus rebels, the State versus terrorism. Modern people become victims of something—not a supernatural agent or an ancestor—but a source of evil defined by a secular moral authority. Meanwhile, violence perpetrated in the name of the State is morally justified.

However, from multiple non-Western perspectives, it is the *real* manifestations of secular forms of moral authority which might seem opaque, arbitrary, or "irrational." The collective memories of the violence and terror of the process of colonialization (Richards, 1996; Taussig, 1987) might have jeopardized the image of Western modern states as a moral authority. In some instances the "public ethic of the State is bankrupt," and the State is experienced by its subjects as a predator, a source of Evil (Devisch, 1995).

The categories of Good and Evil of the Western tradition are not taken for granted. Increased attention to the historical legacy of colonial and neocolonial violence (Shohat, 1992) in non-Western cultures, together with a self-awareness characteristic of the Western *post*modern culture, point at notions such as "State terrorism," "chronic crimes against humanity perpetrated by State business associations," "the ghostly inner spaces of the national security States," and the "culture of secrecy" that surrounds Evil carried out in the name of the State (Lutz, 1997).

In this light, secular moral discourses appear multiple, manipulable by different interest groups, and often arbitrary. In the wake of extreme events, lay people (in consultation with experts) label illnesses and suffering with a particular diagnosis. In doing so, they reinsert themselves into a moral order, replacing their shattered assumptions about justice, Good, and Evil. In many situations, elements of the modern secular discourse as well as the traditional moral culture are offered. In considering their respective value for establishing long-term processes of rehabilitation or interrupting a cycle of violence, Western citizens should be wary of *idealizing* their own taken for granted moral culture and consider the values that traditional moral cultures can display outside episodes of cultural destabilization in more *ideal* circumstances.

The Subtle Balance Between Remembering and Forgetting: A Product of Culture?

Focus on Remembering

A contemplation of "trauma and culture" does not lead only to questions about the moral cultures in which diagnosis and rehabilitation are embedded, but it also brings up the central question of "memory and culture." In other words, do people from non-Western cultures remember (and by extension forget) in the same ways Euro-American people do? Within the Western tradition, an individual can say "I am traumatized," "I have traumatic memories." The discourse on trauma refers equally to "traumatized communities and societies" (see section VII) and includes the discourse of politicians claiming that a whole nation is "traumatized." On one hand are the memories of an individual person; on the other hand are the collective memories, the memories shared by a family, a community, and a nation. It is at the interface between the individual and the collective memory that questions about "memory and culture," and by extension "traumatic memory and culture" can be posed.

Anthropologists investigate the ways in which a collective memory is built from the conglomerate of individual memories. Or, in the case of "traumatic memories," which social and cultural processes are responsible for the fact that a community suppresses certain individual memories of extreme events from its collective memory. Conversely, the question emerges to what extent personal memories of extreme suffering depend upon these collective and culture-specific ways of dealing with the past. It is in this pendular movement between personal and collective memory that the factor of culture plays its role.

The discourse on trauma most frequently addresses individual memories, with the evolving neurobiology of traumatic stress being its prototype. A traumatic memory is defined as a (not yet) removable scar in the neurophysiology or microanatomy of the brain (see Chapters 19 and 22). Within this research tradition, the subject's memory is observed as an isolated entity, a discrete mental property, a mental space in which information is stored (following the Platonic and Aristotelian models of memory; see Küchler, 1987).

Following Halbwachs (1950), one can leave this tradition of isolating the individual's memory aside and refrain from conceiving of personal memory as absolutely separate from the collective memory. Then the two research questions—how does a person and how does a society preserve and rediscover memories—cannot be separated. Each individual memory depends in its essence upon the sociocultural practices and institutions that precipitate certain modes of recollection. Thus memory construction and remembering can be approached as a social and cultural process (Küchler, 1987).

In the analysis of memory systems across cultures, much attention is paid to the nonverbal ways of establishing continuity with the past. In some cultures, memories are mainly passed on in a nontextual, nonnarrative, or nondeclarative way. Through repetitive daily acts and the performance of rituals, memories are transmitted from one generation to the next. Through a lot of "practice," values and traditions are made "habits" of the body (see Bourdieu, 1977). "Knowledge" of ancient traditions is "incorporated" in the repertoire of bodily techniques (Connerton, 1989), in the body's memory (Casey, 1987). Then "memory" depends very much on recurring events and actions, cycles, and rhythms. For example, the repetition and rhythm of oral verse, participation in an annual ritual cycle or in "therapeutic" rites (de Sardan, 1994; Lawrence, in press), or periodical engagement with material objects (Argenti, 1998, 1999; Küchler, 1987; Rowlands, 1993) form a type of memory system.

"Memories" also depend on an awareness of time, the experience of a flow of time that is culturally conditioned to a certain extent (Gell, 1992). A cyclical perception of time, where life is a series of cycles or where each life forms part of the cycle of rebirth, does not lead to the "life history" or "chronological narrative" Euro-American people are so used to (Connerton, 1989).

Apart from the "cultural traditions" as we commonly understand them, other factors also influence time perception and memory. Connerton (1989) argued that people from "cultures" of extreme deprivation and poverty might depend less on past history, memory, sense of future, and linear progress of time to present themselves than members of elite groups. Some people's time perception takes the form of a curriculum vitae with multiple points of reference (from well-determined origins towards the steady accumulation of knowledge, wealth, or influence). However, other people's sense of time is dominated by a cycle of poverty and a repetition of sameness. These differing conceptions of self and time lead to other narrative styles, transfers of memories and patterns of remembering, to another sociocultural formation of "memories" at both the individual and collective level.

Then the obvious question would be to ask whether "traumatic memory," "a traumatic moment in time," and "a traumatized self" are sociocultural realities. Young (1996) states that "traumatic memory is a man-made object" and originates in the scientific and clinical discourses of the nineteenth century. Within Western "psychiatric culture," time is experienced as flowing from an extreme event to the post-traumatic symptoms (Young, 1996). A traumatic event or episode in the past becomes a major point of reference for identity formation or interpretation of unhappiness in the present. Thus, the social practices and institutions that precipitate certain modes of remembering (Halbwachs, 1950) are said to be constituted by contemporary trauma specialists and their institutions.

It is also important to take into account medieval and early modern European cultures, from which the Western notion of "memory" emerged. The Western idea of "memory" is very much tied to a linear conception of time (Yates, 1966). Memory, as a sequence of events that can literally be retraced, has been linked to the spread of literacy and the experience of the durability of memories once written down (Rowlands, 1993). Moreover, the Western notion of personal identity from the seventeenth century onward is intimately linked to a continuity of consciousness, a relationship with the past (Bhabha, 1994).

Western culture gave preference to the visual sense (Classen, 1993; Howes, 1991), and the way Euro-American people relate to themselves (as the consciousness of a past) is analogous to visual perception; an inward- and backward-*looking* mental state so typical of Western culture (Bhabha, 1994; Connerton, 1989; Foucault, 1988). The modern State functions as an important organizer of those memories; public records and national histories give a time consciousness and a uniform sense of the past to the culturally diverse communities they include (Das, 1995).

However, since the advent of the notion of PTSD, the facts that can be narrated and recorded have expanded substantially. Now the transient (or less transient) memories of the body, which would be addressed in other cultures within a nonnarrative, non-declarative memory system, can be recorded. Statistics about the painful bodily memories (PTSD symptoms) of communities and populations are produced, which then constitute an important element of the largely Western collective memory of extreme suffering in recent history.

A specific kind of collective traumatic memory is provided by epidemiologists and trauma specialists (Young 1996). It is a powerful tool for memory formation. A way has been found to systematically inscribe bodily memories in the chronological history of communities and nations. How far this *focus on remembering* will reach depends first of all on the messages that trauma specialists convey to the public and secondly on the way their discoveries will be incorporated in the popular experience of "traumatic memory."

These messages go from speculations upon the durable and indelible character of traumatic memories (for example, Kolb, 1987) to cautious accounts about the possibility of the treatment of PTSD (for example, Solomon et al., 1992), and more optimistic accounts about the upcoming preventive measures against traumatic memories. It is this information that is added to the subtle balance of forgetting and remembering that various cultures and sub-cultures help to provide.

Focus on Forgetting

Some non-Western memory systems allow for continuous strategic acts of erasure and refashioning of "memories" (Küchler, 1987). Systematic ways of "forgetting" sometimes form an essential part of the everyday construction and creation of identities (Carsten, 1995). For Western mental health professionals "forgetting" has mainly negative connotations; they tend to conceive of "forgetting" as a loss, a lack, some knowledge that is absent: "repression," "denial." In a context where communities have undergone repetitive brutal ruptures, knowledge of the past and past relationships might play a less central role in everyday life and rapidly lead to what would be called collective amnesia rather than collective remembering (Carsten, 1995).

The cultural resources and cultural capital that were developed over centuries of living in unstable conditions and violent contexts include some elaborate mechanisms for forgetting that were essential to repetitive cycles of reconstruction. One example demonstrates how new communities and family relationships are created in the present generation and also in previous generations. Narratives rewrite local histories and create new forms of belonging by even adopting *new ancestors* (Richards, 1996). It is equally argued that the body learns to forget in ritual life and that through participation in the very intense multisensorial environments of certain rites, previous bodily states are "forgotten" or rather transcended (Kapferer, 1997).

The culture-specific types of transfer of "memories" between generations or social groups might account for processes of forgetting at the collective level. A complex dynamic develops when differing levels of "forgetting" characterize the interacting groups, such as the local community, the State, humanitarian discourses, the international discourse on trauma, and the discourse of traditional ritual specialists. All too rigid forms of remembering of extreme suffering are associated with recurring cycles of revenge and violence. This issue is addressed in Chapter 8 where the relationship between "traumatization" and the cycle of violence is explored. All too thorough forms of forgetting and fluid strategies for reinventing the self and one's community might be good survival strategies and interrupt the immediate cycle of violence, but are not a good recipe for political action and resistance to chronic oppression in the long term (Shohat, 1992). In many cases the subtle balance between remembering and forgetting is a product of numerous cultures, a complex interplay between local and foreign ways of dealing with the past, the flow of time, identity formation, and "memories." One of the cultural factors in this process is, indeed, the discourse on trauma.

Conclusion: Questions about the Cultural Impact of the Trauma Discourse

> The hero will always have one traumatic experience in the beginning, to which he has flashbacks during moments of stress. Though in the case of "Sudden Death" we have the *surreal* experience of seeing Van Damme go through a traumatic experience as a fireman that he never once has a flashback to! Got ya there! (Aziz, 1996)

Nowadays, the fact that a traumatized hero of the video world does not have one of the major symptoms of PTSD seems surreal to a Sri Lankan urban audience. The notion of trauma is becoming more and more familiar for a large number of people in non-Western cultures. Fragments of Western culture thrive in many places, coexisting with local traditions. Western medicine is often combined with visits to traditional healers; likewise traditional political leaders stay in power under the aegis of Western-style multiparty politics. However, the question is: to what extent does the cultural impact of imported, foreign discourses increase in circumstances of massive destruction, extreme suffering, and concomitant cultural destabilization?

The discourse on trauma of the international community of professional helpers is one such foreign discourse that helps people to reconstruct their life-worlds. The trauma discourse introduces cultural elements that are not mere surface phenomena but core components of Western culture: a secular source of moral authority, a sense of time and identity, and a memory system, as well as mechanisms for forgetting. More and more voices assert the need to approach the introduction of the discourse on trauma in non-Western situations with caution (Bracken et al., 1995; Summerfield, 1996) and to acknowledge the protection of other cultures as a major social responsibility of the international mental health care system (Eisenbruch, 1992).

This might be taken as a call to evaluate the therapeutic value of non-Western healing systems, but in my opinion, the contribution of an ethnographic method goes beyond an evaluation of the effectiveness of local, traditional systems of mental health care and facilitation of their incorporation within the formal mental health care sector (see research agenda in Desjarlais et al., 1995). Ethnographic research questions are not primarily about "therapy" or "mental health." Venturing outside the "therapeutic context" of healer and client leads to an analysis of the negotiation of available moral cultures in situations of cultural destabilization, the ways in which communities establish a relationship with their past, and the manner in which foreign discourses are incorporated within the local culture.

When massive misfortune strikes, the Western discourse on trauma often becomes one of the global cultural influences that eventually plays a role in local long-term processes of rehabilitation. It is in the movement toward an assessment of this role and a critical self-reflection that the contribution of an ethnographic method lies. In other words, it is not too early to inquire into the historical role of the trauma discourse in the geopolitics of global cultural (ex)change.

Acknowledgments. Thanks to Nanneke Redclift, Murray Last, Roland Littlewood, Bruce Kapferer, and Nicolas Argenti. Ethnographic research in Sri Lanka that deals with some of the issues raised in this chapter is funded by the Graduate School, University College London, and a research grant from the Harry Frank Guggenheim Foundation (research for understanding and reducing violence, aggression, and dominance).

References

Abu-Lughod, L., & Lutz, C. (1990). Emotion, discourse and the politics of everyday life. In C. Lutz (Ed.), *Language and the politics of emotion* (pp. 1–23). Cambridge: Cambridge University Press.

Allen, T. (1998). The violence of healing. *Sociologus, 47*(2), 34–52.

Appadurai, A. (1990). Disjuncture and difference in the global cultural economy. *Theory, Culture and Society, 7,* 295–310.

Argenti, N. (1998). Air youth: Performance, violence and the state in Cameroon. *Journal of the Royal Anthropological Institute, 4*(4), 753–781.

Argenti, N. (1999). Ephemeral monuments, memory, and royal sempiternity in a Grassfields kingdom. In A. Forty and S. Küchler (Eds.), *The Art of Forgetting* (pp. 21–52). Oxford: Berg.

Aziz, A. (1996). Van Damme to the rescue. *The Sunday Leader (Sri Lanka),* July 28, p. 6.

Bhabha, H. K. (1994). *The location of culture.* London, New York: Routledge.

Boehnlein, J. K., & Kinzie, J. D. (1992). DSM diagnosis of posttraumatic stress disorder and cultural sensitivity: A response. *Journal of Nervous and Mental Diseases, 180*(9), 597–599.

Bourdieu, P. (1977). *Outline of a theory of practice.* Cambridge: Cambridge University Press.

Bracken, P. J., Giller, J. E., & Summerfield, D. (1995). Psychological responses to war and atrocity: The limitations of current concepts. *Social Science and Medicine, 40*(8), 1073–1082.

Brow, J. (1988). In pursuit of hegemony: Representations of authority and justice in a Sri Lankan village. *American Ethnologist, 15*(2), 311–327.

Brow, J. (1990). Nationalist rhetoric and local practice: The fate of the village community in Kukulewa. In J. Spencer (Ed.), *Sri Lanka: History and the roots of conflict* (pp. 125–144). London: Routledge.

Cantlie, A. (1994). Psychoanalysis and anthropology: Applied or misapplied? *The Psychoanalysis Newsletter, 14,* 2–7.

Carsten, J. (1995). The politics of forgetting: Migration, kinship and memory on the periphery of the Southeast Asian state. *Journal of the Royal Anthropological Institute, 1,* 317–335.

Casey, E. S. (1987). *Remembering: A phenomenological study.* Bloomington, IN: Indiana University Press.

Classen, C. (1993). *Worlds of sense. Exploring the senses in history and across cultures.* London: Routledge.

Connerton, P. (1989). *How societies remember.* Cambridge: Cambridge University Press.

Currer, C., & Stacey, M. (Eds.). (1986). *Concepts of health, illness and disease.* Leamington: Berg.

Das, V. (1995). *Critical events: An anthropological perspective on contemporary India.* Delhi, Bombay, Calcutta, Madras: Oxford University Press.

de Sardan, J. P. O. (1992). Occultism and the ethnographic "I." The exoticizing of magic from Durkheim to "postmodern" anthropology. *Critique of Anthropology, 12*(1), 5–25.

de Sardan, J. P. O. (1994). Possession, affliction et folie: Les ruses de la thérapisation. *Homme, XXXIV*(3), 7–27.

Desjarlais, R., Eisenberg, L., Good, B., & Kleinman, A. (1995). *World mental health: Problems and priorities in low income countries.* New York, Oxford: Oxford University Press.

Devisch, R. (1995). Frenzy, violence, and ethical renewal in Kinshasa. *Public Culture, 7*(3), 593–629.

Devisch, R., & Brodeur, C. (1996). *Forces et signes. Regards croisés d'un anthropologue et d'un psychanalyste sur les Yaka.* Paris: Éditions des Archives Contemporaines.

Eisenbruch, M. (1992). Toward a culturally sensitive DSM: Cultural bereavement in Cambodian refugees and the traditional healer as taxonomist. *Journal of Nervous and Mental Diseases, 180*(1), 8–10.

Evans-Pritchard, E. (1976). *Witchcraft, oracles, and magic among the Azande.* Oxford: Clarendon Press.

Foucault, M. (1972). *The archeology of knowledge and the discourse on language.* New York: Tavistock & Harper Colophon.

Foucault, M. (1988). Technologies of the self. In L. H. Martin, H. Gutman, & P. H. Hutton (Eds.), *Technologies of the self: A seminar with Michel Foucault* (pp. 16–49). London: Tavistock.

Friedman, J. (1990). Being in the world: Globalization and localization. *Theory, Culture and Society, 7,* 311–328.

Gaines, A. (Ed.). (1992). *Ethnopsychiatry. The cultural construction of professional and folk psychiatries.* New York: SUNY Press.

Gell, A. (1992). *The anthropology of time. Cultural constructions of temporal maps and images.* Oxford/Providence: Berg.

Girard, R. (1986). *The scapegoat.* Baltimore: Johns Hopkins University Press.

Halbwachs, M. (1950). *La mémoire collective.* Paris: Presses Universitaires de France.

Hannerz, U. (1987). The world in creolization. *Africa, 57*(4), 546–559.

Harré, R. (Ed.). (1986). *The social construction of emotions.* Oxford: Blackwell.

Heelas, P., & Lock, A. (Eds.). (1981). *Indigenous psychologies. The anthropology of the self.* London: Academic Press.

Helman, C. (1990). *Culture, health and illness.* Bristol: Wright.

Hinton, W. L., Chen, Y. J., Du, N., Tran, C. G., Lu, F. G., Miranda, J., & Faust, S. (1993). DSM-III-R disorders in Vietnamese refugees. Prevalence and correlates. *Journal of Nervous and Mental Diseases, 181*(2), 113–122.

Howes, D. (1991). To summon all the senses. In D. Howes (Ed.), *The varieties of sensory experience. A sourcebook in the anthropology of the senses* (pp. 3–21). Toronto, Buffalo, London: University of Toronto Press.

Kakar, S. (1982). *Shamans, mystics and doctors. A psychological inquiry into India and its healing traditions.* Delhi: Oxford University Press.

Kakar, S. (1985). Psychoanalysis and non-Western cultures. *International Review of Psychoanalysis, 12,* 441–447.

Kapferer, B. (1983). *A celebration of demons. Exorcism and the aesthetics of healing in Sri Lanka.* Oxford, Washington: Berg, Smithsonian Institution Press.

Kapferer, B. (1988). Gramsci's body and a critical medical anthropology. *Medical Anthropology Quarterly, 2,* 426–432.

Kapferer, B. (1997). *The feast of the sorcerer: Practices of consciousness and power in Sri Lanka.* Chicago: University of Chicago Press.

Kolb, L. C. (1987). A neuropsychological hypothesis explaining posttraumatic stress disorder. *American Journal of Psychiatry, 144*(8), 989–995.

Kroll, J., Habenicht, M., Mackenzie, T., Yang, M., Chan, S., Vang, T., Nguyen, T., Ly, M., Phommasouvanh, B., Nguyen, H., Vang, Y., Souvannasoth, L., & Cabugao, R. (1989). Depression and posttraumatic stress disorder in Southeast Asian refugees. *American Journal of Psychiatry, 146*(12), 1592–1597.

Küchler, S. (1987). Malangan: Art and memory in a Melanesian society. *Man, 22*(2), 238–255.

Last, M. (1991). Spirit possession as therapy. Bori among non-Muslims in Nigeria. In I. M. Lewis, Al-SafiA, & S. Hurreiz (Eds.), *Women's medicine. The Zar-Bori cult in Africa and beyond* (pp. 49–63). Edinburgh: Edinburgh University Press for the International African Institute.

Last, M. (1993). Non-Western concepts of disease. In W. F. Bynum & R. Porter (Eds.), *Companion encyclopedia of the history of medicine*, Vol. 1 (pp. 634–659). London, New York: Routledge.

Lawrence, P. (in press). Violence, suffering, Amman: The work of oracles in Sri Lanka's Eastern war zone. In V. Das, A. Kleinman, M. Ramphele, & P. Reynolds (Eds.), *Violence, agency and the self*. Oxford: Oxford University Press.

Levi-Strauss, C. (1963). The effectiveness of symbols. In C. Levi-Strauss (Ed.), *Structural anthropology*, Vol. 1 (pp. 186–205). London: Penguin Books.

Lewis, I. M. (1971). *Ecstatic religion. A study of shamanism and spirit possession*. London: Routledge.

Lewis, I. M., Al Safi, A., & Hurreiz, S. (1991). *Women's medicine. The Zar-Bori cult in Africa and beyond*. Edinburgh: Edinburgh University Press for the International African Institute.

Littlewood, R. (1992). How universal is something we can call "therapy"? In J. Kareem and R. Littlewood (Eds.), *Intercultural therapy. Themes, interpretations and practice* (pp. 38–56). Oxford: Blackwell.

Lutz, C. (1988). *Unnatural emotions. Everyday sentiments on a Micronesian atoll and their challenge to Western theory*. Chicago: University of Chicago Press.

Lutz, C. (1997). The psychological ethic and the spirit of containment. *Public Culture, 9*, 135–159.

Lyotard, J. F. (1979). *The postmodern condition: A report on knowledge*. Manchester: Manchester University Press.

Mbunwe, C. (1997). After ransacking Oku shrines gendarmes go mad, develop swollen testes, tommies. *Cameroon Post*, April 15, p. 1,4.

Mollica, R. F., Wyshak, G., & Lavelle, J. (1987). The psychosocial impact of war trauma and torture on Southeast Asian refugees. *American Journal of Psychiatry, 144*(12), 1567–1572.

Nordstrom, C. (1992). The backyard front. In C. Nordstrom & J. Martin (Eds.), *The paths to domination, resistance, and terror* (pp. 260–274). Berkeley: University of California Press.

Obeyesekere, G. (1981). *Medusa's hair. An essay on personal symbols and religious experience*. Chicago, London: University of Chicago Press.

Obeyesekere, G. (1990). *The work of culture. Symbolic transformation in psychoanalysis and anthropology*. Chicago: University of Chicago Press.

Perera, S. (1995). The reality of post-terror societies. Living with torturers and murderers. In S. Perera (Ed.), *Living with torturers and other essays of intervention. Sri Lankan society, culture and politics in perspective* (pp. 46–55). Colombo, Sri Lanka: International Centre for Ethnic Studies.

Reynolds, P. (1996). *Traditional healers and childhood in Zimbabwe*. Athens: Ohio University Press.

Richards, P. (1996). *Fighting for the rainforest. War, youth & resources in Sierra Leone*. Oxford, Portsmouth: The International African Institute, James Currey, Heinemann.

Rowlands, M. (1993). The role of memory in the transmission of culture. *World Archeology, 25*(2), 141–151.

Schieffelin, E. (1976). *The sorrow of the lonely and the burning of the dancers*. New York: St. Martins Press.

Shohat, E. (1992). Notes on the "post-colonial." *Social Text, 31*, 99–113.

Shweder, R. A. (Ed.). (1988). *Culture theory. Essays on mind, self and emotion*. Cambridge: Cambridge University Press.

Solomon, S. D., Gerrity, E. T., & Muff, A. M. (1992). Efficacy of treatments for posttraumatic stress disorder. An empirical review. *Journal of the American Medical Association, 268*(5), 633–638.

Straker, G. (1994). Integrating African and Western healing practices in South Africa. *American Journal of Psychotherapy, 48*(3), 455–467.

Summerfield, D. (1996). The impact of war and atrocity on civilian populations: Basic principles for NGO interventions and a critique of psychosocial trauma projects. *Relief and Rehabilitation Network, Overseas Development Institute, London, Network Paper 14*, 1–41.

Taussig, M. (1987). *Shamanism, colonialism and the wild man*. Chicago: University of Chicago Press.

Vitebsky, P. (1993). *Dialogues with the dead: The discussion of mortality among the Sora of Eastern India*. Cambridge: Cambridge University Press.

Westermeyer, J., Bouafuely, M., Neider, J., & Callies, A. (1989). Somatization among refugees: An epidemiological study. *Psychosomatics, 30*(1), 34–43.

Wirz, P. (1954). *Exorcism and the art of healing in Ceylon*. Leiden: E.J. Brill.

Yamba, C. B. (1997). Cosmologies in turmoil. Witch finding and AIDS in Chiawa, Zambia. *Africa, 67*(2), 200–223.

Yates, F. (1966). *The art of memory*. Oxford: Clarendon Press.

Young, A. (1993). Description of how ideology shapes knowledge of a mental disorder (post-traumatic stress disorder). In S. Lindenbaum & M. Lock (Eds.), *Knowledge, power, and practice: The anthropology of medicine and everyday life*. Berkeley: University of California Press.

Young, A. (1996). *The harmony of illusions. Inventing post-traumatic stress disorder*. Princeton, NJ: Princeton University Press.

7

Historical and Cultural Construction of PTSD in Israel

ELIEZER WITZTUM AND MOSHE KOTLER

The term trauma has multiple meanings related to the perceived nature of the presenting problem and the frame of reference of the individual involved. The original Greek root refers to a bodily wound or any injury, whether or not the skin is broken (Gaines, 1986). Freud used the term trauma to describe abrupt events in which an individual is overwhelmed by stimuli, particularly noxious stimuli such as loss or threat to life (Freud, 1920). The psychocultural meaning of trauma and its consequences (e.g., traumatic stress, post-traumatic stress disorder) are the subject of this chapter.

Contemporary anthropology defines culture as a set of shared views embodied and enacted within a symbolic system. The symbolic systems include central or key symbols that function as models of experience and social action in religious or secular contexts (Greertz, 1973). Thus culture may be understood as a system of learned, shared, and transmitted meanings, understandings, conceptions, and assumptions that are embodied in symbols. The symbols themselves may represent persons, places, things, events, or ideas, i.e., anything that serves as vehicle for a shared conception (Greertz, 1973).

In the case of trauma and its consequences, striking variations may be observed across cultures in events or situations that are perceived as traumatic. Such differences are grounded in the differing cultures of the individuals (Gaines, 1986).

The history of Israel and its frequent military conflicts, recurrent exposure to traumatic events, and intense cultural mutations constitutes a fertile ground for examining the relationships between psychosocial, cultural, and clinical aspects of PTSD. Hence, lessons from that history will illustrate our analysis of the psychosocial meaning of trauma.

ELIEZER WITZTUM AND MOSHE KOTLER • Mental Health Center, Faculty of Health Sciences, Ben Gurion University of the Negev, Beersheva, 84105, Israel.

International Handbook of Human Response to Trauma, edited by Shalev, Yehuda, and McFarlane. Kluwer Academic / Plenum Publishers, New York, 2000.

Historical Background: The Conception of PTSD as a Clinical Entity

The development of emotional sequelae following traumatic events has generated arguments and discussions among mental health professionals. Historically, this is reflected by frequent transformations of the nosology and the descriptive approach to clinical syndromes that follow such events. The current delineation of PTSD is relatively new (DSM-III, 1980). The concept of trauma-related disorders, however, has a long history that encompasses various cultures and etiologies. Since the nineteenth century, trauma-related terminologies were often used, including "railway spine," "soldier's heart," "war neurosis," "shell shock," "battle fatigue," and "combat reaction." These terms associate specific events with specific mechanisms that reflect the social and cultural conventions of their times.

Along with terminology, various diagnostic approaches have been used that reflect the effect of social constructs on concepts and interpretations. Thus the first two editions of DSM (1958 and 1968) defined the sequelae of trauma as mere reaction to stress (gross stress reaction), a part of the group of transient situational personality disorders that imply a conceptual attitude which holds that if the disorder is not transient and situational, then the diagnosis cannot hold true.

DSM-III was developed in the context of the Vietnam War, in which combatants were exposed to severe combat stress, yet were not welcomed back as heroes and were often vilified as social pariahs. As in previous wars, many Vietnam veterans had severe "stress syndromes," often delayed or chronic. Yet no diagnostic entity could capture their prolonged syndromes. The definition of PTSD in 1980 accommodated such prolonged "stress syndromes" and clearly reflects a renewed recognition of the capacity of traumatic events to provoke extensive and protracted emotional and mental sequelae. The inclusion of such sequelae in a formal nomenclature of mental disorders acknowledged the fact of mental and emotional injury and hence of "mental casualties" of wars and other extreme events.

PTSD in Different Cultures

PTSD was culturally and socially constructed, designed to meet the needs of a specific society at a specific time. It included symptoms that were believed to be common in a given population—the Vietnam War veterans. Therefore, the syndrome's reliability, validity, and universality could be challenged. Indeed, in a recent polemic book, the social anthropologist Allan Young (1995) claimed that the assessment and diagnosis of PTSD are based on culturally mediated assumptions and not on well-defined biological facts. Young argues that traumatic memories, a cornerstone of PTSD, originate within a collectively approved "architecture of traumatic time" that approves of a temporal delay between the occurrence of an event and its recall as traumatic. Underlying PTSD and its treatment, Young finds a discourse that glorifies specific past events, emphasizes intrapsychic turmoil and disruption of the individual's sense of self, and exonerates personal responsibility for disruptive behavior by explaining past events as a cause of bona fide disease.

Young concludes that the nosological category of PTSD is unfounded and unjustified. He also interprets the more recent phenomenological and neurobiological findings in a way that demonstrates the complex interaction between cultural and social issues and this "disorder."

Currently, post-traumatic stress disorder (DSM-IV) is defined as one of the anxiety disorders. The emphasis on anxiety along with other dimensions (e.g., reexperiencing, avoidance, hyperarousal) may also reflect a clinical picture delivered by patients who belong to Western cultures.

When the nosology of PTSD is applied to individuals from non-Western countries, however, distinct content and meanings may emerge and create difficulties in diagnosis and interpretation. Symptoms of PTSD are common among refugees who have endured prolonged threat and severe losses. However, viewing these problems as merely reflecting PTSD may be an oversimplification (Kirmayer et al., 1995).

Studies that attempt to apply DSM PTSD criteria to Southeast Asian and Central American refugees have encountered difficulties (Kinzie et al., 1990; Mollica et al., 1990). In these refugees, somatic symptoms accompany the core symptoms of PTSD, and are also often the cardinal features of the syndrome. Thus, the validity of DSM criteria becomes questionable when applied across cultures. It has been suggested that the plight and affliction of such refugees can, in some respects, be better understood as a form of cultural bereavement (Eisenbruch, 1991; Kirmayer et al., 1995).

According to Eisenbruch, although DSM criteria are measurable in Southeast Asian refugees, they fail to capture the core of their suffering. He proposes the term "cultural bereavement" as a more appropriate descriptor in that it draws the attention to "what the trauma meant to the victims," to their cultural patterns for currently signaling their distress, and to their cultural strategy for overcoming it. Therefore, Eisenbruch suggests that the assessment of a refugee's cultural bereavement be used as a supplementary diagnostic category to PTSD (Eisenbruch & Handelman, 1989; Eisenbruch, 1990, 1991).

Therefore, the social and cultural context within which the events and symptoms of PTSD occur are pivotal and must be taken into account when evaluating individuals or groups.

Cultural and Social Appraisal of Military Trauma in Israel

The protracted military conflict and enduring existential threat, in which the state of Israel has been involved since its establishment, has influenced Israeli ethos, social conventions, and public discourse in a myriad of ways (see Chapter 8). A discussion of the ways in which war-related suffering and PTSD have been construed and dealt with throughout the recent history of Israel clearly illustrate the effect of culture and society on the appraisal of "trauma."

Given the cardinal roles of political, ideological, and social factors, it is not surprising that they had a decisive impact on the perception of combat stress reaction (CSR) and PTSD by Israelis. The core of combat stress reaction is the overwhelming presence of a sense of vulnerability and existential helplessness. These experiences run counter to the sense of safety, mastery, assertiveness, and self control that the founders of Israel and its pioneers strove to inculcate in the native born *sabra*. Such a "new Jew" was to have been liberated from millennia of persecution and humiliation in the Diaspora. The Zionist interpretation of the precariousness of Jewish existence in the Diaspora was clearly substantiated by the Holocaust and later repeated by the persistent threat to Israel's existence posed by its Arab neighbors. It gave birth to strong pressure for heroism and resiliency among Israelis, viewed as a necessary condition to ensure individual and national survival.

Against this background, one can understand how, for the first 30 years of Israel's existence, CSR and PTSD were "forgotten," denied by the military authorities, by society, and even by mental health systems. The state of matters was defined at that time by a former surgeon general, Brigadier General, Dr. M. Kordova: "We do not have this problem and we cannot afford this 'American luxury.'"

A recent survey, based on interviews with historians, senior physicians, and psychiatrists who belonged to the medical services in Israel between 1948 and 1982, revealed a puzzling history of CSR and PTSD (Witztum et al., 1989, 1990, 1996; Levy et al., 1989, 1990, 1991). The current presentation focuses mainly on the findings from the War of Independence (1948), the Yom Kippur War (1973), and the Lebanon War (1982) which had the most significant impact on the genesis and construction of PTSD as an entity in the Israeli culture.

The War of Independence, 1948

According to the national ethos, the War of Independence was heroic. The number of fatalities reached 5,682, almost 1% of the country's Jewish population, which at that time was 649,000. Defeat in this war would have led to the end of the Jewish state (a view that was later transferred to other wars). The war was fought with minimal weapons and poor supplies by men and women with little or no formal military experience. Although some had been trained by the *Hagana*'s underground movement, others were untrained civilians, and some were Holocaust survivors, straight off the boat (Sivan, 1991). It was along with waging this war that the Israeli Defense Forces (IDF) were formed from previous paramilitary bodies, which previously disagreed and even fought one another.

Contrasting with this heroic view, CSR was a serious problem during the War of Independence. Its real dimension is difficult to evaluate because many casualties were not identified and little written documentation remains of those who were. It was apparently widespread enough for the army to establish special treatment units shortly after the war started. As in all wars, one can assume that beyond those who were treated in these units, many untreated cases existed as well.

The Medical Corps of the IDF was formed on the basis of the Medical Service of the *Hagana*, a service which had been established after the Arab riots in 1929 and was geared to care for people who were injured in these and other attacks. It was a small service designed to meet limited needs. In 1947, with the war clearly on the horizon, the Medical Service was expanded to include 4,500 hospital personnel and became part of the IDF and its regular army upon the declaration of the State of Israel in 1948.

As attested by senior physicians and Medical Corps commanders who were interviewed, the Medical Service did not deal with psychiatric issues that existed before the war. A Commander of the Medical Corps, for example, said that he knew vaguely about the existence of "battle shock," but all he remembered was "that they would bring these people to the hospital and give them sedatives to try and calm them down, and that the policy was always to evacuate to hospital, far from the battle front."

Shortly after the beginning of the war, psychiatric problems became widespread and could not be ignored. Therefore, the IDF began to provide mental health services, and South African psychiatrist Louis Miller was appointed to establish a psychiatric service. Miller, henceforth Israel's first Chief Military Psychiatrist, brought with him rich combat experience from World War II and tried to implement the best available expertise in the field. It was believed that the casualty had to be treated close to the front in a situation similar to that in which he had broken down, and with the expectation of being sent back to the front (Salmon, 1919).

Three units were set up to treat psychiatric casualties. Treatment principles included creating a supportive group atmosphere, keeping the patients active (they were required to perform maintenance duties), and maintaining their military identity (they had to wear uniforms). The first unit, P-1, was headed by an English psychoanalyst (Norman Cohen), who had served as a general physician in the British Army during World War II. The emphasis was on group support rather than on individual psychotherapy, although that was also carried out as well. The average length of treatment was about three months. Cohen had the clear impression that the casualties with roots in the country recovered more rapidly than immigrant patients.

Another ward (13A) was set up in a hospital in the north of the country and was headed by psychiatrist Gerald Caplan, who had extensive experience in treating bereaved patients and victims of other catastrophes. The unit admitted soldiers as well as civilians. The staff, which included psychiatrists, social workers, and nurses, were all military personnel. The casualties arrived in waves after large battles. Among them were many Holocaust survivors and volunteers from English-speaking countries. The casualties were described as "severely neurotic" and "mildly psychotic." Those diagnosed as "severely psychotic" were sent to another hospital. A third unit (P-2) was a closed psychiatric ward and treated seriously disturbed mental patients. Although the three units were separate entities with no direct professional communication, two implemented a group and community approach.

A major influence on the therapists seems to have been the psychoanalytic approach advocated by Grinker and Spiegel's *Men under stress* (1945). Grinker and Spiegel recommended abreaction as the treatment of choice for CSR. A drawback of the treatment program was that only few of the patients who recovered were sent back to the front. This was partly due to technical difficulties and in part to therapists' conviction that it was better to discharge the patients from the service. As to casualties who did not recover, the authorities were slow to recognize their plight, and many were stigmatized and received recognition and compensation as disabled years later, following humiliating struggles with the authorities.

Overall, the treatment of war casualties during the War of Independence reflected a humane approach to trauma and was conducted according to principles that represented the state of the art of their time. Three articles published in the journal of the Israel Medical Association, between 1948 and 1949 communicated the experience of treating war casualties by Israeli doctors (Halperin, 1949; Kalmus, 1949; Wollman, 1948). However, the senior professionals in charge were unlikely to have read these articles because of the delay in publishing and because some of them were new immigrants who did not speak Hebrew. Their historical importance is significant, as they depict a view of combat reactions. These descriptions are short and structured. They emphasize therapeutic suggestion and abreaction in accordance with contemporary practice. Their outlook, however, is often very judgmental and describes casualties as "weaklings," unfit, fearful, psychopathic hypochondriacs eager to evade the service.

After the 1948 war, little trace was left of either the fact that there were cases of CSR or the rich therapeutic experience gathered in treating them. There was little documentation, and that which existed was lost, as were the knowledge and skills. Most therapists left the armed services. Some of them left Israel; none wrote about their experiences,

P-1 was shut down at the end of the war, and the other units were disbanded soon after without provision for reopening.

Although a pattern of "lessons learned and forgotten" recurs in the area of traumatic stress (Mangelsdorff, 1985, p. 239; Chapter 2, this volume), specific factors proper to the newly established State of Israel clearly affected the fact of forgetting (about) trauma.

One such factor is that after the war the nation was facing one of its hardest moments. As noted earlier, Israel's scarce resources were drained by the war, and the remaining were channeled to defending survival, absorbing immigrants, and building the nation. Little, if any, were left for dealing with psychological problems.

The young army was, similarly, in a phase of organization. There was considerable disarray as the previous underground movements were molded into a national force (which did not proceed without some resistance). Record keeping was generally poor, and again, there were immediate needs to see to before addressing states of mind, let alone emotions. As attested to by our interviewees, both the General Army Command and the Medical Corps assigned the lowest priority to handling combat stress. Hence, little was done to conserve the actual facilities, write therapy manuals, train therapists, provide guidelines for commanders, or point to the dimensions of the problem in any way.

Undoubtedly, the prevailing social views of that time also affected the attitudes toward psychological casualties. The medical literature (Halperin, 1949; Kalmus, 1949; Wollman, 1948) mentions the contrast between disciplined, battle-ready *sabras* and unstable new immigrants who "had not freed themselves from their tragic past." Implicitly it was assumed that the former were less prone to develop CSR and that combat breakdown had to do with cowardliness, hysteria, or desire for compensation.

When such assumptions exist, there is clearly no point in documenting the symptoms of breakdown, learning from experience, or planning treatment programs for the future. Doing so would also have implied that combat breakdown was to be expected in future wars, a suggestion that questioned the endurance and the motivation of the Israeli soldier. It would also question the widely accepted view that immigrants became *sabras* only in the second generation.

The 1973 Yom Kippur War

This war broke out on October 6, 1973 on the holy fast day of Yom Kippur. It was a complete surprise, and the IDF had to fight simultaneously on several fronts against advancing enemy forces. Later, the Israeli troops counterattacked and fighting moved back to enemy territory. The cost in lives of this war reached almost 2,600, and 7,000 were wounded, most of them during the initial stages of the war.

The impact of the 1973 war on Israeli society was shocking. The surprise attack, the number of losses, and the total failure of the Israeli Intelligence shattered the belief in Israel's complete military superiority. The enormous toll of this war led to deep demoralization and loss of confidence in the military as well as in the civilian leadership. The Yom Kippur War remains a massive trauma and an open wound in the nation's consciousness. It also destroyed the public perception of the combat stress reaction. The toll of CSR in this war was heavy and painful. Official reports labeled 10% of all physical casualties as CSRs, although some professionals claim that the prevalence of

CSR was closer to 55% of all casualties (Noy, 1991). Indeed, CSR casualties were not identified and did not reach frontline treatment facilities. Casualties with delayed reactions were omitted from the count and were listed later as chronic psychiatric patients.

Several clinical presentations of acute reactions were described (Moses & Cohen, 1984; Arielli, 1974):

1. the shocked-stupor casualty who had typical symptoms of severe dissociation and was extremely detached from the surrounding environment;
2. the agitated, anxious casualty characterized by overwhelming anxiety and restlessness;
3. various mixed presentations.

These immediate presentations gave way to subacute conditions characterized by physical and mental exhaustion, exaggerated startle response, amnesiac symptoms, anxiety, and depressive complaints.

The Yom Kippur War finally made the Israeli psychiatric establishment aware of CSR (as World War II did to the American psychiatric community). The vulnerability of the nation as a whole and particularly that of native-born Israeli warriors became a reality that had to be dealt with and did not allow further repression or denial. Following the 1973 war, the Department of Mental Health of the Medical Corps was enlarged, and its functions were expanded to include special frontline units for the care of CSR casualties in future wars. The following years were dedicated to building a treatment approach to be shared by headquarters and implemented in field exercises. A practical test was, indeed, to face the country less than a decade ahead.

The 1982 Lebanon War

The 1982 war was the first elective and planned war in the history of Israel, which the IDF launched with the intent to put an end to the Palestinian Liberation Organization's (PLO) threat in the northern regions of Israel. This "operation" was meant to have limited targets, extend no more than 40 km into Lebanon, and remove the PLO terrorists within a few days. On the ground the situation was very different. A cease-fire was not signed before two months of warfare and the fighting reached Beirut, 100 km from the border. In contrast with other wars, the 1982 war was controversial, with open public debate and harsh criticism regarding the rationale behind the whole operation. For the first time in Israel's history, anti-war demonstrations took place resembling those held during the Vietnam War in the United States. By the end of the occupation of central Lebanon, this military operation has taken the lives of 700 soldiers.

Not surprisingly, nearly a quarter of all casualties were cases of CSR, and their number doubled after the war when previously unidentified and delayed-onset cases became known. According to the Surgeon General (E. Dolev) who lead the Medical Corps during the war, the Department of Mental Health had "somewhat of a stress reaction" when news of the war broke. Nevertheless, within two weeks, it mobilized three first-echelon treatment companies, and others became available during the war.

Difficulties in implementing the principles of frontline treatment, however, led to poor delivery and execution of therapy. Only 7% of all psychiatrically injured soldiers received full frontline treatment. Therapists did not always implement the principles of "return to battle." Medical Corps personnel used to airlift psychiatric casualties to the rear instead of evacuating them to frontline treatment facilities. Mental health teams were not properly introduced to the local military personnel, and their interaction with mental health headquarters was problematic.

Despite these difficulties, the Lebanon War experience contributed significantly to the development of comprehensive treatment models based on the frontline approach. Following that war, CSR was fully recognized in its acute and prolonged forms (PTSD), and intensive research took place which extended for years thereafter (Solomon, 1993).

The typical clinical picture of the post-traumatic sequelae among Israeli veterans of the Lebanon War (Solomon, 1993) is characterized by the following profile:

1. intensive intrusion and avoidance symptoms
2. relatively little guilt
3. intense anger and hostility
4. considerable anxiety and depression

Symptoms of intrusion and avoidance are common to all forms of exposure to heavy and intensive combat. The limited expression of guilt following the Lebanon War, however, contrasted with a greater expression of guilt following the 1973 Yom Kippur War. Particular effort invested in preventing harm to civilians during the Lebanon War may explain the lower levels of guilt about acts committed during that war. The lack of survivor guilt may be due to fewer human losses during the Lebanon War (whereas major losses were inflicted on some military units in 1973). The serious public dispute regarding the war and the intense criticism of the war right from its beginning, along with cultural norms allowing direct expression of anger, constitute a contextual background for feelings of anger and hostility.

Concluding Remarks

Although many cases of psychological breakdown were identified and treated during the 1948 war, the lack of official documentation from that period reflects a desire to ignore the fact of psychiatric casualties. Secrecy around psychiatric units helped isolate the victims from the rest of the army and from society in general. Most casualties were released from service following their recovery and later experienced difficulty in gaining official recognition as handicapped war veterans. Most significantly, as soon as the war was over, the military hastened to dismantle its psychiatric units. As a whole, these attitudes reflected a nationwide trend to overlook the fact of psychological vulnerability. It is in such a social context that the myth of the hardy Israeli soldier was born.

In the following 1956 and 1967 wars, therefore, no lessons of the 1948 war were available to learn from, and it was only the massive occurrence of CSR and PTSD in 1973 that forced a medical corps, totally devoid of theoretical concepts and an organizational infrastructure, to face and cope with psychic trauma. The Lebanon War further illustrates the effect of interacting social, political, and cultural factors on the perception of traumatic stress and its consequences.

To illustrate these effects, the case of Mr. Israeli, a real individual, follows. This repeatedly traumatized PTSD patient has been labeled, successively, as suffering from personality disorder, anxiety, and malingering, and had to fight for recognition as a war casualty. His case illustrates the shifting social conventions, as well as the cumulative effects of recurrent exposure to trauma.

The Case of Mr. Israeli

Mr. Israeli is a 50-year-old single man who has worked only sporadically in the last few years. His main complaints are somatic: "waves of heat and cold," breathlessness, and chest pressure. He is also afraid to leave his home, startles as the telephone rings, and has terrifying nightmares. Occasionally, he would have "failures of memory."

Past History. Born in Iraq, he came to Israel on his own at the age of 14 in 1960. He is the eldest of five siblings (three boys and two girls). His father was a businessman, and his mother a housewife. He attended a course in car mechanics, worked in the Israeli aircraft industry near Tel Aviv for a year, then moved to Jerusalem near his parents' home, and worked in a military industry plant.

Army Service. Mr. Israeli enlisted at the age of 17 and passed his medical checkup without any findings. His military service included assignments to actual combat service, which Mr. Israeli performed as a driver in the Engineering Corps. His regular (3 year) service passed without incident, apart from minor wounds in an accidental explosion—an incident to which he relates little importance. He went on to add a year's service in the regular army (i.e., with pay) in a border patrol unit.

History of Trauma

The Six Day War, 1967. Mr. Israeli was called up as reservist, was sent to Jerusalem, and participated in the battle along the road from Jerusalem to Jericho. During a chase within Jericho, the vehicle he was in entered an ammonia factory, which was then bombarded. The half-track began to burn, and he was choked by smoke and fumes of ammonia. The smell accompanies him since, as well as sight of soldiers' bodies, a dear elderly Arab killed in the bombardment, and a sheep, tethered to its master, licking the body. Mr. Israeli's unit was then transferred to the Golan Heights and he witnessed other war scenes. Most vivid among these were the killing of one of the cooks by a shell in the toilets and scenes of burned bodies.

The War of Attrition—1968–70. Between 1968 and 1970, Israel was involved in what has been called the War of Attrition, during which Israeli forces, stretched along a lengthy frontline, suffered repeated shelling and sniper attacks. On numerous occasions, Mr. Israeli, who still served as a reservist, was under heavy bombardment by artillery and mortars. He recalls "... a buddy getting a bullet right between the eyes, just next to me and his brain spewed out and he just lay there jerking and gurgling until he died." The dying friend gasped and Mr. Israeli held his hand, unable to help, feeling helpless. The picture haunted him for years in flashback memories and nightmares.

Yom Kippur War—1973. Mr. Israeli was called up a day after the outbreak of hostilities and again found himself in the Golan Heights. He was again confronted by scenes of burned and blackened bodies, especially that of a Yemenite soldier with a skullcap (*Kippa*). He reports having also witnessed the death of prisoners of war in bombardments, a scene which shocked him deeply, especially when the bodies were bulldozed into a communal grave. He broke down when the buses he and his compatriots had just left were hit by a pair of Syrian MiG jet fighters. He clearly recalls being petrified with fear. The next day he began to feel strangely detached and confused, his head feeling "... awfully heavy, with grimaces on my face."

He was evacuated to a hospital near Tel Aviv and relieved of further duties on medical grounds. He was examined by an experienced psychiatrist in the hospital and diagnosed as being in a "state of chronic anxiety in a patient with a personality disorder." The psychiatrist also emphasized "with no connection to the war!"

In 1974 Mr. Israeli left Israel for the United States, where he stayed for 13 years. He reported feeling better as time passed, especially as he was "far away from the news broadcasts." He spent three years in New York and ten in Miami, working as a salesman or shop manager. Sporadically, he would have periods of nightmares and anxiety. He had some psychotherapy and occasional pharmacological interventions with benzo-diazepines and phenelzine.

He returned to Israel in 1988 and began suffering anew from fears, anxiety, and sensations of hot flushes and cold waves. He remained unmarried, attributing his bachelorhood to fears and anxieties, as "no woman could possibly desire a man like me."

Psychological Evaluation

Psychodiagnostic tests were performed, showing that the patient was "... suffering from severe anxiety, flooded by sexual impulses, and guilt feelings about killing. The anxiety and guilt are related to the post-traumatic state, whereas flooding with sexual impulses is apparently related to the partial impotence from which he suffers."

The psychological report goes on to detail other findings as follows:

"**Self-Image.** The patient sees himself as a victim. He is extremely sensitive to criticism, flooded by fear of failure.... Mr. Israeli sees himself as a wounded, vulnerable and weak man, who seeks to recover and return to the way he was as a youth."

"**Ego Functioning.** Mr. Israeli developed coping patterns based on techniques of self-relaxation and talking to himself. In spite of this, his ego is damaged, with a high level of disinhibition and impulses that are expressed in nascent form, without refining. In fact, one may say that Mr. Israeli's defenses have crumbled and have not been able to recover."

"**Emotional Structure.** Two main emotions predominate in Mr. Israeli's life: sadness (depression) and fear (anxiety), along with a sense of frustration. These are compensated for by a tendency to grandiosity, ostensibly. Effectively he suffers from instability, especially shifts between depression and hypomania, accompanied by constant anxiety."

In the psychologist's opinion "... judging by his functioning until the ages of 20–22 he possessed adequate ego strengths and coped well with environmental pressures, including the Six Day War. At the time of the examination he is suffering ... at a level of a chronic patient although there is no evidence of psychotic processes."

The psychologist bases his observations also on previous tests performed in 1990 in which post-traumatic features were clearly observed, as well as feelings of guilt. He concludes that Mr. Israeli suffers from recurrent post-traumatic disorder, which did not receive adequate therapy.

Summary

Mr. Israeli is nonfunctional at present and shows severe and chronic post-traumatic syndrome, with predominant anxiety. His life history includes repeated exposure to war trauma. Despite this, this Israeli's PTSD was not recognized by medical authorities as such and he was successively considered a malingerer or a case of chronic anxiety and personality disorder.

This case demonstrates the manner in which cultural and social attitudes distort what should have been coherent clinical judgment regarding trauma in a manner rarely seen in other illness.

References

Arielli, A. (1974). Combat neurosis in an army field hospital. *Harefuah, 87,* 572–577 (Hebrew).

Eisenbruch, M. (1991). From PTSD to cultural bereavement: Diagnosis of southeast Asian refugees. *Social Science and Medicine, 33,* 673–680.

Eisenbruch, M. (1990). The cultural bereavement interview: A new clinical research approach for refugees. *The Psychiatric Clinics of North America, 13,* 715–735.

Eisenbruch, M., & Handelman, L. (1989). Development of explanatory model of illness schedule for Cambodian refugee patients. *Journal of Refugees Studies, 2,* 243–256.

Freud, S. (1955). Beyond the pleasure principle. In *The standard edition of the complete psychological works of Sigmund Freud,* Vol. 18 (pp. 3–143), London: Hogarth Press. (Original work published, 1920).

Gaines, D. A. (1986). Trauma: Cross cultural issues. *Advance in Psychosomatic Medicine, 16,* 1–16.

Granek, M., Witztum, E., Levy, A., & Kotler, M. (1990). Combat reactions, Israel 1948–1973. E: The Yom Kippur War. *Sihot—Israel Journal of Psychotherapy, 5,* 53–59 (Hebrew).

Greertz, C. (1973). *The interpretation of cultures.* New York: Basic Books.

Grinker, R. P., & Spiegel, J. P. (1945). *Men under stress.* Philadelphia: Blakistan.

Halperin, L. (1949). Neuropsychiatric observations in the war of Jerusalem. *Harefuah, 36,* 11–13 (Hebrew).

Kalmus, A. (1949). War neurosis. *Harefuah, 36,* 43–44 (Hebrew).

Kirmayer, L.J., Young, A., & Hayton, B. C. (1995). The cultural context of anxiety disorders. *The Psychiatric Clinics of North America, 18,* 503–52.

Kinzie, J. D., Boehnlein, J. K., Leung, P., Moore, L., Riley, C., & Smith, D. (1990). The prevalence of PTSD and its clinical significance among southeast Asian refugees. *American Journal of Psychiatry, 147,* 913–917.

Kinzie, D., & Goetz, R. (1996). A century of controversy surrounding Post-traumatic stress syndromes: The impact of DSM-III and DSM-IV. *Journal of Traumatic Stress, 9,* 159–179.

Levy, A., Witztum, E., Granek, M., & Kotler, M. (1989). Combat reactions, Israel 1948–1973. A: Introduction. *Sihot—Israel Journal of Psychotherapy, 4,* 60–64.

Levy, A., Witztum, E., Granek, M., & Kotler, M. (1990). Combat reactions, Israel 1948–1973. D: The Six Day War. *Sihot—Israel Journal of Psychotherapy, 4,* 217–221 (Hebrew).

Levy, A., Witztum, E., Solomon, Z., & Kotler, M. (1991). Combat reactions, Israel 1974–1982. G: Lebanon War 1982. *Sihot—Israel Journal of Psychotherapy, 6,* 82–92 (Hebrew).

Levy, A., Witztum, E., & Solomon, Z. (1996). Lessons relearned—when denial become impossible: Therapeutic response to combat stress reaction during Yom Kippur War and the Lebanon War (1982). *Israel Journal of Psychiatry, 33,* 89–102.

Mangelsdorff, A. D. (1985). Lessons learned and forgotten: The need for prevention and mental health interventions in disaster preparedness. *Journal of Community Psychology, 13,* 239–257.

Mollica, R. E., Wyshak, G., Lavelle, G., Troung, T., Tor, S., & Yang, T. (1990). Assessing symptom changes in Southeast Asian refugee survivors of mass violence and torture. *American Journal of Psychiatry, 147,* 83–88.

Moses, R., & Cohen, I. (1984). Understanding the treatment of combat neurosis. In H. J. Schwartz (Ed.). *Psychotherapy of the combat veteran: The Israeli experience* (pp. 269–303). New York: Spectrum.

Noy, S. (1991). Combat stress reactions. Tel Aviv: Ministry of Defense Publications, (Hebrew).

Salmon, T. W. (1919). The war neuroses and their lessons. *New York State Journal of Medicine, 59,* 16–22.

Sivan, E. (1991). The 1948 generation: Myth, profile and memory. Tel Aviv: Ministry of Defense (Hebrew).

Solomon, Z. (1989). A three year prospective study of post traumatic stress disorder in Israeli combat veterans. *Journal of Traumatic Stress, 2,* 59–73.

Solomon, Z. (1993). *Combat stress reaction.* New York: Plenum.

Solomon, Z., Mikulincer, M., & Benbenishty, R. (1989). Combat stress reaction—clinical manifestations and correlates. *Military Psychology, 1,* 35–47.

Witztum, E., Levy, A., Granek, M., & Kotler, M. (1989). Combat reactions, Israel 1948–1973. B: Independence War. *Sihot—Israel Journal of Psychotherapy, 4,* 65–70 (Hebrew).

Witztum, E., Levy, A., Granek, M., & Kotler, M. (1990). Combat reactions, Israel 1948–1973. C: The Sinai Campaign 1956. *Sihot—Israel Journal of Psychotherapy, 4,* 139–141 (Hebrew).

Witztum, E., Levy, A., & Solomon, Z. (1996). Lessons denied: A history of therapeutic response to combat stress reaction during Israel's War of Independence (1948), The Sinai Campaign (1956), and Six Day War (1967). *Israel Journal of Psychiatry, 33,* 79–88.

Wollman, B. (1948). Problems in mental hygiene and military psychiatry. *Harefuah, 35,* 39–41 (Hebrew).

Young, A. (1995). Reason and cause for post-traumatic stress disorder. *Transcultural Psychiatric Research Review, 32,* 287–298.

Young, A. (1995). *The harmony of illusion: Inventing post-traumatic stress disorder.* Princeton, NJ: Princeton University Press.

8

Cultural Identity and Demonization of the Relevant Other

Lessons from the Palestinian–Israeli Conflict

DAN BAR-ON

Cultural Background: Trauma and Its Recognition

Trauma in the Middle East is deeply associated with the bitter struggle during the last hundred years between Arabs and Jews. We will concentrate in this paper on the trauma associated with the Palestinian–Israeli conflict. The Jewish population immigrated to Palestine (after 1948—Israel) from all over the world but mainly from Europe and from the Arab countries in Asia and Africa. Most of the Palestinians* had lived in Palestine whereas some immigrated to it from neighboring countries.† The Jews viewed their immigration (named Aliya in Hebrew, which means "going up") as an act of reviving their national home destroyed two thousand years ago by the Romans. The Palestinians viewed the Jewish immigration as an intrusion by an alien group, similar to previous intrusions of conquerors or colonialists (Crusaders, Mamelukes, British, and French).

The Israeli and Palestinian national groups differ in historical heritage, religious belief, cultural linkage, socioeconomic status, and community setup. They share, however, some similarities. Though they both come from ancient cultural and religious traditions, they both lack a modern, independent heritage of statehood. This means that they have had to develop the tradition of statehood during and to some extent,

---

*Though the Palestinian national entity is composed of a Muslim majority and a Christian minority, it is referred to as one entity in the present discussion.

†This simple issue—how many Palestinians have lived here for ages and how many immigrated in the last century from neighboring countries is an ongoing dispute between Israeli and Palestinian social scientists. This demonstrates how politics and the interpretation of historical facts are deeply enmeshed.

DAN BAR-ON • Department of Behavioral Sciences, Ben Gurion University of the Negev, Beersheva, 84105, Israel.

International Handbook of Human Response to Trauma, edited by Shalev, Yehuda, and McFarlane. Kluwer Academic / Plenum Publishers, New York, 2000.

through the violent struggle with the rival national group.* Psychologically, therefore, they both defined themselves as victims of their enemy, that is, by referring to a "relevant Other."

The Jews viewed the Palestinians as part of the hostile Arab world, supported from 1954–1989 by the Communist bloc, and the Palestinians viewed the Jews as a powerful hostile group, supported by the Western world. Although the Jewish population enjoyed wide support from the Jewish Diaspora after World War II (mainly in America), the violent conflict created a Palestinian Diaspora that slowly gained impact in the West and in Arab countries such as Lebanon, Jordan, and Kuwait. The Palestinians have been manipulated by the Arab countries both during the power struggle with Israel and in the power struggle among themselves (Portugali, 1996) but tend to see Israel as their sole enemy.

Both national entities fought for recognition by trying to eliminate the rival group. The conflict has spread to different spheres of life, such as threats to personal safety, ownership of land, housing and territory, education and cultural autonomy, control over scarce resources such as water, international recognition, and trade. Psychologically, each group addressed the other as the aggressor and saw itself mainly as the victim. For forty years (1949–1989) this situation was manipulated by the struggle between West and East, thereby reinforcing the clear-cut conflict as perceived by each group. Only after the fall of the Communist bloc in 1989 and the lack of military resolution (during the Intifada) did the leaders of both sides finally decide to put aside ideas of elimination and to try and move toward recognition and coexistence.

The Jewish population which arrived in this region prior to World War II was selective and idealistically oriented toward Zionism. They believed in the secular revival of Jewish national identity in the ancient homeland after many generations of exile and Diaspora. This had been the dream and subject of daily prayers of religious Jews throughout the years of exile. Now it became a modern, secular vision in the light of the pogroms in Eastern Europe at the turn of the century and the disappointment with assimilation in Western European countries. The Zionist movement brought with it the revival of Hebrew as a spoken language (not only as the language of the Holy Scriptures) and the vision of a new, strong Jew who could cultivate his land and defend himself.† This vision was the negation of the weak Jew of the Diaspora who did not live on his own land and could not defend himself. This image is thought to have reflected an internalization of the anti-Semitic perception and hatred of the Jewish middleman (Aronoff, 1989; Segev, 1992).

One of the first heroes who exemplified this modern, Zionist vision was Joseph Trumpeldor, a Russian-Jewish officer who had lost his hand in the Russo–Japanese War at the turn of the century. He later immigrated to Palestine and settled at Tel Hai, (paradoxically representing the Hebrew words of both *ruins* and *hill* of *life*) at the northern edge of the Jewish settlement. He fulfilled the ideal of working hard, cultivated the land during the day, and guarded the settlement at night. He was severely injured by an Arab mob in 1917 and became known for saying shortly before he died, "It

---

*The 1948 war was defined as the "War of Independence" by the Israelis (and clearly very differently by the Palestinians). The Intifada (1987–1993) was similarly identified as a national struggle by the Palestinians but as an "uprising" or "unrest" by the Israelis.
†In the texts of the early Zionist ideologists, such as May Nordeau and Theodore Herzl, the role of the new Jew, who represents the antithesis to the Diaspora Jew, is closely associated with the male figure (Glozman, in press).

is good to die for our country." The collective myth which developed around this sentence can teach us quite a lot about the atmosphere of those early days. The Jewish Israelis are surrounded by enemies and have to struggle physically and mentally for our existence. We can succeed only if we are willing to sacrifice a lot, even our lives (Zrubavel, 1986).

This myth of the new secular hero was not a new notion in the Jewish heritage. It was, in a way, a natural continuation of earlier heroes and heroes to come, for example, Bar Kochba—the Jew who rebelled against the Romans after the destruction of the Second Temple—or the heroes of Masada who committed suicide rather than fall into the hands of pagan Roman captors (Zrubavel, 1986). To these were later added other heroes, the Warsaw Ghetto fighters and the sabra* of the 1948 war. It is interesting to see how heroism can be reinterpreted over time. Bar Kochba was redefined during the late seventies by an Israeli general and historian, Yehoshafat Harkabi (Harkabi, 1983). He wrote of Bar Kochba as a fanatical leader who, through his rebellion, caused the destruction of the Jewish population in Judea and the death of about a million peaceful Jewish farmers. He wrote this thesis at a time when fanaticism again threatened to take over, this time within modern Israeli society after the shock of the 1973 war. He was part of the moderate Israeli leadership which looked for symbols to warn us about self-destruction (Zrubavel, 1986). This issue will be discussed later in this chapter.

In the early days of Zionism, Bar Kochba was only a clear-cut symbol of heroism. Then, there was little room for emotional expressions of fear or helplessness. Those who could not cope and left the new settlements (or even returned to their European homeland) were seen as traitors. Some even committed suicide. Only recently have we learned that during the War of Independence, battle shock was not acknowledged. Clearly, the know-how was there from World War I; physicians wrote about it in a local medical journal, but very few of the Palmach or Hagana† soldiers were formally treated for battle shock or PTSD (Levi & Wiztum, 1989).

In a recent study, we interviewed more than one hundred war veterans of the War of Independence. It was found that about a third of our interviewees still believe in 1996 that there was no battle shock in 1948 (Rom and Bar-On, in preparation). Another third could, in retrospect, recall several incidents which belong to some category of battle reactions, and the rest could tell of events which they themselves had suffered. Still, those who suffered from such phenomena had to cope with it by themselves throughout the years. Some were given labels, such as "degenerates," "cowards," or even people who "vanished," never to return to the battlefield. In a few cases there are reports of battle reaction and fatigue which was covered up by comrades, enabling the inflicted people to return to their units unnoticed.

A similar Spartan spirit also existed in the early kibbutzim, which were the backbone of Israeli pioneering society before the establishment of the State of Israel. Children were brought up in children's houses in harsh conditions, under an educational ideology which emphasized physical strength and saw the expression of emotions, especially fear, as weakness (Niv & Bar-On, 1992). Psychological clinical services

---

*Sabra is a nickname for the Israeli born. It is the Arabic name for a wild fruit which has thorns on the outside but is juicy and soft inside. This reflected the public image of the new Jew.
†Names of the Israeli armed forces before the State of Israel, which were illegally trained and emerged as the basis for what became the Israeli Defense Forces (IDF) after May 15, 1948.

were developed relatively late, mainly to answer the needs of children who did not adjust to this harsh and sometimes extreme lack of emotional support.

To these internal and external conditions, one has to add the effect of World War II and the Holocaust. Suddenly, the European families of those who had immigrated to Palestine from Poland or Russia, as well as other European countries, vanished in the catastrophe, the magnitude of which became known only after it was over. People could not imagine what was going on under the Nazi regime and thought of the events in terms of another pogrom (Porat, 1986). When the first survivors arrived in the late forties, many people were in shock and reacted with guilt, shame, and mistrust: "How come you survived and so many died?" "Why did you go like sheep to the slaughter and did not try to fight?" They were trying to make some sense of events, projecting their current self-image onto the European context. These were also the days before the establishment of the State of Israel, during violent conflict with the Arabs, and there was not much room for understanding and working through these differences (Segev, 1992).

A deep cleavage of pain and misunderstanding developed between the two groups (the sabras and the Holocaust survivors), which has taken two generations to surface (Bar-On, 1995). For example, two of my students at Ben Gurion University researched the early period of a kibbutz in which one of the students lived (Keren & Almaliach, 1994). They found that the kibbutz was composed of two groups, a group of about forty sabras who had started the kibbutz and a group of similar size of young survivors of the Holocaust who joined the kibbutz shortly before the 1948 war. The two groups fought together during the war and were taken into captivity by the Jordanian army. During the period of captivity, the survivors were due to be granted full membership in the kibbutz (after a year of being candidates). However, the sabra veterans voted against the change in status because the Holocaust survivors "were not good enough for that."

"They were good enough to fight and to be together in captivity," write Keren and Almaliach (1994), but not to become full members of the kibbutz because they came from **there** (the Holocaust). This traumatic experience was formally corrected only long after they returned from captivity and reestablished their kibbutz. Informally, the survivors were still feeling "not good enough" in the late eighties and early nineties, when they already had children and grandchildren. This is an extreme example of the kinds of emotions that were not acknowledged between subcultures within the dominant Ashkenazi Jewry. But this was only part of the story of the **tribal-ego** system which evolved in Israeli society during its early days.

The establishment of the State of Israel changed many things. A massive Aliya (wave of immigration) brought hundreds of thousands of Jews to the young State, mainly from the Arab countries (North Africa and Asia). This was not an idealistically oriented immigration and came from a very different cultural and socioeconomic background. These were mostly Sephardic Jews who differed from the Ashkenazi Jews culturally and religiously. The new immigrants embraced the young idealistic society which was determined to impose its own values and ideals, quite different from those of the immigrants. Some of the newcomers were placed in outposts near the borders and had to learn to practice modern agriculture. Others were recruited into the army. Some of the wealthy and honored heads of large families found themselves planting trees or unemployed and living on Social Security. The continuous military and economic struggle for survival demanded the primacy of a strong collective identity and mission, and these were interpreted within the dominant discourse of Eastern European Jewry

(Shorris, 1995). Sometimes some of the feelings of humiliation and anger surfaced, but most of the feelings dissonant to the ethos of the sabra had to be repressed and have been denied or overlooked by the dominant Zionist culture for many years (Ram, 1995).

The Yom Kippur War of 1973 created a manifest crisis in the ethos of the sabra. The surprise of the attack and the initial success of the Egyptian and Syrian armies found many young soldiers in the position of begging for their lives, rather than dying for the common cause. This, in retrospect, suggested that survival, in contrast to fighting, may have been legitimate within the context of the Holocaust. This was accompanied by a crisis of trust in the Labor government and the rise to power of the right wing parties in 1977, supported massively by the Sephardic population. The Sephardic population had felt suppressed by the Labor government, the major representative of the dominant Eastern European culture, and now had begun to find its voice.

The 1973 war and trauma also brought the phenomena of nonphysical injuries in war into the public consciousness. It was the first war in which many soldiers suffered and were treated for battle shock. A special military unit was established to treat the psychological aftereffects (PTSD), and it became legitimate to acknowledge trauma as part of war, not only through physical injury or death in the family (Solomon, 1993). In addition, quite a few soldiers were later identified as suffering from battle shock during the Lebanon War in 1982 (though, objectively speaking, there were fewer military reasons for trauma compared to the 1973 war). Interestingly, the 1987–1993 Intifada again created an adverse effect in this respect. Again, no soldiers were recognized as suffering from mental trauma. It became a political dispute (for and against acknowledging the rights of the Palestinians), and psychologists were accused of misusing their professional role when they claimed that soldiers were suffering emotionally by participating in military actions against the Palestinian uprising (Bar-On, 1992; Bar-On et al., 1996).

Today Israel is loaded with layers of trauma that have been transmitted intergenerationally (Bar-On, 1995). At each of these critical points—the Holocaust, the War of Independence, the mass immigration during the fifties, the 1973 war, the Lebanon War and the Intifada—new sources of loss, pain, and trauma were created and had to be acknowledged and worked through. They nourished the struggle between the legend of life and survival, on the one hand, and the myth of death and dying, on the other. But the world outside the Middle East has changed in the meantime, and the latter myth receives less and less external support. Finally, the peace process in the Middle East called for a reevaluation of the relationship between these two myths.

The Peace Process: A New "Trauma" or a "Relief?"

What was the impact of the peace process on the question of trauma and its relief in Israeli society? The process actually began in 1977 with the visit of Sadat to Jerusalem and the Camp David Agreement between Egypt and Israel. It reached an unimaginable climax with the Oslo Accord between Rabin and Arafat in 1993. Suddenly, bitter enemies began to see each other as potential partners. The Palestinian-Israeli Declaration of Principles of September 1993 and the subsequent agreements initiated a major shift in the attitude of the leaders of the two peoples who have been in bitter conflict over this small piece of land known as Palestine and Israel for more than a hundred years. The leaders of both national entities decided to recognize the other's right to exist and to search for a compromise that would enable each group to begin living in freedom and peace alongside the other. This dramatic shift in the formal attitude of the leaders of Israel and the Palestinians clearly reflected the hope of the majority of the Palestinian and Israeli people, but it was not accepted without severe resistance on both sides.

The peace process brought about two main forms of discourse within both societies. The first, a euphoric kind of discourse, emphasized new possibilities for coexistence and peace between peoples who have lived through years of conflict and bloodshed. The second, a pessimistic discourse, claimed that nothing has changed in the relationship between the two societies. There was no open dialogue between these two kinds of discourse. Both reveal the limited readiness of the wider population to acknowledge the difficulty of moving out of the long phase of violent conflict, with its accompanying fantasies of a total victory for one side and total submission of the other, into a new and more open approach of risk-taking for a painful but pragmatic compromise. Such an approach requires acknowledging the other and realistically testing the possibility of coexistence. Such "soft" ideology, however, contradicts the dominant principles of the Zionist worldview, which emphasizes security, settlement, and redemption (Ram, 1995).

The paradox is that the Oslo agreement was created by leaders of both nations who sounded more optimistic than the average person in the Israeli or Palestinian streets. In addition to the top-down political process which was taking place, a bottom-up social and psychological process became crucial for successful implementation of the peace process. In that respect, it has become clear that there are still influential groups within both national entities who were not willing or able to make this shift and continue to ignore the legitimate existence of the other national entity. These strong attitudes are best represented by religious-nationalist Jewish groups (Gush Emunim), on the one hand, and by religious-nationalist Islamic groups (the Hamas and Jihad), on the other.

These groups have done their best to sabotage the first stages of the peace process through reciprocal acts of terror and delegitimation. This activity reached a climax with the assassination of Israeli Prime Minister Yitzhak Rabin on November 4, 1995 by a young extremist of a Jewish religious-nationalist group, the Goldstein massacre in Hebron, and the latest terrorist attacks in Jerusalem and Tel Aviv by Palestinian extremist groups. These assassins hoped that their acts of violence would stop the peace process.

Still, resistance was not exclusively the property of the extreme fundamentalists. Within the Israeli public, there is a real fear of the ambiguity created by the peace process (Biran, 1994). This came to international attention with the elections of June 1996, when the right-wing parties, which originally opposed the Oslo Accord, gained national support and won the elections. But even the change of political leadership in Israel has not totally reversed the process begun in Oslo. Prime Minister Netanyahu had declared that he would abide by the Oslo agreements and met with Arafat. But clearly, the momentum of the peace process, launched by Rabin and Peres, came to a halt.

How can we understand how people who have been enmeshed in conflict for so long, who have carried such a load of unresolved traumas, can resist the hopeful prospect of the peace process? Is it not a paradox that when the dream becomes a reality, people begin to be frightened and hesitant? It probably depends on which perspective one holds of such events. Economists or lawyers may not have a rational explanation for such a trend, but psychologists do have a ready-made perspective for such paradoxical trends. The responses to the peace process within the populations suggest that many Israeli and Palestinian people are not yet ready for mutual acts of dialogue and reconciliation (Biran, 1994; Bar-On, 1995a). They are still too involved in the conflict on all levels: emotions, cognition, and behavior.

Further, Israeli society, being so committed to its struggle for life and living through death and dying, **is undergoing a severe crisis of identity**. It is the first time since the destruction of the Second Temple and the exile into the Diaspora that Jewish identity may not center around the struggle with enemies, around the struggle for survival. This is not an easy transformation for a young nation that has been so deeply involved in its fight for survival. From the myth of "good to die for our country," it has now to address a new myth of "good to live for our country" (or, ourselves) which is very different in its demands on the collective and the individual (Bilu, 1994).

This is a shift far more complex than one would expect. It is difficult enough to develop an approach toward the Other as a partner instead of, or at least in addition to, continuously seeing the Other as an enemy. It may suggest that part of the Israeli identity constructions relied too heavily on the continuation of this conflict and its accompanying myth of death and dying. This identity was defined, negatively, through hatred of the enemy, rather than positively through what they are in their own right, irrelevant of the definition of the Other. Suddenly, all the tribal-egos, which were suppressed for the sake of the overriding goal of the struggle with the Arabs, are allowed to demand attention, as could be seen during the 1996 elections.

Following the Oslo Accord, Israeli people were asked about their fantasies concerning war and peace, and the response of some was that they wanted it "done once and for all." In Hebrew there is an expression for it: "Zbeng vegamarnu." This means "one blow and we are finished with it" (never mind the price or the outcome). Similarly, while talking with people after a new move toward the next round of peace talks or following the latest assault on an Israeli by an Arab (or vice versa), one heard familiar expressions of fantasies or anger and frustration, but very few new expressions or discourse related to more moderate and realistic expectations. This is interpreted here as the difficulty people exhibit in disassociating themselves from their past perspective of warfare.

Certain interviewees spoke openly about their pain: their life span invested in warfare, those who were killed, all of which seemed suddenly as "wasted effort and time" which did not "materialise into the expected positive outcome" (Bar-On, 1995a). Another reaction we identified was that of "floating anxiety": Fantasies about "them" ("how will they react to us after all that we have done to them?"), fears about one's own people ("we will never be able to integrate into the Middle East society because we are strangers here"), even some fear concerning oneself ("who am I if I am not the brave Israeli fighting against our enemies"). Fears were usually associated with a lack of trust in the negotiating parties who may "try to solve some issues and leave us to live afterwards with all the problems." One person reported dreams of doomsday, in which "all this (peace process) will turn suddenly back on us, but we will not be able any more to defend ourselves, the way we could until now, as we already have given up our control of the territories."

As in PTSD (Figley, 1986; Solomon, 1993), there is a realistic aspect in each of these attitudes and emotions. However, they are viewed as traumatic when they control one's perspective and do not enable a more relaxed form of reality testing. The main problem is to envision the possibility that "the future will slowly become different from the past (warfare) and from the present (ambiguity)." This intermediate twilight period has its own stresses, just like periods of war and conflict. Therefore, it may be identified here as a prepeace stress reaction, which should be considered separately from the more familiar PTSD wartime reactions (Bar-On, 1995a).

As examples of such a prepeace traumatic reaction, some of our interviewees projected their anger at the political leadership involved in the negotiations. Certain interviewees spoke of "the betrayal of the leadership which is tired of wars." Others accused them of their lack of courage to admit past mistakes: "After all, it is the same political leadership which has claimed all these years that they will never sit together with Arafat at the same table." Both groups actually expressed the feeling that the leadership has not assisted them in constructing adequate expectations to help them cope better with the ambiguity of the intermediate phase. "In the past the leaders preached that peace will emerge *only as a result* of each side's strength and victories. Now we are expected to take the perspective of the Palestinians into account."

Some argued that only the previous leadership could help the Israeli public go through this change. However, others would argue that this only adds to the stress of the situation. They believed that only fresh political leadership, disassociated from the "collective memory" of the past, could help the public accommodate the new changes and the ambiguity of the intermediate state. Similar projections were made toward the media and the role they play in accommodating the peace accord. They have been accused of being "pro-PLO" and "anti-PLO" by different interviewees, relating to the same programs from opposite perspectives. It seems that certain parts of the media suffer from an additional difficulty during the ambiguous intermediate phase. It is the part of public media which tends to reinforce simplification, attempting to improve their ratings by presenting clear-cut news and sensationalism. They do not view it as their task to help the public cope better with the intermediate "gray zone" of war and peace.

One could ask if there are more specific reasons or conditions that have made the Israeli public more vulnerable to the intermediate stage, that is more than the usual human difficulty of accommodating change and living with ambiguity. In striving for peace for many years, Israelis have had to face many realistic hazards which, manifestly, could be associated with a future state of peace. Israel has had (and may have again in future negotiations) to give up territories, a fact which in some future scenarios could endanger its existence. Israel is still surrounded by totalitarian regimes and strong fundamentalist movements. "They" are many and "we" are few. "They" have natural resources upon which the world depends.

There are, however, other more latent psychological hazards in a future peace. Many Israelis will have to question and let go of the part of their self-definition that has been achieved mainly through the negative use of the Other. Such self-definition is, psychologically speaking, more easily achieved than a positive self-determination with no available and negative Other. As mentioned earlier, Jews have been used to defining themselves by experiencing the Other as persecutory (Keen, 1987). Hence, this peculiar combination of the myth of life and living and the myth of death and dying.

Let us examine some normative rituals to which the Israeli public is still exposed, for example, the education we provide to our children in relation to the relevant Other. They learn from a very young age that our festivals are associated with the Other who endangered our existence during different eras. The Jewish calendar year of celebrations in the kindergarten and elementary schools starts with Hanukkah (around

Christmas), the festival commemorating our success in stopping the ancient Greeks from taking over the First Temple. It continues with Purim (usually, in March) which celebrates our success in preventing the extermination of the Jews by the Persians. Then comes Passover (in the spring), when we succeeded in liberating ourselves from the Egyptian oppressors, followed immediately by Holocaust Day (the Germans) and Independence Day (the Arabs), each a week apart from the other. Last on the list is the Ninth of Av, the day of the destruction of both Temples (by the Babylonians and the Romans) which happens, unfortunately, during the summer holidays.

An anecdote (bitter or funny, depending on one's perspective) that illustrates this general trend was shown on TV during the first school day, September 1, 1993. The Israeli Minister of Education during that time, Professor Amnon Rubinstein, was shown visiting a kindergarten in Jerusalem. He asked the kids if they knew about the peace process and with whom are were trying to make peace. A few of the kids reacted spontaneously: "Of course we know." One spoke about the Germans, the other about Egyptians. Only one said "with the Palestinians."

We are not the only people who were threatened by the loss of "the enemy." Russia is moving through a painful transition in which they lost not only their enemy but also their own ideological identity and their status as a superpower (Zizek, 1989). The American people lost their traditional enemy after the collapse of the Communist bloc in 1989. Though these enemies were imagined rather than real, they did, however, preoccupy people's imagination in both countries for quite a few decades. In a sense, this is a stressful situation because one has to face oneself, one's unresolved problems, after being accustomed for many years to define oneself through negative and relevant Others. In the Israeli case, this kind of danger is not yet so acute. Even if the peace process continues, certain Others may still be counted on to assume the role of the enemy: the Iranians, Hamas, the Hezbollah. Still, the fear of losing the overriding uniting goal that the enemy provided is already a reality and brings with it the fear of falling apart as a united people because of internal conflicts (religious-secular; ethnic groups; political orientations).

There are specific groups within our society (and probably also within the Palestinian society) who may not only suffer from the latent danger of "losing an enemy" but whose stressful situation is real and practical. Some people have been economically linked to the production of weapons (Kimmerling, 1993). Others are directly linked to maintaining our security. For these groups, a future peace may mean personal uncertainty or loss of career. In addition, there is a whole section of Israeli society that moved to the Golan Heights, to the West Bank, and to Gaza for ideological and religious reasons (different from those who went there for economic reasons). For them, even the first steps of the intermediate phase of peace and war have been very stressful. They may have to take into account that the following stages of the peace process will endanger their existence in these places and/or their sense of security.

An additional group concerns the people in charge of the helping professions. Within or right after the intermediate phase, those who suffer from latent PTSD stemming from one of the previous wars and especially those who experienced it during the Intifada, may suddenly show overt PTSD symptoms. Perhaps some of the reactions quoted earlier from the interviews are early signs of this pattern. Now these people will be able to express the traumatic experiences that they had to deny when the political conflict around the Intifada was still full-fledged and did not enable them to relate to their own experiences (Bar-On, 1992). They may find themselves alone with their trauma in the future because their commanders and the politicians who supported their activity during the violent activities, might be more than happy to forget their responsibility for that period.

Another group which may face additional stress in the intermediate phase of war and peace are those families who lost members during the long period of warfare with the Arabs. For them the justification for their loss was that one day peace would come and compensate the living for the dead who thus would not have died in vain. However, this justification was based on the illusion or fantasy of "total peace," not on the ambiguous and complex intermediate phase of peace and war. Such a phase may cause them to question the former justification and feel the meaninglessness of the loss: "Did our dear ones die for this kind of peace?" Again, some of the reactions I have quoted before relate to this aspect.

It is usually seen as the task of the political and social leadership to assist the vulnerable groups in the society, as well as the society as a whole, to accommodate the delicate and complex demands of such an intermediate phase between war and peace. They have to help the public confront previous unrealistic expectations which they may have helped develop during earlier stressful and frustrating years of warfare. However, in many cases the leadership itself is stuck in the same prepeace syndrome (Bar-On, 1995a). Can many leaders state openly, for example, that they sent people to live in outposts for the purpose of national security but now they should leave those places for the same reason because the perspective of national security has drastically changed?

It is not easy to suggest what they should actually do to help the public cope with this ambiguity (Tetlock, 1987). For example, should they prefer to present every new act or situation as an error or as a coincidence, rather than as an anticipated part of a larger process? This may help some people and perhaps distress others. It would help those who cannot cope with the whole process at once, although it may hamper the effort of others who could gain from a wider interpretive map which would help them reduce uncertainty (Lanir, 1990). Some people prefer to receive difficult knowledge about the change in bits and pieces, or even wish it to be presented as involuntary acts, for example, as concessions to American pressure. Because the leaders cannot predict the outcome of the process that they are leading, they may prefer to limit their own perspective and that of others, rather than show a clear direction and be punished if this fails at some point in the future.

The PTSD concept can be applied to other social contexts in which a sudden collapse of the role of the enemy or an intermediate phase of war and peace can be identified. This is true of the countries that were deeply involved in the cold war (such as the United States, Germany, and Eastern Europe). Other societies that are suffering from long and exhausting conflicts (such as Northern Ireland, Bosnia, Cambodia, South Africa) and are trying to move toward resolving the conflict will experience a similar intermediate phase like that described earlier. However, in each social context, these factors and possibly others have to be assessed separately according to the specific characteristics of that context.

References

Aronoff, M. J. *Israeli visions and divisions: Cultural change and political conflict.* New Brunswick: Transactions.

Bar-On, D. (1992). A testimony on the moment before the (possible) occurrence of a massacre: On possible contradiction between the ability to adjust and the maintaining of human moral values. *Journal of Traumatic Stress, 5*(2), 289–301.

Bar-On, D. (1995). *Fear and hope: Life-stories of five Israeli families of Holocaust survivors, three generations in a family.* Cambridge, MA: Harvard University Press.

Bar-On, D. (1995a). Peace intermediate stress syndrome: The Israeli experience. *Palestine-Israel Journal, 2*(1), 69–79.

Bar-On, D., & Selah O. (1991). The "vicious cycle" between current social and political attitudes and attitudes towards the Holocaust among Israeli youngsters. *Psychologia, 2*(2), 126–138 (Hebrew).

Bar-On, D., Yizhaki-Verner, T., & Amir, S. (1996). "The recruited identity": The influence of the Intifada on the perception of the peace process from the standpoint of the individual. *Journal of Narrative and Life History, 6*(3), 193–223.

Bilu, Y. (1994). The image of the enemy: Cracks in the wall of hatred. *Palestine-Israeli Journal, 4,* 24–28.

Biran, H. (1994). Fear of the other. *Palestine-Israeli Journal, 4,* 44–51.

Figley, C. R. (1986) (Ed.). *Trauma and its wake,* Vol. II. *Traumatic stress, theory, research and intervention.* New York: Brunner/Mazel.

Gal, R., & Miesles, O. (1992). *Anticipating chemical warfare during the Gulf war.* Zichron Yaakov: The Carmel Institute for Military Research.

Glozman, M. (in press). The urge for heterosexualism: Zionism and sexuality in Altnewland. *Jerusalem. Theory and Criticism.*

Grumer, K. (1996). *Athena or Aphrodite? Israeli young women talk about their friends' involvement in the Intifada.* Beer Sheva: Ben Gurion University, unpublished manuscript.

Hadar, Y. (1991). The absolute good and bad in the eyes of Holocaust survivors and their descendants. Presentation at *The 8th Family Therapy Conference,* Bat-Yam.

Harkabi, Y. (1983). *The Bar-Kochba syndrome: Risk and realism in international politics.* New York: Rossel Books.

Keen, S. (1987). *Faces of the enemy: Reflections of the hostile imagination.* Weinheim: Beltz.

Keren, N., & Almaliach, D. (1994). A community under siege. In D. Bar-On & D. Fromer (Eds.), *The second reader—after-effects of the Holocaust on second and third generations.* Beer Sheva: Ben Gurion University, Mifal Leshichpul (Hebrew).

Kimmerling, B. (1993). Militarism in the Israeli society. *Theory and Criticism, 4,* 123–140 (Hebrew).

Lanir, Z. (1990). *A young kibbutz in a conceptual crisis.* Hakibbutz Hameuchad: Yad Tabenkin (Hebrew).

Levi, A., & Wiztum, E. (1989). Battle reactions in Israeli wars 1948-1973. *Sichot, 4*(1), 60–70 (Hebrew).

Morris, B. (1996). *Israeli border wars, 1949–1956.* Tel Aviv: Am Oved (Hebrew).

Niv, A., & Bar-On, D. (1992). *The size dilemma of the kibbutz from a system learning perspective.* Greenwich, CT: JAI Press.

Porat, D. (1986). *An entangled leadership: The Yishuv and the Holocaust.* Tel Aviv: Am Oved (Hebrew).

Portugali, Y. (1996). *Implicated relations: Society and space in the Israeli-Palestinian conflict.* Tel Aviv: Hakibbutz Hameuchad (Hebrew).

Ram, U. (1995). *The changing agenda of Israeli sociology: Theory, ideology and identity.* Albany, NY: SUNY Press.

Rom, E., & Bar-On, D. (in preparation). *Battle shock during the war of independence: The social role of silencing the phenomena.* Department of Behavioral Sciences, Ben Gurion University of the Negev.

Segev, T. (1992) *The seventh million.* Jerusalem: Keter (in Hebrew).

Shorris, S. (1995). Jews without Yiddish. *Forkroads, 1*(1), 28–34.

Solomon, Z. (1993). *Combat stress reactions: The enduring toll of war.* New York: Plenum.

Tetlock, P. (1987). A value pluralism model for ideological reasoning. *Journal of Personality and Social Psychology, 50*(4), 819–827.

Zizek, S. (1989). *The sublime object of ideology.* London: Verso.

Zrubavel, Y. (1986). The holiday cycle and the commemoration of the past: Folklore, history and education. *Ninth World Congress of Jewish Studies,* Magnes 4, 111–118.

Part III

The Victimization of Women and Children

In the previous section, we highlighted cultural differences. Yet what seems to be maintained across culture is the propensity of societies to victimize their most vulnerable members. Although the debate about the plight of women in some societies has become enmeshed with social agendas of political correctness and hence has sometimes become intellectualized, the brutalization of women and children is in fact all too concrete. Ironically, beyond their thin veneers and ideologies, all cultures have failed to protect women and children from victimization, and indeed some societies may tacitly condone or even actively promote such brutalization. In this section commonalties in the fate of women and children across different societies are highlighted. However, although similar types of sexual and physical traumatization are described, we also stress differences in the social structures that enable this victimization. For example, the experience of rape may be quite different when performed in the context of domestic violence versus ethnic cleansing.

Sexual victimization and domestic violence appear to be particularly insidious events. Paradoxically, these events are associated with the highest level of psychological consequences but also the highest levels of social denial. They appear in the context of units which are meant to convey safety and security, such as in the family. These chapters, coming from remote areas of the world, describe the different ways in which women and children become particular targets for violence and often do not have the social provisions to protect themselves.

Dora Black and Martin Newman provide a comprehensive and erudite summary of the literature on domestic violence to women and children. They point to the shocking frequency of these events and tackle the most often asked questions about domestic violence, particularly relating to its causes, and the various responses of women who are victimized in this manner. They also address the effects of domestic violence on children and the way in which children may be helped. The important conclusion that is reached by these authors is that it may be more appropriate, and eventually feasible, to prevent domestic violence in the future rather than treat its psychological fallout.

Given the capacity for denial of domestic violence, it is critical that strategies be developed to document and appraise the prevalence and effects of domestic violence. Specific observations must ultimately be generalized so as to become scientific evidence. Gwenneth Roberts discusses the inherent difficulties in systematically studying one of the most frequent forms of abuse to women and children—domestic violence and its consequences. She points to the need to characterize the different forms of

aggression that can be expressed in families to assess their occurrence and consequence, and discusses different ways in which healing can take place. Although this
discourse is about objectifying the facts and may be seen as another way to intellectualize
the problem, it is also the beginning of a necessary process that will ultimately lead to
universal standards that allow women to appraise their victimization from a more
objective perspective that does not depend on the cultural mores.

Drawing on a sample of help-seeking women survivors of sexual abuse, Sahika
Yüksel addresses the frequency and the nature of childhood sexual abuse in Turkish
families. She describes the traditional family structure in which men are heads of the
households and provide all or most of the income. Such a structure prevents women
from freely accessing help or distancing themselves or their daughters from a perpetrator within the family. As such, her discussion is as much about the way society colludes
to perpetuate silence about child abuse and amplifies the helplessness of victims. One
can only admire the bravery and courage to be writing about such a society from within.
Yüksel teaches us that the first stage in combatting victimization is thorough documentation of the problem and providing services to the few who can come forward.

Sue Robinson points to a response that has been seen primarily in traumatized
women. The types of traumatic events inflicted on women that are described in this
section directly involve violation of body boundaries. Hence, beyond the purely psychological responses, such as being reminded of the trauma or having intrusive images of
it, at a very concrete level many women may experience perversions of normal bodily
routines, such as sexual relations or eating habits. Whether therapies that are mainly
designed to grapple with meaning and memories of the trauma are sufficient to restore
these violated body routines is the central issue of this chapter. Robinson extends her
observation to theory and then provides an outline for treatment designs to address the
body and the impact of body violations on the soul and psyche.

As long as societies maintain their internal structures, traumatization of women
and children remain individual cases. When societies disaggregate into civil war, women
and girls become special targets for racial and aggressive tensions. Libby Arcel has been
involved in helping sexually violated Muslim victims of the recent racial cleansing in
Bosnia. She describes the different circumstances in which individual or systematic rape
has occurred and the ways in which such acts become more than simply expressions of
male aggression but rather carry the symbolic message of conquering, dominating, and
humiliating another race or faith. It is hard to believe that such horrors are permitted
in Europe in the late twentieth century. Not believing may be part of the denial that has
allowed the perpetuation of such acts in history, including the relatively recent Nazi
Holocaust. One comes to understand how easy it is to engage in denial and disbelief.

Denial and disbelief are at the core of a major controversy in the United States
regarding the accuracy and historical veracity of accounts of childhood sexual abuse by
adult survivors. Laura Brown provides a historical overview of the False Memory
Movement and then attempts to summarize current scientific understanding about
delayed recall of traumatic events. Again, historical, political, and scientific ideas are
bound together to produce a debate that is difficult to resolve because of antagonistic
social forces. In essence, what happens to women in the United States who come
forward with claims of sexual abuse is that they, as well as their therapists, are confronted
with disbelief. This bodes poorly for women in all corners of the world. Hence, discussing this debate is universally relevant.

9

Children: Secondary Victims of Domestic Violence

DORA BLACK AND MARTIN NEWMAN

A woman, a horse and a hickory tree
The more you beat 'em the better they be.

(old American song, quoted in Greenblat, 1983)

Witnessing domestic violence as an influence on children's development and child psychopathology received little attention until relatively recent times. Now, however, increasing attention is being paid to this subject and to the effects that witnessing or experiencing domestic violence may have on children in the short term and on their longer term development and psychological adjustment.

What is Domestic Violence?

Domestic violence is defined as the physical, sexual, emotional, and mental abuse of women by male partners or ex-partners (Victim Support, 1992). Women can abuse men, too, although they resort to violence or to sexual abuse much less often. For example, men are ten times as likely to kill their spouses or partners than women are (FBI, 1975–1991; Harris et al., 1993). This is partly related to the fact that they are physically less strong but also has complex links with the way girls and boys are differentially socialized (Miedzian, 1991).

Domestic violence involves the abuse of power. Although these are acts of the strong against the weak, they seem to be acts carried out by abusers to compensate for their perceived lack or loss of power. One result of the psychological manipulation common among all types of family abuse is the tendency among victims to blame

---

*This article was first published in *Clinical Child Psychology and Psychiatry*, 1996, *1*(1), 79–88. Reprinted with permission of the Editor.

DORA BLACK • Traumatic Stress Clinic, London, W1P 1LB, England. **MARTIN NEWMAN** • St. George's Hospital, London, SW17 0RE, England.

International Handbook of Human Response to Trauma, edited by Shalev, Yehuda, and McFarlane. Kluwer Academic / Plenum Publishers, New York, 2000.

themselves. Other common patterns among abuse victims are a sense of shame and humiliation, a wish to keep the abuse a secret from others, and a feeling of entrapment (Finkelhor, 1983). Here, we are not discussing the effects on children of being direct victims of physical or sexual abuse but are reviewing the effects on children of witnessing domestic violence between parents and what can be done to help these children, the "other" victims, injured not in body, but in mind.

When considering the subject of domestic violence, we must consider whether a child's social and emotional functioning are altered significantly by family violence and, if so, whether there is a link between the child's disrupted development and the expression of psychological adjustment later on. Then the mechanism of the association needs to be elucidated.

Defining what constitutes significant domestic violence is difficult and Greenblat's study (1983) shows that opinions about what is acceptable between spouses and in society vary widely. There have also been secular changes. For example, in the United Kingdom, wife-beating was considered a husband's duty as late as Victorian times (in the nineteenth century), to keep the wife in order. Until recently, what went on within a marriage was considered private, and police were reluctant to interfere in a domestic dispute. The very term *domestic violence* has trivial, almost cozy connotations, causing it to be almost ignored by the police, politicians, and the general public.

Domestic violence can range from an occasional slap to regular beating with or without an implement, choking, strangling, threatening or injuring with a knife or gun, rape and other forced sexual acts, and can end in death. In about 50 families a year in the United Kingdom, the mother is killed by the father (Cameron & Frazer, 1987; Harris Hendriks et al., 1993).

How Common is Domestic Violence?

In the United Kingdom, domestic violence is the second most frequent type of crime reported to the police, comprising more than 25% of all reported violent crime. Reported incidents are probably the tip of the iceberg. One survey estimated that there are 530,000 assaults on women by men in the home each year. It is estimated that between 90 and 97% of all domestic violence is directed toward women by men (NCH, 1994). One-third of all reported crimes against women result from domestic violence (Victim Support, 1992).

All forms of abuse appear to be higher in the lower socioeconomic strata and more common in families where unemployment and economic deprivation are serious problems. It is not clear to what extent the presence of one form of abuse is a good predictor of the presence of another (Finkelhor, 1983). In Western societies, domestic violence may be a hidden problem because it generally occurs in the home and because many women are too ashamed or frightened to seek help. It has been estimated that one in a hundred marriages are characterized by severe and repeated violence and up to one-third of marriages experience some violence within them (Borkowski et al., 1983).

Our study of children of uxoricide (wife killing) (Harris Hendriks et al., 1993) found that there was a fivefold increase in the incidence of uxoricide in Asian immigrant families compared with indigenous ones. Although factors common to all immigrants (poverty, housing problems, unemployment) play a part in this increase, factors pertaining to the role of women in Asian families are also relevant, particularly the belief that adulterous wives are deserving of death.

Causes of Domestic Violence

The various explanations of the causes of domestic violence include individual pathology (personality disorders and mental illness, including alcoholism and drug abuse); factors in the social structure; and feminist explanations. Some writers suggest that the economic dependence of women may be an important factor. Jealousy, including morbid jealousy, and conflicting expectations about appropriate behavior for women were also found to be causes of violence in relationships (see Finkelhor et al., 1983, for a full discussion of the causes of domestic violence). The role of alcohol and drugs is unclear, but alcohol, which causes disinhibited behavior in relatively low doses, is implicated in some cases of impulsive aggressive behavior. This may be part of a more pervasive personality disorder and may be linked with cerebral biochemical mechanisms (Coccaro et al., 1993; Dodge, 1993; Herbert, 1993).

Why Do Women Stay in Abusive Relationships?

For many women, especially those with dependent children, financial hardship and lack of anywhere else to go are decisive factors. In one survey, this accounted for over half of the women (Mooney, 1993). Nearly one-fifth feared further violence if they left, and this fear is a reality (see below). We have seen families where the woman is relentlessly pursued and can find little protection from society. Injunctions without penal clauses attached have little teeth. For many women (one-quarter of Mooney's subjects), there is always hope that their partner will change, a phenomenon that Goldner et al. (1990) describe as being "hooked on remorse."

Why Do Women Leave Abusive Partners?

For many women, there appears to be a "last straw" which can be the extension of abuse to a child, the threat or fear of being killed, a recognition that the children are being harmed by witnessing the violence, or a realization that her man will never change (NCH, 1994). In a few cases, a new relationship develops but, in many cases, morbid jealousy on the part of the husband forces him to imagine infidelity where none exists. Threatening to leave is a dangerous move, and 22% of women were killed for that reason (Harris Hendriks et al., 1993).

If the woman does pluck up courage and leave, there is, in the United Kingdom and elsewhere, a marked shortage of refuges, and if she returns to her parents, the old adage, "As ye make your bed, so shall ye lie in it," is one that the families of origin may quote as they send her back. In any case, the woman may feel ashamed to return to her parents and tell them of her poor choice of a partner. In many of our uxoricide cases, the maternal family had no idea that there was unhappiness and domestic violence in their daughter's life.

The NCH study (1994) found that many children were confused as to why their mothers had left, although nearly as many were relieved by the move. Many missed their fathers, or were upset about leaving home, school, and friends.

How Frequently Are Children Involved?

The ways in which children witness violence range widely. They may listen to the violence from their bedrooms, at one extreme, to being forced to watch the mother being assaulted, raped, or even killed by their father at the other. One survey suggests that in 90% of cases of wife abuse, children are in the same or an adjacent room (NCH, 1994). Other children may not directly see the violent acts but may be aware of their mother's fear either directly from her or by inference, see her wounds, or experience the disruption that follows when their mother seeks refuge.

Arguments between parents about child-rearing methods and children's behavior are a major precipitating crisis that leads to violent episodes (Strauss et al., 1980). One study (Dobash & Dobash, 1979) found that almost half of domestic violence attacks take place in front of others and that three-fifths of the observers were the couple's own children.

Effects on Children

When studying children's reactions to emotionally laden situations, their cognitive interpretations of such events need to be considered. Children under 8 years old tend to interpret most events in relation to the self. For example, younger children may be more likely than older children to attribute maternal anger to themselves, blaming themselves for "causing" the displeasure. In addition, they may have distorted concepts of causality as a result of their immature reasoning abilities—events are causally linked if there is a temporal association.

Children's responses to witnessing violence to their mother will vary according to their age, sex, stage of development, and role in the family. Many other factors also play a role, such as the extent and frequency of the violence, repeated separations and moves, economic and social disadvantage, and personality characteristics of the child (Jaffe et al., 1990).

From infancy, children seem to be aware of the emotions of those close to them and show an emotional response. Very young children exposed to angry interchanges simulated in the laboratory show distress, suggesting the possibility of direct emotional effects on children of witnessing parental conflict (Cummings et al., 1985; Cummings, 1987).

Various studies (summarized in Fantuzzo & Linquist, 1989; Peled et al., 1995; Smith, 1989) have found a significantly increased incidence of childhood emotional conduct and learning problems, as well as psychosomatic disorders, in children who witness domestic violence compared with control populations. Their self-esteem is lower, and they show less empathy with others. Emery (1989) found an increase in both internalizing and externalizing symptoms in children of divorce who experienced violence, compared with those who did not.

Children of battered women, who witness violence at home, may learn that violence is an acceptable behavior which is an integral part of intimate relationships or that violence and fear can be used to exert control over family members. They may suffer significant emotional trauma and experience fear, anxiety, confusion, anger, and disruptions in their lives (Jaffe et al., 1985). Children who witness repeated or extreme domestic violence, including rape and uxoricide, have a higher incidence of posttraumatic stress disorder (PTSD) than those who do not witness it (Garmezy & Masten, 1994; Masten et al., 1990; Pynoos & Nader, 1988). Our study of 95 children of uxoricide found that nearly all the children who witnessed the killing developed symptoms of PTSD. Of those who did not witness, but developed the syndrome, most had been exposed to chronic domestic violence (Harris Hendriks et al., 1993). PTSD is a chronic and troubling psychiatric disorder, characterized in children by repetitive nightmares and other sleep disorders, flashbacks, traumatic play, and avoidance of the traumatic situation. It can profoundly affect all areas of functioning, including attachment and learning, and is very difficult to treat, although it may be possible to prevent.

As Jaffe and his colleagues (1990) point out, children who are raised in an environment of wife abuse may suffer in a number of ways. These include

experiencing an inability to rely on their parents for safety and nurturance;
a disruption of attachments (as battered women leave the family home and return, or the mother is hospitalized for a period);
disturbed eating and sleeping routines;
being accidentally hit, pushed, or dropped during a violent outburst;
fear, anxiety, and helplessness, waiting for the next attack and being powerless to prevent it.

They may have to take on a parenting role within the family, protect younger siblings during violent episodes, and offer support and reassurance after an episode of violent behavior. Such effects may have other consequences, for example, school attendance and performance may be adversely affected. These children may feel unable to leave their homes because they feel they have to protect mother or siblings or find ways to prevent the violence.

Leaving home may be no protection for the battered wife; more women are seriously injured and even killed during or after separation than before (Barnard et al., 1982; Langan, 1986). Based on clinical observation of children in shelters for battered women, Davidson (1978) and Alessi & Hearn (1984) describe the primary characteristics of different age groups of children. Infants who witness violence are often characterized by poor sleep, poor sleeping habits, and excessive screaming (all of which may contribute to further violence to their mother by an enraged father). Among preschoolers, there may be signs of terror (as evidenced by yelling, irritable behavior, hiding, shaking, and stuttering). Younger children also appear to be more likely to experience somatic complaints and to regress to earlier stages of functioning (Wolfe et al., 1985).

As children get older, initial sympathy for a battered mother may be replaced by anger and overt hostility toward her (Hilberman & Munson, 1987). Older children and adolescents are often more guarded and secretive about violence at home and may deny it. Adolescents from violent families may use aggression as a predominant form of problem-solving or may project blame onto others and exhibit a high degree of anxiety (Alessi & Hearn, 1984; Davidson, 1978). Adolescents may become manipulators of the family system, not allowing the mother to leave or blaming her for the family problems. Running away is also common among this older age group, especially among males, and 10% of adolescents in women's refuges are actively suicidal (Hughes, 1986). Ambivalent feelings toward either or both parents may develop.

Gender-related differences in children's reactions to chronic family violence also begin to emerge by school age. Males are frequently described as being disruptive, acting aggressively toward objects and people, and throwing severe temper tantrums. Females are often reported to have an increasing assortment of somatic complaints or to show withdrawn, passive, and clinging behavior (see Jaffe et al., 1990). As they get older, adolescent girls may develop an extreme distrust of men and express negative attitudes about marriage, whereas boys more often side with their fathers and may also abuse their mothers.

There is evidence of an intergenerational continuity in the experience of being a victim and an aggressor (Widom, 1989). There may also be genetic links because psychopathic and alcoholic parents are likely to have conduct-disordered children. Although there is research evidence that children are profoundly affected by domestic violence, many studies contain methodological problems, including a failure to define the nature and extent of the violence witnessed by the children, lack of control groups, using mothers to report the effects on the children, sample bias, and failing to control for other relevant variables, such as poverty and unemployment or the presence of child abuse and neglect (NCH, 1994).

The factors that enable some children to cope also need definition. The presence of a good relationship with a parent and the support of peers and adults outside the family, especially teachers, is shown to mitigate the effects of stress (Rutter, 1983).

Disclosure of Violence

Children are most likely to disclose at a time of crisis, such as a police intervention, or after a traumatic event such as witnessing mother's killing. Interview technique needs to be appropriate (see Arroyo & Eth, 1995; Harris Hendriks et al., 1993; Pynoos & Eth, 1984) with arrangements in place to provide or refer for ongoing support. There may be adverse consequences if no treatment is offered after the disclosure of severe violence (Pynoos & Eth, 1984). Disclosure may be inadvertent, spontaneous, or in reaction to classroom material or discussions. Children may express their fears or worries directly to adults with whom they feel safe, or indirectly through play and drawings. Children may need several interviews to disclose what has been or is going on.

Our experience is that children who have been affected by witnessing violence, especially if inflicted on someone to whom they are attached, are often ready to describe what they have seen to a receptive listener. The recent research about the processing of traumatic images indicates that these images dominate the child's cognitions in an intrusive and disturbing way (Terr, 1991). The interview devised by Pynoos & Eth (1986) is a very effective way of helping children to describe these intrusive images and take the first therapeutic steps to heal the scars left by them. It involves the therapist inviting the children to draw a picture. Inevitably they draw the intrusive image. Then the children are helped to understand the perceptions they had, one sensory modality at a time, and time is taken to help them to understand that it was not their fault and they could not have stopped what happened.

Helping Children and Adolescents

Mental health clinics, schools, social-services departments, and voluntary agencies are at the threshold of developing programs to help children affected by domestic violence. These programs are better developed in the United States and Canada than in the United Kingdom. The Children's Hospital in Boston, Massachusetts, developed an advocacy program in a pediatric health care setting for battered women and their abused children, called AWAKE (McKibben et al., 1989; Newberger et al., 1993) that combines health care with legal representation and protection for women and children in violent relationships. Several clinics, specifically for children who have been traumatized by witnessing violence, exist in the United States (Black, 1994). In the United Kingdom, the first such clinic was started in 1993, initially at the Royal Free Hospital in London and now under the auspices of the Camden and Islington Community NHS Trust with support from the Department of Health (Harris Hendriks et al., 1995). The aim is to offer swift assessment and preventive and treatment services to children exposed to trauma from witnessing violence of all kinds—domestic, from war, civil conflict, and mass disasters.

Vulnerability to later stressful events and the need for treatment are indicated by the number of children who experience different forms of violence without treatment and end up with the psychiatric diagnostic labels of "borderline personality" and "multiple personality" (Herman et al., 1989). Overwhelming life experiences greatly impact on children, and van der Kolk (1987) points out that a major focus of treatment relates to helping children regaining some sense of mastery in their lives.

An innovative project in New Haven, Connecticut (U.S.) involves the Yale Child Study Center and the police in a joint venture to try to help children who are present at the scene of a violent crime. When the police arrive, one of them will work immediately with any child witness to try to help them cope with their fear, bewilderment, and distress. All the police in the town are trained and supported by the child-study team, who also accept referrals from the police of children who need more intensive or expert help (Marans & Cohen, 1993).

A recently published book (Peled et al., 1995) details several programs in the United States, Canada, and Israel for battered women and their children, ranging from group and individual psychotherapy for the children in refuges (shelters) to school programs to teach coping skills. Matthews (Peled et al., 1995) describes parenting groups for battering fathers, but most of these schemes have yet to be evaluated. Treating the mothers who may be depressed, suffering themselves from PTSD after years of abuse, bowed down by poverty and fear of being found and forced to return to the abusive partner, will inevitably benefit the children. To be effective, any program must include treatment for the mother, too.

Mental-health measures must go hand in hand with measures to protect the child and battered mother from further abuse, and mental-health workers need to work closely with the police, solicitors, social services, and voluntary agencies, such as Victim Support and Women's Aid. Extensive changes are needed in the administration and structure of the legal system in the United Kingdom, if children are to be properly protected. An Inter-Agency Working Party convened by Victim Support (1992) made far-reaching recommendations which, if implemented, will do much to aid this process. The suggestion that each local authority convene Domestic Violence Forums along the lines of Child Protection Committees is currently being explored by the U.K. government.

Prevention of Domestic Violence

Most injured women who attend accident and emergency departments of general hospitals are not asked how they came by them (Smith, 1992). Similarly, Stark et al. (1979) found that a history of domestic violence was identified in only 1 of 25 battered women attending a hospital emergency clinic. We could make a start in preventing secondary battering if those in health services (general practitioners, health visitors, and accident and emergency department staff) became more curious about their patients' injuries and referred battered mothers to sources of help. To lower the incidence of primary battering, we have to change underlying attitudes and behaviors that condone and promote violence among family members, a task outside our competence to cover. Part of that change needs to come from agents of social control, including government ministers, the judiciary, and the police, as well as the media (Black & Newman, 1995). We need to find ways of raising awareness in school about violence in intimate relationships and to teach alternative forms of conflict resolution (e.g., Carlsson-Paige & Levin, 1992). Appropriate professional training and support for social workers and health-care workers and social engineering, including attention to the creation of jobs, control of alcoholism, the provision of parenting classes and neighborhood initiatives to combat isolation, would all contribute to a reduction in wife battering.

In recent years, a major change in public attitude took place toward smoking in the United Kingdom, which led to a marked reduction in the number of the population who smoke. What is needed to reduce the incidence of domestic violence is similar public condemnation of intrafamilial (or indeed other) violence as a method of communicating or solving problems.

References

Alessi, J. J., & Hearn, K. (1984). Group treatment of children in shelters for battered women. In A. R. Roberts (Ed.), *Battered women and their families* (pp. 49–61). New York: Springer.

Arroyo, W., & Eth, S. (1995). Assessment following violence-witnessing trauma. In E. Peled, P. Jaffe, & J. Edleson (Eds.), *Ending the cycle of violence* (pp. 27–42). Thousand Oaks, CA: Sage.

Barnard, G. W., Vera, H., Vera, M. I., & Newman, G. (1982). Till death do us part: A study of spouse murder. *Bulletin of the American Academy of Psychiatry and the Law, 10,* 271–280.

Black, D. (1994). Winston Churchill Travelling Fellowship to USA to study trauma services for children. *Psychiatric Bulletin, 18,* 565–566.

Black, D., & Newman, M. (1995). Television violence and children. Annotation. *British Medical Journal, 310,* 273–274.

Borkowski M., Murch, M., & Walker, V. (1983). *Marital violence—the community response.* London: Tavistock.

Cameron, D., & Frazer, E. (1987). *The lust to kill.* London: Polity Press; New York: New York University Press.

Carlsson-Paige, N., & Levin, D. E. (1992). Making peace in violent times: A constructivist approach to conflict resolution. *Young Children, 47*(3), 4–13.

Coccaro, E. F., Kavoussi, R. J., & Stehle, S. (1993). Serotonin and impulsive aggression: Relationship to alcoholism. In C. Thompson & P. Cowen (Eds.), *Violence: basic and clinical science* (pp. 62–75). Oxford: Butterworth-Heinemann.

Cummings, E. M. (1987). Coping with background anger in early childhood. *Child Development, 58,* 976–984.

Cummings, E. M., Iannotti, R. J., & Zahn-Waxler, C. (1985). Influence of conflict between adults on the emotions and aggression of young children. *Developmental Psychology, 21,* 495–507.

Davidson, T. (1978). *Conjugal crime: Understanding and changing the wife beating pattern.* New York: Hawthorn.

Dobash, R. E., & Dobash, R. P. (1979). *Violence against wives.* New York: Free Press.

Dodge, K. (1993). Studying mechanisms in the cycle of violence. In C. Thompson and P. Cowen (Eds.), *Violence: basic and clinical science* (pp. 19–34). Oxford: Butterworth Heinemann.

Emery, R. E. (1989). Family violence, special issue: Children and their development: Knowledge base, research agenda and social policy application. *American Psychologist, 44*, 321–328.

Fantuzzo, J. W., & Lindquist, C. U. (1989). The effects of observing conjugal violence on children: A review and analysis of research methodology. *Journal of Family Violence, 4*, 77–94.

Federal Bureau of Investigation (FBI) (1975–1991). *Uniform crime reports.* Washington, DC: U.S. Department of Justice.

Finkelhor, D. (1983). Common features of family abuse. In D. Finkelhor, R. J. Gelles, G. T. Hotaling, & M. A. Straus (Eds.), *The dark side of families—current family violence research* (pp. 17–28). Beverly Hills, CA: Sage.

Finkelhor, D., Gelles, R. J., Hotaling, G. T., & Straus, M. A. (Eds.). (1983). *The dark side of families—current family violence research.* Beverly Hills, CA: Sage.

Garmezy, N., & Masten, A. S. (1994). Chronic adversities. In M. Rutter, E. Taylor, & L. Hersov (Eds.), *Child and adolescent psychiatry: Modern approaches,* 3rd ed. (pp. 191–208). Oxford: Blackwell Scientific.

Goldner, V., Penn, P., Sheinberg, M., & Walker, G. (1990). Love and violence: Gender paradoxes in volatile attachments. *Family Process, 29*(4), 343–364.

Greenblat, C. S. (1983). A hit is a hit is a hit ... or is it? In D. Finkelhor, R. J. Gelles, G. T. Hotaling, & M. A. Straus (Eds.), *The dark side of families* (pp. 235–260). Beverly Hills, CA: Sage.

Harris Hendriks, J., Black, D., & Kaplan, T. (1993). *When father kills mother: Guiding children through trauma and grief.* London: Routledge.

Harris Hendriks, J., Black, D., & Morris-Smith, J. (1995). *The first year of the Children's Trauma Clinic, Royal Free Hospital, London.* Presented at the *4th European Conference on Traumatic Stress,* Paris, May 9, 1995.

Herbert, J. (1993). The neuroendocrinology of aggression: Roles of steroids, monoamines and peptides. In C. Thompson & P. Cowen (Eds.), *Violence: basic and clinical science* (pp. 37–61). Oxford: Butterworth-Heinemann.

Herman, J. L., Perry, J. C., & van der Kolk, B. A. (1989). Childhood trauma in borderline personality disorder. *American Journal of Psychiatry, 146*, 490–495.

Hilberman, E., & Munson, K. (1987). Sixty battered women. *Victimology, 2*, 460–470.

Hughes, H. M. (1986). Research with children in shelters: Implications for clinical services. *Children Today, 15*(2), 21–25.

Jaffe, P. G., Wolfe, D. A., Wilson, S. K., & Slusczarzck, M. (1985). Similarities in behavior and social maladjustment among child victims and witnesses to family violence. *American Journal of Orthopsychiatry, 56*, 142–146.

Jaffe, P. G., Wolfe, D. A., & Wilson, S. K. (1990). *Children of battered women.* Newbury Park, CA: Sage.

Langan, P. A. (1986). Preventing domestic violence against women. (Bureau of Justice statistics special report). Washington, DC: U.S. Department of Justice.

Marans, S., & Cohen, D. J. (1993). Children and inner city violence: Strategies for intervention. In A. L. Lewis & A. F. Nathan (Eds.), *Psychological effects of war and violence on children.* Hove, Sussex: Lawrence Erlbaum.

Masten, A. S., Best, K. M., & Garmezy, N. (1990). Resilience and development: Contributions from the study of children who overcame adversity. *Development and Psychopathology, 2*, 425–444.

McKibben, L., De Vos, E., & Newberger, E. H. (1989). Victimization of mothers of abused children: A controlled study. *Pediatrics, 84*(3), 531–535.

Miedzian, M. (1991). *Boys will be boys: Breaking the link between masculinity and violence.* Garden City, NY: Doubleday.

Mooney, J. (1993). The hidden figure: Domestic violence in North London. Islington Council.

NCH Action for Children (1994). *The hidden victims—children and domestic violence. 85,* Highbury Park, London N5 IUD.

Newberger, C. M., Geremy, I. M., Waternaux, C. M., & Newberger, E. H. (1993). Mothers of sexually abused children: Trauma and repair in longitudinal perspective. *American Journal of Orthopsychiatry, 63*(1), 92–102.

Peled, E., Jaffe, P. G., & Edelson, J. L. (1995). *Ending the cycle of violence: Community responses to children of battered women.* Thousand Oaks, CA: Sage.

Pynoos, R. S., & Eth, S. (1984). The child as witness to homicide. *Journal of Social Issues, 40*(2), 87–108.

Pynoos, R. S., & Eth, S. (1986). Witness to violence: The child interview. *Journal of the American Academy of Child Psychiatry, 25*, 306–319.

Pynoos, R. S., & Nader, K. (1988). Children who witness the sexual assaults of their mothers. *Journal of the American Academy of Child and Adolescent Psychiatry, 27*, 567–572.

Rutter, M. (1983) Stress, coping and development: Some issues and some questions. In N. Garmezy & M. Rutter (Eds.), *Stress, coping and development in children* (p. 142). New York: McGraw-Hill.

Smith, L. (1989). Domestic violence: An overview of the literature. Home Office Research and Planning Unit Report (Home Office Research Study number 107). London: HMSO.

Smith, S. (1992). Adult domestic violence. *Health Trends, 24*, 97–99.

Stark, E., Flitcraft, A., & Frazier, W. (1979). Medicine and patriarchal violence: The social construction of a private event. *International Journal of Health Services, 9*(3), 461–493.

Strauss, M. A., Gelles, R. J., & Steinmetz, S. K. (1980). *Behind closed doors.* New York: Anchor Press / Doubleday.

Terr, L.C. (1991). Childhood traumas—an outline and overview. *American Journal of Psychiatry, 148*, 10–20.

van der Kolk, B. A. (1987). The psychological consequences of overwhelming life experiences. In B. A. van der Kolk (Ed.), *Psychological trauma.* Washington, DC: American Psychiatric Press.

Victim Support (1992). *Domestic violence. Report of a national inter-agency working party.* London: Cramer House.

Widom, C. S. (1989). Does violence beget violence? A critical examination of the literature. *Psychological Bulletin, 106*(1), 3–28.

Wolfe, D. A., Jaffe, P. G., Wilson, S. K., & Zak, L. (1985). Children of battered women: the relation of child behavior to family violence and maternal stress. *Journal of Consulting and Clinical Psychology, 3*, 657–665.

10

Evaluating the Prevalence and Impact of Domestic Violence

GWENNETH LILIAN ROBERTS

Methodological Issues in Domestic Violence Research

> Spouse abuse presents a challenge to epidemiology because its parameters are not well defined, its severity is highly subjective, its causes are poorly understood and its psychosocial consequences are often linked in very complex ways to physical events. This helps explain why a problem that may affect as much as 20% of the adult female population and that results in more than three times as many injuries as auto accidents has been largely neglected by health researchers, including those specializing in injury. (Stark & Flitcraft, 1991, p. 125)

In spite of the burgeoning interest and the increased number of journals that include articles on domestic violence, there remain numerous methodological inadequacies in the area of domestic violence research.* Many early research initiatives in domestic violence were poorly designed, were unrepresentative of a particular population, and lacked control groups. Measurement instruments were often not validated, and their psychometric properties were inadequate. Nonparametric or descriptive statistics replaced inferential statistics and experimental rigor. A particular difficulty which has been noted in psychiatric epidemiology is the measurement of post-traumatic stress disorder (PTSD) in the face of an ongoing stressor, such as domestic violence.

Recently there have been improvements in the design of domestic violence research. More studies have used control groups, and researchers have used more precise statistics, such as multivariate analyses. Few studies of post-traumatic stress disorder have investigated domestic violence victims. Most studies have concentrated on war

---

*In this paper domestic violence refers to physical, emotional, or sexual abuse of an adult (16 years or older) during or after a family or close relationship, e.g., legal marriage, de facto, boyfriend/girlfriend, where one partner is afraid of and/or being physically hurt by the other. The term "victim" refers to females because prevalence studies in the hospital Emergency Department have shown that women are three times more likely to experience adult domestic violence than men and five times more likely to experience both child and adult abuse than men (Roberts et al., 1993).

GWENNETH LILIAN ROBERTS • Department of Psychiatry, University of Queensland Child and Youth Mental Health Service, Fortitude Valley, Queensland 4006, Australia.

International Handbook of Human Response to Trauma, edited by Shalev, Yehuda, and McFarlane. Kluwer Academic / Plenum Publishers, New York, 2000.

veterans and victims of natural disaster. However, there is increasing attention to the diagnosis of post-traumatic stress disorder for victims of prolonged, repetitive, cumulative trauma perpetrated by intimates, and victims of domestic violence have recently been included in this group.

An important issue in domestic violence research relates to the interpretation of findings and causality. Even where strong associations of factors have been identified with domestic violence, it has been difficult to establish a temporal sequence because most studies have been descriptive and retrospective and longitudinal studies have not been conducted. Therefore, it has been difficult to specify causal pathways with any certainty and to establish whether the association was a risk factor or an outcome. After analyzing 15 years of empirical research on wife assault, Hotaling and Sugarman (1986) found few risk markers that identified women at risk of violence in close relationships. Only witnessing violence in the wife's family of origin was consistently associated with being victimized. A risk marker refers to an attribute or characteristic that is associated with the risk of being victimized by husband-to-wife violence and is not necessarily a causal factor.

Several reasons may be put forward for these methodological inadequacies. The first was the absence of a knowledge base, e.g., lack of representative studies or lack of accurate recording of domestic violence incidents in medical or police records. This lack of a knowledge base may have served to excuse flawed designs and less than ideal dependent measures. Secondly, this was a difficult population to study, and this included the investigation of a population of aggressive and violent partners. Abusive spouses were frequently reluctant to participate in either treatment or research; the unstable nature of these relationships and the transience of the abusive population created difficulties when researchers attempted to assess the outcome of follow-up studies. Interpartner unreliability of reporting with respect to the occurrence of violence has threatened well-designed studies. The third difficulty relates to ethical issues in domestic violence research. Longitudinal studies of domestic violence would require control groups of victims and nonvictims of domestic violence. It would be unethical to withhold intervention from those who disclosed domestic violence in these studies. Therefore it would be difficult to follow the natural course of this phenomenon, and the only possibility in this type of research would be to evaluate different interventions and their effect on the outcome of domestic violence incidence.

Another problem in domestic violence research has been sociopolitical bias. Both sociopolitical biases and methodology problems could impact negatively on the understanding of the etiology and dynamics of domestic violence. When the first research in family violence was published in 1974 (Gelles, 1987) the battle lines were drawn between feminist researchers who explained spouse abuse as a function of patriarchy versus the social-structuralists who took a more traditional middle-range theoretical approach. Although they have often been critical of each other, feminist explanations and social-structural explanations are not necessarily antithetical despite their different paradigms for theory building. Both use eclectic methods, although their emphases may be different. Feminist researchers place greater emphasis on historical and anthropological analysis whereas social-structuralists prefer survey methods and analyses of contemporary social structures. The difference in method is that social-structuralists start by constructing a model of interrelated variables, whereas feminist researchers identify the variables only after studying the specific contexts within which the violence occurs (Smith, 1989). Feminists have objected to generic terms such as "family violence" used by social-structuralists because they believed that these terms obscured the dimensions of gender and power which were fundamental to understanding the abuse. Rosenbaum (1988) maintained that the extent to which political considerations intruded on design and interpretation of results could be discussed and minimized. Although the tensions between feminists and social-structuralists remain part of domestic violence research, there is a need for a more fully integrated theoretical explanation of the high incidence of domestic violence within society.

In this chapter I will argue that there are two methodological issues in domestic violence research that are interlinked: definitional problems of the dependent measure, namely, how domestic violence is defined, and definitional issues related to the diagnosis of post-traumatic stress disorder for those who experience domestic violence. This will lead into a general discussion about the difficulties of measuring PTSD domestic violence victims. Illustrations of the problems will be given from studies which the author has conducted at the Emergency Department of a major public hospital in Brisbane, Australia.

Definitional Problems

A study by Geffner, Rosenbaum, and Hughes (1988) examined a representative sample of domestic violence investigations and found that only 16.0% described the criteria used to define the abused sample. Even among those who met the criteria, there was substantial variability. In the research there have been two major problems: how should violence (or abuse) be defined, and which relationships should be included as domestic? Definitions that have been used range from physical abuse in current relationships to inclusion of emotional abuse and sexual abuse in past relationships. Goldberg and Tomlanovich (1984) asked subjects whether they had ever been pushed around, hit, kicked, or hurt by a boyfriend or husband, to classify them as abused, whereas Coleman et al. (1980) required serious or repeated injury at the hands of the partner, to consider them abused. Dalton and Kantner (1983) left the operational definition of the classifying terms "battered" or "abused" to the subjective opinion of the subjects.

The second part of the definitional problem relates to which relationships have been included in domestic violence. The broadest definition of domestic violence in intimate sexual relationships has included legal marriage, de facto relationship, boyfriend or girlfriend. The term "marital violence," which has often been used in studies, is a misnomer. Few studies required a legal marital relationship and, in reality, "spouse," "wife," and "husband" have been used generically to refer to a man or woman involved in an intimate marriage-like relationship. Lack of definitional agreement had implications for subject selection, and this has resulted in a variety of estimates of incidence and prevalence rates. Stark & Flitcraft (1988) have argued that domestic violence may involve from 5.0 to 20.0% of the population of the United States, depending on the criteria used for the definition.

Definitions of domestic violence are reflected in the measures which have been used in domestic violence research. The gold standard for the measurement of domestic violence has been the Conflict Tactics Scale (CTS) first published in 1973. The original scale was based on conflict theory and could be used to measure child abuse, wife beating, and husband beating (Straus, 1979). The CTS measures three factorially separate variables: reasoning, verbal aggression, and violence or physical aggression.

The scale was criticized first because it was originally designed to measure conflict rather than abuse. It asked respondents to think of situations in the past year when they had a disagreement or were angry with a specified family member and to indicate how often they engaged in each of the acts included in the CTS. Researchers have argued that partner abuse against women is coercive in nature rather than arising out of conflict which does not necessarily precede abuse (Yllo, 1993; Candib, 1989). Therefore, some violence related to conflict may have been missed. Second, the scale concentrated mainly on physical abuse which is defined as an act carried out with the intention, or perceived intention, of causing physical pain and injury to another person. However intention was not indicated in the measure. It omitted sexual abuse and had only limited measures of verbal aggression (Dobash & Dobash, 1992; Kurz, 1993). Physical and emotional abuse are often associated, and anecdotally, a number of victims state that emotional abuse is worse than physical abuse. A 73-year-old woman in the author's study (Roberts et al., 1993) stated that there is nothing to show people you have been abused with mental cruelty and wished she had been hit so as to show others what was happening. She was forced to have sex against her wishes, and only realized years later that it was rape. She thought that this was part of marriage.

A third criticism of the CTS was that it may have contributed to measurement error in quantitative studies because it did not take into account the intensity and impact of various types of violence on the victims. The lack of information on the consequences of an action meant that some items were classified as minor, e.g., slapping, which has the potential to cause severe injury when perpetrated by a male. A study by Berk et al. (1983) showed that the violence of men against women is more severe and results in greater physical injury than the violence of women toward men. Finally, individual acts of physical violence did not necessarily equate to the broader definition of partner abuse which includes emotional and sexual abuse.

The CTS was used in many studies, and its psychometric properties were well tested, and resulted in some variability. A literature review of selected overseas and Australian studies conducted in English-speaking countries (Table 1) revealed that those studies which used the CTS as their measure showed a pattern of results that was fairly uniform, resulting in lifetime prevalence rates of 20 to 25% (Hegarty & Roberts, 1997).

A later measure, the Revised Conflict Tactics Scale (CTS2) with a theoretical base of conflict memory similar to the original scale addressed some of the aforementioned issues. It included a new sexual abuse scale and an injury scale which would give some indication of the consequences of the physical acts (Straus et al., 1996).

Not all violent behavior between partners constitutes domestic violence, and it has been argued that there are two forms of violence against women (Johnson, 1995). One consists of occasional outbursts of violence from either husbands or wives during conflicts (common couple violence), whereas other families are terrorized by systematic male violence (patriarchal terrorism) and other families may experience both. Mostly quantitative, family violence perspective researchers have used the first definition, whereas the second definition has been used by mostly qualitative, feminist perspective researchers. The latter definition has not been used in survey research on community populations because there has not been a well-validated tool to measure such abuse.

While the CTS2 has broadened the scope of the measurement of domestic violence, its weakness is that it attempts a measure of gender equivalence of individual acts. Each item, e.g., I went to a doctor because of a fight with my partner, is asked first what the participant has done. The higher rates of female domestic victims who go to general practitioners is known (Hagerty & Roberts, 1977), but our own research has shown that very few male victims want to speak to any health professional about being a domestic

TABLE 1. Prevalence of Domestic Violence in Selected Community Samples (Hegarty & Roberts, 1997)

Country	Sample Size (Response Rate)[a]	Sample Type (Method)	Definition Used[b]	12 Month (%)	Lifetime (%)
U.S.A. (Straus et al., 1981)	2,143 couples (65%)	National random probability sample (interview)	CTS physical abuse against wives severe (kicked, bit or hit with a fist, hit or tried to hit with something, beat up, threatened with or use of knife or gun)	12.1 3.8	30 (of couples)
U.S.A. (Straus & Gelles, 1986)	3,520 married or de facto couples (84%)	National random probability sample (telephone)	CTS physical abuse against wives severe (as above)	11.6 3.4	28 (of couples)
Canada (Rodgers, 1994)	12,300 women (not stated)	Random digit dialing (telephone)	CTS physical abuse threatened to hit threw something pushed, grabbed, or shoved slapped kicked, bit, or hit with fist hit her with something beat her up choked her threatened or used a knife/gun Sexual assault	3.0	29 19 11 25 15 11 6 9 7 5 8
Canada (Ratner, 1993)	516 women (78.7%)	Random digit dialing (telephone)	Physical abuse Emotional abuse	10.6 23.0	NA[c]
New Zealand (Mullen et al., 1988)	1,516 women (73.9%)	Random probability sample (interview)	Physical abuse "hit and physically abused"	NA	16.2
Australia (McLennan, 1996)	6,300 women (78%)	Random interview electoral role sample (questionnaire)	CTS physical violence (physical assault includes pushed, slapped, hit, choked, beaten, stabbed, shot, and threatened or attempted assault) Sexual violence (sexual assault or threat) Emotional abuse (insulted with intention to humiliate, damaged property, prevent access to money, car, telephone, family, friends, threat to children or pets)	2.4 CR[d] 0.3 CR NA	22.5 7.6 (CR) 1.0 CR 8.8 CR
Australia (Ferrante, 1996)	1,511 men 1,550 women (52.7%)	Random digit dialing community sample (telephone)	"Attacked, hit, pulled, pushed or punched in an aggressive or threatening manner," and incidents involving stealing by threat or force, personal attack, threat with force, and sexual assault	0.2 men 2.1 women	NA

Note: a) This figure represents estimated eligible rather than all the other figures which have excluded non contacts, non English speaking, or otherwise hard to interview respondents. (b) Unless otherwise stated, frequency of abuse is at least once. (c) NA = not available. (d) CR = Percentage of abused women in current relationships.

violence victim (Roberts et al., 1993). Items such as fear, dominance, and social isolation, which are common features of domestic violence for women, but not for men, are omitted from the CTS2. Men and women may define domestic violence very differently, and this indicates a need for gender-specific reporting.

Crime victim surveys in Australia have obtained figures as low as 3.0% of women assaulted in the 12-month period prior to interview, but these have used assault in the legal sense as the definition (Women's Policy Unit, Qld. Gvt., 1992). Crime victim reports are of limited value in assessing the scope of violence against women because the crimes reported to police were likely to have differed in important ways from the crimes that were hidden.

It is clear from the discussion that there is a need for well-validated measurement instruments which reflect the definitions used for domestic violence and which take into account the frequency, intensity, meaning, and impact on the victims of various types of violence and the context in which the violence takes place.

PTSD and Domestic Violence

The definitional problems of domestic violence which have been discussed in the first section of this paper impinge on the definitional problems of the measurement of PTSD. Which definition of domestic violence fits the criterion for measuring PTSD? Is it "common couple violence," "patriarchal terrorism," or both?

The first criterion (Criterion A) for measuring PTSD is that the person has been exposed to a traumatic event in which both of the following were present: (1) the person experienced, witnessed, or was confronted with an event or events that involved actual or threatened death or serious injury or a threat to the physical integrity of self or others; (2) the person's response involved intense fear, helplessness, or horror (American Psychiatric Association, 1994).

Inclusion of domestic violence in Criterion A for PTSD raises two aspects of domestic violence, involving investigation of the objectivity and subjectivity of the traumatic event/s experienced. First, the objectivity of the event/s requires measuring the extent (frequency and severity), the length and type of domestic violence experienced, including the victim's perception of a life-threatening traumatic event, whereas the subjective aspects address the impact of the traumatic events on the victim.

In the PTSD literature the debate continues as to whether the objectivity or subjectivity of the traumatic event is more critical to the criterion that the stressor is outside the range of usual human experience. A study of battered women in shelters found that the reported subjective distress during or immediately after the battery experience had stronger correlations with presence and degree of PTSD, intrusion, depression, anxiety, and general psychopathology than the objective characteristics of the extent (frequency and severity) of battery and the length of the battering relationship (Kemp et al., 1991). In this study battery was defined broadly to include minimal physical aggression through to attempted murder. The investigators used this definition because they considered that the definition of trauma was not clearly defined.

Studies with rape victims and combat veterans have supported the stronger relationships of subjective stress to the degree of symptomatology compared to the objective characteristics of the event (Kilpatrick et al., 1985; Girelli et al., 1986; Solomon et al., 1987). However, a study of the Beverley Hills Supper Club fire (Green et al., 1985) found that the objective characteristics of the event were more strongly related for survivors of a fire. Kemp et al. (1991) suggested that a possible explanation for these inconsistent findings relates to the nature of the stressor. In rape and combat the trauma is interpersonal, whereas in a fire it is impersonal.

In an attempt to objectify the concept of a stressor, Kilpatrick et al. (1993) devised a measure, the Potential Stressful Events Interview, to systematically assess whether the subject had been exposed to any traumatic incidents that would qualify as an event that met the DSM-III-R criterion A guidelines for PTSD (American Psychiatric Association, 1987). This interview asks each subject specific behavioral screening questions to determine whether they were exposed to "low magnitude potential stressors," e.g., financial problems, marital separation, or divorce. This precedes a lifetime history of the following "high magnitude" stressors: completed rape, other sexual assault, serious physical assault, other violent crime, homicide death of family members or close friends, serious accidents, natural or man-made disasters, and military combat.

Because domestic violence may be described on a continuum from low-level "common couple abuse" to extreme "patriarchal terrorism," it is argued that the events that are likely to fulfill Criterion A would be on the more severe end of the spectrum where the abuse is coercive, repetitive, and cumulative, regardless of the more objective criteria of the type of abuse. However, no studies have differentiated the impact of the subjective distress of the minor stressors of domestic violence from the objective stressors of severity and frequency by using validated measures.

The severe end of the spectrum of domestic violence has been described as "battering." Battering of a woman is an event that poses serious threat or harm to that individual's life and/or may cause death as a result of the physical assault (Woods & Campbell, 1993). It refers to the etiology of a range of health problems that follow the initial episode of abuse. Stark & Flitcraft (1991) identified a battering syndrome among abused women. From a medical standpoint, the syndrome is established by an initial assault (abuse) followed by a history of injury, often including sexual assault, general medical complaints, psychological problems, and persistent help-seeking. In addition to being accompanied by a history of adult trauma, battering may present through chronic (and frustrated) help-seeking; complaints of somatoform pain; injury during pregnancy; fear or anxiety associated with family conflict; isolation; and multiple psychosocial problems related to the stress of living in a violent home, including substance abuse, child abuse, attempted suicide, and mental illness. No process comparable to battering has been observed among abused men.

Battered women's syndrome has been proposed as a subclassification of PTSD, although there has been little research on the adequacy or accuracy of this proposal (Walker, 1991). Most of the studies on post-traumatic stress disorder have been conducted with war veterans or survivors of natural disasters, and the investigation of PTSD in battered women is a very recent field of research. Studies of battered women used small samples who came mostly from women's shelters and lacked control groups. They found that rates of PTSD among help-seeking battered women varied between 40 and 80% (Houskamp & Foy, 1991; Kemp et al., 1991; Astin et al., 1993).

Researchers have recognized that PTSD coexists with other psychiatric diagnoses (Tomb, 1994). Green (1994) considered that PTSD was too narrow an outcome upon which to focus when studying survivors of traumatic events. In studies of battered women, the most common diagnoses that were comorbid with PTSD were depression and anxiety (West et al., 1990; Kemp et al., 1991; Saunders, 1994). Studies have shown the strong association among anxiety and depression and PTSD in rape victims who constitute the largest single group of PTSD sufferers (Steketee & Foa, 1987). Because the majority of rape and sexual assault occurs in intimate relationships, these effects must be included in studying battered women (Russell, 1990, p. 67) An example of marital rape was given in our studies by a 62-year-old woman who said that her husband made her abort her first child and raped her right after the procedure. She used to fantasize about killing her husband. Her husband would demand sex, and she would state that she was too tired. He would rub his fingers along a piece of furniture to collect dust and state "you can't be too tired, you haven't done much today." He used to place coins high in a room to check if they were adequately dusted. Her husband controlled the money and used it as a method to gain sex. She was repeatedly raped but normalized it as a part of marriage.

High rates of dissociative symptoms have been found in samples of subjects with PTSD (Saxe et al., 1993) and in subjects with histories of childhood abuse (van der Kolk et al., 1991). Because numerous studies have shown that a risk factor for adult domestic violence is childhood abuse (Roberts et al., 1993), the relationships among childhood abuse or repetitive trauma, PTSD, and dissociation need further clarification. Researchers have argued that the impact of childhood sexual abuse takes place over a period of time instead of as a circumscribed event and therefore results in a different set of problems (Finkelhor, 1990; Herman, 1993). Studies have also shown the strong associations among dissociation, somatization, and abuse, particularly the association of amnesia with somatization (Pribor et al., 1993). A 22-year-old woman in our studies did not remember her childhood experiences of incest by her half brother at age 6, rape at age 6 by a babysitter for 3 months, or rape at 8 by her father's friend, although she had gained this knowledge from other sources. It has been noted that making the appropriate diagnoses in chronically traumatized patients had a dramatic beneficial effect on their long-term prognosis (van der Kolk, 1996).

Difficulties of Measuring PTSD

One of the difficulties in measuring PTSD in domestic violence victims has been that the traumatic events described are often not single circumscribed events but multiple incidents. Several respondents in the author's current study reported repeated rapes and beatings by their husbands and could not differentiate which was the worst event. The same problems related to the reporting of incest, where a victim described incest from ages 4 to 12 and could not differentiate which was the most stressful event. Individuals who have been subjected to repeated abuse, although not involved specifically in a traumatic event at the moment, may know a constant anxiety that is based, in part, on past personal experiences within the violent relationship.

The worst fear of any traumatized person is that the moment of horror will recur, and this fear is realized in victims of chronic abuse. The repetition of trauma amplifies all the hyperarousal symptoms of post-traumatic stress disorder, and chronically traumatized people are continually hypervigilant, anxious, and agitated. This may be adaptive when faced with ongoing and unpredictable assaults. Hence the difficulty of measuring PTSD for an ongoing stressor, such as domestic violence.

In our studies we found difficulties in using the Composite International Diagnostic Interview (World Health Organization, 1993) schedule which lists extremely stressful events, such as rape, sexual assault, or incest, on the same line. Many women reported their experience of all three events. A 63-year-old woman reported multiple events of serious physical assault by her husband which would climax in rape. She decided to combine both to measure PTSD, given the strength of the connection.

Herman (1994) stated that the prolonged, repeated trauma of domestic violence was similar to that of other people in captivity, such as prisoners in concentration camps and slave labor camps. Captivity creates a special type of relationship, one of coercive control, and this is equally true whether the victim is rendered captive primarily by physical force, e.g., prisoners, or by a combination of physical, economic, social, and psychological means, e.g., battered women and children. The psychological impact may have many common features, whether it occurs in the public sphere or in the private sphere of domestic relations. Herman (1994) reviewed the evidence for the existence of a complex form of PTSD in survivors of prolonged, repeated trauma. She considered that the current diagnostic formulation of PTSD derived primarily from observations of survivors of relatively circumscribed traumatic events, combat, disaster, and rape, and suggested that this formulation failed to capture the protean sequelae of prolonged, repeated trauma. Other clinicians have invoked the need for a diagnostic formulation that followed upon prolonged, repeated trauma, and manifested a constellation of symptoms not fully captured by the reexperiencing, arousal, and avoidance symptoms that comprise PTSD (Krystal, 1968; Kroll et al., 1989).

Diagnostic confusion and debate over the issue of repetitive, cumulative trauma have ensued and have been encapsulated in a paper "Posttraumatic stress in battered women: Does the diagnosis fit?" (Woods & Campbell, 1993). Recently, a new concept called "Disorders of Extreme Stress Not Otherwise Specified" (DESNOS) or "Complex PTSD" was proposed (Herman, 1992). DESNOS symptoms were clustered into five categories: alterations in affective arousal, alterations in attention and consciousness, somatization, chronic characterological changes, and alterations in systems of meaning.

DESNOS criteria were examined in the five-site Field Trial for DSM-IV, 1991–1993 (van der Kolk, 1993). In this trial PTSD and DESNOS were investigated as two distinct syndromes. One of the goals of the DSM-IV Field Trials was to determine empirically the prevalence of the range of trauma-related psychological problems mentioned in the research literature that are not currently captured in the PTSD definition. The Field Trials were designed, in part, to establish how the various trauma-related psychiatric symptoms reported in the research literature are related to each other, as well as to the current diagnostic construct of PTSD.

A Structured Interview for Disorders of Extreme Stress (SIDES) was developed and administered to 520 subjects as part of the DSM-IV Field Trials (Pelcovitz et al., 1997). A list of 27 criteria often seen in response to extreme trauma and not addressed by DSM-IV criteria for PTSD were generated, based on a systematic review of the literature and a survey of 50 experts. Subjects were divided into three groups: early-onset interpersonal abuse, late-onset interpersonal abuse, and disaster. The findings were that people who had been traumatized at an early age tended to have problems in all of the categories. The older the victims were and the shorter the duration of the trauma, the more likely they were to develop only the core PTSD symptoms; the longer the trauma and the less protection, the more pervasive the damage. Trauma was found to have its most profound impact during the first decade of life (van der Kolk, 1996). Although the study yielded data to support the reliability, content, and face validity of the interview, the investigators considered that the construct validity of the measure needed to be further investigated. This could be done by comparing endorsement of DES symptoms across different types of trauma populations. They hypothesized that victims of interpersonal trauma would be particularly likely to present with the symptoms measured by the scale.

The outcome of the DSM-IV Field Trials was that DESNOS was incorporated under the "Associated Features and Disorders" section (American Psychiatric Association, 1994, p. 488). The ICD-10 created a separate category to accommodate enduring personality changes after catastrophic experience (World Health Organization, 1992, pp. 136–138).

Earlier research has shown that trauma has a different impact on psychological adaptation at different stages of development and that earlier trauma affects subsequent maturational processes (Cole & Putnam, 1992). Research with rape victims (Burgess & Holmstrom, 1974), battered women (Walker, 1984), and concentration camp survivors (Krystal, 1968) has shown the long-term impact that trauma can have in the areas of self-regulation and personality development. Trauma literature suggests that the profound impact of traumatic experiences on self-regulation, self-concept, and interpersonal functioning would be most pronounced in younger victims (Cole & Putnam, 1992; Pynoos, 1993) and when the source of the trauma is interpersonal assault as opposed to natural disasters, e.g., earthquakes or hurricanes (Davidson & Smith, 1990).

Other writers have argued that the specific vulnerability to PTSD associated with severe, chronic childhood trauma is merely a risk factor for later PTSD (Tomb, 1994). Nevertheless, this issue remains unclear because the evidence shows that the pathology resulting from early or extremely severe trauma often bears scant resemblance to PTSD (Herman, 1992). The relationship between early and severe trauma and PTSD remains to be clarified.

Another difficulty in measuring PTSD and domestic violence is the effect of psychological or emotional abuse, including constant verbal abuse, threats to kill, and other serious threats to the victim. A major component of the trauma may involve emotional abuse and betrayal. Trauma at any age, but particularly trauma inflicted by caregivers, generally has a profound effect on the capacity to trust (van der Kolk, 1996). A woman who experiences relatively low levels of physical violence may develop higher levels of PTSD symptomatology if she also experiences emotional abuse. A 29-year-old woman said that she did not class her physical domestic violence as serious but said verbal abuse was worst. She did not include physical assault on the PTSD Criterion A measurement scale.

Other areas of trauma and character development which need to be investigated in battered women are the capacity to attribute responsibility properly, resulting in self-blame, shame, and guilt. Prevalence studies conducted by the author in the Emergency Department showed that these three characteristics were the main reasons why women did not disclose domestic violence to their doctors (Roberts et al., 1993, 1996). Identification with the aggressor results in negative effects on identity and failure to maintain a personal sense of significance, competence, and inner worth (van der Kolk, 1996). Research has shown that once people have been victimized, they are at risk of being victimized in the future (Widom, 1987; Roberts et al., 1993, 1996).

Conclusion

Given the high rates of domestic violence in the community (McLennan, 1996) and the high rates of PTSD among rape victims, many of whom are the victims of intimate perpetrators, the problems which have been raised in this chapter indicate the need for further research with domestic violence victims and survivors. First, the need for validated measurement instruments that capture the frequency, severity, meaning, and impact of different types of domestic violence victims has been demonstrated. To measure PTSD, further investigation is necessary to determine which definitions of domestic violence fulfill the requirement for a traumatic event in which both of the following were present: (1) the person experienced, witnessed, or was confronted with an event or events that involved actual or threatened death or serious injury or a threat to the physical integrity of self or others; (2) the person's response involved intense fear, helplessness, or horror.

A number of areas of PTSD research remain to be clarified across a range of traumatic incidents, e.g., the inclusion of the objective or subjective aspects of the stressor in Criterion A. Particular areas that apply to victims of repetitive, cumulative trauma need to be addressed in research with victims of domestic violence. These pertain to the reexperiencing, avoidance, and arousal core symptoms, as well as to a wider range of symptoms that have been described in the trauma literature, e.g., alterations in affect, somatization, characterological changes, and alterations in systems of meaning. Some of the core symptoms such as avoidance may not constitute a disorder but may be a protective mechanism that the victims use to avoid further violence. Depression, anxiety, somatization, and dissociation have been found to be significantly comorbid with a diagnosis of PTSD. How do these other diagnoses fit with the diagnosis of PTSD? Are they able to discriminate victims of repetitive, cumulative trauma from victims of circumscribed traumatic events?

Little is known about the impact of prolonged trauma perpetrated in an intimate relationship. How do victims of interpersonal trauma differ from victims of impersonal trauma such as natural disasters? Will the prevalence rates of PTSD and specific symptoms related to domestic violence be different for men and women?

Although information about the prevalence of PTSD in battered women may be useful, the description of specific symptoms resulting from their experiences is likely to be of greater use. The similar and distinctive consequences of acute episodes of battering and those of ongoing, chronic incidents need to be determined both in cross-sectional and longitudinal studies. Is it a question of dose-response relationships or does familiarity with the threat or event alter the response over time and impact on the development of specific symptoms in those who experience domestic violence?

As Green (1994, p. 357) says, "We need to move away from simply documenting the presence of PTSD and other diagnoses following traumatic events, to studies of ... basic [psychological] processes that will enhance our understanding of how human beings struggle to adapt to severely adverse environments. ... Further, we should strive to understand those individuals who are able to adapt without help to enhance our appreciation of those personal and environmental variables that protect." The nature of PTSD as a protective mechanism or a survival technique in battered women needs to be explored.

References

American Psychiatric Association (APA). (1987). *Diagnostic and statistical manual of mental disorders*, 3rd ed., Revised. Washington, DC: American Psychiatric Press.

American Psychiatric Association (APA). (1994). *Diagnostic and statistical manual of mental disorders*, 4th ed. Washington, DC: American Psychiatric Press.

Astin, M. C., Lawrence, K. J., & Foy, D. W. (1993). Post-traumatic stress disorder among battered women: Risk and resiliency factors. *Violence and Victims*, 8(1), 17–28.

Berk, R. A., Berk, S. F., Loseke, D. R., & Rauma, D. (1983). Mutual combat and other family violence myths. In D. Finkelhor, R. J. Gelles, G. T. Hotaling, & M. A. Straus (Eds.), *The dark side of families* (pp. 197–212). Newbury Park, CA: Sage.

Burgess, A. W., & Holmstrom, L. L. (1974). Rape trauma syndrome. *American Journal of Psychiatry*, 131(9), 981–986.

Candib, L. M. (1989). Violence against women: No more excuses. *Family Medicine*, 21(5), 339–341.

Cole, P., & Putnam, F. W. (1992). Effect of incest on self and social functioning: A developmental psychopathology perspective. *Journal of Consulting and Clinical Psychology*, 60, 174–184.

Coleman, K., Weinman, M. C., & Hsi, B. P. (1980). Factors affecting conjugal violence. *American Journal of Psychology*, 105, 197–202.

Dalton, D. A., & Kantner, J.E. (1983). Aggression in battered and non-battered women as reflected in the hand test. *Psychological Reports*, 53, 703–709.

Davidson, J., & Smith, R. (1990). Traumatic experiences in psychiatric outpatients. *Journal of Traumatic Stress*, 3, 459–475.

Dobash, R. E., & Dobash, R. P. (1992). Knowledge and social change. *Women, violence and social change* (pp. 251–284). London: Routledge.

Ferrante, A., Morgan, F., Indermaur, D., & Harding, R. (1996). *Measuring the extent of domestic violence*. Sydney: Hawkins Press.

Finkelhor, D. (1990). Early and long-term effects of child sexual abuse: An update. *Professional Psychology: Research and Practice*, 21, 325–330.

Geffner, R., Rosenbaum, A., & Hughes, H. (1988). Research issues concerning family violence. In V. B. Hasselt, K. L. Morrison, A. S. Bellack, & M. Hersen (Eds.), *Handbook of family violence* (pp. 457–481). New York: Plenum.

Gelles, R. J. (1987). *The violent home*. Newbury Park, CA: Sage.

Gelles, R. J., & Straus, M. A. (1988). *Intimate violence*. New York: Simon & Schuster.

Girelli, S., Resick, P., Marhoefer-Dvorak, S., & Hutter, C. (1986). Subjective distress and violence during rape: Their effects on long-term fear. *Violence and Victims*, 1, 35–46.

Goldberg, W. G., & Tomlanovich, M. C. (1984). Domestic violence victims in the emergency department. *Journal of the American Medical Association*, 251(24), 3259–3264.

Green, B. L. (1994). Psychosocial research in traumatic stress: An update. *Journal of Traumatic Stress*, 7(3), 341–362.

Green, B. L., Grace, M., & Gleser, G. (1985). Identifying survivors at risk: Long-term impairment following the Beverly Hills Supper Club fire. *Journal of Consulting and Clinical Psychology*, 53, 672–678.

Hegarty, K., & Roberts, G. (1997). How common is domestic violence against women? Issues in the definition of partner abuse in prevalence studies. *Australian & New Zealand Journal of Public Health* (in press).

Herman, J. L. (1992). Complex PTSD: A syndrome in survivors of prolonged and repeated trauma. *Journal of Traumatic Stress*, 5(3), 377–391.

Herman, J. L. (1993). Sequelae of prolonged and repeated trauma: Evidence for a complex post-traumatic syndrome (DESNOS). In J. R. T. Davidson & E. B. Foa (Eds.), *Post-traumatic stress disorder: DSM-IV and beyond* (pp. 213–228). Washington DC: American Psychiatric Press,

Herman, J. L. (1994). *Trauma and recovery*. London: Harper Collins.

Hotaling, G. T., & Sugarman, D. B. (1986). An analysis of risk-markers in husband to wife violence: The current state of knowledge. *Violence and Victims*, 1(2), 101–123.

Houskamp, B. M., & Foy, D. W. (1991). The assessment of posttraumatic stress disorder in battered women. *Journal of Interpersonal Violence*, 6(3), 367–375.

Johnson, M. P. (1995). Patriarchal terrorism and common couple violence: Two forms of violence against women. *Journal of Marriage and the Family*, 57, 283–294.

Kemp, A., Rawlings, E. I., & Green, B. L. (1991). Post-traumatic stress disorder (PTSD) in battered women: A shelter sample. *Journal of Traumatic Stress*, 4(1), 137–148.

Kilpatrick, D. G., Resnick, H. S., & Freedy, J. R. (1993). A description of the posttraumatic stress disorder field trial. In J. R. T. Davidson & E. B. Foa (Eds.), *Posttraumatic stress disorder: DSM-IV and beyond*. Washington, DC: American Psychiatric Press.

Kilpatrick, D., Veronen, L., & Best, C. (1985). Factors predicting psychological distress among rape victims. In C. R. Figley (Ed.), *Trauma and its wake* (pp. 113–141). New York: Brunner/Mazel.

Kroll, J., Habenicht, M., Mackenzie, T., Yang, M., Chan, S., Vang, T., Nguyen, T., Ly, M., Phommasouvanh, B., Nguyen, H., Vang, Y., Souvannasoth, L. & Cabagou, R. (1989). Depression and post-traumatic stress disorder in Southeast Asian refugees. *American Journal of Psychiatry, 146,* 1592–1597.

Krystal, E. (Ed.). (1968). *Massive psychic trauma.* New York: International Universities Press.

Kurz, D. (1993). Physical assaults by husbands: A major social problem. In R. Gelles & D. R. Loseke (Eds.), *Current controversies on family violence* (p. 88). Newbury Park, CA: Sage.

McLennan, W. (1996). Women's Safety Australia. Canberra: Australian Bureau of Statistics.

Mullen, P., Romans-Clarkson, S., Walton, V., & Herbison, G. (1988). Impact of sexual and physical abuse on women's mental health. *The Lancet,* 841–845.

Pelcovitz, D., van der Kolk, B., Roth, S., Mandel, F., Kaplan, S. & Resick, P. (1997). Development of a criteria set and a Structured Interview for Disorders of Extreme Stress (SIDES). *Journal of Traumatic Stress, 10*(1), 3–16.

Pribor, E. F., Yutzy, S. H., Dean, T., & Wetzel, R. D. (1993). Briquet's syndrome, dissociation, and abuse. *American Journal of Psychiatry, 150,* 1507–1511.

Pynoos, R. S. (1993). Traumatic stress and developmental psychopathology in children and adolescents. In J. Oldham & A. Tasman (Eds.), *Review of psychiatry* 12 (pp. 205–238). Washington, DC: American Psychiatric Press.

Ratner, P. (1993). The incidence of wife abuse and mental health status in abused wives in Edmonton, Alberta. *Canadian Journal of Public Health, 84*(4), 246–249.

Roberts, G., O'Toole, B., Lawrence, J., & Raphael, B. (1993). Domestic violence victims in a hospital emergency department. *Medical Journal of Australia, 159,* 307–310.

Roberts, G. L., O'Toole, B. I., Raphael, B., Lawrence, J. M., & Ashby, R. (1996). Prevalence study of domestic violence victims in an emergency department. *Annals of Emergency Medicine, 27*(6), 747–753.

Rodgers, K. (1994). Wife assault: The findings of a national survey. *Statistics Canada Catalogue, 14*(9), 1–21.

Rosenbaum, A. (1988). Methodological issues in marital violence research. *Journal of Family Violence, 3*(2), 91–104.

Russell, D. H. (1990). *Rape in marriage.* Indianapolis: Indiana University Press.

Saunders, D. G. (1994). Posttraumatic stress symptom profiles of battered women: A comparison of survivors in two settings. *Violence and Victims, 9*(1), 31–44.

Saxe, G., van der Kolk, B. A., Hall, K., Schwartz, J., Chinman, G., Hall, M. D., Lieberg, G., & Berkowitz, R. (1993). Dissociative disorders in psychiatric inpatients. *American Journal of Psychiatry, 150*(7), 1037–1042.

Smith, L. J. F. (1989). *Domestic violence: an overview of the literature.* London: HMSO Publications Centre.

Solomon, Z., Mikulincer, M., & Hobfoll, S. (1987). Objective versus subjective measurement of stress and social support: Combat-related reactions. *Journal of Clinical Psychology, 55,* 577–583.

Stark, E., & Flitcraft, A. (1988). Violence among intimates: An epidemiological review. In V. V. Hasselt, R. Morrison, A. Bellack, & M. Hersen, (Eds.), *Handbook of family violence* (pp. 293–316). New York: Plenum.

Stark, E. & Flitcraft, A.H. (1991). Spouse abuse. In M. L. Rosenberg & M. A. Fenley (Eds.), *Violence in America: A public health approach* (pp. 123–157). New York: Oxford University Press.

Steketee, G., & Foa, E. B. (1987). Rape victims: Post-traumatic stress responses and their treatment. *Journal of Anxiety Disorders, 1,* 69–86.

Straus, M. A. (1979). Measuring intra-family conflict and violence: The Conflict Tactics (CT) Scales. *Journal of Marriage and the Family,* February, 75–88.

Straus, M. A., & Gelles, R. J. (1986). Societal change and change in family violence from 1975 to 1985 as revealed by two national surveys. *Journal of Marriage and the Family, 48,* 465–479.

Straus, M. A., Gelles, R. J., & Steinmetz, S. K. (1981). Violence in the home. *Behind closed doors. Violence in the American family* (pp. 4–28). Newbury Park, CA: Sage.

Straus, M. A., Hamby, S. L., Boney-McCoy, S., & Sugarman, D. B. (1996). The Revised Conflicts Tactics Scale (CTS2)—development and preliminary psychometric data. *Journal of Family Issues, 17*(3), 283–316.

Tomb, D. A. (1994). The phenomenology of post-traumatic stress disorder. *Psychiatric Clinics of North America, 17*(2), 237–250.

van der Kolk, B. A., Roth, S., Pelcovitz, D., & Mandel, F. (1993). *Complex PTSD: Results of the PTSD field trials for DSM-IV.* Washington, DC: American Psychiatric Association.

van der Kolk, B. A. (1996). The complexity of adaptation to trauma: Self-regulation, stimulus discrimination, and characterological development. In B. A. van der Kolk, A. C. McFarlane, & L. Weisaeth (Eds.), *Traumatic stress* (pp. 182–213). New York: Guilford.

van der Kolk, B. A., Perry, C., & Herman, J. L. (1991). Childhood origins of self-destructive behavior. *American Journal of Psychiatry, 148,* 1665–1671.

Walker, L. E. (1984). *The battered woman syndrome.* New York: Springer.

Walker, L. E. (1991). Post-traumatic stress disorder in women: Diagnosis and treatment of battered woman syndrome. *Psychotherapy, 28*(1), 21–29.

West, C. G., Fernandez, A., Hillard, J. R., Schoof, M., & Parks, J. (1990). Psychiatric disorders of abused women at a shelter. *Psychiatric Quarterly, 61*(4), 295–301.

Widom, C. S. (1987). The cycle of violence. *Science, 244,* 160–165.

Women's Policy Unit. (1992). Women's experience of crimes of personal violence. A gender analysis of the 1991 Queensland Crime victims Survey: Office of the Cabinet, Queensland Government.

Woods, S. J., & Campbell, J. C. (1993). Posttraumatic stress in battered women: Does the diagnosis fit? *Issues in Mental Health Nursing, 14,* 173–186.

World Health Organization. (1992). *ICD-10: International Statistics Classification of Diseases and Related Health Problems,* 10th rev. Geneva: WHO.

World Health Organization. (1993). *Composite International Diagnostic Interview—Version 1.1.* Geneva: WHO.

Yllo, K. (1993). Through a feminist lens: Gender, power and violence. In R. J. Gelles & D. R. Loseke (Eds.), *Current controversies on family violence* (pp. 47–63). Newbury Park, CA: Sage.

11

Collusion and Denial of Childhood Sexual Trauma in Traditional Societies

SAHIKA YÜKSEL

Adult Sequela of Child Sexual Abuse

During the past decades, child sexual abuse (CSA) has emerged as a subject of public and professional concern. The incidence of CSA in non-Western countries remains unknown. Yet, there are widespread prejudices, based on the assumption that sexual abuse is rare in these societies. Very few studies have addressed the effect of race, ethnicity, or religion on CSA and its consequences. The stigma of sexual abuse, however, may be greater in some groups and therefore could affect the resulting psychopathology. Russell (1986) noted that 83% of Latin victims reported extreme trauma as a result of incest, compared with about half of Asian and White victims. Wyatt (1985) compared Afro-American with Caucasian women and found that the effects of childhood sexual abuse were longer in the latter, who also tended to blame themselves for their victimization.

Until very recently, the prevalence of domestic violence and CSA in Turkey was largely unknown, and such was also the case for other Muslim societies. Possibly, this gap in our knowledge was due to denial of the problem and its impact by the public and by professionals. The few articles that had been published were restricted to describing clinical cases, in which such situations were presented as a rare "illness." As Korbin (1991) states, however, "the absence of published cases of child maltreatment does not necessarily mean the absence of the problem." Furthermore, from clinical practice, personal experiences, and anecdotal information, we strongly suspected that the actual incidence of CSA in Turkey was much higher than assumed. Moreover, most of the women whom we have seen had been abused by their own fathers (Yüksel, 1993, 1997; Yüksel et al., 1996).

SAHIKA YÜKSEL • Istanbul-Psychosocial Trauma Programs, Department of Psychiatry, University of Istanbul, Topkapi, Istanbul, Turkey.

International Handbook of Human Response to Trauma, edited by Shalev, Yehuda, and McFarlane. Kluwer Academic / Plenum Publishers, New York, 2000.

Many sexually abused children develop mental health problems, such as post-traumatic stress disorders (PTSD), depression, eating disorders, and sexual problems, that may bring them to consult with mental health professionals (Briere, 1988, Finkelhor et al., 1984; Goodwin, 1990; Herman, 1981). A history of CSA, therefore, is frequently observed among psychiatric patients, e.g., in 42% of female outpatients and 22% of female inpatients (Jacobson & Richardson, 1987). Hence, a search for a life history of sexual abuse among mental health patients is a reasonable way to learn about the magnitude of the problem in the population at large. Moreover, in Turkey, there are almost no institutions for victims of sexual abuse as such. Consequently, protective shelters or specialized treatment are rarely available. In this study, therefore, the occurrence and the nature of CSA in Turkey were investigated in help-seeking patients to evaluate the dimensions of the problem and to help those who survived. The information obtained from these patients reflects a larger psychosocial reality.

Method

Participants

The study's participants included patients referred for psychiatric treatment who reported a history of CSA before the age of 16. The patients were evaluated at the Psychosocial Trauma Program, Medical School, Istanbul University. The entry criterion was that the participant had experienced sexual abuse in a kinship relationship before the age of 16. The information collected is based upon the victims' own testimony. However, in the case of psychosis or mental retardation, the story is reevaluated at different times and, if available, information coming from relatives is taken into account. Cases with insufficient information were excluded, as well as male subjects and subjects under the age of 14. One hundred ten applicants fulfilled the entry criterion, but fourteen were excluded, leaving 96 women for the study group. This study, therefore, includes what Finkelhor et al. (1984) defined as "cases known to professionals but not officially reported to child protective services."

Procedure

The cases were evaluated in terms of sociodemographic features, histories of physical and sexual trauma, patterns of family relationships, psychopathology, and other long-term adjustments problems. Clinical diagnoses were made on the basis of DSM III-R (1987) criteria. Beyond formal diagnoses, other adjustment problems were also investigated.

CSA was defined as the "occurrence of a sexually inappropriate act including acts of exposure, genital fondling, oral/vaginal/anal intercourse taking place before the age of 16." If the abuse was committed by a person who was five or more years older than the victim; the one initiating the sexual act is regarded as exploiting the child in question.

Physical abuse was defined as inflicting injury, such as bruises, head injuries, fractures, internal injuries, lacerations, or any other form of physical harm lasting at least 48 hours (Walker et al., 1988). Physical neglect is defined as an act of omission in which the child is not properly cared for in terms of nutrition, safety, education, medical care, etc. Emotional neglect is defined as failure to bond, lack of affection, love, support, nurturing, or concern.

Results

The average age of the study population was 21 ± 7.28 years (range 14 to 45). About half of the sample (48%) consisted of adolescents (aged 14 to 20), 30% were between 21 and 30, and the remaining were between the ages of 31 and 45. Thirty-two percent of the sample finished primary school, 44% finished high school, and 17% were university graduates. Sixty-four percent of the subjects were single, 29% were married, and 7% were widowed. Most of the girls (85%) grew up with both parents, in 8% the mother was absent, in 4% the father was absent, and 3% were raised with no parent. About half of the subjects came from a low economical level, one-fourth had experienced poverty, and the remaining third was raised with a high income level. Thirty-seven percent were the only daughters, 22% had one sister, 28% two sisters, and 7% belonged to families with four sisters or more.

Most applicants (70%) asked for help long after the incident. Only 12% came during the time of abuse, and 15% in the three months following it. Usually they referred themselves to hospitals (77%), but some sought help in women's shelter consultations. More than half of the clients sought help directly related to sexual abuse. In 41% of the cases, help was sought for mental problems. Interestingly, most individuals were accompanied to their first interview, most frequently by mothers (45% of all cases) and sisters (24%).

The characteristics of the incest are shown in Table 1. The mean duration of abuse was 4.9 ± 3.28 years (range 1–17 years). Nearly 70% had been abused for more than 3 years. The onset of abuse was at an average age of 9.1 ± 9 (range 3–17). The

TABLE 1. Traumatic Antecedents

	Number	%		Number	%
Number of perpetrators			Duration years		
Single	80	83	Shorter than one year	16	17
Multiple	16	17	1–2 years	16	17
Relationship with abusers			3–5 years	27	27
Father	47	56	6–8 years	21	21
Stepfather	6	6	9+	14	15
Brother	14	17	Unknown	2	
Uncle (father's side)	7	8	Pattern of sexual abuse		
Other relatives	19	20	Nontouching	2	3
Child's age at onset			Nonpenetrative sexual abuse	59	62
3–7	30	31	Intercourse	24	25
8–11	45	47	Anal intercourse	10	10
12–17	21	22	Repetition with sister		
Age at termination			Yes	28	29
6–11	24	25	No	17	18
12–17	57	60	No available sisters	35	37
18–+	14	15	Unknown	16	16
Unknown	1		Severity of physical abuse		
			Absent	35	41
			Moderate	26	31
			Severe and frequently	24	28
			Unknown	11	

average age of termination of abuse was 13.9 ± 4.24 years (range 4–29) years. In some cases the abuse involved more than one sister, in which case both sisters would sometimes come together. Other girls sought help after the treatment of their sisters.

Most of the abused girls' mothers were housewives; the others were unskilled workers. Those mothers who did work, however, could scarcely earn enough for a living. The mothers were either uneducated or primary school graduates (only 10% had graduated high school). Most mothers (55%) knew about their daughters' trauma, yet many (31%) were not aware of it. Of the 55% who knew about the incest, only one-third were able to create efficient strategies to protect their daughters.

The abused girls' fathers tended to have higher educational levels than the mothers (50% finished primary school and 30% finished secondary school), and most of them had regular jobs. We have not recorded any addiction problem besides alcohol, which 25% of the fathers used regularly. One out of four fathers could be defined as "problematic," i.e., used physical violence against the mother or the children, did not carry out his responsibility toward his family, or caused some other problems in the family. Twelve fathers sexually abused more than one daughter. Thirteen fathers were invited to interviews, but only five complied, all of whom were trying to prevent a divorce triggered by the abuse.

Discussion

Sexual abuse in the family is commonly denied in Turkey. The victims of CSA do not know that they can be protected by telling people of their abuse. Therefore, they tend to deny the incident and come to seek help with ambivalent feelings (Yüksel et al., 1996). Nevertheless, the results presented suggest that the extent of the problem is significant.

Importance of the First Interview

Several authors suggested that disclosure is much more complex and costly for a person who has been involved in long-standing abuse and who worries about her responsibility toward her biological father to whom she feels strongly tied. She is also aware that revealing the abuse will cause major turmoil within the family (Herman et al., 1989; Sazier, 1989; Schatzow & Herman, 1989).

Indeed, the first interviews with CSA patients are extremely critical. A significant portion of the applicants requested help either during the process of abuse or a few months later. They came hesitantly and often had unrealistic expectations. More than half of the women spoke directly about their sexual abuse. The rest of them, however, disclosed preliminary signs as they expressed other psychological and somatic problems. This interview was aimed at strengthening their motivation to continue the contact rather than allowing ventilation of feelings.

Patterns of Childhood Sexual Abuse: Similarities and Differences among Studies

The patterns of CSA in Turkey resemble those previously observed in other countries. For example, the ages at which CSA begins and ends in our sample, as well as the fact that abusing fathers often started by abusing the oldest daughter and then continued to other daughters, are very consistent with those previously reported (Herman, 1981, 1992b).

The first noticeable difference is that most of the abusers in this sample were biological fathers. Stepfathers are less involved because of the low rates of divorce in Turkey. Moreover, nearly all of the victims were living with their natural fathers at the time of the abuse. There is a consensus among researchers that sexual relations between fathers and daughters are more damaging to the victims of CSA (Herman & Hirschman, 1984; Schetky, 1990).

The second difference is related to virginity. The types of abuse were divided into three groups based on the degree of violence on the body, that is, penetrative sexual abuse, nonpenetrative sexual abuse, and abuse involving no physical contact. The results indicate that although one-third of the children suffered from penetrative sexual abuse, i.e., vaginal and anal intercourse, most of the girls experienced nonpenetrative sexual abuse, such as different degrees of touching, petting, and masturbation. Among penetrative sexual abuse, one-fourth of this group had sexual abuse that destroyed the hymen.

The importance of this issue in terms of culture should be discussed (Kennedy & Manwell, 1992). Except for three individuals, the group consisted of Muslims, whereas other studies consisted of Christians or Jewish populations. In her work *Sexual Abuse in Nine North American Cultures*, Fontes (1995) points out the importance of cultural differences:

> Our ethnic cultures shape our attitudes toward our bodies, physical contact, virginity, gender roles, sexuality, shame and help-seeking and these impact our experiences of sexual abuse. Prevention and treatment programs that are tailored to the needs of specific groups are likely to be more effective. As we learned to acknowledge the impact of culture on our clients and ourselves, we must also acknowledge that characteristics of our clients may result from their experiences of oppression and not their culture.

Traditions in Turkey vary from one region to another. The importance of virginity is generally very high, especially in the traditional region. In many places the absence of virginity may mean that a young girl loses her chance for marriage. If the situation is known, she loses her prestige within the family as the family loses it in their close neighborhood. The exclusion of vaginal penetration in sexual relationships between young people is, therefore, common. Sexual abusers seem to pay attention to this issue, and some girls are threatened with "losing their hymen" which explains nonpenetrative sexual abuse. On the other hand, the first reaction of the nonoffending parent and other relatives is to take the child or young girl for an examination of her virginity, when they find out about the abuse. If the hymen is left intact, the sexual abuse cannot be proved, and this makes the denial easier for the family. Professionals, therefore, emphasize the fact that the presence of the hymen does not preclude sexual abuse.

The type of sexual activity changes with the victim's age. Sexual intercourse is more frequent toward adolescence. In the meantime, the young girl's perception of sexual abuse changes as she grows older. The denial she could have once employed becomes insufficient and she starts taking actions to stop the abuse. When abuse continues at the age of 16–17, psychopathology becomes more apparent and becomes severe in those cases whose sexual abuse continued up to or beyond 18 years of age. In our sample, psychotic episodes, borderline personality disorder diagnoses, as well as comorbidty and sexual problems were most frequent. This is consistent with Herman et al.'s (1989) description of prolonged abuse.

Diagnosis

Table 2 presents the various Axis I diagnoses in this study. Alarming rates of psychopathology have been reported for sexually abused children by different authors (Blanchard et al., 1986; Briere, 1988; Herman, 1992a; Silverman et al., 1995; Stone, 1989). A study of hospitalized patients in Turkey found that 15% of women patients have an incest story (Tutkun, Sar, Yargýç, Özpulat, Yanýk, & Kýzýltan, 1998). On the other hand, Herman and Schatzow (1987) reported that half of all incest victims in a community sample considered themselves to have recovered well, and only 27% reported severe consequences. The abuse histories reported in our sample, however, are more severe and include a much higher proportion of incestuous involvement with the father. The high rate of paternal abuse observed among our patients does not necessarily mean that paternal abuse is widespread in our society. It may simply represent the rate of paternal abuse among help-seeking patients who have severe psychopathology.

PTSD

As expected in a sample of trauma survivors, PTSD was the most frequent diagnosis in our sample. PTSD, however, does not account for the complexities in the patients

TABLE 2. Psychopathology and Related Problems

	Number	%		Number	%
Number of diagnoses			Eating problems		
None	4		No	58	60
Single	35		Anorexia/bulimia	10	11
Comorbidity	56		Anorexic behaviors	16	17
Two diagnoses	40		Obesity	6	6
Three diagnoses	16		Unknown	6	
Unknown	1		Relational problems		
Distribution of diagnoses[a]			Good/moderate	22	23
Complicated PTSD	41		Not close contact	35	37
Anxiety disorders	19		Problems	27	28
Depressive disorders	40		Unknown	12	12
Borderline personality	15		Sexual dysfunction		
Somatoform disorders	7		Satisfactory	12	15
Psychotic	3		Single/mild problem	49	63
Dissociative disorders	12		Multiple/severe problems	17	22
Sexual disorders	31		Unknown	18	
Mental retardation	2		Type of sexual dysfunction[a]		
Others	2		Hypoactive sex desire disorder	23	
Missing	1		Sexual aversion disorder	33	
Hospitalization			Anorgasmia	23	
Only outpatient	84	87	Sexual pain disorder	3	
Inpatient	12	13	Promiscuity	5	
Suicide attempts					
No	53	55			
Only single attempt	18	19			
Multiple attempts	21	22			
Unknown	4				

[a]The number is higher than 96 because of the comorbidity.

seen here, many of whom have experienced prolonged, repeated, man-made traumatic incidents. In fact many symptoms of "complex PTSD" have been observed, including somatic symptoms, dissociation, changes in relationships to others, alterations in systems of meaning, and alterations in self-perception. As a result, although the leading diagnosis has been PTSD, comorbidity has been a rule.

PTSD symptoms wax and wane with periods when avoidance or numbing symptoms are at the frontline, particularly when depression and amnesia of the traumatic event are present. Therefore differential diagnosis of PTSD may require that the clinician accomplish a thoughtful, creative tracing of the impact of traumatic stress longitudinally on the patient's personality and all realms of mental and social functioning (Blank, 1994).

Anxiety Disorders

Several authors pointed out that there is a particular association between CSA and anxiety disorders. Epidemiological studies also support the relationship between CSA and the subsequent development of anxiety disorders. A recent study (Silverman et al., 1995) confirmed this association. In these studies CSA was higher among women with anxiety disorders (45%) than among a women's comparison group (15%) and was higher among women with panic disorder (60%) than among women with other anxiety disorders (30%) (Herman, 1992a; Schetky, 1990). In this study, because the PTSD and anxiety symptoms overlapped, anxiety disorder diagnoses were relatively rare (Blank, 1994; Blanchard et al., 1986; Herman, 1992a,b; Turner et al., 1996).

Depression

Depressive symptoms are frequently reported in survivors of trauma. Disturbance of self-esteem are common sequels of trauma. In the case of CSA, secrecy is a rule, and such secrecy reinforces the victim's guilt, isolates her from sources of support, and decreases her self-esteem. It has been reported that suicide attempts are a common sequel to sexual abuse at a rate between 33 and 66%. Our finding, which was 41%, fell into this range (Herman, 1981; Schetky, 1990). Morrison (1989) reported that 55% of women with somatization disorder experienced sexual abuse before the age of 18. In our study, it was observed that somatization disorders were common.

Self-Mutilation

It was reported that self-mutilative behavior (SMB) and CSA are highly correlated. Eating problems are similarly observed in survivors of CSA. Because obesity is frequently observed among women in Turkey, one tends to suggest that antecedents of CSA should be looked for in women presenting with severe obesity and self-neglect (Baral et al., 1998).

Interpersonal and Sexual Difficulties

Difficulties in interpersonal relationships are a common complaint among incest survivors. This may have been the reason that some women came for treatment (Herman, 1992b; Stone, 1989). About 65% of women presented problems, such as distrust and feelings of detachment in interpersonal relationships.

Obviously, CSA is likely to distort the development of an association between pleasure and sexual activity. The consequences of such an effect vary from complete avoidance of sexual activity to avoidance of all close interpersonal relationships. Other manifestations include sexual pain disorder and promiscuity (Steele & Alexander, 1985). The most commonly stated problem in our sample was the recall of the abuse during sex. Additionally, flashbacks were reported, as well as feelings of disgust with sexual life and its complete avoidance. Except for two lesbians, the sexual orientation observed was heterosexual. Finally, most women who reported having satisfactory sexual lives were still uncomfortable with some types of sexual behavior, such as sudden touches or touching from behind by a partner. Sexual difficulties associated with difficulties in interpersonal relationships, in general, were mostly mistrust and feelings of detachment.

Principles of Intervention in CSA

The first step in any intervention in a sexual abuse case is to make sure of the security of the young girl (Herman, 1992b; Stone, 1989; Waites, 1993). To this end, we have to clearly identify the family picture. The abused and the abuser share the same space. The offender is often the head of the family, and the mother and children economically depend on him. There is no way of living alone. Hence, key people must be present whom the abused girl can trust and who would protect her—sometimes protect her life, when needed. Such providers of psychological and social support have to be the mediators of a change in the victim's life.

The most available resources are often the mother, sisters, and brothers. They sometimes know about the situation but may not want to believe; else they may believe but not know what to do. Nonoffending parents are often threatened by the abuser and sometimes also by society, in which case they may be traumatized themselves. Hence, it is very important to know who the mother is and in what kind of psychological state she finds herself. Most mothers in our sample were housewives with low education and low personal income. For a women of such a background, listening to her daughters' confessions initiates a complex process which includes confusion, denial, anger, and attempts at adaptation. In despair, some mothers come to specialized consultations with their daughters, expecting us to solve the problem.

Obviously, no one can solve a problem that embraces the whole family simply with words. However it has been observed that if the mothers receive adequate counseling and support for themselves, they become much more supportive to their daughters. Often it is the mother–daughter relationship that becomes the object of therapy, and older problems of mutual confidence become the core issue. Even mothers who would not openly acknowledge the full extent of the abuse took some necessary precautions, such as sending their daughters to one of their relatives. Other women manage to create "safe space" in the households. For example, a woman who could not go anywhere with her four children and was also accused of being "bad" by her mother-in-law had to continue to live with her husband in the same place. Because she could not talk of the incident to her own family, she organized a new space at home by separating her bedroom and sharing her bed with her daughter during the one-year period she received the therapy.

The social pressure on mothers who attempted to get divorced was particularly strong and had to be dealt with. However family relatives, especially from the abused mother's own family, were often very supportive, and such relatives should be contacted and brought into the supportive network (Yüksel, 1997). Unfortunately, we did not observe collaborative attitudes in fathers, even when the abuser was from another family. An abused girl is often unwilling to share her situation with her father, and only few fathers actually joined the therapy of their female family members.

Conclusion

The results of this survey, along with its limitations, may be summarized as follows: Women of different ages participated in this study, that is to say, we have included both adolescents, whose CSA could manifest itself quickly and whose problems were acute, and adults, who had long-standing, late sequelae.

Participants were help-seeking patients, and as such do not represent society at large. However, this indirect approach allows us to undercut the social taboos concerning CSA and provide some information bearing on the problem.

The study group is composed only of women, yet sexual abuse of boys is also occurring. Because the number of male applicants was very low, we excluded them from the study. This finding is in conformity with the finding which shows that female children have a higher risk of CSA (Finkelhor, 1994; Russell, 1995; Waites, 1993). Despite these shortcomings, our findings confirm the association between CSA and long-term consequences in a range of areas, including psychological, sexual, and interpersonal behavior.

In Turkey, secrecy about CSA and the effort to cover up the incidents within the family and the society are widespread. Seemingly, such is the case in most societies, in which, in some way or another, personal issues and mental health issues are linked with social and political attitudes (Bloom, 1996). First among human rights, the right of a safe childhood makes the prevention of CSA and its treatment one of the highest priorities of human society across cultural and geographic boundaries. This work taught us that CSA is frequent in Turkey, and it has taught us ways to support traumatized individuals within the specific constraints of our own culture.

References

American Psychiatric Association (1987). *Diagnostic and statistical manual of mental disorders*, 3rd ed., Rev., DSM-III-R. Washington, DC: American Psychiatric Press.

Baral, I., Kara, K., Yüksel, S., & Sezgin, U. (1997) Self-mutilative behavior among sexually abused girls: An experience from Turkey. *Journal of Interpersonal Violence, 13*, 427–437.

Blanchard, E. B., Gerardi, R. J., Kolb, L. C., & Barlow, D. H. (1986). The utility of the anxiety disorder interview schedule in the diagnosis of post-traumatic stress disorder in Vietnam veterans. *Behavior Research Therapy, 24*, 577–580.

Blank, A. S. (1994). Clinical detection, diagnosis, and differential diagnosis of post-traumatic stress disorders. *Psychiatric Clinics of North America, 17*, 351–384.

Bloom, S. L. (1996). Every time history repeats itself, the price goes up: The social reenactment of trauma. *Sexual Addiction & Compulsivity, 3*, 161–194.

Briere, J. (1988). The long-term clinical correlates of childhood sexual victimization. *Annals of the New York Academy of Science, 528*, 327–334.

Finkelhor, D., Hotaling, G. T., & Lewis, I. (1984). Sexual abuse in the National Incidence Study of Child Sexual Abuse and Neglect: An appraisal. *Child Abuse and Neglect, 8,* 23–32.

Finkelhor, D. (1994). The international epidemiology of child sexual abuse. *Child Abuse and Neglect, 18,* 409–417.

Fontes, L. A. (1995). *Sexual abuse in nine American cultures.* London: Sage.

Goodwin, J. M. (1990). Applying to adult incest victims what we have learned from victimized children. In R. P. Kluft (Ed.), *Incest related syndromes of adult psychopathology.* Washington, DC: American Psychiatric Press.

Herman, J. L. (1981). *Father daughter incest.* Cambridge: Harvard University Press.

Herman, J. L. (1992a). Complex PTSD: A syndrome in survivors of prolonged and repeated trauma. *Journal of Traumatic Stress, 5,* 377–392.

Herman, J. L. (1992b). *Trauma and recovery.* New York: Basic Books.

Herman, J. L., & Hirschman L. (1984). Father–daughter incest. In P. P. Ricker, & E. H. Carmen (Eds.), *The gender gap in psychotherapy* (pp. 237–258). New York: Plenum.

Herman, J. L., & Schatzow, E. (1987). Recovery and verification of memories of childhood trauma. *Psycho-analytic Psychology, 4,* 1–14.

Herman, J. L., Perry, J. C., van der Kolk, B. (1989). Childhood trauma in borderline personality disorder. *American Journal of Psychiatry, 42,* 490–495.

Jacobson, A., Richardson, B.(1987). Assault experiences of 100 psychiatric inpatients: evidence of the need for routine inquiry. *American Journal of Psychiatry, 144,* 1426–1433.

Johnson, J. T. (1984). *Mothers of incest survivors.* Bloomington: Indiana University Press.

Kennedy, M. T., & Manwell, M. K. C. (1992). The pattern of child sexual abuse in northern Ireland. *Child Abuse Review, 1,* 89–102.

Korbin, J. E. (1991). Cross-cultural perspectives and research directions for the 21st century. *Journal of Child Abuse and Neglect, 15* (Suppl. 1), 67–77.

Loewenstein, R. J. (1990). Somotaform disorders in victims of incest and child abuse. In R. P. Kluft (ed.), *Incest related syndromes of adult psychopathology* (pp. 75–111). Washington, DC: American Psychiatric Press.

Morrison, J. (1989). Childhood sexual histories in women with somatization disorder. *Journal of American Journal of Psychiatry, 146,* 239–241.

Russell, D. E. H. (1986). *The secret trauma: Incest in the lives of girls and women.* New York: Basic Books.

Russell, D. E. H. (1995). The prevalence, trauma, and sociocultural causes of incestuous abuse of females. In R. J. Kleber, C. H. Figley, & P. R. Gersons (Eds.), *Beyond trauma: Cultural and societal dynamics* (pp. 171–186). New York: Plenum Press.

Sazier M. (1989). Disclosure of child sexual abuse. *Psychiatric Clinics of North America, 12,* 455–470.

Schatzow, E., & Herman, J. L. (1989). Adult survivors disclose to their families. *Psychiatric Clinics of North America, 12,* 337–350.

Schetky, D. H. (1990). A review of the literature on the long-term effects of childhood sexual abuse. In R. P. Kluft (Ed.), *Incest related syndromes of adult psychopathology.* Washington, DC: American Psychiatric Press.

Silverman, A. B., Reinherz, H. Z., & Giaconia, R. M. (1995). The long-term sequel of child and adolescent abuse: A longitudinal community study. *Journal of Child Abuse and Neglect, 20,* 709–723.

Steele, B. F., & Alexander, H. (1985). Long-term effects of sexual abuse in childhood. *Sexually abused children and their families* (pp. 233–234). Elmsford, NY: Pergamon.

Stone, M. H. (1989). Individual psychotherapy with victims of incest. *Psychiatric Clinics of North America, 12,* 237–256.

Turner, S. W., McFarlane, A. C., & van der Kolk, B. A. (1996). The therapeutic environment and new explorations in the treatment of posttraumatic stress disorder. In B. A. van der Kolk, A. C. McFarlane, & L. Weisaeth (Eds.), *Traumatic stress: The effects of experience on mind, body, and society* (pp. 537–558). New York: Guilford.

Tutkun, H., Sar, V., Yargýç, L. I. Özpulat, T., Yanýk, M., & Kýzýltan, E. (1998). Frequency of dissociatif disorders among psychiatric inpatients in a Turkish university clinic. *American Journal of Psychiatry, 155,* 800–805, 1905.

Waites, E. A. (1993). *Trauma and survivor.* New York: Norton.

Walker, C. E., Bonner, B. L., & Kaufman, K. L. (1988). *The physically and sexually abused child.* New York: Pergamon Press.

Wyatt, G. E. (1985). Sexual abuse of Afro-American and White American women in childhood. *Child Abuse and Neglect, 9,* 507–519.

Yüksel, S. (1993). Identification and management of incest. *Archives of Neuropsychiatry, 30,* 352–357.

Yüksel, S. (1997). Working with mothers in father daughter incest. Presented in Fifth European Conference on Traumatic Stress. Maastricht, Netherlands.

Yüksel, S., Sezgin, U., & Baral, I. (1996). How families in Turkey become aware of childhood sexual abuse. II. *World Conference of the International Society of Traumatic Stress Studies,* Jerusalem.

12

Body Image and Body Recovery

SUE ROBINSON

This chapter explores the psychological aspects of bodily recovery and body image. My thinking developed from my work with women who survived sexual abuse and/or who suffer from eating disorders. It is predicated on the idea that improved bodily self-esteem can enhance physiological and psychological recovery. The material presented here provides ways to think about the mind and body in relation to trauma and body image. Different traumas violate the body in different ways. Surviving incest is not the same as surviving an accident; each has its own particular process of physical and psychological recovery. What I think may be the same, whatever the kind of trauma, is the emotional response. The raw emotions activated are probably akin to those evoked in early infancy if only the *recovery template* could be pinpointed. Visceral responses to trauma leave residues in which the obvious, the obscure, the visible, and the invisible are all merged. Weir Mitchell's (1872) classic account of phantom limbs and reflex paralysis, based on work with patients injured in the American Civil War, exemplifies the visible, noticeable traumas, whereas Terry Waite (1994), a British hostage held in Beirut, wrote after his return of the "lingering sense of isolation." Each speaks to the over-whelming sense of disassociation induced by trauma.

What is Body Image?

Body image is a kind of internal image, an image in the mind about one's body. This image has many components. Raphael-Leff (1994) writes of the totality of body image including

1. Body schema: the body as sensory register and processor; source of biological needs, reflexes; closely related to neurological process.
2. Body concepts and precepts: a private world of cognitive bodily images of body appearance, size, competence, gender, experience, and memories.
3. Body ideal: the concept against which these are measured.
4. Body self: the body as self-stimulus and instrument of purposive action.

SUE ROBINSON • Institute of Psychiatry, London and Heathlands Mental Health Trust, London W6 7HH, England.

International Handbook of Human Response to Trauma, edited by Shalev, Yehuda, and McFarlane. Kluwer Academic / Plenum Publishers, New York, 2000.

5. Body-image affect: derived from the body as an expressive instrument and social stimulus to others.
6. Body-image attitude: ideas and rules that organize our view of our physical self.
7. Personal dominion: the psychic extension or intrusive projection of the self into internal objects or bodies in the surrounding space beyond body boundaries.

In terms of clinical work, these elements are not always easy to recognize or distinguish. For instance, how should patients who are complaining that they feel "displaced, isolated or ugly" be classified in this schema? Should such statements, which are not uncommon in those suffering from low bodily self-esteem, be viewed as an amalgamation of body image totality? If so, how should questions be formulated to understand the nature of underlying fears, repulsion or rejection of the body self? Nonetheless, the concept of body image totality is valuable in that it underlines the complexity of thoughts and feelings about the body. Raphael-Leff's taxonomy is just an outline of the different ways body image may be conceptualized.

The Body and the Body Self

Freud (1927) told us that, "The ego is first and foremost a body ego; ultimately derived from bodily sensations, chiefly those springing from the surface of the body." Without always realizing, we observe and detect levels of bodily and physical self-esteem from the way individuals approach food, touch, exercise, gesture, sexuality, breath, voice, tone, skin, complexion, hair, methods of protection, positioning, orientation, and proximity. There are a host of other ways of gleaning information about body sensations and feelings.

Sherrington (1940) coined the term proprioception, our "secret or sixth sense," that describes the continuous but unconscious sensory flow from the movable parts of our bodies (muscles, tendons, joints) by which position, tone, and motion are continually monitored and adjusted. Concepts such as kinesthesis (awareness of body movement or position) and coenesthesis (awareness of the body) can be considered related notions. Proprioception is so automatic that it passes almost without notice. It is indispensable to our sense of ourselves because proprioception makes our bodies our own property. This concept of proprioception can be understood in the idea that we can sometimes feel our body self, almost like sensing when someone is standing behind us.

Sacks (1985) elaborated the idea of proprioception in a clinical case study of an acute polyneuritis. A common form of polyneuritis, such as Guillain–Barre syndrome, has overwhelming motor impairment, but in Sack's case study the patient had an almost purely sensory neuritis that affected the sensory roots of spinal and cranial nerves throughout the neuraxis (i.e., nerves affecting the muscle, tendon, or joint sense). He characterized this patient as the "disembodied" lady because she described her self being "pithed like a frog" and that her body was "not hers" because it was "blind and deaf to itself ... a body without a sense of self." He suggested that this patient had lost her sense of proprioception, the fundamental, organic mooring of identity, or at least of corporeal identity. Many survivors of sexual abuse or sufferers with eating problems mention similar feelings without the actual physical symptoms prevailing in the case described by Sacks. Comments such as these are common: "I was watching what happened to me," "It did not feel like my body," "I was elevated above myself looking down." The term "proprioception" permits us both separation and reconnection of mind and body.

Kreuger (1989) also tried to integrate mind and body by listening to the body-derived experiences in the associative material to recognize how basic they are to the core of cognitive-affective life. A slip of the tongue can provide verbal imagery for emotional experiences. Metaphor describes the immediate self-state and often reveals physical state and bodily perception, as well as the emotional experience of the moment "I feel tight"; "I feel like I am falling"; "I feel disconnected inside." He also drew attention to the spontaneous metaphor accessible in everyday language, suggesting that it is a condensation of forgotten experience and can reveal the psychophysical origin of present psychic experience. Metaphor provides information about instinctual tension.

Sharpe (1940) saw metaphor developing concurrently with the control of body orifices. The emotions that originally accompany bodily discharge find substitute channels and expression via metaphor. The child's competence with feeding, walking, and sphincter control usually occurs in tandem with the development of language and words. The first sounds emitted are often words like "mmmh," "mummm," "yummh," depicting feeding experiences. Perhaps this has partly created the confusion that Stern (1988) pinpoints—that

> feeding is a vital activity for emergent relatedness for many reasons. It is one of the first major recurrent social activities, an occasion that repeatedly brings parent and infant into intimate face-to-face contact, during which the infant cycles through various states, including alert inactivity. (The newborn sees things best at a distance of about ten inches—the usual distance from a mother's eyes to the eyes of the infant positioned at her breast.) The feeding activity thus assures that the infant, when in an appropriate state to be attentive and attracted to stimulation, will be offered an engagement at appropriate distances with the full array of human stimulation, in the form of parental social behaviour that generally accompanies feeding experiences.

Stern continues,

> None of this has anything directly to do with eating or consummatory acts, although these are what brought the social occasion into being. What, then, about the fact and feelings of hunger and satiation? The role and place of hunger–satiation experience has loomed very large as a metaphor for much theory-building. Its importance is unquestionable in the light of both common observation and the prevalence of oral symptomatology and fantasy in many clinical circumstances. A relativistic perspective is instructive, however.

Sandler and Dare (1970) link the visual and oral, providing a bridge between the ways taste, incorporation, or absorption mediate the outside world. They comment,

> Observation of children in the first year of life has shown the biological function of "grasping" is transferred, as development proceeds, to both the hand and the eye. Thus the visual "taking in" may have a direct psychobiological connection with earlier oral incorporation. ... This does not mean to say, however, that the process of visual perception is accompanied by, or is derived from, infantile fantasies of incorporating the mother's breast, although the impression that this is so may be gained from some psychoanalytic literature. It is probably true, on the other hand, that the pleasures gained by the infant in developing perceptual and motor achievements are developmentally related to the pleasures of eating, and this is a field well worth exploring further.

Anzieu (1990a) has focused on other elements of bodily vibrations, in particular the skin. "The body is the bedrock of the mind. ... The surface of the body allows us to distinguish excitations of external origin from those of internal origin." He suggests further that

> tactile experience has the peculiarity in comparison with all other sensory experiences of being at once endogenous and exogenous, active and passive. I touch my nose with my finger: my finger gives me an active sensation of being touched by something. This double sensation, passive and active, is peculiar to the skin. Tactile sensation procures the basic distinction between "inside" and "outside," and it is only the skin that can provide it; the other senses can only do it by reference to tactile sensation. ... A proof, what is more is that you find human beings who suffer from blindness or deafness or no sense of smell, and this does not prevent them from living, nor from succeeding in communicating, perhaps in a somewhat more complicated way but they do communicate. By contrast, there is no human being without a virtually complete envelope of skin. If one-seventh of the skin is destroyed by accident, lesion or burns. ... The skin is so fundamental its functioning is taken so much for granted, that no one notices its existence until the moment it fails.

Anzieu makes links between skin and body image, and this could extend Raphael-Leff's totality to include skin image or body skin. In relation to trauma and body image, Anzieu's thinking heralds paradoxes of fusion and division in terms of what separates and joins the body and the images held about it. One paradox is configured in the questions about how sensory motor processes influence and affect mental processes. For example, assaults to the visual and auditory senses, as well as the imagination, wreak as much if not more anguish than actual physiological injury or loss. Garwood (1996) observes that "being forced to be totally passive and helpless in the face of the Holocaust was perhaps the most devastating experience of the survivor." More recently, Danieli (1999) has developed this thinking in terms of the experience of second and third generation survivors and Tauber (1999) specifically with reference to survivors of the Holocaust who work as therapists.

Paradoxes with Traumas and Images

There is also a paradox in relation to the ideas about body image and the blind or partially sighted. Wagner-Lamp and Oliver (1988) have sought to bring imagery into the world of the visually impaired by distinguishing different kinds of imagery, including the eidectic, involuntary, voluntary, imagery for desensitization, and guided imagery. They describe how "imagery with memory and imagination opens the inner eye and brings the light of an inner vision into ... darkness." McFarlane (1989) expands on this in relation to blindness and anorexia nervosa. Blagden (1997) shows how certain concepts, such as "yellow," "transparent," "outline," "glimmer," require extra explanation for those with impaired vision but feelings and visions about body images can be accessed and vocalized in creative ways. Her theory, co-authored in Blagden and Everett (1992), is neatly encapsulated in their title, "What colour is the wind?"

Assessment of Body Image

In the world of eating disorders, there is an interesting controversy about the measurement of body image and its significance in relation to recovery. Some researchers (Fernandez-Aranda, 1995; Probst, 1995) have concluded that the sense of anguish about the body and its image cannot easily be measured or quantified. Yet it is still used as an indicator of bulimia in psychiatric assessments such as DSM-IV (American Psychiatric Association, 1994). Thomson, Penner, and Altabe (1990) summarize many available measures to assess body image, which include scales; questionnaires; computer body mapping; the distorting video image; and the light beam method (where subjects estimate the width of their body with lights). Methods of measurement and evaluation have become so complex that before selecting their method, clinicians need to be clear initially about their purpose in making the assessment. Most clinicians who diagnose body image disturbance have developed their own individual methods of assessment, sometimes by amalgamating different body-image assessment scales. Cash and Pruzinsky's (1994) work demonstrates how even the most sophisticated methods of diagnosis do not cohere into a consistent schema for DSM-IV diagnosis. Such a codified system would eclipse the advantages of a variety of techniques to diagnose and treat body image disturbance. Even so, the information about the benefits and shortcomings of the different methods are rarely available to the patients or users before they embark on treatment. Robinson, Dare, Lieberman, and Curry (1998) have analyzed the issue of preliminary preparation before treatments—specifically with regard to body image and bodily recovery—and shown how patients rarely approach their troubled feelings about their bodily image from the standpoint of a quest for body image therapy.

Body-Image Therapy

Presupposed in body-image therapy is the question of the appropriateness of the treatment for the type of body-image problem. Clinicians mostly consider that their general remit includes the enhancement of bodily self-esteem. They aim to integrate this into whatever realms of therapy they implement. Yet the wide diversity of ideas on what constitutes disrupted or distorted body image is steeped in the underlying confusion about the nature of bodily self-esteem. Later in this chapter some delineations are drawn of the various constituents of bodily self-esteem, to begin clarifying how they may be used in clinical and research methods.

Cash (1991) developed a cognitive technique, "body image therapy," that uses questionnaires, tapes, scales, and imaginative fantasy. His body image program starts with a body-satisfaction assessment and a "situational inventory of body-image distress and automatic body-image thoughts." His treatments proceed through to desensitization logs, defeating, self-defeating, and affirming behaviors, and finish with private body talk, new self-reflections, corrective thinking, cognitive errors, and preventative maintenance.

Conger (1994) challenges the separation of verbal and bodywork therapies by integrating Reich's concepts of "character armoring" with psychoanalytical and Jungian theories. Broom (1997) advocates that disease or illness is a language in itself. He says, "in a patient's choice of disorder it is often possible to discern a statement or a language of the body. Illness (or some illnesses) seen from this perspective is construed as a form of communication."

Other methods of body-image therapy include the psychodynamic and the Feldenkrais. The latter is a unique psychophysical approach that uses movement exercises, similar to yoga, to retrain the nervous system in enhancing body image and promoting embodiment. Marcia Hutchinson (1994) developed it into a type of program specifically for body-image therapy. Two comments are particularly illuminating in her approach. "Since image is the language of the unconscious and of feelings, the focused use of imagery is also appropriate for accessing primary-process material and affective memories." She continues, "a single image can symbolise and arouse an entire constellation of meanings, which can then be explored." She then sketches a time-limited and structured body-image therapy program, based on her theory of recovery. As has been mentioned already, disrupted bodily self-esteem does not necessarily have exterior indications, and in this respect the relationship between body image and sexual abuse should be considered. The literature in this field has at times become ensnared in controversy about causation rather than exploring possible connections. It is easy to leap to the conclusion that patients who have been sexually abused develop eating disorders, which may not always be the case, as Fairburn (1992) argues.

Connections between Body Images and Sexual Abuse

Sexual abuse probably has an impact on body image, but there is little in the relevant literature that documents this. Even Herman's (1992) findings (an exception) mention body image only in passing. Hardly researched is the impact on the sense of the body engendered by isolation, the loss of loved ones in war, or political troubles. Freund (1990) suggests that emotional modes of being connect our embodied selves to social relationships in ways which fundamentally shape our ability to achieve bodily well-being. Similarly, van der Kolk, McFarlane, and Weisaeth (1996) say "A person's bodily response of fear can be mitigated by safety of attachments, by security of meaning schemes, and by a body whose reactions to environmental stress can be predicated and controlled. One of the mysteries of the mind is that as long as trauma is experienced in the form of speechless terror, the body continues to conditioned stimuli as a return of trauma, without the capacity to define alternative courses of action." The type of violations that occur to the body in sexual abuse are likely to have an impact on feelings about appearance and body image, although connections between sexual abuse and symptoms of anorexia and bulimia are not fully researched. Pope and Hudson (1992) have questioned whether there *are* links between bulimia nervosa and sexual abuse. But Vanderlinden and Vandereycken (1996), in their critique of this position, draw parallels between the statistics indicating the levels of those surviving sexual abuse and bulimia and the levels of abuse in the general population rates. They conclude, "there is no reasonable argument to question our conviction that sexual/physical abuse in childhood places adults at special risk for developing crises." Some writers, such as Schmidt, Tiller, and Treasure (1993) suggest that "childhood adversity" can contribute to the form of eating disorder that later develops and 65% of their study of bulimic patients had suffered abuse as children. Herzog et al. (1993) also found similarly that 65% of those in their study of eating-disordered women reported childhood sexual abuse. Other studies, such as Folsom et al. (1989), Calam and Slade (1989), Beckman and Burns (1990), and Gregory-Bills (1990), report similar findings.

Pyle (1992) supplies evidence that shows that treatment failure can be linked to histories of abuse, especially when the abuse has not been addressed. Leon et al. (1987) found that negativity toward sexuality predicted poor psychological status at the end of treatment, especially influencing patient's measures of body image. Studies of differing racial groups, such as Ahmad et al. (1994), pinpoint more positive body image among Caucasian and Hindu adolescents than among Muslims. How attitudes toward body image foster the building of immunity systems when traumas have been experienced has not been researched. This highlights the confusion between body and mind or the split between psyche and soma. Costin (1996) says, "The separation of the psychological self from the body self is an overriding feature of eating-disorder patients and those with sexual abuse histories, and the most extreme cases are those who have both. How the body/mind separation becomes manifest is crucial and points to the need for the body self to be directly part of the treatment." She suggests that manifestations include disassociation, numbness, somatization, reenactment, and repetition. Anzieu (1990b), quoting Pankow, suggests that the two functions of body image are to provide spatial form and to gain experience of dynamic contents endowed with meaning. By concentrating on the function of body image, its role in bodily recovery may become clearer.

Bodily Recovery

Given these findings, how should clinicians think about bodily recovery? Van der Kolk (1999) has undertaken research into language development and the evolution of stress modelling, as well as affect regulation. He suggests "early attachment relations are critical because they help individuals construct the world. These maps determine how people see themselves and their significant others ... the more one is capable of modifying feelings with thought, the more flexibility one has in responding to a given challenge." van der Kolk's work (1996) epitomizes his thinking about body processes and he outlines the use of images in "exposure therapy" but he merely mentions in passing the topic of body image as an entity in itself. Herman's (1992) three stages of recovery can be applied to physical and bodily recovery.

Stage One: Safety and the Establishment of Control

At this stage, bodily symptoms are most intense and out of control. Physical behaviour can be risky and destructive and can include self-harm. Sufferers can feel that their bodies do not belong to them because of the disassociation and splitting from the mind. Nightmares (and sometimes night sweats) can be important elements. Other features comprise disoriented sensations; vacillating feelings about bodily touch; hearing noises, like breathing or imagining footsteps; and frequent physical problems, such as headaches, allergies, stomach problems, tiredness, dizziness, and vaginal infections. Bodily boundaries are hard to draw. There may be oscillating desires for closeness and withdrawal, substance abuse, sexual problems, and disassociation. Herman uses the metaphor of the marathon because it captures the strong behavioral focus of conditioning the body, as well as the psychological dimensions of determination and courage. Distortions in the image of the body are probably most magnified at this point. How these distortions of body image commonly manifest themselves has rarely been researched, but in terms of typical body functioning, Cash and Pruzinsky (1990) suggest that hatred of buttocks, thighs, and stomach is most common for women, whereas for men, one area, such as a paunch, bald head, or scar is the focus of preoccupation.

Stage Two: Remembrance and Mourning

Remembrance

Keane (1991) stresses that witness must be borne to the bodily disruptions and "sensations like smells, heart racing and muscle tension will be avoided because they are so aversive." A narrative devoid of traumatic imagery and bodily sensations is incomplete; the goal is to put the story and its imagery back into words. Testimony has both private and public dimensions that enlarge the patient's individual experience. Posttraumatic symptoms such as flashbacks and nightmares are also valuable routes to memory, and these begin to become more controllable at this stage and need to be harnessed through a "sequestered back channel of communication."

Mourning

There may be grief about the effects and ravages of real or imagined corporeal trauma. Individuals may struggle to find ways of living with the limitations of their bodies. The future can seem bleak when the insight first dawns that eating, sex, or some physical impairment may always be a problem with which to be contend throughout life. There may be sadness about time lost, impairment to physical development, and the ill effects on relationships. In terms of body image, feelings of despair and disorientation are at their most chaotic. They are no longer disembodied or divorced from the self and the full reality of the physical trauma begins to be assimilated.

Hornyak and Baker (1994) used "guided imagery" in their work with bulimics and anorexics: the client is asked to imagine her mother pregnant with her sitting with father at a holiday family gathering. The mother begins to daydream about the baby inside. She imagines the gender she would prefer and how she wants the baby to look. Father also daydreams. Their client's perceptions of the mother and father's ideal conformed to patterns in which the mother daydreams admiringly of a baby but not an adult body, and the father dreams of a baby boy. Orbach (1978) used similar "imaging" techniques with compulsive eaters. These techniques, devised to help sufferers of eating problems, can be modulated and reformulated to apply to other visceral violations. This can be accomplished by careful imagining the body before and after the trauma and contemplating one small change to improve feelings of bodily self-esteem.

Stage Three: Reconnection and Communality

Old beliefs and images about the physical self begin to be reframed into a new sustaining faith, and strategies start to be devised to grapple with the feelings and circumstances that engender negative body images. Patients in my working contexts speak of feeling that they can enjoy sexual relations or celebrate having curves or the resumption of menstruation. They are also confronted with trepidations and fears of different kinds. Where the bodily damage is more permanent, such as harm to the reproductive system, damage to the vagina, or loss of limb, there is a quest to find resolution by recognizing the loss or by trying to find alternative remedies to the physical harm. These remedies can be physical and psychological. Some reconciliation must be established between the self and the body-self. The sustaining bonds of body-image totality (attitude, affects, and ideals) must be integrated into a new schema. This involves reconnection between the body and the self. Individuals talk of "watching themselves being abused, and it feeling like an out of body experience." Being able to speak about the splits between the mind and the body helps to reintegrate them, so that after a time a familiarity with divisions moves towards greater integration of the mind and body. Familiarity with embodied connections starts to increase and there tend to be fewer "out-of-body experiences."

Hutchinson (1994) uses body-restoration techniques that map the landscape of self-feelings, memories, thoughts, inner voices, sensations, and intuitions as an antidote to feelings of emptiness. She describes being embodied as experiencing the "body as the centre of existence. Everything we think and feel must register in our bodies." The solidarity of a group can re-create a sense of belonging by helping those involved to recognize that everyone has dissatisfactions with their body. Negative feelings about appearance dehumanizes but a group can restore humanity. Rejoining the wider world and forming connections with a broader range of people is the last stage of recovery. The "specialness" of identity begins to be relinquished, as through the reduction of isolation survivors start to envisage their tragedy as embracing the human condition.

Boal (1995) uses body-drama, a technique akin to sculpting in family therapy and he founded a street theater, entitled the Theatre of the Oppressed. He developed games and other techniques for what he calls "spect-actors" who are both audience and players. This theater was and is used as a political force for change both in individuals and communities and he evolved it in the context of political oppression in South America. In his drama the "spect-actors" are all part of the performance and they decide the form of the production. The joker, or facilitator, must follow their wishes. Boal's principal ideas are epitomized in his creations of the "Cop in our heads" and the "Rainbow of desires" whereby different "spect-actors" play out different repressions or various desires. He uses sculpting, groups, games, and other body techniques to enact these internal processes partly as part of his Theatre of the Oppressed, partly as therapy, and partly as a perspective or insight to the oppressed. Some of the body techniques include the idea of repetitive sounds and movements that convey particular oppressions.

Harvey (1990) identified seven criteria for the resolution of trauma:

1. Physiological or bodily symptoms have been brought within manageable limits.
2. Ability to bear feeling associated with traumatic memories.
3. Authority over memories has been established: the person can elect to remember or not.
4. Memory of the traumatic event is a coherent narrative linked with feeling.
5. Damaged self-esteem has been restored.
6. Important relationships have been re-established.
7. A coherent system of meaning and belief has been reconstructed that encompasses the trauma.

The stages mentioned mark the lines of development that can alter ideas about bodily self-esteem, but they do not characterize the components or constituents of bodily self-esteem.

Bodily Self-Esteem

Bodily self-esteem is an ephemeral idea that sounds straightforward, "feeling good about the body," but such a formulation is deceptive. Among survivors, disassociation, suppression, denial, psychosomatic communications, and some of the other body–mind disjunctions mentioned already evince the need for caution about the accuracy of self-reported bodily esteem. Bruch (1982) claimed that the denial stage in anorexia nervosa is frequently the period when destructive behavior toward the body is at its zenith. Many authors refer to the notion of bodily self-esteem as if its components are agreed or understood by implication. Promoting healthy or good feelings about the body, its image, and recovery may or may not be articulated clearly by the sufferer. Questions inquiring into care, nurture, indulgence, and so on can yield responses that give the clinician benchmarks as to the areas of confidence and weakness about bodily self-esteem. Often these feelings are computed into the mind without conscious recognition. This lack of conscious recognition introduces complicated thinking about bodily processes into the arena. Some psychoanalysts have been assiduous in their attention to visceral responses.

McDougall (1989), for instance, inferred that bodily self-esteem is expressed in the language of the body, implying that each person's body language is unique in terms of psychosomatic process. Her illuminating clinical case studies are rich in the detail of the psychosomatic process. Yet her theories are difficult to summarize because of their intricacy. The quotes below afford some interesting highlights. She hypotheses,

> 1. Certain allergic, gastric, cardiac, and other such reactions may be a somatic expression of an attempt to protect oneself against truly archaic libidinal and narcissistic longings that are felt to be life-endangering, much as a small infant might experience the threat of death.
>
> 2. To achieve this purpose, the psyche in moments of danger sends, as in infancy, a primitive psychic message of warning to the body which bypasses the use of language. Therefore, the danger cannot be thought about.
>
> 3. This may result in psychosomatic dysfunctioning, such as the urgent need to empty the body of its contents (as in ulcerative colitis), to hold one's breath (as in bronchial asthma), or to produce violent skin reactions (as in excema and urticaria). Alternatively the psychic message might result in increased gastric secretion, heightened blood pressure, quickened pulse rate, and so on. Or again, the message may give rise to disturbances of such normal bodily functions as eating, sleeping, eliminating etc.

She further proposes that psychosomatic maladies can unconsciously serve a protective function, such as defining one's body limits. Fears of merging when in an affective interaction with others recalling unconsciously a disturbed mother–infant relationship, and the fear of being engulfed or abandoned, are alleviated by the somatic process or condition. Pines (1993), another psychoanalyst, also portrays a vision of bodily recovery. In relation to body image in particular she says,

> Biological puberty necessitates a change of body image from that of a child to that of an adult woman capable of bearing a child herself. The girl's awareness of her developing adult body not only revives previous conflicts about her identification with her mother but also intensifies bodily feelings and stimulation. A young woman's alive body establishes adult status but also enables her to split off and deny painful emotional states by substituting bodily sensations ... a sexual act which, to the outside world, appears to be an act of adult, genital sexuality, may unconsciously become a means of satisfying unfulfilled preoedipal longings for the mother and for being mothered.

Leff et al. (1982) used techniques for observing and measuring families with highly expressed emotion. Highly expressed emotions could be applied to bodily self-esteem. This could be developed into a method which characterizes the way bodily recovery processes operate after traumas.

Different authors accentuate their own favored aspects of body image but there is a consensus that feelings about body image are embedded in the five senses because the senses mediate the boundaries between the exterior world and the internal and external body self. In themselves such processes of mediation are also part of the function of body image. Formulating an explicit checklist of indexes pertaining to bodily self-esteem in order to provide pointers to decipher how these mediations translate themselves into aspects of self-esteem and to take steps toward finding ways to vocalize and sculpt the images on the *inner templates of recovery*. The following is in no way meant to be an exhaustive list; merely a starting point for conceptualizing indexes of bodily self-esteem according to my main working contexts at this time. Readers will want to evolve their own indicators of bodily self-esteem according to their working environments.

The components of bodily self-esteem I devised include appearance, boundary space, proprioception, expression, gesture intonation, and attitudes to bodily excreta. This categorization codifies material incorporated in the ideas of body-image totality. Codifying the nature of body image, bodily recovery, and bodily self-esteem in these ways may enhance the clinician's observational acuity and also may improve the chances of measuring and quantifying such material, thereby making it more accessible to research formats in future.

1. **Appearance**: Clothes are important. Dress makes statements. Anorexics, for instance, use clothing to attract attention or to hide a skinny body with lots of layers. Rosen et al. (1994) use the dysmorphic disorder examination, a series of questions about appearance over a given monthly period, to evaluate body image as an indicator of body-image therapy. Neziroğlu and Hsia (1999) have begun to research the relationships between sexual abuse and body dismorphic disorder and found correlations.

2. **Boundary-Space**: Space and boundaries contour the scars of the trauma. Torture marks or medical appliances can be concealed in the contortions of hunches, stoops, clothes, and so on. Individuals have a kind of personal boundary-space around them. How is this space shaped? This can give clues as to how the trauma was survived. Individuals can be helped to draw their own boundaries by learning how to voice their anger and planning how to say "no."

   Ellis (1982) observed that young offenders tended to have an extended sense of vulnerability at the back of the neck which was greater than the average vulnerability space of eight to ten inches. Argyle and Henderson (1985) used the statistical technique of cluster analysis to divine cultural variations in the anatomy of relationships and showed how relationships could be grouped into "high, moderate, and nonintimate clusters" according to cultural differences and similarities. Their work showed a cross-cultural consensus about appropriate behaviors across some clusters but not others. There seems to be no reason why a similar cluster analysis could not be developed to apply to different boundary-space issues that emerge in the stages of recovery for the survivors of trauma. This could include presentation, protection, proximity, and movement, and indices could be evolved along the lines mentioned below.

   a. *Presentation.* The body has its own presence. The way individuals carry themselves gives important clues to their internal body state. For instance, a neatly presented exterior, masked in makeup or carefully groomed clothes is often an indication that there is something intolerably messy and chaotic inside, indicating that one coping mechanism is to present a false self to the world. Hair gives a distinctive message. For example, alopecia (hair loss) is often associated with trauma.

b. *Protection and Proximity.* The tension that abuse instils is often held in the body. Stiff, hunched shoulders can hold many injuries. The boundary space also manifests itself in the ways closeness and relationships are negotiated. What proximity or closeness is permitted? What determines comfortable boundary spaces for individuals in their networks of family and friends? How are intimate and distant relationships positioned?

c. *Movement* can be overcontrolled or disorganized. When sexual abuse has occurred, often the way the secrecy about the trauma was maintained determines the patient's movements; for instance, in families where the traumas took place in an emotional vernacular that was tempestuous and volatile, the abuse is frequently subsumed beneath the general fracas and malaise. Compulsive exercising is often a means for anorexics and bulimics to reestablish control by purging and expunging negative feelings from their bodies.

3. **Expression** applies particularly to the face, as well as to verbal articulation. Skin gives important clues about internal communications from the heart of the person. Psychosomatic complaints like eczema and psoriasis are often indications of suppressed aggravation and aggression. Bulimics can be recognizable by the translucent pallor of their bloated skin (edema) and their poor teeth that have become vulnerable from the effects of reverse saliva after bingeing and vomiting. Expression would also allow for the submerged nature of trauma over generations as Tauber (1999) has implied in her idea of a compound personality where second and even third generation holocaust survivors can keep traumatic experiences deeply submerged over long periods. Similarly, Schützenberger (1998) has shown how trauma experienced as far back as five previous generations can be both somatically experienced or become the focus of preoccupation and anxiety or as she puts it, "mind-body connection." In one of her clinical examples, she instances the trauma of the 1915 Armenian genocide. At the age of only 7 years, the grandmother of her patient witnessed three relatives (the great grandmother, or the grandmother's mother, and the grandmother's two sisters or great-great-aunts) being carried off "impaled on lances as if their brains were dripping out." This patient whose daughter had died after a head injury, was one of a generation of several generations of hairdressers, who sought to "pretty-up heads," and several generations of offspring with what the patient described as "serious head problems." These problems included "neck-braces," birth with the cord round the neck, or birth with herniated cervical disk (depicted as "brains dripping from their head").

Kreuger (1989) suggests (in relation to movement and body image) scrutinizing for the following characteristics:

1. symbolic content;
2. unity of movement, affect, and words;
3. position and interrelationships of the body, e.g., hands and feet;
4. coordination of movement, e.g., timing, intensity, and change;
5. associations of client to movement; and
6. patterns in transference.

4. **Gesture** is an important visceral communication from the corporeal self. The levels of animation, depression, composure, and so on give important signals about internal feelings toward the body persona. This is often linked with

the disassociation between the body and emotion that occurs during trauma or "double think." If no resistance occurred, guilt can lead to body currents that are numbing, submissive, and compliant.

5. **Intonation**: The modulation and tones in the voice and responsiveness to sounds in the environment can become an intense focus of preoccupation as a way of disassociating the pain of the trauma. Robinson (in press) has shown more body parameters, such as the emblems of sighing, gasping, and fluctuations in inhalations and exhalations, in the inventory of breath.

6. **Attitudes to bodily excreta** from sexuality, menstruation, ejaculation, and food: all give off important messages about the way people assimilate and form their bodily self-esteem and identity.

7. **Proprioception**: this sixth sense that Sherrington (1940) described can often be confirmed by a bodily movement, like an angry flashing in the eye or a half-twitching, half-kicking foot. The atmosphere and the prevailing feelings and projections can usually be connected with specific body communications that will affirm diagnostic hunches and intuitive instincts.

Conclusion

Whatever the debates about the definition, form, or assessment methods of body image, most theorists agree that an enhanced sense of bodily self-esteem will help furnish bodily recovery. The components of bodily recovery are rarely made explicit or consciously calculated in the analysis of bodily self-esteem, but scrutinizing them carefully brings the idea of *inner templates of recovery* closer into vision. By amalgamating theories from the literature on the affects of eating disorders on body image with ideas about recovery from the writings on trauma, a new synthesis could begin to be developed, highlighting and isolating possible components of bodily self-esteem, such as gesture, intonation, and proprioception.

References

Ahmad, S., Waller, G., & Verduyn, C. (1994). Eating attitudes and body satisfaction among Asian and Caucasian adolescents. *Journal of Adolescence, 17*(5), 461–471.

American Psychiatric Association. (1994). *Diagnostic and statistical manual of psychiatric disorders, 4, DSM-IV* (p. 236). Washington, DC: American Psychiatric Association.

Anzieu, D. (1990a). Formal signifiers and the ego skin. In D. Anzieu (Ed.), *Psychic envelopes* (pp. 1–55). London: Karnac.

Anzieu, D. (1990b). *Skin for thought: Interviews with Gilbert Tarrab.* London: Karnac.

Argyle, M., & Henderson, M. (1985). *The anatomy of social relationships.* London: Penguin Books.

Beckman, K. A., & Burns, G. L. (1990). Relation of sexual abuse and bulimia in college women. *International Journal of Eating Disorders, 9,* 487–492.

Blagden, S., & Everett, J. (1992). *What colour is the wind?* Bristol: NSEAD.

Blagden, S. (1997). Personal communication with author.

Boal, A. (1995). *The rainbow of desire.* London: Routledge.

Broom, B. (1997). *Somatic illness and the patient's other story.* London: Free Association Press.

Bruch, H. (1982). *The golden cage:The enigma of anorexia nervosa.* Cambridge, MA: Harvard University Press.

Calam, R., & Slade, P. (1989). Sexual experience and eating problems in female undergraduates. *International Journal of Eating Disorders, 8,* 391–397.

Cash, T. (1991). *Body image therapy: A programme for self-directed change.* New York: Guilford.

Cash, T., & Pruzinsky, T. (1990). *Body images: Development deviance and change.* New York: Guilford.

Conger, J. (1994). *The body in recovery.* Berkeley, CA: Frog Ltd.

Costin, C. (1996). Body image disturbance in eating disorders and sexual abuse. In M. Schwartz & L. Cohn (Eds.), *Sexual abuse and eating disorders* (pp. 109–128). New York: Brunner/Mazel.

Danieli, Y. (1999). *International handbook of multigenerational legacies of trauma.* New York: Kluwer Academic/ Plenum.

Ellis, M. (1982). Personal communication with author.

Fairburn, C. G. (1992). Sexual abuse and eating disorders. Presented at the *11th National Conference on Eating Disorders,* Columbus, Ohio.

Fernadez-Arranda, F. (1996). Does additional body-image therapy improve the treatment of anorexia nervosa? A comparison of two different approaches. Presented at *European Council for Eating Disorders,* Dublin.

Folsom, V., Krahn, D. D., Canum, K. K., Gold, L., & Silk, K. R. (1989). Sex abuse: Role in eating disorders. *New research program abstracts: 142nd Annual Meeting of the American Psychiatric Association.* Washington, DC: American Psychiatric Association.

Freud, S. (1927). Footnote added to *The ego & the id (1923).* In *On metapsychology: The theory of psychoanalysis* (p. 364). London: Pelican.

Freund, P. (1990). The expressive body: A common ground for the sociology of emotions and health and illness. *Sociology of Health and Illness, 12*(4), 454–477.

Garwood, A. (1996). The Holocaust and the power of powerlessness: Survivor guilt an unhealed wound. *British Journal of Psychotherapy, 13*(2), 243–259.

Gregory-Bills, E. T. (1990). Eating disorders and their correlates in earlier episodes of incest. Unpublished doctoral dissertation, University of Houston.

Harvey, M.(1990). An ecological view of psychological trauma. Unpublished manuscript, Cambridge Hospital. Cambridge, MA.

Herman, J. (1992). *Trauma and recovery.* New York: Basic Books.

Herzog, D. B., Stanley, J. E., Carmody, S., Robbins, W. M., & van der Kolk, B. A. (1993). Child sexual abuse in anorexia nervosa and bulimia. *Journal of American Academic Child and Adolescent Psychiatry, 32*(5), 962–966.

Hornyak, L., & Baker, E. (1994). *Experiential therapies for eating disorders.* New York: Guilford.

Hutchinson, M. G. (1994). Imagining ourselves whole: A feminist approach in treating body image disorders. In P. Fallon, M. Katzman, & S. Wooley (Eds.), *Feminist perspectives on eating disorders* (pp. 152–168). New York: Guilford.

Keane, T. (1991). Interview, January 1991. In Herman (1992).

Kreuger, D. (1989). *The body self and the psychological self.* New York: Brunner/Mazel.

Leff, J., Kuipers, L., Berkowitz, R., Eberlein-Fries, R., & Sturgeon, D. (1982). A controlled trial of social intervention in the families of schizophrenics. *British Journal of Psychiatry, 141,* 121–134.

Leon, G. K., Lucas, A. R., Ferdinand, R. F., Mangelsdorf, C., & Colligan, R. C. (1987). Attitudes about sexuality and other psychological characteristics as predictors of follow up status in anorexia nervosa. *International Journal of Eating Disorders, 6*(4), 477–484.

McDougall, J. (1989). *Theaters of the body.* New York: Norton.

McFarlane, A. C. (1989, June). Blindness and anorexia nervosa. *Canadian Journal of Psychiatry, 34*(5), 431–433.

Neziroğlu, F., & Hsia, C. (1999). *Incidence of abuse in person with body dismorphic disorder.* Paper presented in Istanbul 1999 ESTSS (European Society for Traumatic Stress Studies).

Orbach, S. (1978). *Fat is a feminist issue.* London: Arrow.

Palmer, R. L., Oppenheimer, R., Dignon, A., & Chaloner, D. A. (1990). Childhood sexual experiences with adults reported by women with eating disorders: An extended series. *British Journal of Psychiatry, 156,* 699–703.

Pines, D. (1992). *A woman's unconscious use of her body.* London: Virago.

Pope, H. G., & Hudson, K. I. (1992). Is childhood sexual abuse a risk factor for bulimia nervosa? *American Journal of Psychiatry, 149,* 455–463.

Probst, M. (1995). Treatment and research on body image experience. Presented at *European Council for Eating Disorders,* Dublin.

Pyle, R. L. (1992). Physical and sexual abuse in bulimia nervosa. Track Workshop presented at *11th National Conference on Eating Disorders,* Columbus, Ohio.

Raphael-Leff, J. (1994). Imaginative bodies of childbearing: Visions and revisions. In A. Erskine & D. Judd (Eds.), *The imaginative body.* London: Whurr.

Robinson, S. *The inventory of breath* (in press).

Robinson, S., Dare, C., Lieberman, S., & Curry, A. (1998). Counting the cash. In W. Vandereycken & P.

Beumont (Eds.), *The treatment of eating disorders: Personal, ethical & legal issues in the treatment of eating disorders*. London: Athlone Press.

Rosen, J., Reiter, J., & Orosan, P. (1994). Assessment of body image in eating disorder with the body dysmorphic examination. *Behavioural Research Therapy, 33*(1), 77–84.

Sacks, O. (1985). The disembodied lady. In *The man who mistook his wife for a hat*. London: Picador.

Sandler, J., & Dare, C. (1970). The psychoanalytic concept of orality. *Journal of Psychosomatic Research, 14*, 211–222.

Schmidt, U., Tiller, J., & Treasure, J. (1993). Setting the scene for eating disorders: childhood care, classification and course of illness. *Psychological Medicine, 22*(3), 663–672.

Sharpe, E. (1940). Psychophysical problems revealed in language: An examination of metaphor. *International Journal of Psychoanalysis, 21*, 201–213.

Sherrington, C. S. (1940). *Man on his nature*. Cambridge: Cambridge University Press.

Shützenberger, A. A. (1998). *The ancestor syndrome*. London: Routledge.

Stern, D. (1988). *The interpersonal world of the infant*. New York: Basic Books.

Tauber, Y. (1998). *In the other chair: Holocaust survivors and second generation therapists as clients*. Jerusalem: Gefen.

Tauber, Y. (1999). Personal communication based on paper *Who tells the story? Compound personality in child survivors*. Paper presented at Mästericht in 1997.

Thomson, J. K., Penner, L. A., & Altabe, N. M. (1990). Procedures, problems in the assessment of body images. In T. F. Cash & D. Pruzinsky (Eds.), *Body images development, deviance and change*. New York: Guilford.

van der Kolk, G. (1989).The compulsion to repeat trauma: Re-enactment, re-victimisation and masochism. *Psychiatric Clinics of North America, 12*(2), 235–248.

van der Kolk, G. (1999). The development of affect regulation. Paper presented at *6th European Conference on Traumatic Stress*.

van der Kolk, G., McFarlane, A., & Weisaeth, L. (1996). *Traumatic stress*. New York: Guilford.

Vanderlinden, J., & Vandereycken, W. (1996). Is sexual abuse a risk factor in developing an eating disorder? In M. Schwartz & L. Cohn (Eds.), *Sexual abuse and eating disorders* (pp. 17–23). New York: Brunner/Mazel.

Wagner-Lampl, A., & Oliver, G. W. (1988). Bringing imagery into the world of visual impairment. *Journal of Visual Impairment and Blindness*, Nov., 373–377.

Waite, T. (1994). *Taken on trust*. London: Coronet.

Waller, G. (1992). Sexual abuse and bulimic symptoms in eating disorders: Do family interaction and self esteem explain the links? *International Journal of Eating Disorders, 12*(3), 235–248.

Weir Mitchell, S. (1872). *Injuries of nerves* (Drover, repr. 1965), cited in Sacks, O. (1985). The disembodied lady. In *The man who mistook his wife for a hat*. London: Picador.

Wooley, S. (1994). Sexual abuse and eating disorders. In P. Fallon, M. Katzman, & S. Wooley, *Feminist perspectives on eating disorders*. New York: Guilford.

Wooley, S., & Kearney-Cooke, A. (1986). Intensive treatment of bulimia and body image disturbance. In J. C. Hansen & J. E. Harkaway (Eds.), *Eating disorders: Physiology, psychology, and treatment of obesity, anorexia and bulimia*. New York: Basic Books.

13

Deliberate Sexual Torture of Women in War

The Case of Bosnia-Herzegovina

LIBBY TATA ARCEL

Women and men have been tortured sexually by all sides in the wars in Croatia and Bosnia-Herzegovina (1991–1995). However, all documentation proves that systematic rape was committed mainly upon Bosnian Muslim women by Bosnian Serb and Serb militia, military personnel, and other persons in authority, often as a weapon in "ethnic cleansing." Health and mental health professionals may play an important role in documenting rape in war, as well as in the treatment of survivors. The first section of this chapter presents data on 55 sexually tortured women who were included in the Danish psychosocial treatment programme Boswofam.*

On the basis of the 55 stories, an analysis of specific patterns and characteristics of the war rapes is presented. The second section critically discusses feminist conceptualizations of war rape, and the author puts forward alternative explanations. The rapes in Bosnia-Herzegovina have led to a change in the appraisal of war rape, especially in its legal aspects. From being understood as a sexually motivated "by-product" of wars, war rape is now defined as a politically motivated act, and this constitutes sexual torture.

Introduction

> A nation is not conquered until the women's hearts lay on the ground. Only then is this nation finished. This regardless of how brave its men are or how strong its weapons are.
> (Cheyenne Indian saying)

The goal of war is to defeat the enemy by military means and also to break down the morale of the civilian population. A sure way of affecting morale is to target women

---

*This study focuses on the war rape of Bosnian–Muslim and Bosnian–Croat women. For the rapes of Serb women, see UN Report S/1994/674/Add.2 (Vol. V).

LIBBY TATA ARCEL • International Rehabilitation Council for Torture Victims, DK-1014 Copenhagen K, Denmark; and Institute of Psychology, University of Copenhagen, DK-2300, Copenhagen S, Denmark.

International Handbook of Human Response to Trauma, edited by Shalev, Yehuda, and McFarlane. Kluwer Academic / Plenum Publishers, New York, 2000.

and children. Sexual torture as mass weapon in war, a "privilege" of the conqueror, injures mentally and stigmatizes socially the female victim and also her whole family, even the whole nation. Woman is symbolically connected with the earth, the territory. Hence, rape of women is equated with rape of the territory, and violent occupation of territory is often equated with rape, e.g., the expressions the "Rape of the Hun" (the violation of Belgium during World War I), the "Rape of Bosnia," but also the "Rape of Nanking,* etc.

When we in Europe, as well as the international community, heard with astonishment and incredulity about the systematic rape of women in the war in Bosnia-Herzegovina in 1992, we assumed that we were witness to an *unprecedented* use of systematic sexual torture as a weapon of war. As mental health professionals, we believed that we contributed to drawing international attention to these horrific acts *for the first time in history*. Very soon we learned that sexual torture of women has always been an instrument of terror in war (Card 1996). Despite that fact, war rape has until recently been a neglected and underreported aspect of armed conflict.

The societal and individual silence meant that we knew very little about the extent and the patterns of war rape in different wars, and even less about the way women, their families, and the community reacted to psychosexual trauma. What Henry Krystal calls "the conspiracy of silence" with respect to atrocities (1968) was, and still is, valid, in society and also among mental health professionals, contributing in many areas, to stigmatize, rather than protect, the survivor. This issue will be considered later in the chapter.

Brownmiller (1975), Feig (1981), Hoerning (1988), and Tanaka (1996) present data on historical examples of systematic and widespread rape involving Belgian, Jewish, Polish, and Soviet women by the Nazis, German women by the Soviet army, Italian women by Moroccan mercenaries in the French Army, Korean and Chinese by Japanese, Vietnamese by both Americans and Thai boat pirates, Greek-Cypriot women by Turkish-Cypriots and Turkish soldiers in 1974 (Blatt, 1992), and Bengali women by Pakistani soldiers in 1971.

In fact, the story of Bosnian women was not the first to receive international attention, but rather that of women in Bangladesh. It is estimated that at least 200,000 Bengali women were raped, with 25,000 subsequent pregnancies. They were later declared "war heroines" by religious leaders in an effort to avert stigmatization, marginalization, and even the murder of many by their own families. Yet, at that time we in the Western world could distance ourselves from these stories "from an obscure war in an obscure corner of the globe" (Brownmiller 1975, p. 86) as something that could not happen in our "civilized world."

The terror of unarmed Bosnian women, facing armed men sexually torturing them, while living in Europe, 800 to 2,000 km from our own homes was too close to be denied. Their fate concerned us, their suffering touched us, and, wilfully or not, we became witnesses. Consequently, the war-rape crimes in Bosnia are better investigated and documented than any other occurrence in history. They were documented by the media focus and human rights organizations, such as Helsinki Watch (1992), Amnesty International (1993, 1994), and Physicians for Humans Rights (Swiss & Giller, 1993),

---

*The "Rape of Nanking" refers also to the mass rape, killing, and looting of tens of thousands of Chinese women by Japanese soldiers who conquered Nanking in 1937.

and also by intergovernmental agencies, such as the United Nations (1994/674), the European Union (1993), and the International Criminal Tribunal for the former Yugoslavia.

The United Nations Commission of Experts developed methods to document the extent of rape and collected individual testimonies (1993). The International Criminal Tribunal has performed hundreds of investigative interviews concerning rape to prosecute the perpetrators of this war crime. The feminist consciousness of many professionals, both women and men, as well as of female decision makers and the humanitarian sector in the former Yugoslavia and internationally, have played a decisive role in charting war rape in Bosnia.* The author of this chapter was a witness when she visited Croatia and Bosnia in late 1992 and early 1993 as an expert member, representing Denmark, of an investigative mission for the European Commission of the European Union (at that time EEC) (Report of Warburton mission, EEC, February 1993. UN DOC. S/25240 February 1993). She was there for the second time when leading a psychosocial treatment program in Zagreb for Bosnian torture and war victims. The following is an account gathered by the author:

> Ajnusha was 25 years old and newly married shortly before the war. She was sexually tortured during the war. When asked in the Karlovac refugee transit centre, Croatia, in 1992, if she felt shame or guilt because of what happened to her, she answered:
>
> "The shame is theirs, not mine. And it is they, not I, who will have a bad conscience sometime in the future. It is true that they took everything from me, my house, my cattle, my body—but *I gave them nothing*, they took everything by force."
>
> Ajnusha was one of the few women who had the ability to differentiate between herself as an object of violence and herself as a subject without any complicity in what happened. Unfortunately, this was not the case with many others, whose feelings of guilt burdened them.

Health and mental health professionals may play an important role in documenting rape during war, as well as in treating survivors. This chapter is an attempt to bear witness for those whose voices have remained silent in this war as in many wars before because of fear of stigmatization and the torturers' death threats. Although a number of men were also sexually tortured in the Bosnian war, the focus in this chapter is on women. For patterns of sexual torture of men, see Loncar (1998).

Definition of War Rape

A strict definition of war rape is as follows:

> Forcible penetration or near penetration of a woman's body openings by body parts of or any instrument used by a person who acts in an official capacity during armed conflict with the purpose of manifesting aggression and causing physical and psychological damage.

This definition is narrower than that of sexual assault, which, besides rape, includes other forms of forced sexual activities, e.g., forced impregnation, forced prostitution,

*However, an unknown number of rapes were committed by the other parties, especially by Bosnian Croats during the expulsion of Muslims in Herzegovina and by Croats during the expulsion of Serbs in Krajna. The fragile coalition between Muslims and Croats in Bosnia required a "toning down" of their crimes against each other.

forcing the woman or man to take part in perverse sexual relations (e.g., with animals), inflicting pain on the genitals with different materials (stimulation of the erogenous zones), forced witnessing of rape and unnatural sexual relations, being forced to masturbate or to masturbate others, being forced to perform fellatio and oral coitus, exposure to a general atmosphere of sexual aggression that arises from being molested, forced to be naked, derogatory remarks, and death threats. I will use the terms rape and sexual assault interchangeably throughout the chapter.

Method

War-Raped Refugees

During the armed conflict in Croatia and Bosnia-Herzegovina, two million people were deported or otherwise relocated, especially to neighboring countries. Croatia, for example, received approximately 250,000 refugees. A Danish psychosocial program, Boswofam (Arcel, ed., 1998), provided psychosocial help, health, and mental health services to Bosnian women, war victims, and their families through four small counseling offices in cooperation with local professionals and with two women's organizations, B-H Women and Biser. The program provided various interventions to all war victims with special focus on sexually tortured survivors. The interventions included social support, medical treatment, counseling, psychotherapy, pharmacotherapy, and material help. Data on survivors who were included in the program are presented below.

The survivors seen by Boswofam were living as refugees in Zagreb during the years 1993–1995. They referred themselves to Boswofam for treatment, hence they constitute a selective (not random) group. The program field workers did the first screening and recorded sociodemographic information, trauma history, and presented symptoms and problems. Then they were referred, if they so wished, to doctors or psychologists for medical or psychological treatment. Problems in psychotherapy of war-raped women are discussed in Arcel (ed., 1998).

Data collection from refugees during war is always difficult because of the great mobility within the population, the unusual settings of help (refugee collective centers and small counseling places), the ethical considerations of asking traumatized people to disclose themselves, and the widespread suspicion in refugee groups. In the case of sexually assaulted refugees, we had to employ extreme caution with any kind of examination, registration, or mental health testing. Many of them were not resettled and had only limited residence permits, which made them feel unsafe. They were very suspicious of all kinds of "papers," and they hid and disappeared from the program at the least imaginary hint that their stories could be used for any purpose other than getting help. Even the professional custom of taking notes during an interview could threaten them.

Our contact with some of them was, at times, elusive. They came to the counseling centers one day, stayed away for some time, returned for some time, and stayed away again until they were completely sure that they would not be pressed into any kind of confession or examination. There were several reasons for this suspicion. First, they were afraid to be victims of inappropriate curiosity and public exposure as part of the international attention to the Bosnian conflict. Croatia and Bosnia were overrun during 1991–1995 by professionals from all trades who were interested in talking with "some raped women." Rape survivors in refugee camps found themselves suddenly confronted with TV cameras or journalists pressing them to tell their stories, with no control over what was to be broadcasted. Second, most women had been threatened by the perpetrators not to tell anybody what happened, else they or their families in other parts of Bosnia would be killed. Many expressed profound (and unrealistic) fear of being found in Zagreb by the perpetrators and raped again. Third, many women had told nobody, or very few persons, about what had happened to them, and they were afraid that the fact of seeking psychological help would reveal to the whole world that they had been raped. After receiving medical help, many disappeared for some time until the pressure of psychological problems brought them back again.

Therefore, the rule in Boswofam was that no woman should be pressed to tell her story if she did not want to disclose it herself, and no woman should be tested for mental health unless it was necessary for diagnostic reasons.

Table 1 compares the findings on sociodemographic data for 55 sexually assaulted survivors with a group of 1,894 nonsexually assaulted persons who received help in Boswofam.

Sociodemographic Data

Compared with the large client population, the group of raped survivors tended to be younger. However, almost 25% of the raped women were more than 40, supporting the hypothesis of indiscriminate raping. There was a tendency for a higher educa-

TABLE 1. Sociodemographic Data

		Controls (N = 1894) (%)	Sexually Abused (N = 55) (%)
Sex	Female	76.7	94.5
	Male	23.3	5.5
Age	0–18 years	9.7	8.0
	19–40 years	40.4	68.0
	41–60 years	32.1	18.0
	61–90 years	17.7	6.0
Education	0 years	9.5	–
	1–4 years	22.7	17.2
	5–8 years	34.5	48.3
	9–12 years	23.5	20.7
	13–16 years	9.2	13.8
	17+ years	0.6	–
Marital status	Single	20.3	29.1
	Married	62.7	47.3
	Extramarital community	0.1	–
	Divorced	1.7	1.8
	Separated	0.6	3.6
	Widowed	12.4	16.4
	Undetermined	2.1	1.8
Accommodation before leaving	Town	50.6	23.3
	Village	49.4	76.7
Present accommodation	Private	50.8	67.7
	Collective center	49.2	32.3

tional level in the group of raped survivors, probably connected with their younger age. The proportion of Muslim women among those raped was higher than that of Muslims in the Bosnian population. Most Bosnian Muslim survivors lived before the war in the area of Prijedor (northwestern Bosnia). This confirms many other reports that Prijedor was the area most mercilessly cleansed ethnically. There were more married women than single women in the assaulted group, and a few older widows were assaulted as well. Women previously living in villages largely outnumbered those from towns. Again the explanation is unclear. Town dwellers might have had more resources and perhaps did not seek help as much as the villagers. Else it could also have been easier to hide from the enemy in towns. Generally town dwellers left their homes earlier than the villagers who were bound to their land and cattle (Arcel et al., 1998). Finally, most raped survivors lived in private accommodations on the outskirts of Zagreb. This possibly reflects the family's wish to get the raped family member away from questions and from the inappropriate curiosity of countrymen and others. Families with raped members had a definite tendency to isolate themselves.

Data on the Assault

Almost all women (N = 52) were raped during 1992. By far the largest group had been assaulted while in captivity in a Serbian detention camp (Omarska, Trnpolje, Keraterm, Jaice); one took place in a Croatian camp. This result also confirms the findings of the Commission of experts who found that 80% of the rapes had occurred during captivity (1993). The second most frequent place of rape was the woman's own home. The remaining cases were raped in noncustodial settings. Captivity (N = 32) lasted between one day and one year (mean, 81 days). The most frequent duration of captivity fell into two groups, either two days or two months.

Almost 10% of the women became pregnant as a result of the assaults and there were three abortions and two deliveries. One woman kept the baby and the other gave it to be adopted immediately after delivery. If we include only women of fertile age, (N= 44; cutoff 45 years), the percentage of pregnancies is 11.3%. This percentage is high compared with estimates established in medical studies, which show that a single act of unprotected intercourse results in pregnancy in 1–4% of cases (Swiss & Giller, 1993). The most likely explanation is that pregnancy after rape is an additional trauma for a woman, so she will have a higher tendency to seek professional help.

As a rule, the women were very secretive about their sexual torture. For 12 women, it was only the adults in the family who knew about the torture, for 8 only the therapist and a few other persons, and for 4 only the children. Five of the 26 married women kept it secret from their husbands. In other words, none of the women we have treated is identical with the many Bosnian women who have stepped forward for the mass media and other investigations and talked either in public or with foreigners about the torture. In describing the number of persons who knew about their rapes, the women did not include the actual witnesses of the assault itself. So in reality more persons knew about it, but they did not belong to the immediate social circle. Given the general atmosphere of secrecy, the fact that so many survivors opened up in connection with their treatment shows, once more, the importance of the role mental health professionals have in documenting war rape and other human rights violations.

The attitude of families toward the assault varied considerably. The assaulted woman was accepted in 14 families, but the rape was absolutely taboo so that nobody, including the woman, ever talked about it; six families did not have this taboo and showed open acceptance and caring for the suffering woman or girl; six families showed indirect rejection by hiding away and constantly criticizing the assaulted family member for other reasons; and three families rejected the assaulted woman, and the husbands divorced their wives when they learned about the rape. One of these marriages was of mixed nationality with hostile in-laws, and the other two had been dysfunctional for many years before the war.

As a general rule, the Bosnian family, being basically European, did not ostracize a raped family member. Another general rule was the protective attitude the family members had toward each other. They took care to an unusually high degree, at least for a west European psychologist not to burden each other with their own problems. A special painful silence and restraint of emotional expression was the rule concerning rape. Two women who had been raped together, say two sisters, a mother and daughter, a daughter-in-law and mother-in-law, could sit in separate rooms and cry, remembering the terrible experiences, and still not communicate the pain to one another. Shame, concern for others, social taboo, fear of putting the pain into words, and chaotic feelings prohibited them from communicating with each other, and great emotional isolation resulted. Exactly for this reason they may have felt relief in talking to a field-worker or a professional they could trust.

Patterns of Rape and Sexual Assault

The patterns, aims, and functions of war rape/sexual assault vary from war context to war context and require concrete investigation and analysis in each instance. The analyses in this chapter result partly from the cases treated and partly from other investigations (Commission of experts, 1993). The illustrative cases refer to women who received treatment in Boswofam. Some details of the stories are changed to protect anonymity. The rapes in ex-Yugoslavia fall mainly into the five following patterns:

1. Rape before fighting reaches a region

Before armed conflict reached a region, small groups of soldiers or militia often broke into houses, plundered, intimidated, threatened, and terrorized the inhabitants, urging them to leave the town; the women were raped, regardless of age.

2. Rape in connection with capture of towns and villages.

When a town or village was captured, the population was driven out of their houses, gathered, and prepared for deportation. All valuables were stolen, and the men were killed or arrested and taken away. The women were raped in their own houses, often in front of other family members.

3. Rape of captive women in detention before final deportation

After a town or village was captured and the men were executed or sent to detention camps, the women and children were taken to various detention places. These could be small transitional detention places (a garage, mill, school, sports hall, or restaurant) in which they were kept for a short time before deportation. Others stayed in larger concentration camps for longer periods. In such circumstances, soldiers, camp guards, police officers, and paramilitary personnel would pick women, night after night, and rape them in separate rooms when the detention place was large, or rape them during the day in front of others when the detention place was small. In camps where men were detained, some were also subjected to sexual abuse. The women were sometimes raped in the presence of or by the camp commander.

4. Rape in "rape camps" or "brothels"

Some women were detained in houses, "pensions" (e.g., a pension in Sarajevo called Sonja's Kon-Tiki restaurant), or huts in the woods for up to 6 months, alone or with their children, apparently for no other reason than sexual abuse, and served the soldiers regularly. If they became pregnant, they were detained until it was too late to obtain an abortion.

Elements Common to All Rape Situations

Rapes and sexual assaults in the Croatian and Bosnian war had certain common characteristics.

Widespread Rape Was Part of the Early War Phases

Systematic rape occurred mainly during the early phases of the war (1992 and early 1993), through all the stages of displacement of the civilian population in areas that were crucial for military aims, from the first stage of national discrimination and plundering of homes of non-Serbs, to the middle stage of captivity in transitional detention places and large detention camps, and to the final deportation of the civilian population. Rape occurred in the later phases of the war, but to a greatly lesser extent.

Violent Gang Rape

Most rapes were done by groups of 2–10 men. Larger groups operated in detention camps, where officials were seemingly not afraid of punishment. Gang rape with spectators (family or strangers) turns one of the most private and intimate human acts into a public affair, exposing the woman (or man) to maximal humiliation and traumatization. Smaller groups, comprising paramilitary and military personnel, operated in the homes. The group structure shows that the rapes were not casual acts committed by a "few black sheep"; a certain degree of planning and group organization was required. Even though the rapes were a "public secret" for everybody, the victims were often threatened with death if they reported what happened. Rapes were often accompanied by gun or knife threats. Wounds, bleeding, inflammations, hormonal disturbances, and pregnancies were the most usual physical sequelae (see articles by Boswofam gynecologists in Arcel, 1998).

Sadistic Rape

Rape in detention camps often involved other forms of physical torture, such as knife cuts, cigarette burns, abuse with bottles, guns, and other objects. The physical torture was accompanied by psychological torture, e.g., the forced singing of Serb songs, saying Christian prayers, etc. Sexual torture of men was committed in the larger detention places. The larger the abusing group, the worse the dehumanization of the victims, who were eventually killed.

Expressed Motive of Expulsion

Rape/sexual assaults that occurred systematically during the early phases of attacks in the homes and transitional detention places were directly connected by the perpetrators themselves with a motive of expulsion: "You must leave now or we will come back and rape you again."

Expressed Motive of Transgenerational Revenge and Punishment

The narratives of rape revealed feelings of revenge for acts committed against Serbs during World War II or during the 450-year Ottoman occupation of the Balkans. Phrases, such as "You, Ustasha whore, killed my father" (addressed to a Bosnian Croat woman), or "You, Turkish whore, now ask Alja (Izetbegovic, the President of Bosnia) to come and help you" (addressed to women who were not even born during World War II), show that the perpetrators saw them as representatives of a powerful enemy (World War II Fascism, Turkish Islam). Through the rape, such an imagined enemy was made powerless and humiliated.

Genocidal Mentality and Nationalistic Superiority

Genocidal mentality is reflected by the constant idea that sexual penetration was somehow transforming non-Serb women into Serb women by that of forced impregnation. Standard phrases after rape were: "Now you are a Chetnik woman." "Now you will get a Chetnik baby." The worst derogatory words were used for the *Muslim* women, Balija (slime), and for the Croats, Ustasha (the Fascist Croatian movement during World War II).

Misogyny

The perpetrators' acts and narratives expressed a high degree of misogyny and rage against women. Degrading sexual references to the victim and the victim's mother were standard during the assault. The traditional dress, "Dimije" (a kind of baggy trousers worn by older Muslim village women), was ripped violently with a knife before rape.

Perpetrators and Victims

The perpetrators of rape could be paramilitary personnel, regular soldiers, police officers, camp guards, in rare cases camp commanders, and other persons in office. No estimate has been made of how many men were involved in the crime of rape. Irregular militia groups and younger, poorly educated soldiers were most likely to be willing to rape. Victims could identify specific rapists and torturers in the camps and provide full names and personal biographies. The victims sometimes recognized neighbors, colleagues, and former school teachers among the perpetrators. Serbs proper were described by the victims as more cruel and merciless than Bosnian Serbs. Estimates of the number of women who were raped range from 12,000 (Swiss & Giller, 1993), to 20,000 (Warburton Mission, 1993), to 50,000 (Bosnian Government). Many victims reported that one or more Serb civilians or Serbs in office helped them, at great risk to themselves (Vranic 1996).

Goals of War Rapes in Bosnia

Our observation is in line with other reports that describe the primary aim of the systematic mass rape in the Bosnia as a war strategy, designed to hasten the expulsion and deportation of non-Serb nationals from some areas, i.e., as an instrument of ethnic cleansing. Spreading terror and fear ensured that people would leave the area, fearing rape and impregnation of their females. It also ensured that they would never return, having experienced the humiliation and social stigmatization of being raped.

The Final Report of the UN Commission of Experts concluded:

> The presence of these factors strongly suggest that a systematic rape and sexual assault policy exists but this remains to be proved. It is clear that some level of organisation and group activity is required to carry out many of the alleged rapes and sexual assaults. One factor in particular that leads to this conclusion is the large number of allegations of rape and sexual assault which occur in places of detention. (UN DOC S/1994/674/ Annex IX p. 13)

The undermining of the enemy's familial, social, and national bonds by humiliating females and males, by creating scars in woman's and man's body and mind, and by socially stigmatizing women, comprises psychological warfare and is thus hurting the enemy's masculine pride and boosting their own pride. In a patriarchal society, each rape symbolizes military defeat and the impotence of the defeated man to protect his family's females. All of the men in the families of the women whom we treated, especially fathers of young daughters, felt guilt for not having been able to protect their women.

Secondary aims of rape activities were sexual services for soldiers, as a way to boost their morale and feeling of masculinity, boost their feeling of national superiority, or reward irregulars and regulars for their fighting spirit. The few perpetrators who were interrogated claimed that they obeyed orders, were victims of war propaganda, were afraid of being sent to the front line if they disobeyed, were afraid to lose their houses or to endanger their own families, or wished to revenge the loss of soldier mates or relatives (Drakulic, 1993; Stiglmeyer, 1994). Group pressure played an important role. Individuals who would not rape during war are called sissies by their comrades.

Military Masculinity and Nationalism in War Rape

Feminist conceptualizations, e.g., Hague (1997) define the strategy of mass war rape in Bosnia as genocidal rape, claiming that certain masculine ideals (e.g., men enjoying a position of sexual dominance, masculine identity being reinforced by humiliation, subjugation, and submission) are behind the perpetration of rape. Brown-miller (1975) believes that rape in war "reveals the male psyche in its boldest form without the veneer of chivalry or civilisation." Hague claims that, in the case of Serb perpetrators, such masculinity went hand in hand with the construction of nationalist identity:

> By raping and impregnating women and girls, watching men rape each other in prison camps, and assuming the power position of "masculine" in all rapes, the Bosnian Serb military and its allied irregulars proved to themselves their own identities as powerful, manly and, crucially, Serbs. The policy equation of Serb national identity to the powerful masculine position in the perpetration of genocidal rape, asserted the dominance of Serb and Bosnian Serb men across the Balkans. (Hague 1997, p. 56)

These descriptions of rape characteristics confirm that nationalist feelings and superiority played an important role. Such feelings contribute to motivation for torture and sexual torture of groups perceived as "lower" human beings. However, although masculine constructions and nationalist identities both constitute powerful motivations for war rape, one must be cautious in proclaiming them as *causes* of war rape. With due respect for Brownmiller's (1975) great pioneer work on rape and war rape, I do not share her essentialist view, according to which war rape reveals "*the male psyche in its boldest form*" (my italics). I believe, in fact, that the "male psyche" is the wrong place to seek the whole truth about war rape and that greater differentiation is required. In the following I present a preliminary hypothesis on war rape, based on reflections from my experiences in a war area between 1992 and 1995.

Sexuality in the Service of Fascist and Racist Warfare

It is my hypothesis that issues of masculinity and nationalist identity are exploited in racist military wars, yet may not be expressed as sexual crimes in other wars. For example, Vietcong soldiers rarely raped during the Vietnam war, and if they did, they were punished by public execution. Possibly the presence of women among the Vietcong helped prevented the sexual humiliation of other women. Hague's conceptualization, although challenging, makes problematic generalizations that equate Serb nationalism and masculinity with war rape. In the same sense that masculinity, which is boosted by rape, is perverted masculinity (in peace as in war), nationalist identity that endorses "ethnic cleansing" and genocide is also perverted nationalism, more deserving the label of Fascism and racism than nationalism.

Even though the extent of rape was horrific, one can claim that, in the same sense that the raped and sexually assaulted women, even in the largest governmental estimate of 50,000, do not represent all Bosnian women, so the estimated number of Bosnian Serb and Serb paramilitary and military personnel who raped do not represent all nationalist Bosnian Serb and Serbian men in office. Furthermore, it was a rule that a single rapist raped a greater number of women. This, naturally, does not rule out the existence of a deliberate policy of war rape, nor does it free the individual perpetrators from their accountability. The point, however, is that the main responsibility lies with those identified leaders and their followers who conceived and allowed war rapes, thereby cultivating and releasing a perverted sexuality and perverted nationalism. Permissive military and political leadership and social anomie during war lower the borders of acceptable behavior, change the norms, and corrupt and exploit many men, especially the young and poorly educated, in acts they would not commit during peace. As stated before, perpetrators tended to belong to the lowest military hierarchy, yet they had the tolerance of the higher hierarchies.

Going further, Hague's and similar conceptualizations would have difficulty in explaining the rape of Serbian and Muslim women in the very same territory by Bosnian Croats and Croats, of Serbian women by Bosnian Muslims, and of Serbian women in Croatia by Croats (UN DOC S/1994/674/Add. 2 (vol. V)). Should they also be explained by a masculine/nationalist identity construction in the Croat or Bosnian military, and, if the answer is yes, then what differentiates Serb rapists from other rapists? I believe that the scientific discourse on war rape needs more differentiated knowledge about the context and circumstances. Such differentiated knowledge is the precondition for facilitating the development of strategies of prevention.

Therefore, I suggest the following four dimensions as putative explanations of war rape.

War Rape Happens Because It Is Allowed

Bewildered and distressed by the extent of rape in Bosnia-Herzegovina and being in Oslo in 1993, I asked the late Leo Eitinger, pioneer in research on concentration camp survivors, what he thought was the background for the rapes. His answer was simple. They happen because they are allowed. He mentioned a historical example of martial rape of Yugoslav women by Soviet soldiers on their way to Germany during World War II, which stopped after Stalin, out of loyalty to Tito, prohibited the rapes with punishment of those who disobeyed (Eitinger, 1993, personal communication).

A high-standing European military officer in Zagreb, whom I asked about the reasons for war rape, suggested two "functional" explanations. First, rape was, logistically, a cheap way to induce expulsion. It does not need sophisticated or expensive weaponry, and it does not leave the attacker with dead bodies. Second, anxiety and physiological tension which accumulate before combat activities may be released in the form of rape. Accordingly, it takes a very disciplined military corps and harsh punishment to prevent rape. Notwithstanding their validity, such explanations suggest that impunity of perpetrators is an important mechanism behind the occurrence of war rape (see also Roth-Arriaza, 1995; Niarchos, 1995).

War Rape Happens Because of Misogyny, Especially in Military Institutions

Another factor that may make some men, without resistance and even with pleasure, engage in sexual humiliation of females (and males) during war, when allowed, is the latent misogyny that thrives in patriarchal societies and its institutions, such as the military. When perverted masculinity is defined as objectification and contempt of females, under certain circumstances the sexual maltreatment of females releases a feeling of power that boosts the masculine identity of certain males.

Some years ago Danish newspapers reported that during a NATO exercise in Jutland soldiers were running and shouting a drill song from the bottom of their hearts: "Rape! Burn! Kill!" Officers confronted with the information made light of the drill song, saying that "it was only for fun."

War Rape Happens Because of a Genocidal Mentality and Nationalistic Superiority

In the context of the conflict in Bosnia, systematic rape was clearly related to the policy of "ethnic cleansing" and thus received implicit permission or at least the tolerance of the military and political leadership. Questions for future study are, how is the connection created between the institutional level and the individual person's feelings? What is the link between archaic conceptions of Purity and Impurity on the one hand and sexuality as a transformation process? By what mechanisms are these fantasies cultivated, and under what circumstances are they actualized?

War Rape is An Act of Transgenerational Revenge

As mentioned before rape symbolically actualized revenge for atrocities committed decades and even centuries ago. Such may be the case in other regions in which cultural groups have been struggling continuously for territorial hegemony. Collective trauma is transferred between generations (e.g., Danieli, 1993), and thus can be reactivated under certain circumstances. A question for future studies is (Kordon et al., 1988) what role does the impunity of the perpetrators play in the transgenerational trauma? A Bosnian politician told me that it was necessary for the perpetrators to be punished by the International Tribunal, "otherwise the burden remains on our shoulders, so we have to take revenge sooner or later."

The Process of Dehumanization and Merger of Aggression and Sexuality

Above and beyond the previously mentioned factors, dehumanization of the other is possibly the one necessary condition without which war rape would not be possible. Orchestrated demonization of the enemy and cultivation of aggression to the point of being able to kill requires a psychological process of dehumanization and objectification of the enemy. Loss of empathy with the sufferings of those on the opposite side is the precondition for killing, as well as for the sexual torture. An interpretation of the "physiological release" hypothesis of rape mentioned before suggests the existence of hidden anxieties in warriors, related to the fear of death. Such fear may then be counteracted by aggressive sexuality. In this context, the contention "Now you will have a Chetnik baby" can be seen as a perverted expression of a wish to continue one's own life. Aggression and sexuality are merged into one destructive force in such circumstances.

Societal Responses and Individual Consciousness

Undoubtedly, rape is an act of destruction that results in physical and mental trauma (Allodi & Stiasny, 1990; Hanson, 1990; Holmes & Lawrence, 1983; Filice et al., 1994), so much more in the context of war, when violent sexual acts rarely stand alone and are always followed by humiliating and degrading language, psychological torture, and sometimes sadistic acts of cutting and beating. The importance of the societal response to such is substantial. Attitudes towards peacetime rape have changed during the last two decades in the Western world. A similar development has happened to the conceptualization of war-rape. From being understood as "a byproduct of war," it is now defined also in a legal setting as a politically motivated act defined as sexual torture. Although no woman who was raped had any doubt that she was subjected to destruction (Hoerning, 1988), many preferred to remain silent because they fear victimization and lacked adequate protection.

Such has also been the case in the ex-Yugoslavia. It is the author's impression that in both Catholic and Muslim communities it is shameful to admit a rape. Women are to be mute and suffer in silence, and such silence represents a "dignified position." Nobody forgets, nobody forgives, but most practice silence. Few women from ex-Yugoslavia have broken the silence, stepped forward, and spoke publicly about their sufferings.

The role of mental health professionals in the "conspiracy of silence" is hard to evaluate. Seemingly, Croat and Bosnian mental health experts were culturally unprepared to treat sexual assaults at the beginning of the wars. Until then, sexual assault was taboo, and research regarding women and mental health was undeveloped in socialist Yugoslavia. Personal communications from colleagues suggest that male and female psychiatrists and psychologists feel embarrassed when talking about sexual torture with a patient who has been raped. Krystal and Niederland interpreted this attitude as a defense designed to minimize the traumatization of the interviewer. With regard to rape, Krystal himself admits that, acting for three years as an examiner of Holocaust survivors, he did not specifically enquire about rape, and no case was reported. When he changed the examination procedure, five women in one year reported rape (Krystal, 1968, p. 341).

The societal consciousness of war rape has definitely had an impact on the work of all the help professions in the former Yugoslavia, bringing more openness to the question and greater protection for the women. Since 1992, almost all countries have given high priority to asylum-seeking war-raped women from ex-Yugoslavia, considering them victims of torture, rather than nontortured victims. Treatment and rehabilitation programs in Bosnia and all over the world are ready to receive and treat them without stigmatization and suspicion. Now they meet sympathy instead of contempt, understanding instead of victimization. The women of the former Yugoslavia were unfortunate in that it was their fate that redefined war rape as sexual torture for the international community. The psychological meaning of this redefinition for the victims themselves remains to be investigated.

References

Allodi, F., & Stiasny, S. (1990). Women as torture victims. *Canadian Journal of Psychiatry, 35*, 144–148.
Amnesty International (1993). *Bosnia-Herzegovina—rape and sexual abuse by armed forces.* London (EUR 63/01/93): AI.
Amnesty International (1994). *Amnesty international report 1994.* London: AI.
Arcel, L. T. (Ed.). (1998). *War violence, trauma and the coping process. Armed conflict in Europe and survivor response.* Nakladnistvo Lumin, Zagreb: International Rehabilitation Council for Torture Victims, Rehabilitation Center for Torture Victims, Institute of Clinical Psychology, Copenhagen.
Arcel, L. T., Folnegovic-Smalc, V., Kozaric-Kovacic, D., & Marusic, A. (Eds.). (1995). *Psycho-social help to war victims: Women refugees and their families.* Nakladnistvo Lumin, Zagreb: International Rehabilitation Council for Torture Victims.
Arcel, L. T., Folnegovic-Smalc, V., Tocijl-Simuncovic, G., Kozaric-Kovacic, D., & Ljubotina, D. (1998). Ethnic cleansing and post-traumatic coping—war violence, PTSD, depression, anxiety, and coping in Bosnian and Croatian refugees. A transactional approach. In L. T. Arcel (Ed.), *War violence, trauma and the coping process. Armed conflict in Europe and survivor response.* Copenhagen: IRCT, RCT, ICP.
Blatt, D. (1992). Recognizing rape as a method of torture. *Review of Law & Social Change, XIX*, 821–862.
Brownmiller, S. (1975). *Against our will—men, women and rape.* New York: Ballantine Books.
Burgers, J. H., & Danelius, H. (1988). *The United Nations convention against torture—a handbook on the convention against torture and other cruel, inhuman or degrading treatment or punishment.* Dordrecht, The Netherlands: Martinus Nijhoff.
Card, C. (1996). *The unnatural lottery: character and moral luck.* Philadelphia: Temple University Press.
Danieli, Y. (1993). *Diagnostic and therapeutic use of the multigenerational family tree in working with survivors and children of survivors of the Nazi Holocaust.* New York: Plenum.
Drakulic, S. (1993). *Balkan Ekspres—Glimt fra krigen i os selv.* Copenhagen: Spektrum.

European Community. Danish Mission (1993). European Community Investigative Mission into the treatment of Muslim women in the former Yugoslavia. Submission to the United Nations Security Council. UN Doc S/25240.

Feig, K. G. (1981). *Hitler's death camps. The sanity of madness.* New York: Holmes & Meier.

Filice, I., Vincent, C., et al. (1994). Women refugees from Bosnia-Herzegovina: Developing a culturally sensitive counselling framework. *International Journal of Refugee Law, 6*(2), 207–226.

Hague, E. (1997). Rape, power and masculinity: The construction of gender and national identities in the war in Bosnia-Herzegovina. In R. Lentin (Ed.), *Gender and catastrophe* (p. 50). London: Zed Books.

Hanson, K. R. (1990). The psychological impact of sexual assault on women and children: A review. *Annals of Sex Research, 3*(2), 187–232.

Hartman, C. R., & Burgess, A. W. (1988). Rape trauma and treatment of the victim. In F. M. Ochberg (Ed.), *Post-traumatic therapy and victims of violence.* New York: Brunner/Mazel.

Helsinki Watch (1992). *War crimes in Bosnia-Hercegovina.* Human Rights Watch.

Hoerning, E. M. (1988). The myth of female loyalty. *The Journal of Psychohistory, 16*(1).

Holmes, M. R., & St. Lawrence, J. S. (1983). Treatment of rape-induced trauma: Proposed behavioral conceptualization and review of the literature. *Clinical Psychology Review, 3,* 417–433.

Kordon, D. R., Edelman, L. I., Lagos, D. M., Nicoletti, E., & Bozzolo, R. C. (1988). *Psychological effects of political repression.* Buenos Aires: Talleres Edigraf.

Krystal, H. (Ed.). (1968). *Massive psychic trauma.* New York: International Universities Press.

Lentin, R. (Ed.). (1997). *Gender and catastrophe.* London: Zed Books.

Loncar, M. (1998). Sexual torture of men in war. In L. T. Arcel (Ed.), *War violence, trauma and the coping process.* Nakladnistvo Lumin, Zagreb: IRCT/RCT/ICP.

Niarchos, C. N. (1995). Women, war, and rape: Challenges facing the International Tribunal for the former Yugoslavia. *Human Rights Quarterly, 17*(4), 649–690.

Richter-Lyonette, E. (Ed.). (1997). *In the aftermath of rape—women's rights, war crimes and genocide.* Givrins: The Coordination of Women's Advocacy, Ancien Collège.

Roht-Arriaza, N. (Ed.). (1995). *Impunity and human rights in international law and practice.* New York: Oxford University Press.

Stiglmayer, A. (Ed.). (1994). *Mass rape. The war against women in Bosnia-Herzegovina.* Lincoln: University of Nebraska Press.

Swiss, S., & Giller, J. E. (1993). Rape as a crime of war—a medical perspective. Journal of the American Medical Association, *270,* 612–615.

Tanaka, Y. (1996). *Hidden horrors—Japanese war crimes in World War II.* Boulder, CO: Westview Press.

United Nations. General Assembly and Security Council (1993). Report of the team of experts on their mission to investigate allegations of rape in the territory of the former Yugoslavia from 12 to 23 January 1993, Annex II, UN Doc. A/48/92, S/25341.

United Nations. Security Council (1994). Final Report of the Commission of Experts established pursuant to Security Council Resolution 780 (1992), Annex 241 n.65, UN Doc. S/1994/674.

Viseur-Sellers, P. (1997).The gender policy of ICTY. In E. Richter-Lyonette (Ed.), *In the aftermath of rape—women's rights, war crimes and genocide.* Givrins: The Coordination of Women's Advocacy, Ancien College.

Vranic, S. (1996). *Breaking the wall of silence—the voices of raped Bosnia.* Zagreb: Izdanja Antibarbarus.

Wilson, J. P., & Raphael, B. (Eds.). (1993). *International handbook of traumatic stress syndromes.* New York and London: Plenum.

14

The Controversy Concerning Recovered Memory of Traumatic Events

LAURA S. BROWN

Before 1992, the field of trauma studies appeared to consider unremarkable the notion that memories for traumatic events could at times be delayed in their recall. Clinicians who observed trauma survivors, beginning with World War I "shell-shock" patients had noted that exposure to trauma frequently led to either hypermnestic or amnesiac disturbances in recall. Recall of trauma was commonly accompanied, in addition, by disturbance in affect and evidence of either numbing or emotional intensity was commonly present. Observation indicated that the process of remembering traumatic events often differed from that of remembering the everyday, and trauma presented itself as unintegrated into the personal narrative of autobiographical memory.

Different terms were used by different writers to describe the phenomenon of delayed or impaired recall for trauma, depending upon the particular author's theoretical perspectives, and terms including post-traumatic amnesia, dissociative amnesia, and repressed memory appeared at various points in the scholarly literature. But there was little debate among students of trauma over the principle that this particular manifestation of traumatic stress was real and observable across the range of traumatic events. Some trauma survivors had insufficient "forgettery"; others could remember only when the circumstances of their lives shifted in some manner so as to allow consciousness of the painful materials.

Since March of 1992, however, the question of how trauma affects memory has ceased to be a matter of unremarkable observation and clinical consensus among trauma researchers and therapists. Instead, beginning with the founding of an organization called the False Memory Syndrome Foundation, there has been a remarkable flurry of highly politicized debates, frequently played out in the popular media of the United States and other English-speaking nations, as to whether all such delayed recall of trauma is merely an iatrogenic phenomenon arising from poorly conducted, sugges-

LAURA S. BROWN • Seattle, WA 98015-4801.

International Handbook of Human Response to Trauma, edited by Shalev, Yehuda, and McFarlane. Kluwer Academic / Plenum Publishers, New York, 2000.

tive psychotherapy, the position advanced by the FMSF and its various supporters. Most of the debate has centered on whether long-delayed recall of sexual abuse in the childhoods of certain psychotherapy patients is real or is confabulated material created in response to suggestion. Adherents of the false memory position have asserted that the phenomenon of intrusive recall represents the sole expectable manifestation of traumatic memory (Loftus & Ketcham, 1994) and have also argued at times that most child sexual abuse is not traumatic to children and could not possibly be affected by traumagenic memory dynamics (Ceci et al., 1994). Despite the fact that the locus of the debate has been around memories of childhood abuse, the questions raised by the debate have sharpened the focus of the field of trauma studies on the relationship of trauma to memory because the underlying questions are those that would apply to any delayed recall of trauma, irrespective of the content of the index event.

In this chapter, I explore the social and political movements that have created this public debate because we theorize that it is impossible to comprehend this phenomenon absent an understanding of the social milieu that gives rise to it. Then I will briefly examine current knowledge regarding the impact of trauma on memory and the questions raised by the so-called "false memory" movement regarding iatrogenic creations of false beliefs about childhood trauma. Finally, I briefly examine a variety of theoretical models for delayed recall of trauma. It is my working hypothesis that trauma, as an event or process leading to altered states of affective arousal, cognition, and information processing, cannot *not* have an effect on the way the memory for the trauma is stored, retained, and recalled. Basic research on human learning has long established that the level of physiological arousal at the time of learning mediates recall and retention. By their very definition, traumata are not ordinary events, but rather events in which persons experience profound distortions in their levels of arousal. Although the ordinary rules of memory creation, storage, retention, and retrieval likely apply to recollection of trauma, the trauma itself, with its impact on consciousness and physiology alike, interacts with those rules to produce outcomes different from those for memories of ordinary experiences. Additionally, emerging brain research indicates that brain involvement in perception, storage, and retrieval of traumatic events differs from that involved in perceiving ordinary nontraumatic experience.

I am aware that therapeutic malpractice exists and that rarely such malpractice includes iatrogenic induction of false beliefs that are coconstructed by therapist and client as memories of childhood abuse (Pope & Brown, 1996). But I view this line of the discussion as a red herring that focuses attention away from the more basic questions of the way trauma affects memory.

A Brief Historical Overview of the Debate

Confusions of Meaning

The use of the term "false memory" is itself somewhat misleading in the light of current research and theory about memory. Memory, in general, tends toward a mixture of the accurate and inaccurate in all circumstances, given that human memory is a reconstructive phenomenon that is continuously undergoing transformation via rehearsal, retelling, and the addition of new input. Current cognitive science construes memory not as a sort of video or still camera, but rather as an interactive process that occurs within social and interpersonal contexts and is subject to suggestion, errors of inference, and variability over time.

Additionally, a review of the research on the topic of "false memories" finds a confusion of meanings. A "false memory" in one study refers to the inclusion of the wrong word in a list (Roediger & McDermott, 1995; Schachter et al., 1996), whereas another might describe an unusual, although not traumatic, event, such as being lost while shopping or going to the hospital in the middle of the night with an earache, that has been deceptively suggested to a research participant by a family member or friend (Loftus & Pickrell, 1995; Hyman et al., 1995; Pezdek & Roe, 1994), and in yet another, a lengthy or complex series of traumata at the hands of a family member such as incest, has been suggested by a therapist to a psychotherapy patient (Loftus & Ketcham, 1994). An examination of discussion sections of journal articles in which these memory phenomena have been described suggests that the choice to describe any of these phenomena as a "false memory" or the interpretation of capacity to produce such a belief as evidence that it is simple to generate "false memories of sexual abuse" often reflects the standpoint of the writer in the context of the current political debate. This variability in the use of terminology and willingness to extrapolate from certain kinds of laboratory findings to the complex process of psychotherapy indicates that an author's choice of terminology reflects struggles over the control of meaning-making in a particular social, political, or familial milieu. This confusion of meanings itself makes it difficult to sift through the controversy to its core.

The False Memory Movement

Despite this vast imprecision among scientific discussion of memory phenomena, the concept of "false memories" and a "false memory syndrome" have become part of public parlance in the English-speaking world, even finding increasing acceptance in forensic settings. This acceptance of the concept of a false memory syndrome is largely due to the successful public education efforts of the false memory movement, and in particular its lead organization, the U.S.-based False Memory Syndrome Foundation (FMSF). The FMSF was created in March of 1992 by Peter Freyd, a man who alleges that he was falsely accused of committing incestuous abuse; his wife, Pamela (who has been the Executive Director of the FMSF since its inception); and Ralph Underwager, a psychologist with a lengthy history of testifying on behalf of men accused of perpetrating sexual abuse on children. The founding members created the concept of a False Memory Syndrome (FMS) to describe what they believed was occurring in young adults who were reporting recovery of sexual abuse memories from childhood. Although empirical evidence for an FMS has yet to be uncovered (Pope, 1995), the concept has been formally defined as a diagnosis similar to a personality disorder (Kihlstrom, 1996), its detection and prevention are discussed at continuing education workshops for mental health professionals, and it is included in some of the standard undergraduate psychology texts now being produced in the United States (Tavris & Wade, 1995).

The FMSF and related groups such as the British False Memory Society have generated and framed a public debate over memory for trauma. Its gist is as follows:

- Traumatic events are always remembered because they are too painful to forget.
- There is no scientific support for the concept of repressed (also known as delayed, recovered, or dissociated) memory.

- Allegations that a traumatic event from childhood has been recalled after a long delay cannot be accurate. Instead, they are confabulations (Loftus, cited in Goldstein & Farmer, 1994).
- Most allegations of delayed recall of childhood sexual abuse arise from suggestive influences. These suggestive influences include self-help books for sexual abuse survivors, most notably the volume *The Courage to Heal*, in which one sentence in the original edition suggests that people who have the symptoms associated with some cases of childhood sexual abuse must have been abused, as well as a form of psychotherapy defined by the false memory movement as "Repressed Memory therapy, or RMT (Kihlstrom, 1995).
- Most individuals accused of sexual abuse by their adult offspring are falsely accused.

Several corollary premises arise from these core assertions of the false memory movement. For example, the FMSF has filed amicus curiae briefs in a number of state and appellate courts in the United States urging that courts allow no testimony on delayed recall of trauma, arguing that there is no scientific support for the concept of recovered memory. FMS proponents have attacked certain diagnoses, especially the diagnosis of dissociative identity disorder (Piper, 1994), on the grounds that such manifestations reflect therapist iatrogensis alone. The contribution of trauma as a risk factor for a range of human psychopathology has been challenged (Pope & Hudson, 1995) by the argument that most emotional distress is biologically based and determined by temperament. In the United States, groups associated with the false memory movement have attempted to limit the practice of psychotherapists in a variety of ways and have encouraged the parents of adults in therapy to file third-party lawsuits and complaints against those therapists, frequently resulting in the revelation of therapy records to the complaining parents. Such complaints have been construed by advocates of the false memory movement as the sole avenue for preventing the sort of risky therapies that they believe must have led to clients' delayed recalls of trauma. Some therapists (including the author) have been the targets of picketing and harassment (Calof, 1996).

The Incest Survivor Movement

On the "other" side of this debate, as it were, are two parties. The first consists of a grassroots, loosely organized phenomenon, the incest survivor movement. In the United States, and to some extent in other industrialized nations, the 1980s saw the growth of consciousness about the prevalence of sexual abuse of children, particularly in their families. Feminist commentators (Armstrong, 1978; Butler, 1978; Rush, 1980), therapists (Herman, 1981), and other critics of the mental health professions (Masson, 1984) began to write and speak of the hidden and silenced crimes against children, and adults who had experienced sexual abuse began to come forward with first-person accounts (Bass & Thornton, 1983; McNaron & Morgan, 1982) of such abuse, including first-person accounts of delayed recall of such trauma. In 1988, Ellen Bass and Laura Davis, who had been conducting self-help groups for sexual abuse survivors, published *The Courage to Heal*, much of which consisted of first-person accounts of surviving sexual abuse, with suggestions about ways to successfully get through the process and maintain emotional well-being. A number of self-published newsletters by and for sexual abuse survivors began to appear in the United States, and in the early 1990s, various celebrity figures exposed their personal histories of sexual abuse and, in the case of some, delayed recall in the popular media. The incest survivor movement appeared based on the premises that incest is relatively common, frequently citing Russell's (1986) 38% statistic. Psychotherapy, particularly therapy in which memories could be recalled, processed and integrated into a personal narrative was valued. This movement also credited as generally accurate all accounts of sexual abuse, including those delayed in their recall and those with content that was unusual or difficult for some to believe, such as stories of ritualized or satanic abuse.

Research in Trauma

Another party in this debate is the scholarly field of trauma studies. As noted in the introduction to this chapter, clinicians and researchers in the field of trauma had long been aware of the impact of trauma on memory. Frequently, trauma scholars derived their understandings of human trauma response from the experiences of adults with delayed recall of childhood sexual abuse (e.g., Herman, 1992). Additionally, traumatologists had found what appeared to be robust links between experiences of trauma and later manifestations of psychopathology, although such links were rarely described as directly causal. Although there was not a universal agreement as to the mechanism underlying delayed recall of trauma, its scientific acceptance was not perceived as being in doubt.

Particularly in regard to memories for childhood sexual abuse, trauma scholars appeared to be united on the notion that although it was not necessary that each and every memory of abuse be sought out and excavated (Harvey & Herman, 1994), it was valuable for people abused as children to remember and make sense of what had happened to them (Briere, 1989; Courtois, 1988; Herman, 1992; Ochberg, 1988) and to integrate these experiences into a coherent personal narrative. The field of traumatology also referred to a growing number of studies indicating that significant percentages of adults who reported being victims of childhood sexual abuse also reported having had delayed recall of this trauma (Briere & Conte, 1993; Elliott & Briere, 1995; Feldman-Summers & Pope, 1994; Herman & Schatzow, 1987; Loftus et al., 1994). Additionally, one large-scale prospective study of adults whose child sexual abuse experience was known to authorities found that after a delay of 17–20 years, more than 35% of the survivors had no recall of the index event, even when such factors as offset of infantile amnesia were taken into account (Williams, 1994, 1995). The data suggested that delayed recall of the trauma of child sexual abuse was not uncommon across vastly differing populations.

These conflicting perspectives on memory for trauma arising from the false memory movement, on one hand, and the incest survivor movement and the field of trauma studies, on the other, create the sociopolitical frame for the examination of scientific data. Next we turn to questions of the way memory functions and how it is affected by trauma.

Current Knowledge Regarding Memory of Trauma

For an event to be remembered, it must pass from working memory into long-term storage. Several factors influence this process of storage. They include the opportunity for rehearsal or repetition of the event; the familiarity of the event, allowing for an established cognitive framework or schema in which to code it; and the level of arousal at the time of the event experience and the retention. The ability of the remembering person to focus attention on the event or experience will similarly play a part in whether it is stored in long-term memory. The developmental level of the remembering person plays a part; children's ability to accurately represent and code events into memory differs from that of adults and also changes across early development. Finally, the social and interpersonal contexts appear to play a part in whether events are remembered, and social support plays an important role in improving event retention (Goodman et al., 1994; Tessler & Nelson, 1994).

Not everything that is remembered or stored is recalled, however. Much of what we remember is simply not salient to usual functioning or has become so implicit and automatic that it is not perceived as a memory per se. For instance, our knowledge of how to drive a car or place a phone call is in fact a memory, yet few people would describe "today I remembered how to place a long-distance call." Memories are often recalled from long-term storage when something in the intra- or interpersonal environment makes them salient. Thus, memory is considered to be state-dependent, and recall is frequently contingent on the re-creation of certain internal or external cues associated with the original event or experience.

Because the states of affective arousal associated with trauma are frequently unique and demarcated from those of ordinary life, they serve an important function in the storage and later retrieval of memory for the traumatic event. A certain level of high arousal, such as is experienced by some persons at the time of the trauma, may be helpful in retaining the event in long-term memory (Christianson, 1992). However, as Marmar and his associates (1994) have noted, some traumatees experience a *decrease* in affective arousal at the time of trauma. This numbing peritraumatic dissociation, as Marmar and colleagues have labeled it, can have a converse impact on how the event is stored into long-term memory. When the traumatic event is accompanied by both hyperarousal and peritraumatic dissociation, the stage is set for distortions, deletions, or gaps in the material that is retained in long-term memory.

Once material is stored, it does not remain static. New, related experiences, the acquisition of new data, and the process of recall per se all have an affect on what is stored. Loftus (1988) argued that new versions of events transform and also erase the original memory trace. New personal narratives place a new slant on stored data; as a story is retold, the relative importance and salience of certain events changes, as does what is stored in memory. Time itself leads to decay of certain memory traces, and recall for some very remote events becomes less clear. Additionally, various insults to the brain can impact memory. The lack of opportunity to remember and thus rehearse an event yet again can also weaken a memory trace. Weaker memory traces may require stronger or more specific cues to elicit recall (Dalenberg et al., 1995), even when an event has been retained in long-term memory, thus leaving individuals with the impression that they had forgotten and then remembered an event that was always technically remembered (i.e., retained in long-term memory), but was difficult to recall to conscious awareness.

Memory and Suggestibility

But no matter how well-stored, memory is also subject to suggestive influences, a fact that has been central in the debate over delayed recall. We will describe two suggestibility phenomena here. The first describes the potential for transforming an already-recalled event, research largely based on the work of Loftus regarding eyewitness memory. The second and more recent research stream concerns whether it is possible to suggest new information to individuals so that they encode it as a memory, even when the event "remembered" can be shown never to have happened in the person's life.

Loftus (Loftus & Davies, 1984; Loftus & Hoffman, 1989; Loftus & Loftus, 1980; Loftus, 1979) has pioneered the paradigm for studying the effects of suggestion on eyewitness memory for events. She reports a quite robust finding in a range of laboratory settings indicating that a clear, although minor, percentage of research participants will report a different memory of the index event (usually a videotaped version of a car accident or a purse-snatching) in the direction of the experimental suggestion. She posits that the memory trace has been permanently changed by the suggestion. Others who attempted to replicate her findings indicate that certain interpersonal demand characteristics of the experimental setting can yield different results. For example, research on actual forensic eyewitnesses indicates that they may be less vulnerable to suggestive influences on memory, suggesting that when the actual stakes for accuracy are higher, suggestibility may decrease (Yuille & Cutshall, 1989; Yuille, 1993).

Additionally, a purely cognitive model of remembering has been critiqued. Social psychologists Spanos and MacLean (1986) argued that the apparent changes to memory are simply changes in reports rendered by subjects who wish to comply with experiments. Some critics argue that memories associated with strong affect are less vulnerable to suggestion and more resilient than more neutral memories, such as those tested in experimental settings (Yuille & Cutshall, 1989; Christianson, 1992; Reisberg & Heuer, 1992), and that the Loftus model does not generalize universally.

Research on children's suggestibility has also yielded conflicting results. Ceci and his colleagues (1987, 1994) developed a paradigm in which children aged three and four are repeatedly read a story about an event that they are supposed to have either witnessed or experienced. He reports a robust suggestibility effect, although it is of interest that his younger, theoretically more suggestible research subjects appear less so than their slightly older counterparts. However, what also appears to be the case is that other researchers who attempted replications and extensions of Ceci's findings found more equivocal results. Smaller percentages of children were open to suggestion (McCloskey & Zaragoza, 1985; Zaragoza et al., 1987; Zaragoza, 1991), and some studies found that children were highly resistant to suggestions, including those with overtones of implied sexual abuse (Goodman et al., 1991; Goodman et al., 1994; Pezdek & Roe, 1994).

Attempts to Experimentally Implant "False" Memories

A research paradigm that has been vigorously pursued since the inception of the debate over delayed recall has been whether it would be possible to implant an entire and false memory of a traumatic event. Although skeptics of the false memory movement have always been willing to concede that it was possible, as Loftus had done, to suggest the presence of a "stop" sign when a "yield" sign had actually been present, they argued that it would be less likely to create an entirely false memory of one, or often many, complex traumatic events that were highly affect-laden, as was argued by the false memory movement. This debate was the genesis of a series of experiments, again pioneered by Loftus and her students and associates, in which attempts were made to induce false beliefs about life history in experimental subjects.

Loftus (1993) described an experiment conducted by Coan (1993), her undergraduate research assistant, in which the latter experimentally induced in his younger brother a false recollection of being lost, as a small child, in a shopping mall. Although some authors have been critical of this initial experiment because it occurred in the absence of usual protections for human research participants, and used young children as the targets of suggestion (Pope, 1995), it provides the basic paradigm for the most recent experimental scientific response to the memory debate. In this paradigm, a research confederate attempts to suggest a false memory to the target subject. The confederate is either an older family member of the target individual or is recounting information alleged to have been reported about the target by an older family member. In all instances, the material being suggested to the target by the confederate is portrayed as something that the *confederate* remembers. Thus, for instance, the target will be asked, "do you remember when ..." and the confederate will tell a story that she/he alleges to have witnessed. The events being falsely suggested can be defined as somewhat unpleasant (e.g., being lost in a shopping mall while a child, having a bad earache and having to go to the hospital in the middle of the night, pulling a punchbowl down off a table at a wedding), and several of them occur at a relatively high base rate.

A number of attempts to replicate and extend the original Loftus and Coan paradigm have produced provocative, yet not necessarily convincing, findings. Hyman et al. (1995), who used a variation in which actual events described by parents of college students were interspersed with false suggestions (earache and punchbowl), found that only approximately 20% of their target subjects were able to adopt the suggestions and that most subjects required more than one exposure to the suggestion. Loftus' own attempts to replicate the study using an over-eighteen group of targets and the original shopping mall story produced a similarly small number who accepted the suggestion. Pezdek (1995) found that when she extended the paradigm by having some confederates suggest a memory of a rectal enema to the targets, she was unable to achieve any adoptions of the false memory, and she interpreted her findings to suggest that subjects were less likely to adopt unfamiliar material into their autobiographical narratives simply due to suggestion.

Hyman (personal communication, 1997) has indicated that those targets who accepted the suggestion tended to score high on the Dissociative Experiences Scale and suggested that individual differences in suggestibility, rather than the simple fact of suggestion itself, may be responsible for the acceptance of suggestions of false memories. This comports with D. Brown's (1995) argument that individual differences in suggestibility, rather than any suggestion or trance techniques, might lead to the creation of inaccurate beliefs about childhood in the population of therapy patients. Others, including this author (Brown, 1996) have argued that the Pezdek study indicates that although it is less difficult to achieve adoption of a suggestion of relatively neutral material such as the lost-in-the-mall or earache stories, that it is more difficult to achieve adoption via suggestion of false stories of extremely painful events that violate a person's beliefs about loved individuals.

Models for Post-Traumatic Amnesia

The cognitive mechanisms by which post-traumatic amnesia may occur are poorly understood at best. We describe two currently posited models that do not depend on adopting any particular metapsychological theory (as is the case for repression as a paradigm) and are potentially empirically testable.

Yates and Nasby (1993) suggested that dissociation, an empirically demonstrable phenomenon with physiological correlates, which has been empirically linked to the trauma response, is the mechanism which is most likely to account for post-traumatic amnesia. Drawing upon Bower's model for the influence of the affect on memory, they propose a mental mechanism of neural and cognitive initiation of memories for trauma in the absence of specific disinhiting environmental conditions or triggers.

More recently, Jennifer Freyd (1995, 1996) proposed a social-cognitive model, "betrayal trauma" (BT), for post-traumatic amnesia and return of memory in the specific case of childhood sexual abuse. She posits that the evolutionary requirement of human children's dependency on adults will lead to an inability to know consciously of memories of sexual abuse/betrayal that are stored in long-term memory until the child is no longer dependent on those caregivers. She argues that the betrayal is what cannot be known, rather than the sexual contact per se, and that dependency renders cognitive "cheater-detectors," as described by Cosmides (1989; Cosmides & Tooby, 1992), inoperative for such children, leading to a requirement that information about the betrayal become unavailable.

In their review and synthesis of research on memory for trauma, Koss et al. (1995) argue that a complex model of memory that integrates understanding of neural phenomena, the meaning of the trauma for the individual, and the relationship of the traumatic experience to the overall personal context is what will be necessary to adequately explain the phenomenon of post-traumatic amnesia. However, they note that even in the absence of an adequate explanatory model, currently available evidence argues against a paradigm of memory for trauma as highly malleable or easily subject to suggestion.

Current Research Findings on How Trauma is Remembered

Experimental research on the actual recall of trauma also provides mixed results. Some themes emerge. Brewin et al. (1992) found that adults performed more accurately in their free recall of painful childhood events than their parents when both sets of recall were matched against concurrent records. Christianson (1992) found that although the quality of recall of a traumatic event was mixed, central details of the events appeared to be well-retained and peripheral details were more fuzzy or less accurate. Elliott and Briere (1995), reporting on a large-scale study of nonpsychiatric patients, found that all traumas had the potential to be delayed in recall, including such events as automobile accidents. One problem with experimental research is that it is frequently difficult to define trauma experimentally to accurately replicate the conditions of horror, terror, helplessness, and fear for life or safety, as well as the shattering of beliefs about the world, that commonly characterize traumatic events in their natural settings. However, the trend appears to be that trauma survivors have incomplete recall for what has happened to them, yet do not suffer deficits in accuracy regarding what has happened when their memories are measured against objective corroborating materials.

Neurobiological Aspects of Memory for Trauma

One of the exciting aspects of the debate over delayed recall is that it has taken place in the context of emerging knowledge of the neurobiological aspects of trauma and the impact of trauma on the brain. Because much of the available data are new and come from small samples, conclusive statements cannot be made from them. However, what does become clear from this body of research is that exposure to traumatic stressors, including sexual abuse in childhood, has an impact on both brain structures and brain neurochemistry, both of which are implicated in the storage, retention, and retrieval of memory for the traumatic events in question.

McGaugh (1992) and his colleagues (Cahill et al., 1994) report that neurohormones released into the brain at the time of a stressful event enhance the brain's consolidation and storage of emotionally laden events. Yehuda and her colleagues (Yehuda, 1994; Yehuda et al., 1995) reported that there are neurohormonal deficits, specifically, changes to the ambient cortisol level, in the brains of persons with both a verified history of trauma and reports of absent, fragmented, distorted or incomplete memories for that trauma. van der Kolk (1992; van der Kolk, van der Hart, & Marmar, 1996) has demonstrated that exposure to trauma leads to changes in the activation of limbic system and amygdala in trauma survivors, compared to a matched normal group. Southwick and colleagues (1994) presented preliminary experimental data suggesting that trauma survivors' noradrenergic response system varies from that of people without a trauma history. Some research (Yehuda, 1994) finds that increased REM phasic activity is associated with either the presence of PTSD or increased PTSD severity, indicating a change in brain neurophysiology in response to trauma. Wright and colleagues (1994) demonstrated diminished EMG and GSR reactivity in survivors of known repetitive childhood trauma. Geise and colleagues (1994) demonstrated impaired gating of the P50 auditory evoked response and evidence of CNS noradrenergic dysfunction in a group of trauma victims. Of particular interest is the work of Bremner and colleagues (1995) who reported decreased hippocampal volumes on one or both sides for child sexual abuse survivors and combat veterans. Putnam found profound biological alterations of the brain stress response systems in a group of sexually abused girls aged 6–15 (1994). This line of research, which is still in its early stages, suggests that there are neurochemical correlates of certain kinds of intense emotional experiences. Such neurochemical changes are posited to impact memory storage and retrieval.

The development of workable and testable hypotheses regarding the specific effect of trauma on memory is still relatively new. There is also debate over the possibility that such neurobiological and neurochemical phenomena are evidence of a biological susceptibility to the development of PTSD and other psychopathology in the wake of trauma exposure, as is argued by Yehuda and McFarlane (1995), or represent the sequelae of the trauma exposure. However, what does appear to be clear is that brain structures that affect memory are changed from the norm in trauma survivors with symptoms of post-traumatic amnesia.

Summary and Conclusions

What conclusions may be drawn from the current state of science regarding trauma and memory? First, we would argue that assertions that all "real" traumatic events will be recalled without delay cannot be supported by the available data. Such assertions should, instead, be regarded as polemics in a highly politicized debate in which appeals to authority are unsupported by the bulk of the evidence. In every study, even those conducted by adherents of the false memory perspective (e.g., Loftus et al., 1994), some percentage of individuals exposed to a known traumatic stressor will report a delay in recalling that event. Some extremely striking personal case examples (e.g., Cheit, 1994; Cutting, 1996; Fitzpatrick, 1994; Van Derbur Atler, 1991) of extensively corroborated delayed recalls of trauma also serve as refutation to the assertion made by many in the false memory movement that "real" trauma is remembered trauma. Particularly in those instances where the meaning of the trauma is such that it threatens important personal relationships or, on occasion, the core sense of self and identity, its recall may be hindered for many years, and it may be accompanied by extreme emotional distress and self-doubt.

This is not to argue that *all* reports of delayed recall of trauma are accurate, however. The popular media have presented us with such spectacles as reports of recall of trauma that occurred at the age of six months, of alien abduction (Mack, 1995), or of past lives. Controversy continues in the field of dissociative disorder treatment over reports of ritualized abuse (Ross, 1995). And even reported delayed recalls of more "ordinary" forms of childhood trauma are not necessarily accurate. Because of developmental differences from adults, children may distort information as it is being stored, leading to inaccurate reports in later life. Additionally, some first-person accounts of abusive so-called therapy experiences indicate that under some conditions, therapists can and have used coercive techniques to induce powerful yet temporary false beliefs in an experience of childhood sexual abuse (Gavigan, 1994; Pasley, 1994). The author has evaluated individuals in the process of suing therapists who have engaged in such behaviors, which included misuse of hypnosis, group coercion techniques, and other cult-like activities by the so-called therapists. The frequency with which this occurs, however, appears to be quite low. Even the false memory movement has been unable to generate significant numbers of reports of such experiences.

Second, I would argue that there is yet to be a conclusive explanatory model for the appearance of post-traumatic amnesia. Arguments over the reality of repression are not useful to our comprehension of delayed recall because they assume adherence to a particular theory of the phenomenon, which I believe is a premature closure of the paradigm. Currently, models that draw upon cognitive science, such as J. Freyd's BT model and those that explore the neurobiological concomitants of dissociation, appear to be the most promising. As it becomes more possible to conduct noninvasive studies of the working brain post-trauma via new imaging techniques, the mechanisms of post-traumatic amnesia and remembering may become more apparent anatomically, thus allowing more precise cognitive models to be developed. However, it is premature for anyone to assert that any one model currently adequately explains this phenomenon.

More of concern are the social and legal implications of this debate. In the United States, Canada, and Great Britain, false memory defenses to current charges of rape, sexual assault, and sexual abuse have already possibly served to obstruct justice in criminal cases, as legal authorities find the notion persuasive that a victim's accusations are confabulated, particularly when the victim is a child. Lawsuits against therapists in the United States by parents of adults who have delayed recall of abuse are proliferating. Because the reality of child sexual abuse challenges most of our deeply held illusions about the safety of children in families, the narrative of the false memory movement, which denies sexual abuse, particularly in white and upper middle class homes, is seductive and appealing. It is far simpler to accuse misguided or politically motivated therapists of implanting memories of abuse, as has been asserted by adherents of the false memory movement (Goodyear-Smith, 1993; Loftus & Ketcham, 1994; Pendergrast,

1995; Wakefield & Underwager, 1994), than it is to recognize the frequency with which abuse occurs in erstwhile, fine, upstanding families from the dominant social group. Because no empirical evidence exists for a False Memory Syndrome (Carstensen et al, 1993; Pope, 1995), the relative ease with which it has been accepted contrasts starkly with the struggles now faced to convince the lay public that post-traumatic amnesia, an empirically well-documented phenomenon, does exist.

However, ultimately this debate has been fruitful for the field of trauma studies. It has generated a large volume of inquiry into the phenomenon of post-traumatic amnesia and has spurred collaborations between traumatologists and cognitive scientists that might never have otherwise occurred. It has affirmed the reality of this long-observed phenomenon and led to the creation of new models for understanding the biological, intrapersonal, and sociocultural sequelae of trauma.

References

Armstrong, L. (1978). *Kiss daddy goodnight: A speakout on incest.* New York: Pocket Books.

Bass, E., & Davis, L. (1988). *The courage to heal: A guide for women survivors of child sexual abuse.* New York: Perennial/Harper Collins.

Bass, E., & Thornton, L. (Eds.). (1983). *I never told anyone: Writings by women survivors of child sexual abuse.* New York: Harper Colophon.

Bower, G. H. (1981). Mood and memory. *American Psychologist, 36,* 129–148.

Bremner, J. D., Randall, P., Scott, T. M., Bronen, R. A., Seibyl, J. P., Southwick, S. M., Delaney, R. C., McCarthy, G., Charney, D. S., & Innis, R. B. (1995). MRI-based measurement of hippocampal volume in patients with combat-related post-traumatic stress disorder. *American Journal of Psychiatry, 152,* 973–981.

Brewin, C. R., Andrews, B., & Gotlib, I. A. (1993). Psychopathology and early experience: A reappraisal of retrospective reports. *Psychological Bulletin, 113,* 82–98.

Briere, J. N. (1989). *Therapy for adults molested as children.* New York: Springer.

Briere, J. N., & Conte, J. (1993). Self-reported amnesia for abuse in adults molested as children. *Journal of Traumatic Stress, 6,* 21–31.

Brown, D. (1995). Pseudomemories: The standard of science and standard of care in trauma treatment. *American Journal of Clinical Hypnosis, 37,* 1–24.

Brown, L. S. (1996). Politics of memory, politics of incest: Doing therapy and politics that really matter. *Women and Therapy, 19,* 5–18.

Butler, S. (1978). *Conspiracy of silence: The trauma of incest.* San Francisco: New Glide.

Cahill, L., Prins, B., Weber, M., & McGaugh, J. L. (1994). B-Adrenergic activation and memory for emotional events. *Nature, 371,* 702–704.

Calof, D. (1996). Notes from a practice under siege. Internet posting, April 27, 1996.

Carstensen, L., Gabrieli, J., Shepard, R., Levenson, R., Mason, M., Goodman, G., Bootzin, R., Ceci, S., Bronfenbrenner, U., Edelstein, B., Schober, M., Bruck, M., Keane, T., Zimering, R., Oltmanns, T., Gotlib, I., & Ekman, P. (1993). Repressed objectivity. *APS Observer,* March, p. 23.

Ceci, S. J., Ross, D. F., & Toglia, M. P. (1987). Suggestibility of children's memory: Psycholegal implications. *Journal of Experimental Psychology: General, 116,* 38–49.

Ceci, S. J., Huffman, M. L. C., Smith, E., & Loftus, E. F. (1994). Repeatedly thinking about a non-event; source misattributions among preschoolers. *Consciousness and Cognition, 3,* 388–407.

Cheit, R. E. (1994, April). Untitled paper presented at the Mississippi Statewide Conference on Child Abuse and Neglect, Jackson, MS.

Christianson, S. A. (1992). Emotional stress and eyewitness memory. *Psychological Bulletin, 112,* 284–309.

Coan, J. A., Jr. (1993). *Creating false memories.* Unpublished senior honors thesis. Seattle: University of Washington.

Cosmides, L. (1989). The logic of social exchange: Has natural selection shaped how humans reason? Studies with the Wason selection task. *Cognition, 31,* 187–276.

Cosmides, L., & Tooby, J. (1992). Cognitive adaptations for social exchange. In J. H. Barkow, L. Cosmides, & J. Tooby, (Eds.), *The adapted mind: Evolutionary psychology and the generation of culture* (pp. 163–228). New York: Oxford University Press.

Courtois, C. (1988). *Healing the incest wound: Adults survivors in therapy.* New York: Norton.

Cutting, L. (1996). *Memory slips.* New York: Basic Books.

Dalenberg, C., Coe, M., Reto, M., Aransky, K., & Duvenage, C. (1995). The prediction of amnesiac barrier strength as an individual difference variable in state-dependent learning paradigms. Presented at a conference, *Responding to Child Maltreatment,* San Diego, CA.

Elliot, D. M., & Briere, J. (1995). Post-traumatic stress associated with delayed recall of sexual abuse: A general population study. *Journal of Traumatic Stress, 8,* 629–647.

Feldman-Summers, S., & Pope, K. S. (1994). The experience of "forgetting" childhood abuse: A national survey of psychologists. *Journal of Consulting and Clinical Psychology, 62,* 636–639.

Fitzpatrick, F. (1994). Isolation and silence: A male survivor speaks out about clergy abuse. *Moving Forward, 3,* 4–8.

Freyd, J. J. (1995) Betrayal-trauma: Traumatic amnesia as an adaptive response to childhood abuse. *Ethics and Behavior, 4,* 307–329.

Freyd, J. J. (1996). *Betrayal trauma theory: The logic of forgetting abuse.* Cambridge, MA: Harvard University Press.

Gavigan, M. (1994). My recovery from "recovery." In E. Goldstein & K. Farmer (Eds.), *Confabulations: Creating false memories, destroying families* (pp. 251–283). Boca Raton, FL: SIRS Books.

Geise, A. A., Adler, L. E., Montgomery, P., Nagamoto, H., Gerhardt, G., McRae, K., & Hoffer, L. (1994, November). *Sensory physiology and catecholamines in PTSD.* Poster presented at the Tenth Annual Meeting of the International Society for Traumatic Stress Studies, Chicago, IL.

Goldstein, E., & Farmer, K. (Eds.). (1994). *Confabulations: Creating false memories, destroying families.* Boca Raton, FL: SIRS Books.

Goodman, G. S., Quas, J. A., Batterman-Faunce, J. M., Riddlesberger, M. M., & Kuhn, J. (1994). Predictors of accurate and inaccurate memories of traumatic events experienced in childhood. *Consciousness and Cognition, 3,* 269–294.

Goodman, G. S., Bottoms, B. L., Schwartz-Kenney, B., & Rudy, L. A. (1991). Children's memory for a stressful event: Improving children's report. *Journal of Narrative and Life History, 1,* 69–99.

Goodyear-Smith, F. (1993). *First do no harm: The child sexual abuse industry.* Auckland, NZ: Benton-Guy.

Harvey, M. R., & Herman, J. L. (1994). Amnesia, partial amnesia and delayed recall among adult survivors of childhood trauma. *Consciousness and Cognition, 3,* 295–306.

Herman, J. L. (1981). *Father-daughter incest.* Cambridge, MA: Harvard University Press.

Herman, J. L. (1992). *Trauma and recovery.* New York: Basic Books.

Herman, J. L., & Schatzow, E. (1987). Recovery and verification of memories of childhood sexual trauma. *Psychoanalytic Psychology, 4,* 1–14.

Hyman, I. E., Jr., Husband, T. H., & Billings, F. J. (1995). False memories of childhood experiences. *Applied Cognitive Psychology, 9,* 181–187.

Kihlstrom, J. F. (1995). *Recovered memory therapy defined.* Unpublished manuscript, Traumatic Stress Listserv, Interpsych.

Kihlstrom, J. (1996). False memory syndrome. *FMS Foundation Brochure* (email version). Philadelphia, PA: FMS Foundation.

Koss, M. P., Tromp, S., & Tharan, M. (1995). Traumatic memories: empirical foundations, forensic and clinical implications. *Clinical Psychology: Science and Practice, 2,* 111–132.

Loftus, E. F. (1979). *Eyewitness testimony.* Cambridge, MA: Harvard University Press.

Loftus, E. F. (1988). *Memory: Surprising new insights into how we remember and why we forget.* New York: Ardsley House. (Originally published 1980).

Loftus, E. F. (1993). The reality of repressed memories. *American Psychologist, 48,* 518–537.

Loftus, E. F., & Davies, G. M. (1984). Distortions in the memory of children. *Journal of Social Issues, 40,* 51–67.

Loftus, E. F., & Hoffman, H. G. (1989). Misinformation and memory: The creation of new memories. *Journal of Experimental Psychology: General, 118,* 100–104.

Loftus, E. F., & Ketcham, K. (1994). *The myth of repressed memory: False memories and allegations of abuse.* New York: St. Martins Press.

Loftus, E. F., & Loftus, G. (1980). On the permanence of stored information in the human brain. *American Psychologist, 35,* 409–420.

Loftus, E. F., & Pickrell, J. E. (in press). The formation of false memories. *Psychiatric Annals.*

Loftus, E. F., Polonsky, S., & Fullilove, M. T. (1994). Memories of childhood abuse: Remembering and repressing. *Psychology of Women Quarterly, 18,* 67–84.

Mack, J. E. (1995). *Abduction: Human encounters with aliens.* New York: Del Ray.

Marmar, C. R., Weiss, D. S., Schlenger, W. E., et al. (1994). Peritraumatic dissociation and post-traumatic stress in male Vietnam theater veterans. *American Journal of Psychiatry, 151,* 902–907.

Masson, J. M. (1984). *The assault on truth: Freud's suppression of the seduction theory.* New York: Farrar, Straus & Giroux.

McCloskey, M., & Zaragoza, M. A. (1985). Misleading postevent information and memory for events: Arguments and evidence against memory impairment hypotheses. *Journal of Experimental Psychology: General, 114,* 1–16.

McConkey, K. M., Labelle, L., Bibb, B. C., & Bryant, R. A. (1990). Hypnosis and suggested pseudomemory: The relevance of test context. *Australian Journal of Psychology, 42,* 197–205.

McGaugh, J. L. (1992). Affect, neuromodulatory systems, and memory storage. In S. A. Christianson (Ed.), *Handbook of emotion and memory* (pp. 245–268). Hillsdale, NJ: Lawrence Erlbaum.

McNaron, T., & Morgan, Y. (Eds.). (1982). *Voices in the nights: Women speaking out about incest.* Minneapolis: Cleis Press.

Ochberg, F. (Ed.). (1988). *Post-traumatic therapy and victims of violence.* New York: Brunner/Mazel.

Pasley, L. E. (1994). Misplaced trust. In E. Goldstein & K. Farmer (Eds.), *Confabulations: Creating false memories, destroying families* (pp. 347–365). Boca Raton, FL: SIRS Books.

Pendergrast, M. (1995). *Victims of memory: Incest accusations and shattered lives.* Hinesburg, VT: Upper Access.

Pezdek, K. (1995). *What types of false childhood memories are not likely to be suggestively implanted.* Presented at the *Annual Meeting of the Psychonomic Society,* Los Angeles, CA.

Pezdek, K., & Roe, C. (1994). Memory for childhood events: How suggestible is it? *Consciousness and Cognition, 3,* 374–387.

Piper, A. (1994). Multiple personality disorder. *British Journal of Psychiatry, 164,* 135–141.

Pope, K. S. (1995). What psychologists better know about recovered memories, research, lawsuits, and the pivotal experiment. *Clinical Psychology: Science and Practice, 2,* 304–315.

Pope, H. G., & Hudson, J. I. (1995). Can individuals "repress" memories of childhood sexual abuse? An examination of the evidence. *Psychiatric Annals, 25,* 715–719.

Pope, K. S., & Brown, L. S. (1996). *Recovered memories of abuse: Assessment, therapy, forensics.* Washington, DC: American Psychological Association.

Putnam, F. (1994). Sexual abuse as a biologically altering experience. In C. W. Portney (Chair). Psychophysiological effects of childhood trauma and their influence on development. Symposium presented at the *Tenth Annual Meeting, International Society for Traumatic Stress Studies,* Chicago IL.

Reisberg, D., & Heuer, F. (1992). Remembering the details of emotional events. In E. Winograd & U. Neisser (Eds.), *Affects and accuracy in recall studies of "flashbulb" memories* (pp. 162–190). New York: Cambridge University Press.

Roediger, H. L. III, & McDermott, K. B. (1995). Creating false memories: Remembering words not presented in lists. *Journal of Experimental Psychology: Learning, Memory and Cognition, 21,* 803–814.

Ross, C. A. (1995). *Satanic ritual abuse: Principles of treatment.* Toronto: University of Toronto Press.

Rush, F. (1980). *The best-kept secret: Sexual abuse of children.* New York: McGraw-Hill.

Russell, D. E. H. (1986). *The secret trauma: Incest in the lives of girls and women.* New York: Basic Books.

Shalev, A., & Peri, T. (1994). A biopsychological perspective on memory in PTSD. In R. Yehuda & A. C. McFarlane (Chairs). Biological basis of traumatic memory regulation. Symposium presented at the *Tenth Annual Meeting, International Society for Traumatic Stress Studies,* Chicago IL.

Southwick, S. M., Krystal, J. H., Bremner, J. D., Morgan, C. A., & Charney, D. S. (1994, November). Traumatic memory and noradrenergic systems. In R. Yehuda & A. C. McFarlane (Chairs) Biological basis of traumatic memory regulation. Symposium presented at the *Tenth Annual Meeting, International Society for Traumatic Stress Studies,* Chicago, IL.

Spanos, N. P., & McLean, J. M. (1986). Hypnotically created pseudomemories: Memory distortions or reporting biases? *British Journal of Experimental and Clinical Hypnosis, 3,* 155–159.

Tavris, C., & Wade, C. (1995). *Psychology in perspective.* New York: Harper Collins.

Tessler, M., & Nelson, K. (1994). Making memories: The influence of joint encoding on later recall by young children. *Consciousness and Cognition, 3,* 307–326.

Van Derbur Atler, M. (1991). Say "incest" out loud. *McCall's,* September, *78,* 80–81, 148–149.

van der Kolk, B. A. (1992). PTSD, memory and noradrenergic dysregulation. In B. A. van der Kolk (Chair), Biological aspects of trauma, Symposium presented at the *First World Conference of the International Society for Traumatic Stress Studies,* Amsterdam, The Netherlands.

van der Kolk, B. A., & Saporta, J. (1991). The biological response to psychic trauma: Mechanisms and treatment of intrusions and numbing. *Anxiety Research, 4,* 199–212.

van der Kolk, B., van der Hart, O., & Marmar, C. R. (1996). Dissociation and information processing in post traumatic stress disorder. In B. A. van der Kolk, A. C. MacFarlane, & L. Weisath (Eds.), *Traumatic stress: The effects of overwhelming experience on minds, body, and society* (pp. 303–327). New York: Guilford.

Wakefield, H., & Underwager, R. (1994). *Return of the furies: An investigation into recovered memory therapy.* Chicago: Open Court.

Williams, L. M. (1994). Recall of childhood trauma: A prospective study of women's memories of child sexual abuse. *Journal of Consulting and Clinical Psychology, 62,* 1167–1176.

Williams, L. M. (1995). Recovered memories of abuse in women with documented histories of child sexual victimization histories. *Journal of Traumatic Stress, 8,* 649–673.

Yates, J. L., & Nasby, W. (1993). Dissociation, affect and network models of memory: An integrative proposal. *Journal of Traumatic Stress, 6,* 305–326.

Yehuda, R. (1994). Stress hormones and memory disturbance in PTSD. In R. Yehuda & A. C. McFarlane (Chairs). Biological basis of traumatic memory regulation. Symposium presented at the *Tenth Annual Meeting, International Society for Traumatic Stress Studies,* Chicago, IL.

Yehuda, R., & MacFarlane, A. C. (1995). The conflict between current knowledge of PTSD and its original conceptual basis. *American Journal of Psychiatry, 152,* 1705–1713.

Yehuda, R., Kahana, B., Binder-Byrnes, K., Southwick, S., Mason, J. W., & Giller, E. L. (1995). Low urinary cortisol excretion in Holocaust survivors with post-traumatic stress disorder. *American Journal of Psychiatry, 152,* 982–986.

Yuille, J. C. (1993). We must study forensic eyewitnesses to know about them. *American Psychologist, 48,* 572–573.

Yuille, J. C., & Cutshall, J. E. (1989). Analysis of the statements of victims, witnesses and suspects. In J. C. Yuille (Ed.), *Credibility assessment* (pp. 175–191). Norwell, MA: Kluwer Academic.

Zaragoza, M. S. (1991). Preschool children's susceptibility to memory impairment. In. J. Doris (Ed.), *The suggestibility of children's recollections: Implications for eyewitness testimony* (pp. 27–39). Washington, DC: American Psychological Association.

Zaragoza, M. S., & Koshmider, J. W. (1989). Misled subjects may know more than their performance implies. *Journal of Experimental Psychology: Learning, Memory and Cognition, 15,* 246–255.

Zaragoza, M. S., McCloskey, M., & Jamis, M. (1987). Misleading postevent information and the recall of the original event: Further evidence against the memory impairment hypothesis. *Journal of Experimental Psychology: Learning, Memory and Cognition, 13,* 36–44.

IV

Studying the Effects of Trauma over Its Changing Longitudinal Course

The previous sections have highlighted the necessary for systematically studying the effects of trauma beginning at the level of the individual. Indeed, this requires evaluating both the past events, the immediate responses to trauma, and the subsequent chronic psychopathology or adaptation. Systematic research involves accurately measuring facts and events. Hence the effect of using accurate instruments cannot be overlooked because inappropriate implementation of measurement can lead to erroneous conclusions which then may be hard to replicate and create confusion.

Several questions emerge. First, what do people remember and how would their remembrance of a traumatic event be captured by asking them to report retrospectively on past events? Second, how can the immediate and evolving effect of traumatic stress or stressful events be documented and quantified? Third, to what extent do post-traumatic reactions remain stable over time? This is particularly important because the fluctuating expression of disorders such as PTSD may make it difficult to correctly attribute current problems to past events.

Looking at the most widely recognized consequence of traumatic stress, chronic PTSD, Barbara Niles, Elana Newman, and Lisa Fisher present the results of a longitudinal study in which they assess the level of PTSD symptomatology in trauma survivors at two times. Their findings—that individual levels can shift dramatically from one evaluation session to the other, while group means at the two times are maintained—are provocative because they challenge the conception that those with chronic PTSD maintain a stable level of symptomatology. This study reveals the extent to which PTSD patients are highly responsive to environmental cues, as well as to protective and stabilizing factors. From a methodological perspective, the findings raise numerous issues about capturing the clinical state of current PTSD in relation to its course.

In evaluating the causes, severity, and chronicity of PTSD, it is imperative to inquire about all possible lifetime traumatic events. Although such inquiry seems simple, in fact accounts of past trauma, even when captured by structured instruments, vary significantly in a given individual between assessment sessions. This is much harder to rationalize than changes in symptom expression, which appear to be related to reactivation and reexposure. Indeed, it is necessary to determine whether traumatic events are in fact remembered in very different ways at different times, and if so, what determines such differences in accessing and/or reporting past traumatic events. Carole Corcoran et al. present a methodology for lifetime trauma assessment and discuss these complex issues. It is possible to speculate that current perspectives of one's past may be influenced by different mood states or life events. However, it is imperative to understand this process because it is often used to invalidate rather than aid trauma survivors. Corcoran et al.'s chapter raises the interesting speculation that perhaps the temporary inaccessibility of traumatic memories is an adaptive mechanism that prevents us from being constantly affected by the past.

Although the presence and accuracy of a traumatic event can be challenged in some survivors, it is much harder to do so in the face of archived historical events, such as the Nazi Holocaust. Moreover, given the length and dimensions of exposure of some survivors, one would expect that memories of traumatic events from the Holocaust would be clearly remembered and not forgotten. To what extent Holocaust survivors can forget what happened to them and what the mechanisms may be for such forgetting is the subject of Onno van der Hart and Danny Brom. Their studies show that even traumatic events as severe as the Holocaust, or some aspects of such events, can be neglected by memory. The authors discuss the different levels of forgetting and different forms in which traumatic materials can become inaccessible to recollection. Obviously, it is extremely difficult to systematically measure the degree to which something has been forgotten. However, forgetting can be implied by "remembering" events upon reexposure. The case reports described in these studies remind us of the fluctuating nature of human memory in general and trauma survivors in particular.

The unreliability of retrospective accounts presents a cogent argument for the necessity of prospectively analyzing both trauma exposure and its evolving effects. Indeed, most of what we know about the effects of trauma has been based on retrospective accounts, and ultimately these observations must be validated by prospective analysis. Sara Freedman and Arieh Shalev discuss the various ways in which the immediate and delayed effect of traumatic stress exposure can be appraised. They focus on the need to identify trauma survivors at high risk for developing PTSD in the immediate aftermath of trauma and present data on different assessment instruments as they may be applied by clinicians and researchers alike. The salient point of this review is to underscore the fact that certain traumatic stress responses may predict longer term pathology. The early identification of survivors at higher risk for subsequent chronic illness may ultimately allow secondary prevention of chronic or prolonged traumatic stress responses.

15

Obstacles to Assessment of PTSD in Longitudinal Research

BARBARA L. NILES, ELANA NEWMAN, AND LISA M. FISHER

Despite the burgeoning literature on the assessment, diagnosis, and treatment of post-traumatic stress disorder, there are few empirical findings to guide clinicians and researchers in anticipating how individuals with PTSD will fare over a time span of years. This chapter first briefly overviews current findings about the course of PTSD and then identifies reasons why longitudinal investigations of PTSD have been largely bypassed by PTSD researchers.

What We Know about the Course of PTSD

Great strides have been made in recent years in developing psychometrically sound instruments to identify PTSD and assess its severity (see Newman et al., 1996, for a review of measures). This sophistication in measuring PTSD has allowed researchers to examine PTSD symptoms in both retrospective and prospective studies. Retrospective investigations have documented that PTSD symptoms can persist for decades following a traumatic event (Green et al., 1992; Kulka et al., 1990). For example, the National Vietnam Veteran's Readjustment Study (NVVRS; Kulka et al., 1990), the largest, most comprehensive study of combat-related PTSD to date, found that 15% of the veterans evaluated had current symptoms of PTSD. An additional 15% of the participants in this study reported that they met criteria for lifetime PTSD (i.e., they had previously experienced such symptoms but did not at the time of assessment).

Several researchers have examined PTSD symptoms prospectively over months following extreme stressors such as rape (Rothbaum et al., 1992), assault (Riggs et al., 1995), motor vehicle accident (Frommberger et al., 1996; Klein et al., 1996), and a bush-fire disaster (McFarlane, 1988, 1989, 1992). These studies suggest that, for the majority of individuals, PTSD symptoms are present immediately following a potentially trau-

BARBARA L. NILES AND LISA M. FISHER • National Center for Posttraumatic Stress Disorder, Boston Veterans Affairs Medical Center, Boston, Massachusetts 02130.   ELANA NEWMAN • University of Tulsa, Tulsa, Oklahoma 74104.

International Handbook of Human Response to Trauma, edited by Shalev, Yehuda, and McFarlane. Kluwer Academic / Plenum Publishers, New York, 2000.

matic event, recede over the subsequent months, and eventually remit after several months. However, for a substantial minority of people, the symptoms persist.

Other research has indicated that PTSD symptoms can be reactivated after periods of relative dormancy. Life stressors, such as retirement, death of a parent, or children leaving home, have precipitated PTSD symptoms in World War II combat veterans (Christenson et al., 1981). Visits to war memorials and other public ceremonies that were reminders of combat have been reported to exacerbate symptomatology in Vietnam veterans (Faltas et al., 1986). Solomon (1993) documented how the 1982 Lebanon War reactivated symptoms in Israeli combat veterans of the 1973 Yom Kippur War.

In a prospective study of veterans' health service utilization, Ronis et al. (1996) found that the use of mental health services by PTSD patients was both persistent and episodic. The investigators concluded that the absence of PTSD symptoms does not mean that the disorder has resolved for these patients.

Thus, research is accumulating which suggests that

- PTSD symptoms develop acutely in many individuals following an extremely stressful or potentially traumatic event;
- PTSD persists and becomes a chronic disorder in a substantial minority of these individuals; and
- symptoms are frequently reactivated after periods of dormancy.

Many questions remain unanswered, however. It is clear that there is considerable individual variability in the chronicity and course of PTSD although the factors that contribute to this variability are largely unknown. Prospective, longitudinal research is needed to inform us when and how the disorder recurs and fluctuates.

Why We Do Not Know More

Although vital to our knowledge about the course of PTSD, longitudinal research in this area is scarce. We will use our follow-up study of Vietnam veterans with PTSD as an illustration of some of the obstacles that have limited research in this area.

Recruitment and Retention Difficulties

Longitudinal or follow-up research on any population is arduous, time-consuming, and expensive. Researchers have bemoaned the low rates of subject retention in longitudinal investigations (e.g., Capaldi & Patterson, 1987). Suggested methods for maintaining contact with study participants and maximizing subject participation (e.g., Twitchell et al., 1992) require extensive resources. As a result, longitudinal studies with high rates of retention are rare.

There is also evidence suggesting that individuals with PTSD may be even more difficult to recruit and maintain in such studies than other populations. Sparr et al. (1993) demonstrated that clients with PTSD and/or substance abuse are more likely to miss psychiatric appointments than clients with other disorders. Niles et al. (1997) found that patients in a primary care clinic who endorsed symptoms of PTSD on a self-report screening form were more than twice as likely to refuse or be unavailable for follow-up telephone interviews than patients who did not endorse PTSD symptoms.

The avoidance symptoms that are elements of the diagnostic criteria for PTSD may contribute to this low rate of follow-up. Because a person with PTSD "commonly makes deliberate efforts to avoid thoughts, feelings, or conversations about the traumatic event (Criterion C1) and to avoid activities, situations, or people who arouse recollections of it (Criterion C2)," (American Psychiatric Press, 1994, pp. 424–425), it follows that such an individual would seek to avoid researchers who attempt to ask questions about the event or probe into reactions to it. A general distrust of authority is a characteristic that is also commonly associated with the disorder (Blake et al., 1990). In the case of combat veterans, who are often skeptical and distrusting of anyone who represents the government, recruitment calls or letters from government researchers may be met with hostility or extreme avoidance.

Problems of homelessness or transience are also common in chronic PTSD cases. For example, in a recent evaluation of U.S. Veterans Administration inpatient treatment for Vietnam veterans with PTSD, 33% of the sample was homeless or living in a hospital (Johnson et al., 1996). These problems further complicate the difficulties of finding and following clients in longitudinal research.

In the study we conducted, all of these factors appeared to contribute to difficulty in follow-up. This study was conducted to examine the course of PTSD symptomatology in veterans who had been evaluated in the Boston Veterans Administration PTSD clinic in the late 1980s (Time One). In 1994 and 1995 (Time Two), the research team attempted to locate, contact, and recruit all 111 Vietnam veterans who had been evaluated for combat-related PTSD at Time One. Thirty-eight (34.3%) completed the follow-up protocol, whereas 19 (17.1%) declined to participate, 14 (12.6%) were identified as deceased, 16 (14.4%) were reached but failed to appear for the evaluation, and 24 (21.6%) could not be located despite extensive efforts, including the use of a national locator service.

One unanticipated factor that limited the number of participants at Time Two was the high number of deaths in this group. The rate of death over the average 6.6 years between Time One and Time Two was more than five times the national average for men of comparable age in the United States (U.S. Bureau of Census, 1994). Thus, one sad finding from this study is that premature death in this population also limits follow-up of the course of symptomatology.

Because follow-up rates are low in this population, another issue to consider is that those individuals who do participate in follow-up studies may not be representative of the entire group. Our follow-up study provided some evidence of this: those who participated at Time Two were shown to have significantly lower (i.e., less impaired) Time One scores on a variety of PTSD and related psychopathology measures than either those who died or those who did not participate. One potential remedy for this would be to use a prospective design, where individuals are approached at the outset of their initial assessment and are asked to participate in a longitudinal evaluation. Such an approach would be likely to boost rates of follow-up participation, but prospective studies can also have high rates of refusal. Therefore, there are important limitations on how much one can generalize the results from follow-up or prospectively designed longitudinal studies of individuals with chronic PTSD.

Overall, it is very difficult to locate and complete evaluations of individuals with PTSD in follow-up studies. Once individuals are successfully located and persuaded to participate, the next obstacle is measurement of changes.

Measurement Difficulties

Current demands on health care providers to demonstrate effective treatment has led to recent emphasis on psychometric instruments designed to demarcate improvements in mental health patients. However, the symptomatology accompanying PTSD is extremely complex, and it is difficult to identify or target specific symptoms with which to measure change. Determining what, how, and when to measure has been a great challenge in research on PTSD (e.g., Bleich et al., 1992; Shalev, 1997).

What to Measure

Aggregated Data and Individual Variability.   Examining differences over time in mean scores on psychometric measures appears to be a useful way to investigate changes for a group. However, using only group means to characterize changes for a number of individuals with PTSD may lead one to draw spurious conclusions about the individuals. For example, Table 1 depicts the mean Mississippi Scale score for the group and the individual scores for the veterans who took part in the Time Two evaluation in our follow-up study of combat veterans. The difference in mean scores between Time One and Time Two indicated very little change over time. At both Time One and Time Two, the mean score was well above the suggested 107 cutoff indicating PTSD for combat veterans (Keane et al., 1988). However, when the individual scores were examined, it

TABLE 1. Comparison of Time One and Time Two Mississippi Scores for Group and Individuals

	Mississippi Scores				Mississippi Scores		
	Time One	Time Two	Difference		Time One	Time Two	Difference
Group mean	123.37	120.91	−2.20	Individual	150	152	2
Individual	142	85	−57	scores	134	139	5
scores	127	89	−38	(*cont.*)	136	143	7
	126	93	−33		106	116	10
	89	57	−32		142	153	11
	134	104	−30		94	105	11
	145	117	−28		140	154	14
	160	132	−28		107	123	16
	97	73	−24		94	113	19
	125	107	−18		120	142	22
	130	112	−18		130	152	22
	132	116	−16		111	134	23
	93	79	−14		100	126	26
	160	146	−14		122	154	32
	92	79	−13		115	151	36
	128	116	−12		99	156	57
	132	123	−9		144	–	–
	145	140	−5		90	–	–
	126	125	−1		145	–	–
	126	126	0				

became apparent that there were dramatic changes in some cases: a few individuals moved three standard deviations up or down in symptomatology, as measured by this scale. Therefore, examination of group means can obscure dramatic individual changes.

Domains and Symptoms.   It seems obvious that measuring of the specific symptoms of PTSD would be the central domain for research on the course of PTSD. One might assume that a focus on the diagnosis of PTSD would be useful in examining its course over time. However, whether an individual's symptoms are sufficient to meet diagnostic criteria is often not a meaningful distinction in chronic PTSD. In severe cases a PTSD diagnosis may be maintained even when symptoms abate substantially. In less severe cases an individual's symptom levels may hover around diagnostic cutoffs, falling below at one point and above at another. In this situation, use of a dichotomous diagnosis variable to represent PTSD can allow minor fluctuations in symptoms to appear greater than they really are.

Measuring the number and severity of PTSD symptoms and how they fluctuate over time might allow for a more sensitive examination of changes. However, even when the units of measurement are quite refined, PTSD symptoms for a group may not change substantially in the chronic phase of this disorder (Johnson, 1997; Shalev, 1997). Comorbid psychopathology, related symptomatology, and quality of life assessment may provide better information about change. Comorbid disorders, especially depression and substance abuse, are pervasive in the veteran PTSD population (Keane & Kaloupek, 1997; Keane & Wolfe, 1990; Sierles et al., 1983) and should be assessed to illustrate a full picture of symptomatology.

Therefore, it is unclear whether the large changes in Mississippi Scale scores shown in Table 1 represent meaningful changes. Close examination of some of these cases has demonstrated that the Mississippi Scale taps PTSD symptoms only and is not a good indicator of overall functioning. For some individuals, great strides may be made in other areas of functioning even when PTSD symptomatology increases. (See Niles et al., 1998 for a case study illustration of this phenomenon.) It is a great challenge to determine the relative importance of various symptoms when individuals present uneven patterns of strengths and difficulties.

Criterion A Events.   When individuals have experienced many potentially traumatic events, it can be difficult to decide which or how many of them contribute to the post-trauma symptomatology. There are several reasons that there may be shifts over time in the way various events affect current functioning. For example, in the case of combat-related PTSD, war-zone experiences are considered the "index events" that are identified as Criterion A for the diagnosis. Many soldiers suffered several traumatic experiences while in the war zone, and the relative significance of these events may change over time for the individual. Also, many veterans experienced nonmilitary traumatic events both before and after their military traumas. In some cases, these additional events may be more distressing for the individual than the identified index event. In longitudinal research, an individual might experience a new traumatic event subsequent to the beginning of the research project. A dramatic increase in PTSD symptomatology may result from such an experience. Finally, subjective appraisal of a specific event may change. Several recent studies have documented that estimation of combat exposure, for example, can change dramatically over time (Niles et al., 1999; Roemer et al., 1998; Southwick et al., 1997). Therefore, when examining the course of

PTSD in longitudinal research, it is important to consider that the differential salience of traumatic events may change over time.

How To Measure

Assessment of symptoms can also be challenging. The most common method of gathering information about psychiatric symptomatology is to ask the individuals to rate their symptoms. Several valid and reliable self-report checklists have been developed to assess PTSD symptoms, and some assess related symptomatology as well. For example, as mentioned before, in our follow-up study the 35-item Mississippi Scale for combat-related PTSD (Keane et al., 1988) was used to assess PTSD symptoms. This scale has been widely used in assessing combat-related PTSD and has performed well as a self-report measure of the disorder (Kulka et al., 1990).

The advantage of self-report assessment measures is that they are cost-efficient and do not require clinician time for administration. In addition, the ratings are not influenced by potential clinician bias. However, an important shortcoming of such instruments is that they have a limited ability to indicate whether the information provided is accurate. Individuals may exaggerate or underestimate on ratings, misunderstand the questions, respond randomly on the questionnaire, and/or be poor observers of their symptoms.

Clinician-administered structured or semistructured interviews have also been widely used for assessment. Two commonly used instruments of this type, the Structured Clinical Interview for DSM-III-R diagnosis (Spitzer et al., 1990) and the Clinician-Administered PTSD Scale (Blake et al., 1990), were used in our follow-up study. In such an interview, a clinician can ensure that all symptomatology is reviewed in detail while allowing interviewees to describe their symptoms in their own words (Newman et al., 1996). The clinician can use both verbal and nonverbal information to evaluate whether the interviewee understands the questions or is responding randomly and can guide the interview accordingly. In addition, a skilled clinician can often detect when an interviewee is overstating or understating symptoms. However, clinician judgment can also be biased or inaccurate. Unfortunately, both self-report and clinician-administered PTSD assessment instruments do not have psychometrically valid and reliable ways to determine the individual's reporting style.

Psychophysiological assessment of PTSD, that is, measurement of physiological reactivity to exposure to cues of the traumatic event, can offer important additional information in a comprehensive assessment. Measures of heart rate, blood pressure, muscle tension, and skin conductance do not rely on either self-report or clinician judgment. This minimizes the impact of response sets or biases. However, psychophysiological reactivity is considered an indicator of PTSD, not a definitive measure. These assessments have good specificity, but the sensitivity is low (Gerardi et al., 1989); reactivity can be influenced by many outside factors, such as psychotropic and antihypertensive medications (Prins et al., 1995). In addition, in many outpatient settings, the resources necessary for such assessments are not available.

Reports from partners, family members, or friends can also provide valuable information in clinical assessment. Collateral assessment of PTSD can bypass some of the obstacles to accurate self-reporting, such as denial, reading comprehension problems, avoidance, or amnesia. However, collateral information is often not accessible to the assessor. When it is, it is also subject to influence from biases and response sets.

All of the measures described above can provide meaningful information in an assessment but are associated with some degree of error. The literature on the evaluation of PTSD has greatly emphasized the importance of combining data derived from self-report interviews, structured clinical interviews, and, when possible, psychophysiological assessment and collateral reports (e.g., Keane & Kaloupek, 1997; Keane et al., 1987, 1996; Kulka et al., 1990). When comprehensive multimodal assessment is used, the strengths of some measures can compensate for shortcomings of others.

When To Measure

A limited number of empirical studies and some clinical illustrations have demonstrated that chronic PTSD is both persistent and fluctuating. The striking persistence of PTSD symptoms has been widely discussed in clinical literature, particularly with regard to combat veterans, in descriptive accounts (e.g., Horowitz, 1986, 1993) and in the emerging treatment outcome literature (e.g., Johnson, 1997; Shalev et al., 1996). In the NVVRS (Kulka et al., 1990), about half of the Vietnam veterans who reported that they ever met diagnostic criteria for PTSD were also diagnosed with this disorder when they were assessed in the late 1980s. The remarkable chronicity and severity of PTSD in Vietnam veterans who seek inpatient VA PTSD treatment has led Shalev (1997) to suggest that long-standing combat-related PTSD in Vietnam veterans may be "treatment-resistant" in many cases. In all, these findings support the conceptualization of PTSD as a chronic, unremitting disorder.

Yet there is also compelling evidence for fluctuation in the symptoms of PTSD. The other half of the veterans in the NVVRS, who were diagnosed as having had PTSD in their lifetimes, reported that their symptoms had decreased to such an extent that full diagnostic criteria for PTSD were no longer met (Kulka et al., 1990). This suggests that at least some symptoms remit over time.

Because there is considerable variability in PTSD symptomatology over time and individual scores on various measures may go up and down considerably, group means may not change substantially. General trends for a group are hard to detect when data are aggregated and when there is a large dispersion of changed scores for individuals. Figure 1 represents some possible scenarios. It illustrates how improvements for a group might not be detected when only two times are examined. Individuals

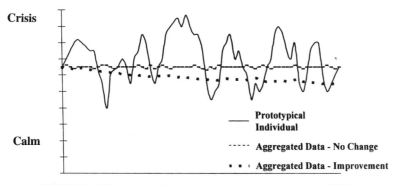

FIGURE 1.   Hypothesized fluctuation of symptoms in chronic PTSD.

may fluctuate up and down, but when data are collapsed or averaged, the line appears relatively flat. Subtle but real changes for the group may be overlooked.

Conclusions

Multimodal assessment, including both observed and subjective reports of improvement or change, is recommended in examining the course of PTSD over time. However, numerous assessment measures can be labor-intensive for both the individuals under study and the investigators: this may limit compliance with follow-up. Nevertheless, it is important to develop a representative picture of individuals who have chronic PTSD so that changes in functioning can be accurately portrayed. In addition, multiple points of measurement in longitudinal research are also needed so that subtle trends can be detected.

A great deal remains unknown about the course of chronic PTSD. Although longitudinal investigations in this area are extremely challenging, this line of research is crucial. Greater understanding of the PTSD symptom course and the impact of variables such as life stressors or social support will provide a necessary base for the systematic development of interventions to control and reduce chronic PTSD.

Acknowledgments

We want to express our appreciation for the contributions of Danny G. Kaloupek and Terence M. Keane, who provided the Time One data set and financial, scientific, and editorial support for this project. We also thank Melissa S. Covington for her help in the preparation of this manuscript.

References

American Psychiatric Association (APA). (1994). *Diagnostic and statistical manual of mental disorders*, 4th ed. Washington, DC: American Psychiatric Press.

Blake, D. D., Weathers, F. W., Nagy, L. M., Kaloupek, D. G., Klauminzer, G., Charney, D. S., & Keane, T. M. (1990). A clinician rating scale for assessing current and lifetime PTSD: The CAPS-1. *The Behavior Therapist, 18*, 187–188.

Bleich, A., Shalev, A., Shoham, S., Solomon, Z., & Kotler, M. (1992). PTSD: Theoretical and practical considerations as reflected through Koach—an innovative treatment project. *Journal of Traumatic Stress, 5*, 265–271.

Capaldi, D., & Patterson, G. R. (1987). An approach to the problem of recruitment and retention rates for longitudinal research. *Behavioral Assessment, 9*, 169–177.

Christenson, R. M., Walker, J. I., Ross, D. R., & Maltbie, A. (1981). Reactivation of traumatic conflicts. *American Journal of Psychiatry, 138*, 984–985.

Faltas, F. J., Sirota, A. D., Parson, S. J., Daamen, M., & Schare, M. L. (1986). Exacerbations of post-traumatic stress disorder symptomatology in Vietnam veterans. *Military Medicine, 151*(12), 648–649.

Frommberger, U., Stieglitz, R., Schlickewei, W., Kuner, E., & Berger, M. (1996). Methodological problems in a prospective study on PTSD in traffic accident victims and work-related trauma. Presented at the *Second World Conference of the International Society for Traumatic Stress Studies*, Jerusalem, Israel.

Gerardi, R., Keane, T. M., & Penk, W. E. (1989). Utility: Sensitivity and specificity in developing diagnostic tests of combat-related post-traumatic stress disorder (PTSD). *Journal of Clinical Psychology, 45*, 691–703.

Green, B. L., Lindy, J. D., Grace, M. C., & Leonard, A. C. (1992). Chronic posttraumatic stress disorder and diagnostic comorbidity in a disaster sample. *Journal of Nervous and Mental Disease, 180*, 760–766.

Horowitz, M. J. (1986). *Stress-response syndromes*, 2nd ed. New York: Jason Aronson.

Horowitz, M. J. (1993). Stress response syndromes; A review of posttraumatic stress and adjustment disorders. In J.P. Wilson & B. Raphael (Eds.), *International handbook of traumatic stress syndromes* (pp. 49–60). New York: Plenum.

Johnson, D. (1997). Introduction: Inside the specialized inpatient PTSD units of the Department of Veterans Affairs. *Journal of Traumatic Stress, 10*, 357–360.

Johnson, D., Rosenheck, R., Fontana, A., Lubin, H., Southwick, S., & Charney, D. (1996). Outcome of intensive inpatient treatment for combat-related PTSD. *American Journal of Psychiatry, 153*, 771–777.

Keane, T. M., Caddell, J. M., & Taylor, K. L. (1988). Mississippi scale for combat-related posttraumatic stress disorder: Three studies in reliability and validity. *Journal of Consulting and Clinical Psychology, 56*, 85–90.

Keane, T. M., & Kaloupek, D. G. (1997). Co-morbid psychiatric disorders in PTSD: Implications for research. In R. Yehuda & A. C. McFarlane (Eds.), *Physiobiology of posttraumatic stress disorder* (pp. 24–34). New York: Annals of the New York Academy of Science.

Keane, T. M., Newman, E., & Orsillo, S. M. (1996). The assessment of military-related PTSD. In J. Wilson & T. Keane (Eds.), *Assessing psychological trauma and PTSD: A handbook for practitioners* (pp. 267–290). New York: Guilford.

Keane, T. M., & Wolfe, J. (1990). Comorbidity in post-traumatic stress disorder: An analysis of community and clinical studies. *Journal of Applied Social Psychology, 20*, 1776–1788.

Keane, T. M., Wolfe, J., & Taylor, K. L. (1987). Post-traumatic stress disorder: Evidence for diagnostic validity and methods of psychological assessment. *Journal of Clinical Psychology, 43*, 32–43.

Klein, E., Arnon, I., & Lavie, P. (1996). PTSD in car accident victims: Time course and prevalence one year after the accident (a longitudinal study). Presented at the *Second World Conference of the International Society for Traumatic Stress Studies*, Jerusalem, Israel.

Kulka, R. A., Schlenger, W. E., Fairbank, J. A., Jordan, B. K., Hough, R. I., Marmar, C. R., & Weiss, D. S. (1990). *Trauma and the Vietnam War generation: Report of findings from the National Vietnam Veterans Readjustment Study*. New York: Brunner/Mazel.

McFarlane, A. C. (1988). The aetiology of post-traumatic stress disorder following a natural disaster. *British Journal of Psychiatry, 152*, 116–121.

McFarlane, A. C. (1989). The aetiology of posttraumatic morbidity: Predisposing, precipitating and perpetuating factors. *British Journal of Psychiatry, 154*, 221–228.

McFarlane, A. C. (1992). Avoidance and intrusion in posttraumatic stress disorder. *Journal of Nervous and Mental Disease, 180*, 439–445.

Newman, E., Kaloupek, D. G., & Keane, T. M. (1996). Assessment of posttraumatic stress disorder in clinical and research settings. In B. van der Kolk, A. C. McFarlane, & L. Weisaeth (Eds.), *Comprehensive text on posttraumatic stress* (pp. 242–275). New York: Guilford.

Niles, B. L., Grace, M., Gibeau, A., & Kaloupek, D. G. (1997). The performance of a 3-item screening measure for PTSD in primary care clinics. Presented at the *Annual Meeting of the Association for Advancement of Behavior Therapy*, Miami, FL.

Niles, B. L., Newman, E., & Fisher, L. M. (1998). Therapeutic follow-up in chronic PTSD: The challenges of measurement. *National Center for PTSD Clinical Quarterly, 8*, 6–10.

Niles, B. L., Newman, E., Fisher, L., Erwin, B. M., Kaloupek, D. G., & Keane, T. M. (1999). Stability and fluctuation of veterans' reports of combat exposure. In L. Williams & V. Banyard (Eds.), *Trauma and memory* (pp. 311–317). Beverly Hills, CA: Sage.

Prins, A., Kaloupek, D. G., & Keane, T. M. (1995). Psychophysiological evidence for autonomic arousal and startle in traumatized adult populations. In M. J. Friedman, D. S. Charney, & A. Y. Deutch (Eds.), *Neurobiological and clinical consequences of stress: From normal adaptation to PTSD* (pp. 291–314). New York: Raven Press.

Riggs, D. S., Foa, E. B., & Rothbaum, B. O. (1995). A prospective examination of symptoms of post-traumatic stress disorder in victims of non-sexual assault. *Journal of Interpersonal Violence, 10*, 201–214.

Roemer, L., Litz, B. T., Orsillo, S. M., Ehlich, P. J., & Friedman, M. J. (1998). Increases in retrospective accounts of war-zone exposure over time: The role of PTSD in symptom severity. *Journal of Traumatic Stress, 11*, 597–605.

Ronis, D. L., Bates, E. W., Garefin, A. J., Buit, B. K., Falcon, S. P., & Liberzon, I. (1996). Longitudinal patterns of care for patients with posttraumatic stress disorder. *Journal of Traumatic Stress, 9*, 763–781.

Rothbaum, B. O., Foa, E. B., Riggs, D. S., Murdock, T., & Walsh, W. (1992). A prospective examination of post-traumatic stress disorder in rape victims. *Journal of Traumatic Stress, 5*, 455–475.

Shalev, A. Y. (1997). Discussion: Treatment of prolonged posttraumatic stress disorder—learning from experience. *Journal of Traumatic Stress, 10*, 415–423.

Shalev, A. Y., Bonne, O., & Eth, E. (1996). Treatment of posttraumatic stress disorder: A review. *Psychosomatic Medicine, 58*, 165–182.

Sierles, F. S., Chen, J. J., McFarland, R. E., & Taylor, M. A. (1983). Posttraumatic stress disorder and concurrent psychiatric illness: A preliminary report. *American Journal of Psychiatry, 140*, 1177–1179.

Solomon, Z. (1993). *Combat stress reaction. The enduring toll of war.* New York: Plenum.

Southwick, S. M., Morgan, C. A., Nicolaou, A. L., & Charney, D. S. (1997). Consistency of memory for combat-related traumatic events in veterans of Operation Desert Storm. *American Journal of Psychiatry, 154*, 173–177.

Sparr, L. F., Moffitt, M. C., & Ward, M. F. (1993). Missed psychiatric appointments: Who returns and who stays away. *American Journal of Psychiatry, 150*, 801–805.

Spitzer, R. L., Williams, J. B., Gibbons, M., & First, M. B. (1990). *Structural clinical interview for DSM-III-R—Patient edition (SCID-P, Version 1.0).* Washington, DC: American Psychiatric Press.

Twitchell, G. R., Hertzog, C. A., Klein, J. L., & Schuckit, M. A. (1992). The anatomy of a follow-up. *British Journal of Addiction, 87*, 251–257.

U.S. Bureau of Census (1994). *Statistical abstract of the United States*, 114th ed. Washington, DC: U.S. Government Printing Office.

16

Conceptual and Methodological Issues in Trauma History Assessment

CAROLE B. CORCORAN, BONNIE L. GREEN,
LISA A. GOODMAN, AND KAREN E. KRINSLEY

An increasing number of psychometrically sound measures of post-traumatic stress disorder (PTSD; American Psychiatric Association, 1994) is available for research and clinical assessment purposes, for example, the Clinician-Administered PTSD Scale (CAPS; Blake et al., 1990) and the PTSD Symptom Scale (PSS; Foa et al., 1993). However, although such measures address the B (reexperiencing), C (avoidance/numbing), and D (arousal) *symptoms* of the disorder, they tend not to address assessment of the A (exposure) criterion independently, and methodology for standardized assessment of trauma history has been relatively neglected. A number of efforts to develop such instruments are underway; however, trauma history instruments that are comprehensive and that have established psychometric properties are the exception. Reliably defining traumatic event characteristics that meet Criterion A of PTSD and obtaining validation for the occurrence of these events pose a serious challenge. Problems with recall, memory, and reporting further complicate assessment of these events. This chapter addresses these issues from the perspective of two efforts to develop such instruments. Although the purposes, formats, and target populations for the two trauma history instruments differ widely, both assess a wide range of traumatic events. Preliminary studies of these two instruments have focused on the stability and validity of reports of these events. Problems with operationalizing definitions of traumatic events that meet Criterion A have been encountered in each study. Even decisions regarding how to go about establishing the psychometric properties of these instruments were

CAROLE B. CORCORAN • Department of Psychology, Mary Washington College, Fredericksburg, Virginia 22401.   BONNIE L. GREEN • Department of Psychiatry, Georgetown University, Washington, DC 20007.   LISA A. GOODMAN • Department of Psychology, University of Maryland, College Park, Maryland 20742.   KAREN E. KRINSLEY • National Center for Posttraumatic Stress Disorder, Boston Veterans Affairs Medical Center, Boston, Massachusetts 02130.

International Handbook of Human Response to Trauma, edited by Shalev, Yehuda, and McFarlane. Kluwer Academic / Plenum Publishers, New York, 2000.

complex and not completely straightforward. The chapter discusses these common challenges and their implications for understanding and assessing trauma history and provides suggestions for future research in this area.

Background

Since the introduction of PTSD into the psychiatric nosology in DSM-III (American Psychiatric Association, 1980), one of the criteria in the diagnosis has been exposure to a traumatic event. In DSM-III and subsequently DSM-III-R (American Psychiatric Association, 1987), this was defined as an event "outside the range of normal human experience" (p. 247). More recently, the stressor criterion (A) for PTSD in DSM-IV (American Psychiatric Association, 1994) has been revised to include two major components. The first, A1, refers to qualitative characteristics of exposure that include "actual or threatened death or injury, or a threat to the physical integrity of oneself or others" (p. 427). The second component, A2, specifies that the individual's response to such events includes "intense fear, helplessness, or horror" (p. 427). Thus Criterion A1 refers to more "objective" descriptive characteristics of a traumatic event, whereas Criterion A2 encompasses subjective responses to these events. Although these newer characterizations of events have helped to clarify which types of events should be covered, they are not precise, and investigators have had to develop their own operational definitions.

The failure to include *exposure* assessment in measures of PTSD earlier is likely due in part to the way the trauma field has developed. Research studies have tended to focus on trauma sequelae within specific populations (e.g., Vietnam veterans, sexual assault and abuse survivors, disaster survivors, etc.), and trauma researchers have tended to develop separate and detailed trauma exposure measures for these discrete target events (Goodman et al., in press). However, recent research suggests that it is common for people to experience multiple traumatic events in the course of their lives (e.g., Kessler et al., 1995; Norris, 1992), that a history of prior trauma may affect a survivor's responses to a later event (e.g., Resnick et al., 1993), and that the effects of traumatic experiences may be cumulative (Follette et al., 1996; Goodman et al., 1997). Thus it is imperative that researchers develop psychometrically sound measures of lifetime exposure to a variety of traumatic events, even for studies that focus on a specific target (traumatic) event. Psychometric evaluations of the two trauma history instruments described in this chapter have made it clear that gathering data about past traumatic exposure is not necessarily as straightforward as collecting data on other more clear-cut characteristics, such as demographic information. Rather, assessment of traumatic exposure is a complex measurement task, involving issues of definition, subtleties of methodology, as well as evaluation of consistency and validity of reporting. Therefore, appropriate psychometric validation of such measures is important and necessary.

The Instruments

The Stressful Life Events Screening Questionnaire (SLESQ; Goodman et al., in press) is a 13-item self-report screening measure designed to provide an initial assessment of lifetime exposure to a variety of traumatic events such as traumatic injury, violent bereavement, and physical and sexual assault and abuse. The instrument was developed in the context of a study that examined differential outcomes associated with a range of traumatic events and dimensions. Respondents are asked to indicate whether or not an event occurred, and if so, additional information (depending on the question) is requested, including the following: the age at which the event occurred; a brief description of the incident, injuries; whether someone died; whether the participant's life was in danger; and the perpetrator. Questions are worded in explicit, behaviorally anchored language. Psychometric support establishing the reliability and validity for the instrument was obtained from a university sample ($N = 126$) who completed the questionnaire and two weeks later were randomly assigned to either a second self-report administration or a twenty minute face-to-face interview, covering the same content, with a trained clinical interviewer. In our SLESQ psychometric study, 72% of the participants reported exposure to at least one traumatic event. The mean number of reported traumas for this college sample was 1.83 (SD = 1.96). In a larger screening study using the SLESQ ($N = 2505$), 68% of the college women reported at least one event, and 43% reported two or more. The mean number of reported traumas was 1.69 (SD = 1.80).

The Evaluation of Lifetime Stressors (ELS; Krinsley et al., 1994) is a protocol consisting of a questionnaire and follow-up interview. It provides a comprehensive, multidimensional assessment of traumatic events across the lifetime. The format provides multiple and varied opportunities to report traumatic experiences using both broad and more detailed questions, varied response formats, and a hierarchical arrangement of questions starting with less emotionally intense questions. For all reported events, information regarding threat, injury, emotional response, frequency, and duration is collected, and additional dimensions are obtained for the worst traumas. Support for the reliability and validity of the instrument has been obtained from double administrations of the ELS with outpatient male Vietnam era veterans in an inpatient substance abuse unit. In early analyses of this sample ($N = 40$), participants' overall mean number of reported traumas was 13, notably higher than that for the nontreatment-seeking psychometric and screening samples with the SLESQ.

Defining Criterion A with the SLESQ and ELS

Given the widely differing purposes of a screening versus a comprehensive measure of trauma history, the SLESQ and ELS have used different approaches to address the difficulties in defining Criterion A events and operationally determining thresholds for "counting" exposure. The SLESQ was developed in the context of a research study that required a comprehensive self-report trauma history screening questionnaire to be administered to a large pool of respondents, a subset of whom would then be followed-up with face-to-face interviews. The purpose of the measure is to identify, as quickly and efficiently as possible, all traumatic events experienced by respondents, while avoiding subthreshold events that would not likely be conceptualized as "traumatic," vis-a-vis the qualitative descriptions in Criterion A1 of the PTSD diagnosis. It does not address Criterion A2 (subjective reaction to the event). Given our goals, we decided, for purposes of designing the questionnaire, to develop conservative definitions of events and to make them explicit. Therefore, we wrote questions requiring that events be life-threatening and/or involve a significant level of violence and/or assault to bodily integrity, and that the event occurred to the respondent or an *extremely* close friend or immediate family member. We recognize that our implicit thresholds are somewhat arbitrary. Although the events covered by the SLESQ overlap significantly with some other measures, the SLESQ places *less* emphasis than other screening measures (e.g., the Traumatic Stress Schedule; Norris, 1990 and the Traumatic Events Questionnaire,

Vrana & Lauterbach, 1994) on disasters and *more* emphasis on behaviorally specific assessment of interpersonal trauma. It does, however, elicit additional information (depending on the item) about important details (e.g., age, duration, level of force used, and injury received) for endorsed events and includes two "catchall" questions for other life-threatening and extremely frightening or horrifying experiences (with examples given that include torture, combat, and living in a war zone) that are not specifically covered, to allow some flexibility. Descriptive information is particularly important for "catchall" questions, and it also enables researchers to use the SLESQ to establish study specific criteria to fit the purpose of their research. On the other hand, we acknowledge that investigators who want to pick up a broader range of events (e.g., natural death of a partner) might find the SLESQ too restricting (Goodman et al., in press).

To determine how successful we were in our own purpose, i.e., to develop a measure targeted to pick up primarily Criterion A events, three judges evaluated each item of a systematically selected subsample of screening questionnaires (every third screening measure with a random start; $N = 46$) against the conservative definition of Criterion A trauma developed for each category. Decisions about trauma thresholds were made by consensus. Respondents endorsed a total of 81 events in the 46 question-naires. Judges rated 85% of these events as meeting our severity threshold for a Criterion A event. The most commonly reported subthreshold items included peer fights, spanking by parents, and non-life-threatening illnesses such as mononucleosis. Thus, by and large, the SLESQ appears to be relatively specific for Criterion A type events, based on our own operationalization. Note that although the analyses just reported helped us to examine the specificity of the SLESQ, all further analyses were based upon all (unscreened) responses.

Because the SLESQ was designed to be a relatively brief screening measure, it does not assess trauma exposure in as much detail as the ELS. Collecting information about objective and subjective dimensions of trauma events is considered a crucial feature of the ELS, based on the growing recognition that assessment of trauma should be more comprehensive and multidimensional (e.g., Sutker et al., 1991; Widom & Shepard, 1996). The ELS aims to provide a structured method for collecting empirical data on lifetime exposure to potentially traumatic events by using a clinically viable format. Because the ELS collects multidimensional information about every trauma, it is possible to examine the impact of various characteristics of the events. For example, at least for this small sample of men, consistency of reporting over time is better for events that meet full criteria A1 and A2 of PTSD (those that are accompanied by fear, helplessness, or horror) than for events that are only potentially traumatic but do not meet the emotional criterion. These results are in concordance with a growing body of literature that suggests that there is more consistent recall for more personally signifi-cant events, lending some support to the importance of an emotional reaction to traumatic events, as used in the DSM-IV. This trend holds with the analysis of the complete data set of 76 participants.

Reliability of Reporting for Traumatic Events

How reliable is recall of traumatic events on these two instruments? The SLESQ appears to have very good test-retest reliability. Over a two-week interval, the correlation between the number of events reported at time 1 and the number reported at time 2 was .89. This figure is similar to the .88 and .91 test-retest correlations reported for the

Traumatic Stress Schedule (TSS; Norris & Perilla, 1996) and the Traumatic Events Questionnaire (TEQ; Lauterbach & Vrana, 1996), respectively. However, except for unpublished data on the Trauma History Questionnaire (THQ; Green, 1996) and the ELS (see below), the SLESQ is the first measure to be evaluated for reliability across individual events. Reported kappas for the occurrence of specifically named SLESQ events ranged from .31 for attempted sexual assault to 1.00 for robbery or mugging (median kappa = .73); deleting attempted sexual assault, the range was .57–1.00. This median kappa for reporting on specific events across administrations of the SLESQ was similar to the .64 figure reported for the THQ and the .74 figure reported for the ELS with regard to the early data analysis in adult male veterans. Not surprisingly, the two "catchall" SLESQ items had among the lowest kappas (.25 and .40). With regard to attempted sexual assault, we hypothesized that the low reliability stemmed from the fact that respondents were required to make a judgment about their perpetrator's frame of mind, that is, attempted assault, by definition, is not completed, and therefore respondents must decide whether the perpetrator actually intended to rape them. Overall, there were no significant differences in the proportion of respondents who reported an event the *first time only* versus the *second time only*. Thus, 33% of participants reported an event during the first SLESQ administration that was omitted on the second administration, and 30% of participants reported a new event during the retest.

Psychometric analysis of the ELS has focused on the double administrations of the ELS interview (ELS-I). The ELS questionnaire (ELS-Q) data are not reported here because the questionnaire functions as a prompt for the interview and is not conceptually designed to be a stand-alone instrument. Using the ELS-I, analyses examined the reliability of events reported at Interview 1 and 2 for eight types of trauma. Early global analyses of the first 40 participants suggest that kappa is highly variable but is higher for more salient events and for more clearly defined categories. Kappas ranged from .32 and .41 for serious illness or injury in adulthood and childhood, respectively, to .90 for childhood accidents and 1.0 for both childhood physical abuse and adult war-zone exposure. Due to its comprehensiveness, the ELS can examine the reliability of reporting events in finer detail, for example, according to their A1 or A1 *and* A2 PTSD determination. Kappas ranged from .14 to .78 for potentially traumatic events and from .31 to .84 for traumatic events that meet both criteria A1 and A2 of PTSD. Thus, not only does the ELS demonstrate adequate test-retest reliability, but as noted earlier, it allows examining the subjective component of the stressor Criterion A.

Although both instruments demonstrated good overall test-retest reliability and excellent reliability for some items, it is just as important to note that kappas for some individual items were far from perfect. Some of the inconsistent reporting may have been due to differential interpretation of questions at the separate administrations, but respondents nevertheless failed to report events as serious as rape until the second administration of the SLESQ, for example. Thus, inconsistent reporting may represent a more general phenomenon and not simply characteristics of a specific instrument.

It is unlikely that factors such as amnesia or dissociation played a significant role in unreliable reporting, given the short time frames (two weeks for the SLESQ and two to ten days for the ELS) between the first and second administrations of the instruments. Nevertheless, these phenomena may well play a role in inconsistent reporting generally because a growing number of studies have demonstrated that individuals can lose and then recover memories of past trauma (Briere & Conte, 1993; Williams, 1995), and amnesia for aspects of an event is a PTSD symptom criterion. Another explanation for potential inconsistencies is that a respondent's state of mind may change across administrations, leading to changes in the ability or motivation to retrieve remote memories at any given time or to shifts in appraising a specific event (e.g., whether a rape had been attempted, whether a situation was life-threatening) which could then influence reporting. It is likely that these explanations apply generally to trauma history measures and not just to our instruments.

Validity Assessment for the SLESQ and ELS

Establishing the psychometric soundness of trauma history measures such as the SLESQ and ELS requires ingenuity and creative methodology to address the many inherent challenges of trauma history validation. For example, with the current SLESQ study, seeking external corroboration of events was not feasible, although this would add to the instrument's overall validity if we are able to address this issue in future studies. As another example, because of the ELS' comprehensiveness, which goes far beyond prior measures, it is not appropriate to compare ELS prevalence rates for Vietnam-era veterans with regional or national probability samples using less comprehensive measures. Once again, the differing formats and purposes of the SLESQ and the ELS led to different strategies for evaluating the two measures.

Concurrent Validity. To establish concurrent validity for the SLESQ, we compared prevalence rates from our own study to those obtained in studies using other instruments. Again, for all analyses, we used *all* responses, whether or not they met the conservative cutoff established for determining specificity. Wording of items, behavioral specificity of questions, definitions, and thresholds for trauma differ across trauma history measures and make comparisons across studies imprecise. However, where possible, prevalence rates for the traumatic events listed in the SLESQ were compared to rates found in prevalence studies using two large probability samples (Kessler et al., 1995 [national]; Norris, 1992 [regional]). Except for robbery, traumatic bereavement, and witnessing death, the prevalence rates for specific events in our college sample were consistent with (e.g., life-threatening accident) or higher than (e.g., child and adult sexual assault and abuse, as well as physical abuse) those reported by either Kessler et al. or Norris (see Goodman et al., in press). With regard to the higher rates for assault/ abuse, our sexual assault questions, for example, included probes about a range of potential perpetrators, specific sexual acts, and situations such as being asleep or drugged. Because avoiding loaded terms such as "rape," including behaviorally specific items, and comprehensive questioning have been shown to have a profound influence on reporting rates, it is not surprising that our prevalence rates were higher than those elicited with Kessler's more loaded question or Norris's more general question. Our sexual assault prevalence rates are consistent with those reported in a national probability sample of college students (Koss et al., 1987) that used a detailed measure of sexual assault which includes behavioral definitions and avoids labels. The lower rates for robbery and traumatic loss may be due to wording, but our questions for those items were heavily based on the TSS (Norris, 1992). Thus, a more parsimonious hypothesis is that the samples in these two studies simply had different opportunities to experience those events based on their age differences.

Construct Validity. Further evidence for the validity of the SLESQ was obtained in a larger study of college women (*N* = 2483) who had also taken the Trauma Symptom Inventory (TSI; Briere, 1995). The total number of events reported on the SLESQ was correlated with the TSI clinical scales. All correlations were significant at $p < .001$, and ranged from .23 for the impaired self reference scale to .41 for the intrusive experiences scale.

Pilot data using an early version of the ELS with male veterans on an inpatient substance abuse unit indicated that over 50% of the men reported histories of severe physical or sexual child abuse (Krinsley et al., 1992). Evidence for the construct validity of the ELS was demonstrated by differences between veterans who did and did not report abuse histories. The veterans who reported childhood trauma reported significantly more severe levels of psychopathology on self-report measures, including significantly elevated scores on the MMPI-2, the Symptom Checklist 90-Revised, and the Mississippi Scale for Civilian PTSD. Childhood traumas were also associated with higher levels of PTSD and a higher incidence of Axis II diagnoses. In the psychometric study of the ELS, trauma severity for the first 40 participants was significantly associated with symptom severity on measures of PTSD such as the CAPS (Blake et al., 1990), thus supporting the validity of the ELS as a trauma-assessing instrument.

Convergent Validity.   Overall, the SLESQ demonstrated good convergent validity with a correlation of .77 between the number of events reported on the screening measure and the number of events reported in an interview two weeks later. Kappas for the occurrence of specific traumatic events ranged from .26 (witnessed death/assault) to .90 (life threatening illness), with a median kappa of .64. Kappas for the two "catchall" items were .08 for other horrifying event and .88 for other life threat. Six items fell below a kappa of .60, and for all of these lower kappa items, the differences in reporting across screen-interview administrations was in the direction of increased reporting in the interview. Indeed, in contrast to the screen–screen condition, many more participants reported an *additional* event in the interview (54%) compared to those who *omitted* an event at the follow-up interview (30%). Similarly, significantly more events were reported for respondents interviewed at the second administration (mean = 2.94 for time 2 interview) compared to the number of events reported at the time 1 screening (mean = 1.89) (Goodman et al., in press).

To explore whether the increased reporting at the time 2 interview (and subsequently lower kappas on particular items) resulted from the interview's relatively greater sensitivity to detect exposure to Criterion A events or from its elicitation of more subthreshold events, we used the event evaluation procedure described earlier with respect to specificity to determine whether the additional events reported in the course of the interview met the Criterion A standard. In addition, to determine whether differential reporting resulted from timing (second administration) versus method (interview), we also evaluated all additional events reported at the time 2 screening but not reported at the time 1 screening. Using this method, we rated 46 (63%) of the additional events reported in the interview condition as subthreshold, compared to only 10 additional events (29%) reported in the time 2 screening condition. Therefore, most of the additional events reported in the interviews were actually events that we did not define as potential Criterion A events and thus did not intend to pick up on the screening questionnaire (e.g., sibling fights and spanking by parents) (Goodman et al., in press).

Collateral Confirmation of Worst Traumas.   In a separate part of the ELS psychometric study, there is an ongoing attempt to document convergent validity by obtaining corroborating reports on participants' two worst traumas, one from childhood and one from adulthood. This task is clearly very difficult, but the attempt was considered important. The goal was to investigate what, if any, additional validation could be found for a wide variety of retrospectively reported traumatic events. For the first 40 participants, 72% of the events were confirmed when a source was available and could be located. However, this involved only 65% of the total cases; when the total number of "worst events" ($N = 77$) was considered, the percent of satisfactorily confirmed cases dropped to 47%. Because relatively few resources were devoted to this aspect of the study, it is not clear whether these results would have improved with greater effort. On the other hand, the fact that even 47% of past traumatic events have some outside confirmation supports the validity of the ELS.

Limitations. We have presented two measures that are presently being used to assess lifetime exposure to traumatic events. However, although the initial work on these instruments is promising, these studies, so far, have been conducted on restricted populations. The ELS has been limited to male veterans, and the SLESQ has been tested only on college students. Therefore, both instruments need additional work of the same type using more general samples. Presently, we are gathering data on the SLESQ in samples of low-income women in the community who are attending family planning clinics. This sample will help us establish the psychometric properties of the SLESQ in a more representative sample. We will also be testing differences associated with its administration as a self-report.

Research Recommendations and Clinical Implications

It seems clear that psychometric evaluation of trauma exposure measures, although difficult, needs to be conducted to advance our understanding of which types and aspects of exposure place individuals at risk for negative outcomes. Although the SLESQ and ELS generally demonstrate good reliability and validity, even with consistent questions and short time periods between measure administrations, reporting of individual potentially traumatic events is not completely reliable. Thus, the reliability problems found with both measures need to be further explored. Changes may be associated with particular events or other characteristics of exposure. For example, are events that occurred in childhood reported more unreliably than those experienced in adolescence or adulthood? Are events involving shame or guilt more unreliably reported, etc.? How do respondents react when we remind them of an omitted event they reported previously? We may be observing more specific and meaningful lapses in reporting than are assessed by simply indicating that an event has been reported on one, versus two, occasions. The kappas, of course, vary by event and give us some of this information. However, more details could be obtained to help address why changes occur.

Another implication of these findings, we believe, is that omnibus traumatic event questions, like those on the Structured Clinical Interview for the DSM-III-R (SCID; Spitzer et al., 1987) are unlikely to provide comprehensive exposure data. If our questioning about specific events did not lead to completely reliable reporting, the likelihood is quite low that one open-ended question about traumatic exposure would produce reliable results. It is already known that these types of questions underestimate exposure. For example, Weaver (1998) asked the open-ended exposure question from the SCID, followed later in the interview by specific, behaviorally worded items assessing separate event types. In her sample of battered women, she found huge increases in reporting with the specific assessments. For example, reports of childhood sexual abuse went up from 7% on the SCID question to 53% with the behaviorally specific item. Childhood physical abuse went from 9% to 74%, and adult rape from 7% to 21% with more specific questions. These findings reinforce the importance of using comprehensive measures, and the work cited herein underscores the need for psychometric work with these more comprehensive measures.

This work has major implications for clinical practice as well. For example, because of inconsistency in reporting, clients may need to be evaluated on more than one occasion to obtain a relatively complete picture of their trauma histories. As noted earlier, because of the frequency and cumulative effects of multiple traumas, even if a client is seeking treatment for a specific trauma or disorder, it is important to obtain a comprehensive assessment of trauma exposure to understand the possible range of influences on current symptoms, feelings, and behaviors.

Despite the DSM-IV general guidelines and even with reliable reporting, investigators may disagree about definitions of exposure to a "traumatic event." Thus, researchers must continue to establish their own threshold criteria, and consensus is likely to be lower at the event-specific level. The extent to which respondents' own appraisals are incorporated into definitions (e.g., whether an encounter was "life-threatening") also varies across studies. Although the respondents' assessments will almost certainly be good predictors of their psychological reactions, they also merge subjective and objective aspects of stressor definitions.

In conclusion, it is clear that whether and how a person experiences a trauma is a complex question, requiring an equally sophisticated response beyond a simple "yes" or "no" answer. We recommend using measures that have been psychometrically evaluated to assess trauma history. Finally, more psychometric evaluations are necessary for existing and future measures.

References

American Psychiatric Association (1980). *Diagnostic and statistical manual of mental disorders*, 3rd ed. Washington, DC: American Psychiatric Press

American Psychiatric Association (1987). *Diagnostic and statistical manual of mental disorders*, 3rd ed., rev. Washington, DC: American Psychiatric Press.

American Psychiatric Association (1994). *Diagnostic and statistical manual of mental disorders*, 4th ed. Washington, DC: American Psychiatric Press.

Blake, D. D., Weathers, F. W., Nagy, L. M., Kaloupek, D. G., Klauminizer, G., Charney, D., & Keane, T. M. (1990). A clinician rating scale for assessing current and lifetime PTSD: The CAPS-1, *The Behavior Therapist*, *13*, 187–188.

Briere, J. (1995). *Trauma symptom inventory professional manual*. Odessa, FL: Psychological Assessment Resources.

Briere, J., & Conte, J. (1993). Self-reported amnesia for abuse in adults molested as children. *Journal of Traumatic Stress*, *6*, 21–31.

Foa, E. B., Riggs, D. S., Dancer, C. V., & Rothblum, B. O. (1993). Reliability and validity of a brief instrument for assessing post-traumatic stress disorder. *Journal of Traumatic Stress*, *6*, 459–473.

Follette, V. M., Polusny, M., Bechtle, A. E., & Naugle, A. E. (1996). Cumulative trauma: The impact of child sexual abuse, adult sexual assault, and spouse abuse. *Journal of Traumatic Stress*, *9*, 25–35.

Goodman, L. A., Corcoran, C. B., Turner, K., Yuan, N., & Green, B. L. (in press). Assessing traumatic event exposure: General issues and preliminary findings for the Stressful Life Events Screening Questionnaire. *Journal of Traumatic Stress*.

Goodman, L. A., Dutton, M. A., & Harris, M. (1997). The relationship between violence dimensions and symptom severity among episodically homeless, mentally ill women. *Journal of Traumatic Stress*, *10*, 51–70.

Green, B. L. (1996). Trauma history questionnaire (self-report). In B. H. Stamm (Ed.), *Measurement of stress, trauma, and adaptation* (pp. 366–368). Lutherville, MD: Sidran.

Kessler, R. C., Sonnega, A., Bromet, E., Hughes, M., & Nelson, C. (1995). Posttraumatic stress disorder in the National Comorbidity Survey. *Archives of General Psychiatry*, *52*, 1048–1060.

Koss, M. P., Gidycz, C. A., & Wisniewski, N. (1987). The scope of rape: Incidence and prevalence of sexual aggression and victimization in a national sample of higher education students. *Journal of Consulting and Clinical Psychology*, *55*, 162–170.

Krinsley, K. E., Weathers, F. W., Vielhauer, M. J., Newman, E., Walker, E. A., Kaloupek, D. G., Young, L. S., & Kimerling, R. (1994). Unpublished document. NC-PTSD—Behavioral Science Division.

Krinsley, K. E., Young, L. S., Weathers, F. W., Brief, D. J., & Kelley, J. M. (1992). Behavioral correlates of childhood trauma in substance abusing men. Presented at the *Annual Meeting of AABT*, Boston, MA.

Norris, F. H. (1990). Screening for traumatic stress: A scale for use in the general population. *Journal of Applied Social Psychology*, *20*, 1704–1718.

Norris, F. H. (1992). Epidemiology of trauma: Frequency and impact of different potentially traumatic events on different demographic groups. *Journal of Consulting and Clinical Psychology*, *60*, 409–418.

Norris, F. H., & Perilla, J. L. (1996). The Revised Civilian Mississippi Scale for PTSD: Reliability, validity, and cross-language stability. *Journal of Traumatic Stress*, *9*, 285–298.

Resnick, H. S., Kilpatrick, D. G., Dansky, B. S., Saunders, B. E., & Best, C. L. (1993). Prevalence of civilian trauma and posttraumatic stress disorder in a representative national sample of women. *Journal of Consulting and Clinical Psychology*, *61*, 984–991.

Spitzer, R. L., Williams, J. B., & Gibbon, M. (1987). *Structured Clinical Interview for DSM-III-R—Non-Patient Version* (SCID-NP). New York: New York State Psychiatric Institute, Biometrics Research Department.

Sutker, P. B., Uddo-Crane, M., & Allain, A. N., Jr. (1991). Clinical and research assessment of posttraumatic stress disorder: A conceptual overview. *Psychological Assessment: A Journal of Consulting and Clinical Psychology*, *3*, 520–530.

Vrana, S., & Lauterbach, D. (1994). Prevalence of traumatic events and posttraumatic psychological symptoms in a nonclinical sample of college students. *Journal of Traumatic Stress*, *7*, 289–302.

Weaver, T. L. (1998). Method variance and sensitivity of screening for traumatic stressors. *Journal of Traumatic Stress*, *11*, 181–185.

Widom, C. S., & Shepard, R. L. (1996). Accuracy of adult recollections of childhood victimization: Part 1. Childhood physical abuse. *Psychological Assessment*, *8*, 412–421.

Williams, L. M. (1995). Recovered memories of abuse in women with documented child sexual victimization histories. *Journal of Traumatic Stress*, *8*, 649–673.

17

When the Victim Forgets

Trauma-Induced Amnesia and Its Assessment in Holocaust Survivors

ONNO VAN DER HART AND DANNY BROM

I want to remember my past
To see before my eyes
The image of my parents
The house in which I grew up
The village in which my family lived for generations
I don't want to remember my past
I fear for what my memory
Might bring before my eyes
I wonder whether I can continue my life
If I'll rescue from oblivion
What I want to recall.
(Itta Benhaiem-Keller, 1996, Holocaust survivor)

People who went through the horrors of the Holocaust struggle with their memories in different ways. Many experience overwhelming and intrusive recollections accompanied by strong emotions, even more so fifty years after the end of the war than earlier. Others have tried to silence their memories by attempts to keep the memories away or by dissociating themselves from the memories. Not much has been written about this other side of the coping process, that is, to what extent do survivors of the Holocaust succeed to distance themselves from their experiences. Forgetting in the form of repression, denial, and dissociation is a common phenomenon in the aftermath of other traumatic instances (Kleber & Brom, 1992), and amnesia has also been demonstrated after combat experiences (Karon & Widener, 1997; Van der Hart et al., 1999).

The purpose of this chapter is to present a systematic overview of the existing

ONNO VAN DER HART • Department of Clinical Psychology, Utrecht University, Utrecht, The Netherlands; and Cato-Polm Institute, Zeist, The Netherlands. **DANNY BROM** • AMCHA, The National Israeli Center for Psychosocial Support of Survivors of the Holocaust and the Second Generation, Jerusalem 93385, Israel.

International Handbook of Human Response to Trauma, edited by Shalev, Yehuda, and McFarlane. Kluwer Academic / Plenum Publishers, New York, 2000.

literature on the subject of trauma-induced amnesia in Holocaust survivors. Although the concept of repression was current in the older clinical literature, we prefer the expression of dissociative amnesia instead, thereby following DSM-IV (APA, 1994) and the currently prevailing view (e.g., Brown et al., 1998; van der Kolk et al., 1996). The DSM-IV describes dissociative amnesia as "an inability to recall important personal information, usually of a traumatic or stressful nature, that is too extensive to be explained by normal forgetfulness" (p. 478). Here we are primarily interested in descriptions of dissociative amnesia as a phenomenon, not whether it should be regarded as a psychiatric disorder or as a part of a disorder.

Relevance of the Subject

In the recent emotionally charged debate on the existence of trauma-induced amnesia and false/recovered memories, in particular with regard to childhood sexual abuse (CSA) (Loftus, 1993; Ofshe & Watters, 1993), the issue of amnesia in Holocaust survivors for their war traumas has become the center of a heated debate. Although some participants in this debate have proposed that psychogenic amnesia, other than normal forgetting, for trauma does not exist at all (e.g., Loftus, 1993; Ofshe & Watters, 1993; Pope & Hudson, 1995), some memory specialists have even stated that no evidence exists for the occurrence of amnesia in survivors for their experiences in the Nazi concentration camps (Wagenaar & Crombag, 1995). This point is taken further by Holocaust revisionists, such as Butz (1991), who claim that testimonies about the Holocaust do not prove that the Holocaust did actually occur.

In the area of CSA, empirical evidence is accumulating that a significant proportion of adult survivors have amnesia (Pope, 1996) for all or parts of their abuse. Thus, Brown, Scheflin, and Whitfield (1999) reviewed 68 data-based studies, both retrospective and longitudinal, that demonstrate that such amnesia is a robust finding across all of these studies. In other fields of traumatic stress there is a body of research showing the occurrence of amnesia (Loewenstein, 1996). However, in documenting the psychological sequelae of the Holocaust in its survivors, the emphasis in ego documents and scientific and clinical publications has mainly been on remembering their sufferings and on how their memories affect their current lives. In a continuing urge to bear witness, the fact that some survivors may be amnesic for all or significant parts of their Holocaust experiences has been relatively neglected. True as this may be, references to this phenomenon are not altogether absent.

Amnesia in Holocaust Survivors: General Remarks

In his book, *Moments of Reprieve*, author and Holocaust survivor Primo Levi (1986) remarked that "it has been observed by psychologists that the survivors of traumatic events are divided in two well-defined groups: those who repress their past en bloc and those whose memory of the offense persists, as though carved in stone, prevailing over all previous or subsequent experiences" (pp. 10–11). Levi went on to say that he, by nature, belonged to the second group. "Of my two years of life outside the law I have not forgotten a single thing. Without any deliberate effort, memory continues to restore to me events, faces, words, sensations, as if at that time my mind had gone through a period of exalted receptivity, during which not a detail was lost" (p. 11). Primo Levi, whose focus was on bearing witness of his own experiences in the Nazi camps, nevertheless noted the existence of massive amnesia in some other survivors.

In Dwork's work on the oral history of child survivors of the Holocaust (1991), the emphasis is also on the phenomenon of hypermnesia, almost by definition ignoring the existence of amnesia. Thus, she quoted Halina Birenbaum (1971), age fifteen when liberated from the concentration camp Neustadt-Glewe, who twenty years later, in the conclusion of her account of her Holocaust experiences confessed her inability to forget. "Everything, down to the most minute details, remained unerased and fresh in my memory, as though it had happened yesterday" (p. 244).

What, then, has been reported on amnesia for such experiences? Apart from the various case descriptions to be presented here, several authors have paid largely unsystematic attention to it. In general, their observations are rather abstract or do not include enough data to be certain about the nature of this presumed amnesia. One of the first was Niederland (1968), who, in his discussion of the symptomatology of the so-called survivor syndrome, mentioned memory disturbances such as amnesia and hypermnesia, disorientation between the present and the period of persecution, as well as dissociative phenomena. In the same year, the psychoanalyst and Auschwitz survivor De Wind (1968) remarked that most former inmates of Nazi concentration camps could not remember anything of the first days of imprisonment. "The experience of reality would be overwhelming and would cause chaos" (p. 19). Allowing chaos and regression was dangerous in the camps, De Wind noted, because one had to remain capable of reacting more or less adequately. In describing disturbances in thought and memory, Musaph (1973) observed that amnesia may exist for certain persecutory experiences, whereas other Holocaust experiences are extremely well remembered. Kluft (1997) stated, "... among the Holocaust survivors I have interviewed, I have not encountered any one who did not recall being caught up in the Holocaust, but I have spoken to many who, despite the inextinguishable recollection of unspeakable horrors, had considerable gaps in their autobiographical memories of their personal ordeals" (p. 50). Hogman (1985), herself a child survivor of the Holocaust, writes about the "arduous, but necessary task" of recovering memories that were lost since the traumatic period.

Trauma-induced amnesia is referred to in Van Ravesteijn's (1976) clinical observations of survivors of the Nazi concentration camps. In reality, he remarked, they feel impotence to remember this episode: most memories have become prey to amnesia. "A smell, a sound, an image evoke fragments of images or emotions, more compelling than current reality, fragments to which all experienced pain, anger, fear, shame and powerlessness have attached themselves. Must a coherent account be given, then it is often painfully apparent that this is impossible. Mostly, the person is unable to present an overview of this period" (p. 195).

In their study of Holocaust-related memories, Mazor et al. (1990) interviewed 15 child survivors of the Holocaust and stated, "Only two individuals said that they repressed their past. For one the war seemed a prehistoric period disconnected from the time after the war. The other person said that he was too young and could not grasp the war period at all ... one person said that he repressed his memories both after the war and 40 years later, and he forgot a lot of his memories" (p. 6). However, the exact nature of this repression remained unclear: did this "repression" refer to true amnesia, or did their observations pertain to conscious efforts to avoid the memories?

The same question can be asked about the observations of Bastiaans (1987), who wrote, "The intensities of repression and of that which was repressed were highly underestimated" (p. 114).

The findings of Lagnado and Dekel (1991) in this regard do seem to imply true amnesia, but the question may be asked here if infantile amnesia, i.e., the loss of memories from early childhood, is what this amnesia is about. In their study of the twins who were abused by Dr. Josef Mengele in his cruel experiments in Auschwitz, these authors reported, "A few of the twins insisted that they had no memories of Auschwitz whatsoever. Instead, they dwelt on the sadness of their postwar adult lives—their emotional upheavals, physical breakdowns, and longings for the dead parents they had hardly known. The younger they were at Auschwitz the less they consciously remembered, the greater their turmoil as adults: That was the rule" (p. 8).

Laub and Auerhahn (1993) more systematically studied trauma-induced amnesia in Holocaust survivors, which they placed within their typology of forms of knowing and not knowing massive trauma (i.e., Holocaust trauma). They organized the different forms of knowing along a continuum according to the mental distance from the traumatic experience.

> The different forms of remembering trauma range from not knowing; fugue states (in which events are relived in an altered state of consciousness); retention of the experience as compartmentalized, undigested fragments of perceptions that break into consciousness (with no conscious meaning or relation to oneself); transference phenomena (wherein the traumatic legacy is lived out as one's inevitable fate); its partial, hesitant expression as an overpowering narrative; to its use as a metaphor and vehicle for developmental conflict. These different forms of knowing, ranging along the continuum of psychological distance from the trauma, also vary in degree of encapsulation versus integration of the experience and in degree of ownership of the memory—i.e. the degree to which an experiencing 'I' is present as subject. (p. 289)

In this chapter we are mainly concerned with the first two forms, which pertain to trauma-induced amnesia with and without dissociative reexperiences (i.e., hypermnesia).

Amnesia in Holocaust Survivors: Case Descriptions

The existing literature reports several cases of Holocaust survivors with amnesia for some or all of their Holocaust experiences. In presenting these cases, we follow the DSM-IV (APA, 1994) classification of dissociative (or psychogenic) amnesia, a traditional classification which was proposed a century ago (e.g., Janet, 1893/1901): localized amnesia, selective amnesia, generalized amnesia, continuous amnesia, and systematized amnesia.

Localized Amnesia

According to the DSM-IV, in localized amnesia the individual fails to recall events that occurred during a circumscribed period of time, usually the first few hours following a profoundly disturbing event. Janet (1893/1901) noted: "The events of which the remembrance is lost are gathered into a common characteristic. They all belong to the same epoch, the same period of the patient's life" (p. 83). Localized amnesias may pertain to events of short duration, e.g., one traumatic event; others may range for longer periods of time. De Wind's (1968) observation, cited before, that most former inmates of Nazi concentration camps could not remember anything of the first days of imprisonment is an example of this circumscribed form of amnesia. However, the Holocaust literature reports cases with amnesia for more extended periods of time.

With regard to more restricted localized amnesia, several authors report amnesia in child survivors for the traumatic separation from their parents.

Daniela. In his study on Jewish war orphans in the Netherlands, Keilson (1979/92) described the case of Daniela, born on May 5, 1935, who was rescued from the "creche," a place for Jewish children waiting for their transport to the camps, in Amsterdam at the age of 8 together with her two older siblings. Commenting on a follow-up interview which he had with her in 1971, Keilson remarked: "Her numerous memories of her childhood and her parents were sharply delineated and accompanied by a strong emotional tone. This made it particularly surprising that the moment of separation from her parents and the train journey to her foster parents accompanied by a strange woman had apparently been erased from her memory" (p. 211).

Katy. In her classic paper on dissociative phenomena in former concentration camp inmates, Jaffe (1968) described a dissociative episode in a female patient manifested during a psychiatric examination and referring to an extremely traumatic experience for which apparently amnesia existed.

> Katy was 24 years old when war broke out. During the psychiatric examination she suddenly turned her head, rose, bowed, made searching movements with her head, covered her eye with her hand, as if to see better into the distance, listened, talked to herself, and burst into laughter which resembled crying. The impression she made on the observer was that of a psychotic patient. After some minutes she regained composure and related that she had heard her sister's voice. Exploration in narcoanalysis revealed that this pantomimic scene is an almost exact repetition of a traumatic situation which she had gone through on her arrival at the railway station of Auschwitz concentration camp. She had arrived there with her 8-year-old son and her younger sister who was the boy's maid. After the journey of several days in a closed cattle van, she had got out exhausted and dazed. When recovering after the first minutes of perplexity and confusion, she saw two columns of people leaving the station in different directions, one consisting of the old and of mothers with children, and the other one of young men and women. She understood from previous experiences that this was a "selection" and that the first column was destined for death. Before she could run after them and take her sister's place in order to save her, she was kicked into the second column of those selected for work. She could hear her sister calling "Katy where are you? Why do you leave me?"

Jaffe calls this phenomenon a dissociative state, in which "formerly suppressed and or hazily experienced events ... still cannot attain to the integrative faculty of the ego" (p. 312). Although Jaffe did not refer to amnesia per se, we believe that the disrupted connection between Katy's personal consciousness and her traumatic memories (explored in narcoanalysis) can be called dissociative amnesia.

Rose. A rather similar state was reported by Hass (1995), who described a woman who was 19 years old in the spring of 1944. Relating her visit to Auschwitz 40 years after liberation, she said: "And then the room filled with children's shoes. That was the hardest thing. I had been repressing something before I saw the children's shoes.... I saw children carried by Nazi soldiers to the Pit and dropping them into the Pit.... At the time I didn't want to believe that was what I was seeing. I hid that in my memory until I saw the shoes" (p. 166).

Misha. In his book *De zoektocht* [*The search*], the Dutch sociologist Durlacher (1991), a child survivor of Maennerlager Birkenau B II D, described his search for and meetings with another twenty child survivors from this camp. Misha, one of them, told him about his youth in Czechoslovakia and about the first years of the war, before he would be transported to the nazi camp Therezienstadt. Durlacher wrote:

> Misha's tempo of narrating slows down. He stares in the air to press the facts from his memory, he looks helplessly at me and admits hesitantly that the period in the camps is wiped out from his brain. The old school notebooks in front of him on the table appear to contain the report which he wrote directly after his liberation, following the advice of the doctors of the sanatorium in the Tatra mountains. With each question regarding the period of December 12, 1942, till May 7, 1945, he admits while feeling embarrassed that he cannot remember anything, and he leafs nervously through the pages written with a child's hand. He shows me his notebooks, and although I am unable to read the Czechoslovakian text, I recognize a great many situations from that time from the simple but revealing pen drawings: barracks, guards and Kapo's, prisoners at "appel", under stick beatings, at the gallows, SS's with whips and guns, a crematorium, barbed wire with isolators, a selection, the gate of Mauthausen. My questions about them die down. Why should I rip that soft coat of forgetfulness? There in that sanatorium during the Spring of 1945 he liberated himself of that poisonous burden. I almost envy him." (pp. 119–120)

In the next conversation, Misha told Durlacher about the time after the war. After having worked extremely hard (in order to numb himself), he went to live in 1951 with a nephew and his family in the United States.

> They were good to me, but I didn't feel happy there. I lived under a bell jar. The world around me seemed unreal. In spite of my dejection, I finished my studies at Columbia University. Suddenly, the loss of my family penetrated vehemently in me. I collapsed, and then a piece of the life in the camps disappeared. "Partial amnesia," the doctor called it. Without my notebooks, those years would have disappeared altogether. (p. 123)

Jindra. Durlacher (1991) described the similar example of Jindra, born in 1931, who was able to give some precise information about his childhood before the Holocaust, but who had to admit that he hardly remembers anything from his years in the camps. One thing he remembered is receiving the tattooed number on his left arm.

> From the winter months of 1944 until just before the liberation in April 1945, only two words stayed with him: Dora and Nordhausen. He mentions them, uncertain about the pronunciation. In a flash I understand his amnesia, and shocked I hold my tongue. Dora was the hell which almost nobody survived, was it not? Underground, without fresh air or daylight, Hitler's secret weapon of destruction, the V-2 rocket, was made by prisoners. Only the dying or the dead came above ground, and Kapo's and guards. (p. 129)

Mark. Kathy Steele (personal communication, August 30, 1996) mentioned her treatment of Mark, a male patient of Dutch Jewish descent suffering from a dissociative disorder. When he was between age twelve and fourteen, Mark had been interned— without his father, who had died before, or his mother—in one of the lesser known Nazi concentration camps. He had received this information from his mother and he reported this as a fact. However, he said that he had absolutely no memory of those two years. Subsequently, he told Steele that he had "caves" in his head, and many memories were stored there. He did not want to open them.

Child Survivor of Auschwitz. Somer (1994) described the treatment of a 58-year-old woman, born in Poland, who survived the Holocaust, amongst others, a year-long internment in Auschwitz. She was 11 years old when she saw the American liberators enter the gates of Auschwitz.

> During the first five sessions the patient's life history was taken.... The diagnostic impression was one of post-traumatic stress disorder, chronic, with dissociative features and psychosomatic correlates. The patient was amnesic to almost the entire duration of her imprisonment in Auschwitz. Fragmentary recall was devoid of any affect. The patient had only scarce memories of the years prior to her internment in the death camp. She felt as if her life began only following her liberation and subsequent immigration to Israel. (p. 57)

In hypnoanalytic therapy this patient managed to recover many memories of Auschwitz and of her separation from her parents.

Helen Landsbury. Auerhahn and Laub (submitted) tell of Helen Landsbury, a survivor who was reported on the ABC news show 20/20 in 1995. She

> has no recollections of her Holocaust experiences. Nor does she recall reunification after war with her two surviving siblings with whom she was persecuted during some of the war years. Instead, she fondly remembers the prewar years of her earlier childhood and her postwar marriage to a non-Jewish British soldier. She left her siblings in Europe to begin a new life in England, where she raised her children as non-Jews and talked to her new family only about the "before," never about the war itself. She had no idea that her siblings, who eventually emigrated to the United States, were still alive and that they continued to search for her for 50 years. By the time they finally located her through the American Red Cross, she was in her 70s and facing ovarian cancer. At that point she was finally able to acknowledge regret and a sense of loss over having given up her ties to Judaism and over the gap in her memories.

Selective Amnesia

In selective amnesia, the person can recall some, but not all, of the events during a circumscribed period of time, e.g., a combat veteran can recall only some parts of a series of violent combat experiences (APA, 1994).

Ava Landy. In Marks' (1995) collection of interviews with hidden child survivors, Ava Landy described her amnesia for most of her experiences during the war, since Yom Kippur 1942, when she was four years of age. Then the SS came to arrest her father, after which she went into hiding in a series of different places.

> So much of my childhood between the ages of four and nine is blank. I have so many questions without answers! I feel like an unfinished puzzle. It's almost as if my life was smashed into little pieces on that Yom Kippur that my father was taken, and I've been spending my life ever since then trying to put the pieces together in a way that make sense. The trouble is, when I try to remember, I come up with so little. This ability to forget was probably my way of surviving emotionally as a child. Even now, whenever anything unpleasant happens to me, I have a mental garbage can in which I can put all the bad stuff and forget it. (p. 188) At night I lie in bed and I try to remember my childhood, but I just can't! I tried hypnosis once. It didn't work at all. Nevertheless I keep hoping and imagining that someday something will bring my memory back. Whenever my sister and I get together, or when I go to Belgium or Israel, we always end up talking about the war. Eventually the reminiscing gets to be competitive. Invariably someone starts to brag, "If you think you know an interesting story, listen to this one!" That's been the ritual, year after year. Well, you know what? I'm the one who knows all the best stories! I know a zillion stories. The trouble is, they're all other people's stories. None of them are mine. (p. 193)

Systematized Amnesia

Systematized amnesia is loss of memory for certain categories of information, such as all memories relating to one's family or to a particular person (APA, 1994). "The patients lose, not all their remembrances acquired during a certain period, but a certain category of remembrances, a certain group of ideas of the same kind, constituting a system. Thus, they will forget what relates to their family or all the ideas relating to such or such a person" (Janet, 1901, p. 79).

Ruth Rubenstein. In Marks's (1995) collection of interviews with hidden child survivors, Ruth Rubenstein reported amnesia for the visits her parents, also in hiding, made to her once a month. Her family fled from East Prussia to Belgium in 1939, when she was one and a half. Shortly thereafter, her father was picked up and sent to a detention camp from which he escaped one year later. Ruth did not recognize him anymore. In 1942 her parents left her with the nuns without giving any explanation. When they were allowed to visit her after six weeks, "I was a wreck! I was practically mute and I kept crossing myself. I wasn't sure who they were. I had lice, impetigo, and bronchitis. I also must have been very angry. When they asked me if I wanted to come home, I said no" (p. 117). Subsequently, she was brought to a childless couple named DeMarneff, with whom she had a good time. "As it turned out, this was my first normal childhood experience. I had children to play with, including two best friends. My parents, who spent the war hiding in a series of different places in Brussels, visited me once a month. Apparently that was the only time they got to eat. Strangely I cannot remember a single one of their visits!" (p. 118). Ruth stayed with the DeMarneff's for two and a half years. "When the war was over, Mami and Papi DeMarneff didn't want to part with me. Once again I don't remember any good-byes" (p. 118).

Judy Cohen. Judy Cohen (personal communication, June 6, 1996) related that her amnesic episodes during the Holocaust seemed to be connected with trains and travel. A survivor of Jewish-Hungarian origin born in 1929, she survived approximately five months in Auschwitz-Birkenau, three months in Bergen Belsen, three months working as a slave laborer in a Junkers Aeroplane factory in Asherleben, and a forced march lasting about ten to fourteen days, she believes. On May 5, 1945, at age 16, she was liberated, together with the pitiful remnants of about 185 from the original 500 at the beginning of the march from Asherleben to possible oblivion. She remembers most of the major events but not specific episodes related to trains and travel. This is not only true today but also for the time directly after liberation.

The trip from Auschwitz-Birkenau to Bergen Belsen is not more than a "blur," although she does have clear memories from Bergen Belsen itself. The same pattern of "forgetting" is present in all of her reporting.

> My memory fails me again when it comes to getting, with 500 other girls, from Bergen Belsen to Asherleben. I have no idea whether the mode of transportation was cattle cars or regular passenger trains, or whether we ate or not. Nothing, zilch.
> And then, finally, after the liberation by the American Armed Forces, we were gathered in a huge refugee center in Leipzig.... This much I recall that the Americans took all of us who wanted to return to Hungary to the Czech border, in huge army trucks. There they put us on trains. And that's it. From here on, my mind is a total blank. I have absolutely no idea how I, along with the others, got to Budapest. How long it took, who provided food, what cities we went through? I remember nothing, absolutely nothing.
> The next thing I recall is being in the office of the Budapest Jewish Community,

which was functioning quite well by then. I remember eating good food somewhere, maybe in a restaurant, and then again being put on yet another train to get back to my hometown Debrecen. The same thing here, too. The trip is a blank.

Bessie K. Laub (personal communication, May 1996) remarked that, among types of amnesia, the phenomenon that struck him most is that of parents who lost their children in the Holocaust and did not "remember" their existence. "I truly believe they did not know of those children. I have seen myself three such patients and heard of many more." In this regard Laub and Powell (submitted) refer also to Langer (1995), who quoted the videotaped testimony of the Holocaust survivor Bessie K. She recalled how she attempted to hide her baby boy while German guards separated men, women, and children in preparation for boarding them into cattle trains.

> But the baby was short of breath, started to choke, and it started to cry, so the German called me back, he said in German, "What do you have there?" Now; I didn't know what to do, because everything was so fast and everything happened so suddenly. I wasn't prepared for it.
> To look back, the experience was—I think I was numb, or something happened to me, I don't know. But I wasn't there. And he stretched out his arms I should hand him over the bundle; and I hand him over the bundle. And this is the last time I had the bundle ...

Soon after, in the Stutthof concentration camp, she met the doctor who had previously treated her while they both lived in the ghetto before the deportation. She continued:

> And when she [the doctor] saw me there she was so happy to see me, and right away she says, "What happened, where's the baby, what happened to the baby?" And right there I said, "What baby?" I said to the doctor, "What baby? I didn't have a baby. I don't know of any baby."

Bessie K. then paused, tapped her brow with a finger, and concluded: "That's what it did to me" (pp. 143–144).

Generalized Amnesia

In general amnesia, failure of recall encompasses the person's entire life (APA, 1994). If we extend this definition to amnesia for one's entire life before the war or until some time after the liberation, then several cases reported in the current literature should be placed under this heading. Janet (1893/1901) observed that in cases of this rare form of amnesia, "the patient, after a series of attacks or sleeps, may have apparently lost entirely all the remembrances acquired in her life. It would seem that she is born a second time, and that she has to learn over again all she has learned in her childhood" (1901, pp. 85–86).

It is perhaps not surprising that, after such massive traumatization as occurred during the Holocaust, this form as compared to the number of other reported kinds of Holocaust amnesias is not exceptionally rare.

Dan. In his follow-up study on the fate of the Jewish war orphans in the Netherlands, Keilson (1979/1992) presented 204 case studies. A few of them showed extended amnesia, which is mentioned only in passing by Keilson. One of the clearer instances concerns Dan, born on October 12, 1930, who fled from Germany to Holland at the age of seven with two older siblings.

He spent the war—separated from his siblings—in ten different hiding places. His second traumatic sequence must be classed as particularly severe. This period is described ... as follows: arrested in several raids, escaped, hiding place guesthouse, dangers, isolated, no schooling, nights on the streets, enuresis, occasional contact with older sister, courier for the resistance movement. After the war Dan stayed in his last foster environment for three months as his siblings were not yet able to take him in. Then came a six-month stay in a Danish convalescent home and return to his siblings. Apart from severe difficulty concentrating and working—he withdrew from the final examination of high school—he had considerable gratitude problems, flight fantasies and persecution dreams. He was inhibited, lacking in initiative, tense and suffered from total amnesia concerning the first ten years of his life; he perspired heavily. Pseudo-adaptation in Jewish settings and associations. Essentially isolated, depressive, difficulty relating to others. (1992, p. 205)

O.K.   Modai (1994) reported the case of O.K., a 58-year-old female hidden child survivor in Israel with total amnesia for her whole childhood including the Holocaust, who sought help for depression. She suffered from inability to function, low self-esteem, lack of concentration, insomnia, suicidal ideation, withdrawal and guilt feelings. O.K. heard some details about her childhood from a cousin in Israel who witnessed her childhood hardships. She was born in Hungary, an only child to a Jewish couple. When she was eight years old, the Germans first took her father, then a few months later, arrested her mother. She was left with her grandmother who died a few days afterwards. The neighbors found her sitting by her dead grandmother and put her in a monastery. There she learned to serve Christianity. After the war, she was collected by her parents who survived concentration camps and sent to a Jewish religious school. When she was 14 years old, she immigrated to Israel with her parents. The immigration ship was arrested by the British authorities and all immigrants were taken to a camp in Cyprus. While getting off the ship, she lost her parents and was found by a British soldier. In Israel she was put in a kibbutz (p. 69).

> She suffered from total amnesia of her childhood in Hungary and of everything that happened to her during the Holocaust. When talking about it in an intellectual manner, no feelings were aroused. She could only cognitively imagine a sad story of another child going through all these hardships but without actually feeling anything. Also, she did not dream about any event that happened to her during these hard times.
>
> The information she received from her cousin did not revive her memory. Childhood was completely dissociated from the course of her life. An attempt to confront her with actual objects from her past, for instance, sending her to visit the immigrant ship, triggered an immediate manic episode followed by a deep depression and a dangerous suicidal attempt. She tried to jump in front of a big truck. (pp. 69–70)

In the course of psychotherapy she did not regain her memory of her childhood.

Child Survivor of Auschwitz.   Simenauer (1968) saw "the complete loss of identity" in numerous survivors of the concentration and extermination camps. Although it is not totally clear what he means by this loss of identity, he clearly refers to the loss of the memory of most of the traumatic period, which allows the person to live as if he had not gone through it. Simenauer describes the case of a 7-year-old boy who was taken to a Polish ghetto with his family. Afterwards he was transferred to Auschwitz. "His only conscious memory of Auschwitz contains heavy work, hunger, cold and disturbed sleep." After the war he "achieved extraordinary adaptive processes" and besides some free floating anxiety "his character formation presents all the signs of an infinitely precarious balance, but up to now no more psychopathological symptoms are forthcoming" (p. 307).

Continuous Amnesia

The DSM-IV defines continuous amnesia as the inability to recall events subsequent to a specific time up to and including the present. We have not found any reference to the occurrence of continuous amnesia in Holocaust survivors.

Research Data

In the research literature on Holocaust survivors we found six studies reporting on amnesia. We should make clear, however, that most of these studies report on amnesia as a symptom, and they generally do not refer separately or specifically to amnesia for traumatic experiences. Two clinical studies use case reports as research material; one used the Structured Clinical Interview for the DSM-III-R, and three empirical studies used the Dissociative Experiences Scale (DES) (Bernstein & Putnam, 1986) in population samples.

The first study of Krystal and Niederland (1968) pertains to symptoms found in the case records of 149 patients who were treated by them. Among the "disturbances of cognition" (which nowadays are more likely to be labeled as dissociative phenomena), they report on 26 cases (19%) suffering from amnesia. The amnesia they observed consisted of

> far-reaching memory defects with total or partial amnesia for various traumatic events, marked vagueness of the capacity to recollect, and the emergency of acute episodes of confusion and anxiety when urged to remember what the events were.... In the most intense panics, we observed episodes of confusion, disorientation, and also dreamlike states in which the patients believed themselves to be back in a concentration camp (7 percent of our patients). (p. 329)

Kuch and Cox (1992) investigated 123 Holocaust survivors, of whom 78 had been in concentration camps for more than one month, 20 had been in an extermination camp and had been tattooed with identification numbers, and 45 had survived the Holocaust after being in labor camps, ghettos, or in hiding. Psychogenic amnesia was reported in 3 (3.8%) survivors of the concentration camps and in 2 (10%) survivors of the extermination camps.

A sample of 100 Holocaust survivors, of whom 70 had been in concentration camps and 30 had been in hiding during the Holocaust, was studied to detect differences in their symptom profiles (Yehuda et al., 1997). Participants were volunteers, and they were interviewed by mental health workers with expertise in evaluating and treating PTSD and additional training in the use of the research measures. Amnesia was measured through the Clinician Administered PTSD Scale (CAPS), which provides a quantified measure of each PTSD symptom on a scale of 0 to 8. The mean amnesia score for the whole group was 1.99 (SD 2.8) and for those who endorsed the amnesia item it was 4.33 (SD 1.79). In 46% of this sample, the amnesia item was endorsed, indicating its presence to some degree.

In three studies the DES, which taps the field of dissociation and includes several

**TABLE 1. Dissociative Symptoms as Measured
by the Dissociative Experiences Scale**

	Total Score		Amnesia		
	M	SD[b]	N	M	SD
Yehuda et al. (1996)					
Survivors with PTSD	18.4	[a]	35	2.89	2.72
Survivors without PTSD	9.5	[a]	25	0.80	1.2
Comparison subjects	5.3	[a]	16	0.0	0.0
Mooren & Kleber (1996)					
Clinical survivors	25	17	63		
Survivors receiving compensation	15	13	272		
Nonclinical survivors	11	11	225		
Nonsurvivors nonclinical controls	7	9	349		
Brom et al. (1996)					
Population sample of child survivors	7	6	34		

[a]The standard deviations are given in square root.
[b]SD = standard deviation.

questions on dissociative amnesia was used. The studies were conducted in the United States on 60 elderly survivors with a mean age of 67 (SD = 4.4) (Yehuda et al., 1996), in The Netherlands on three samples of people who were victimized in the Netherlands Indies during World War II (Mooren & Kleber, 1996), and in Israel on a sample of 34 child survivors of the Holocaust (Cohen et al., 1997). The data from these studies are shown in Table 1.

All of these studies show that dissociative symptoms are present in different samples of survivors of World War II. Although the relationship between general dissociative symptoms and amnesia for traumatic events has not been studied specifically, we can assume that there is a high correlation between them.

Discussion

Paucity of Literature on Holocaust-Related Amnesia

In this article an overview has been presented of the relevant literature—biographies, autobiographies, clinical and research publications—on the issue of amnesia in survivors of the Holocaust. From this overview we may conclude that amnesia for Holocaust experiences has been reported in all of the sources. The phenomenon has existed for many years, but attention to it has been relatively scarce. One reason may be that the use of psychoanalytic concepts such as denial and repression, with their often vague or ambiguous meanings, in clinical writings on Holocaust survivors have obscured the existence of the phenomenon of (dissociative) amnesia itself. It should be added, however, that in the recent psychoanalytic writings of authors such as Laub and Auerhahn (1993) trauma-induced amnesia in Holocaust survivors is receiving explicit attention.

As mentioned before, a second reason for the lack of attention to amnesia in

Holocaust survivors may lie in the socially accepted norms that surround the Holocaust. Kirmayer (1996) eloquently showed the different social demands made on survivors and the influence of this demand on the narrative that has developed concerning the Holocaust, in contrast to the narrative concerning sexual abuse. The relatively low prevalence of amnesia in Holocaust survivors and the high prevalence of amnesia in survivors of child sexual abuse are described by Kirmayer in the context of social norms. The retelling of the Holocaust is experienced as a collective duty, and personal testimony is part of the evolving collective experience. Retelling of childhood abuse involves breaking an accepted image of family life and as a rule is an individual effort. Considering these social norms we may understand in part that amnesia as a phenomenon in Holocaust survivors has been relatively neglected and that hypermnesia has received most attention. Given the massive amount of empirical research on this issue (see Scheflin & Brown, 1996), it is much more expected that CSA survivors will temporarily forget their traumatization and subsequently recover these memories.

Another possible reason for the low incidence of amnesia among Holocaust survivors is the age effect, which seems to influence the prevalence of dissociative phenomena. The question that remains unanswered is what the prevalence of dissociative symptoms has been during the course of the life of the survivors from the war until now. From recent research that indicates that peritraumatic dissociation is a strong predictor for posttraumatic disorders (Marmar et al., 1994; Shalev et al., 1996), we might assume that in those survivors who suffer from posttraumatic symptoms now, dissociation has been stronger in the past.

Almost No Delayed Recall

One obvious characteristic of the examples presented of amnesia for Holocaust-related experiences is that in almost all cases the amnesia still existed at the time of the report. Although survivors of the Holocaust do mention the late recall of previously "forgotten" material, the issue of the recovery of memories has not been often described in this literature. Only in Somer's (1994) case did the use of hypnosis help the patient to recover many of her memories of Auschwitz and of her separation from her parents. In the literature on CSA, the reported amnesia is much more often related to delayed recall, except in studies in which the researchers took a sample of reported instances of CSA and subsequently, i.e., 17 years later, interviewed the former victims (Williams, 1994).

Amnesia and Alexithymia

Another relevant concept in this regard is alexithymia, which refers to the inability to feel or express emotions, fantasy, imagery, or to the defense against such feelings and experiences. Bastiaans (1987) related this concept to the fixation of Holocaust survivors to their most painful experiences during the war, while at the same time being unable to find words for what they went through. We can assume that alexithymia is a phenomenon related to amnesia and that we will actually find amnesia in those reporting alexithymia. Research by Yehuda et al. (1997) on survivors of the Holocaust with and without post-traumatic stress disorder, has shown that there is a relationship between post-traumatic symptoms and the presence of alexithymia.

Other Causes of Amnesia

When we try to determine the origin of the amnesia in Holocaust survivors, we have to cope with several possible explanations. The question of normative childhood forgetting inevitably comes up when we discuss the topic of amnesia. We can only speak about dissociative amnesia if we may expect recall in the given circumstances. One possible competitor as an explanation for the lack of recall is normative infantile amnesia. There are no set rules to determine what one could expect someone to recall from one's early childhood. Verbal memories are unlikely to be available for experiences prior to age two (Loftus, 1993), although a review of the literature on childhood memory (Enns et al., 1995) maintains that memory systems of young children are similar to those of older children or adults and that nonverbal memories of experiences prior to age two may be available and accessible. Infantile amnesia should be considered an alternative when dealing with memories before age four, but with prompting even earlier memories often are accessible (Parkin, 1997).

Another explanation for cognitive disturbances in Holocaust survivors is the physical ordeal they went through. Both the hunger and the other forms of emaciation have had strong influences on the physical and mental well-being of survivors, and some authors have brought up the idea that cognitive problems may have organic causes, such as extreme undernourishment (Thygesen et al., 1970).

Recommendations for Further Study

Amnesia constitutes one of the more complex fields of study because one looks for the void, for the absence of something. In the light of the fact that delayed recall has not been reported frequently in Holocaust survivors, it seems natural that amnesia has remained an underreported phenomenon. Systematic study of amnesia for trauma will have to become more specific, and both general dissociative symptoms and amnesia as symptoms cannot be considered sufficient measures of trauma-induced amnesia. In future studies, measures will have to be developed that can grasp the discontinuity of memory that seems to be an important part of coping with massive trauma.

References

American Psychiatric Association (1994). DSM-IV. Washington, DC: American Psychiatric Press.

Auerhahn, N. C., & Laub, D. Intergenerational memory and the Holocaust. Submitted for publication.

Bastiaans, J. (1987). Difficulties in psychotherapy of victims of man-made disasters. *Acta Neurochirugica, 38,* 114–116.

Bernstein, E. M., & Putnam, F. W. (1986). Development, reliability, and validity of a dissociation scale. *Journal of Nervous and Mental Disease, 174,* 727–735.

Birenbaum, H. (1971). *Hope is the last to die.* New York: Twayne.

Brom, D., Cohen, M., & Dasberg, H. (1996, November). A controlled study on child-survivors of the Holocaust. Presented at the *Annual Conference of the International Society for Traumatic Stress Studies,* Montreal.

Brown, D., Scheflin, A. W., & Hammond, D. C. (1998). *Memory, trauma treatment, and the law.* New York: Norton.

Brown, D., Scheflin, A. W., & Whitfield, C. L. (1999). Recovered memories: The current weight of the evidence in science and in the courts. *Journal of Psychiatry and Law, 27,* 5–156.

Butz, A. R. (1991). A short introduction to the study of Holocaust revisionism. Daily Northwestern, May 13.

Cohen, M., Brom, D., & Dasberg, H. (1997). Child-survivors of the Holocaust 50 years later. Presented at *European Conference on Traumatic Stress,* June, Maastricht.

De Wind, E. (1968). The confrontation with death. *International Journal of Psychoanalysis, 49*, 302–305.

Durlacher, G. L. (1991). *De zoektocht [The search]*. Amsterdam: Meulenhoff.

Dwork, D. (1991). *Children with a star: Jewish youth in Nazi Europe*. New Haven: Yale University Press.

Enns, C. Z., McNeilly, C. L., Corkery, J. M., & Gilbert, M. S. (1995). The debate about delayed memories of child sexual abuse: A feminist perspective. *The Counseling Psychologist, 23*, 181–279.

Hass, A. (1995). Survivor guilt in Holocaust survivors and their children. In J. Lemberger (Ed.), *A global perspective on working with Holocaust survivors and the second generation*. Jerusalem: Amcha/JDC Brookdale.

Jaffe, R. (1968). Dissociative phenomena in former concentration camp inmates. *International Journal of Psychoanalysis, 49*, 310–312.

Janet, P. (1893). *L'Etat mental des hystériques: Les stigmates mentaux*. Paris: Rueff & Cie. English edition: *The mental state of hystericals*. New York: Putnam. (Republished by University Publications of America, Washington, DC, 1977).

Janet, P. (1901). *The mental state of hystericals: A study of mental stigmata and mental accidents*. New York: Putnam.

Karon, B. P., & Widener, A. J. (1997). Repressed memories and World War II: Lest we forget! *Professional Psychology: Research and Practice, 28*(4), 338–340.

Keilson, H. (1979). *Sequentielle Traumatisierung bei Kindern*. Stuttgart: Enke. English edition: *Sequential traumatization in children*. Jerusalem: The Magnes Press/The Hebrew University, 1992.

Kirmayer, L. J. (1996). Landscapes of memory: Trauma, narrative, and dissociation. In P. Antze & M. Lamber (Eds.), *Tense past: Cultural essays and trauma and memory* (pp. 173–198). New York/London: Routledge.

Kleber, R. J., & Brom, D. (1992). *Coping with trauma: Theory, prevention and treatment*. Lisse: Swets & Zeitlinger.

Kluft, R. P. (1997). The argument for the reality of delayed memory recall. In P. S. Appelbaum, L. A. Uyehara, & M. R. Elin (Eds.), *Trauma and memory: Clinical and legal aspects* (pp. 25–57). Oxford/New York: Oxford University Press.

Krystal, H., & Niederland, W. G. (1968). Clinical observations on the survivor syndrome. In H. Krystal (Ed.), *Massive psychic trauma*. New York: International Universities Press.

Kuch, K., & Cox, B. J. (1992). Symptoms of PTSD in 124 survivors of the Holocaust. *American Journal of Psychiatry, 149*, 337–340.

Lagnado, L. M., & Dekel, S. C. (1991). *Children of the flames: Dr. Josef Mengele and the untold story of the twins of Auschwitz*. New York: Morrow.

Langer, L. L. (1995). *Admitting the Holocaust*. New York: Oxford University Press.

Laub, D., & Auerhahn, N. C. (1993). Knowing and not knowing massive trauma: Forms of traumatic memory. *International Journal of Psychoanalysis, 74*, 287–302.

Laub, D., & Powell, D. Psychoanalytic listening to historical trauma: The conflict of knowing and the imperative to act. Submitted for publication.

Levi, P. (1986). *Moments of reprieve*. New York: Summit Books.

Levi, P. (1988). *The drowned and the saved*. London: Michael Joseph.

Loewenstein, R. J. (1996). Dissociative amnesia and dissociative fugue. In L. K. Michelson & W. J. Ray (Eds.), *Handbook of dissociation: Theoretical, empirical and clinical perspectives* (pp. 307–336). New York: Plenum.

Loftus, E. (1993). The reality of repressed memories. *American Psychologist, 48*, 518–537.

Marks, J. (1995). *The hidden children: The secret survivors of the Holocaust*. Toronto: Bantam Books.

Marmar, C. R., Weiss, D. S., Schlenger, W. E., Fairbank, J. A., Jordan, B. K., Kulka, R. A., & Hough, R. L. (1994). Peritraumatic dissociation and posttraumatic stress in male Vietnam theater veterans. *American Journal of Psychiatry, 151*(6), 902–907.

Mazor, A., Gampel, Y., Enright, R. D., & Orenstein, R. (1990). Holocaust survivors: Coping with post-traumatic memories in childhood and 40 years later. *Journal of Traumatic Stress, 3*, 1–14.

Modai, I. (1994). Forgetting childhood: A defense mechanism against psychosis in a Holocaust survivor. *Clinical Gerontologist, 14*(3), 67–71.

Mooren, G. T. M., & Kleber, R. J. (1996). *Gezondheid en herinneringen aan de oorlogsjaren van Indische jeugdige oorlogsgetroffenen: Een empirisch onderzoek*. Utrecht: Utrecht University.

Musaph, H. (1973). Het post-concentratiekampsyndroom. *Maandblad voor Geestelijke Volksgezondheid, 28*, 207–217.

Niederland, W. G. (1968). Clinical observations on the "survivor syndrome." *International Journal of Psychoanalysis, 49*, 313–315.

Ofshe, R., & Watters, E. (1993, March/April). Making monsters. *Society*, 4–16.

Parkin, A. J. (1997). *Memory and amnesia: An introduction*, 2nd ed. Oxford: Blackwell.

Peltz, R. (1994). In the shadow of the empty core: Survival through bearing witness. Opening remarks, panel presentation at *14th Annual Spring Meeting of Division 39 of the American Psychological Association*. Washington, DC. (Quoted by Auerhahn & Laub, work in progress).

Pope, K. S. (1996). Memory, abuse and science. Questioning claims about the false memory syndrome epidemic. *American Psychologist, 51*(9), 957–974.

Pope, H. G., & Hudson, J. I. (1995). Can memories of childhood sexual abuse be repressed? *Psychological Medicine, 25*, 121–126.

Shalev, A. A. Y., Peri, T., Caneti, L., & Schreiber, S. (1996). Predictor of PTSD in injured trauma survivors. *American Journal of Psychiatry, 53*, 219–224.

Simenauer, E. (1968). Late psychic sequelae of man-made disasters. *International Journal of Psychoanalysis, 49*, 306–309.

Somer, E. (1994). Hypnotherapy and regulated uncovering in the treatment of older survivors of Nazi persecution. *Clinical Gerontologist, 14*(3), 47–65.

Stein, A. (1994). *Hidden children: Forgotten survivors of the Holocaust.* Harmondsworth, Middlesex: Penguin Books.

Thygesen, P., Hermann, K., & Willanger, R. (1970). Concentration camp survivors in Denmark. Persecution, disease, disability, compensation. *Danish Medical Bulletin, 17*, 65–108.

Van der Hart, O., Brown, P., & Graafland, M. (1999). Trauma-induced dissociative amnesia in World War I combat soldiers. *Australian and New Zealand Journal of Psychiatry, 33*, 31–36.

van der Kolk, B. A., Van der Hart, O., & Marmar, C. (1996). Dissociation and information processing in posttraumatic stress disorder. In B. A. van der Kolk, A. C. McFarlane, & L. Weissaeth (Eds.), *Traumatic stress* (pp. 303–327). New York: Guilford.

Van Ravesteijn, L. (1976). Gelaagdheid van herinneringen [Layering of memories]. *Tijdschrift voor Psychotherapie, 5*, 195–205.

Wagenaar, W. A., & Crombag, H. F. M. (1995). Verdrongen herinneringen [Repressed memories]. *Nederlands Tijdschrift voor Geneeskunde, 139*, 1275–1279.

Williams, L. W. (1994). Recall of childhood trauma: A prospective study of women's memories of child sexual abuse. *Journal of Consulting and Clinical Psychology, 62*, 1167–1176.

Yehuda, R., Elkin, A., Binder-Brynes, K., Kahana, B., Southwick, S. M., Schmeidler, J. & Giller, E. L. (1996). Dissociation in aging Holocaust survivors. *American Journal of Psychiatry, 153*, 935–940.

Yehuda, R., Schmeidler, J., Siever, L. J., Binder-Brynes, K., & Elkin, A. (1997). Individual differences in posttraumatic stress disorder symptom profiles in Holocaust survivors in concentration camps or in hiding. *Journal of Traumatic Stress, 10*, 453–463.

18

Prospective Studies of the Recently Traumatized

SARA FREEDMAN AND ARIEH Y. SHALEV

Reactions to traumatic events, their course, and their presumed etiology have been studied throughout this century (e.g., Rivers, 1918; Fraser & Wilson, 1918; Grinker et al., 1946), although it is only since these were included in an official nosology that their natural course has been studied systematically. Seventeen years following the inclusion of post-traumatic stress disorder (PTSD) in the psychiatric literature, it seems worthwhile to assess what has been learned from more systematic research and which questions still remain to be answered. This chapter reviews longitudinal studies to date, outlines some of the gaps that remain in our knowledge, and suggests a possible way forward for future research.

The Traumatic Event

PTSD is a unique disorder within psychiatry, in that one of its criteria is also its primary etiologic factor, a traumatic event. It is clear that without this, PTSD cannot be said to exist. Few other disorders include such a clearly defined etiology in their definitions. Despite this clarity, however, many questions regarding the nature of the traumatic event remain, and this is reflected in the changing definitions throughout subsequent editions of the APA's *Diagnostic and Statistical Manual* (DSM). The original definition was a stressor that would "evoke significant symptoms of distress in almost everyone" (APA, 1980). By DSM-III-R, this had changed to "an event outside the range of normal experience and that would be markedly distressing to almost anyone" (APA, 1987). The current definition (DSM-IV, APA, 1994) is an "event that involved actual or threatened death or serious injury, or a threat to physical integrity of self or others" to which the individual's response "involved intense fear, helplessness or horror." These changes reflect better understanding of the types of events that can lead to PTSD. Moving away from combat traumas, researchers began to look for PTSD following other

SARA FREEDMAN AND ARIEH Y. SHALEV • Center for Traumatic Stress, Department of Psychiatry, Hadassah University Hospital, Jerusalem 91120, Israel.

International Handbook of Human Response to Trauma, edited by Shalev, Yehuda, and McFarlane. Kluwer Academic / Plenum Publishers, New York, 2000.

events that affect civilians, such as natural disasters (Green et al., 1985). Later, work moved to events that were much less obviously traumatogenic, in that they did fall within the "range of normal experience," but still seemed to produce the same symptoms, e.g., physical injury (Norman et al., 1991), motor vehicle accidents (Burstein, 1989), and crime (Kilpatrick et al., 1985). The growing awareness that PTSD is to be found after relatively common events has substantially altered views of the disorder. From being perceived as "the normal consequence of an abnormally stressful event" (Wilson & Kraus, 1982), it is now understood to be a pathological reaction that can be triggered by quite common events (Yehuda & McFarlane, 1995).

Predictors of PTSD

With a growing awareness that not all those exposed to a traumatic event would subsequently develop PTSD, researchers began to look for factors identifying those at risk. Studies have examined three areas—factors that occurred pretrauma (e.g., child abuse), during the trauma itself (e.g., intensity of trauma, dissociation during trauma), and post-trauma (e.g., levels of social support, life stressors, psychological symptoms). *Pretrauma variables* that have been shown to be significant predictors include alcohol abuse and an Axis II disorder in victims of motor vehicle accidents (Blanchard et al., 1996). Physical abuse was found to be a predictor of PTSD in Vietnam veterans (Donovan et al., 1996), and child abuse and physical abuse predicted PTSD in battered women (Kemp et al., 1995). McNally & Shin (1995) found that intelligence is predictive in Vietnam veterans. Social economic status was predictive in POWs (Sutker et al., 1990). Finally, a few studies have shown that personality is significant—in Vietnam veterans (Foy et al., 1984) and in World War II veterans (Lee et al., 1995).

Aspects of the trauma itself were traditionally considered crucial to the likelihood of developing PTSD. For example, "there is typically a dose-response relationship between degree of exposure and outcome" (Green & Lindy, 1994). Within the combat population, the extent of combat exposure is a consistent predictor of PTSD (Davidson & Baum, 1993; Donovan et al., 1996; Foy et al., 1984; Lee et al., 1995; McNally & Shin, 1995). In civilian populations, the findings are less consistent, and some studies show no stressor effect (McFarlane, 1992), whereas other have found that it is a good predictor, for instance, in crime victims (Resnick et al., 1992) and police officers (Carlier et al., 1997). Another aspect of the trauma that has latterly been found to be significant is the degree of dissociation experienced during the trauma (Marmar et al., 1994; Koopman et al. 1993; Shalev et al., 1996).

Significant predictors have also been identified in the period that follows exposure. Several studies have shown that *social support* is significant with battered women (Kemp et al., 1995), ferry disaster victims (Joseph et al., 1994; Dalgleish et al., 1996), burn patients (Perry et al., 1992), and Gulf War troops (Sutker et al., 1995). *Symptoms of intrusion and avoidance* have been shown to be important in some studies, for instance in motor vehicle accident victims, avoidance at 1–4 months predicted PTSD at one year, and intrusion and avoidance were significant predictors in ferry disaster victims (Dalgliesh et al., 1996) and in Vietnam veterans (Davidson & Baum, 1993). McFarlane (1992) found that intrusive symptoms, but not avoidance, are a significant predictor of PTSD in firefighters. *Coping style* is predictive with burn patients (Bryant, 1996) and battered women (Kemp et al., 1995). Life events were predictors in Gulf War troops

(Sutker et al., 1995), victims of the Oakland/Berkeley firestorm (Koopman et al., 1994), and battered women (Kemp et al., 1995). Finally, other symptoms such as *irritability* (Blanchard et al., 1996) and *helplessness* (Joseph et al., 1994) have also been significant predictors. The most salient conclusion regarding research on predictors is that rarely has one variable been shown to be the predictor of PTSD, but a combination of pre-, peri- and post-trauma variables is normally found.

The work on predictors looks at the potential, once one is exposed to a trauma, of developing PTSD. Other work, primarily epidemiological, has considered risk factors for being exposed to a trauma. Breslau et al. (1995) report that trauma exposure is more likely for men, for those with lower levels of education, for those with three or more early conduct problems, for those with a family history of psychiatric disorder or substance abuse, and for those who are neurotic and extroverted. Kessler et al. (1995) also found that men were more likely to be exposed to trauma and that also the majority of those who have experienced a trauma have actually been exposed to more than one trauma during their lifetimes.

Course of PTSD

Original conceptualizations understood that the symptoms of PTSD occur in cyclic waves—periods of intrusion are followed by periods of avoidance, that lead to a working through in a normal response, but in the pathological response are more intense and do not lead to resolution (Horowitz, 1986). Other researchers assumed that symptoms were more consistent and became pathological only if they persisted after an unspecified period of time (e.g., Rachman, 1980). Research has shown that the acute phase immediately following the trauma is characterized by high levels of symptoms in most trauma victims. Over time, these slowly dissipate. Rothbaum et al. (1992) describe a gradual decrease in levels of PTSD in rape victims, from 94% at 12 days, to 65% at 35 days, and 47% at 94 days. Similarly, Green et al. (1990) looking at victims of the Buffalo Creek disaster, found a gradual decline of psychological symptoms, with 28% showing PTSD 14 years post-trauma, compared with 44% at 2 years. Blanchard et al. (1996) examined motor vehicle accident victims and found a gradual increase in remittance from 1–4 months post-trauma until 1 year, with 50% recovery at 7 months, and nearly two-thirds recovery by 1 year. After this, little change was seen between 1 year and 18 months. Feinstein and Dolan (1991) also found an improvement in symptoms and a recovery rate of almost 50% between 6 weeks and 6 months. McFarlane found a decline in intrusion and avoidance over time (McFarlane, 1992). Epidemiological data from Kesslar et al. (1995) indicate that most people improve in the first year, after which the rate decreases. Research by Solomon (1989) with soldiers suffering from combat stress reaction showed that there was a gradual decline in symptoms in the first three years post-trauma, intrusion appears in the first two years, and then avoidance. Shalev et al. (1992) found an increase in avoidance symptoms in the 6 months following traumatic events in subjects who developed PTSD. These results differ from the others presented here (where a gradual decline was seen in all symptoms) and are more consistent with Horowitz' original formulation. Bremner et al. (1996a) examined Vietnam veterans and found that symptom onset occurred during the war and increased in the first two years. Then a plateau was reached that stayed at a chronic level. They found that hyperarousal symptoms appeared first, followed by avoidance and intrusions later on. In a population of body handlers for the Gulf War, Ursano et al. (1995) found a decrease in intrusion and avoidance and in PTSD over time, and no increase in depression.

Summary of Longitudinal Studies

It is clear from the above that our original conceptualizations of PTSD have been dramatically altered by the research carried out since 1980. Many people are exposed to traumatic events during their lifetime but do not suffer long-lasting effects. Various factors affect the chance that PTSD will develop, and most improvement takes place shortly after the trauma. There are, however, still many gaps in our knowledge about PTSD. The course of PTSD is still not clear. As can be seen from the studies presented, there are conflicting views regarding the occurrence of symptoms, their order of appearance, and their significance to chronicity. Similarly, despite the advances in understanding the predictors of PTSD, the studies illustrate lack of consensus.

These gaps in our knowledge can possibly be explained by two aspects of the research: the *design* of the studies and the *methodology* used in analyzing the results. These are considered in turn, and some future directions are suggested.

Research Design

There are several ways of designing research studies, and these can be crudely divided into three types. First, are *cross sectional* studies, where subjects are studied at one particular time. The second type of design is *retrospective*, where subjects are studied now, and compared with the way they were at a past time(s). The last type is *prospective* studies, where subjects are followed up at different times. All of these designs can give a sense of changes over time.

The majority of studies in PTSD are cross-sectional or retrospective. As explained before, both designs can give information regarding changes that take place over time. Asking people how they were before their trauma or during it and comparing with the way they are today also gives a sense of changes. Despite the information that can be gained from these types of studies, there are, however, disadvantages with them. For example, retrospective data do not account for the degree to which memory of events is affected by the current state: does someone with PTSD remember the trauma in the same way as someone without PTSD? If not, then the data from retrospective studies are likely to be biased. The knowledge that some people are amnesic about certain aspects of their trauma (Bremner et al., 1995b) and that mood affects memory (Eich, 1995) clearly indicates the need for objective studies that circumvent the problems with cross-sectional and retrospective designs. This is probably achieved only by prospective studies.

Much of the early research on PTSD concentrated on Vietnam veterans. Given that the formal concept of PTSD was not recognized when these veterans returned to the United States, it is not surprising that most of these data are retrospective. Only as the link between traumatic events and their sequelae was better understood and attention moved to other types of trauma did prospective studies become feasible. Although the most expensive type of design in terms of time and resources, they are clearly the best way to learn about the course of a disorder. The difficulties in carrying out this type of research are reflected in the number of prospective studies that exist. A search of the current literature found three studies that had followed subjects from before the time of their trauma to a significant period of time after it (Breslau et al., 1995; Nolen-Hoeksema & Morrow, 1991; Lee et al., 1995). Prospective studies following subjects from some time immediately after the trauma (less than 1 month) to a later time are limited to eight (Feinstein & Dolan, 1991; Karlehagen et al. 1993; Koopman et al., 1994; Malt, 1988; Perry et al., 1992; Rothbaum et al., 1992; Shalev et al., 1993, 1996) and another six where the initial assessment took place more than 1 month after the trauma (Blanchard et al., 1996; Carlier et al. 1997; Fisher & Jacoby, 1992; Hauff & Vaglum, 1994; Southwick et al., 1995; Ursano et al., 1995). Table 1 summarizes the major prospective longitudinal studies.

Data Analysis Techniques

If we consider predictors of PTSD, then a second type of "missing" information is apparent, the applicability of research results to real life settings. A clinician arrives at an ER after a major trauma and finds 100 patients there. Since it is unlikely s/he will have the resources to follow up and treat all of them, how is a decision made on who is most at risk? Being well-read on the current PTSD literature, the clinician may know that certain factors increase the chances of developing PTSD—for instance, high levels of intrusion and avoidance symptoms, low social support available, a defensive coping style. Had our clinician read, or remembered slightly different studies, s/he would have decided that levels of intrusion and avoidance were unimportant, but that trauma intensity, extent of injury, alcohol abuse and child sexual abuse were the important factors. Thus having decided on the important criterion, how does the clinician assess this? Assuming that the same assessment instruments that were used in the research studies are available, how is the "amount" of the factor in question decided upon? In other words, knowing that "more" social support is positive is helpful only if we know how much more and can consequently begin to sort out the 100 trauma victims into those who may need intervention and those who will not.

One of the most common ways in which empirical research has addressed the clinician's dilemma (i.e., to assess the effect of predictors) is with *multiple regression*. This test rests on the assumption that if variables are related consistently, then it is possible to summarize the relationship by a linear approximation. Clearly, if the regression line represents the relationship between the predictor and the outcome, a given value of the predictor can be linked with the outcome (e.g., PTSD symptoms). In the case of multiple predictors, the relative contribution of each variable to the outcome model can also be calculated.

Multiple regression, however, is limited to predicting a continuous measure of outcome, such as intensity of PTSD symptoms. To predict a dichotomous outcome (i.e., whether or not someone has PTSD), different techniques such as *logistic regression* must be used, although the same principles apply.

Multiple regression is widely known and understood and is easily utilized through the more common statistical packages. It provides a straightforward answer to assessing predictors and allows for the individual contribution of each factor, as well as the combination of different factors. However, if we return to our previous query in the ER, the results of multiple regression are less useful to us because they do not give us a "critical amount" of the variable in question.

TABLE 1. Longitudinal Studies of PTSD in Trauma Survivors

Study	Population	Design	Significant Predictors of PTSD	Data Analysis Techniques[b]
Blanchard et al., 1996	Motor vehicle accidents N = 132	Follow-up at 1–4, 7, 13, and 18 months following trauma	PTSD at 6 months: irritability and sense of foreshortened future. PTSD at 12 months: alcohol abuse, Axis II diagnosis, hyperarousal and avoidance	LR; MR
Feinstein & Dolan, 1991	Physical trauma N = 48	4–7 days, 6 weeks, 6 months	Intrusion and avoidance symptoms, alcohol consumption	DFA
Fisher & Jacoby, 1992	Assaulted bus crews N = 22	Within 6 months, 2 years	Severity of assault, family psychiatric illness, initial PTSD, higher initial GHQ[a]	
Hauff & Vaglum, 1994	Vietnamese refugees N = 145	3 months after arrival and 3 years	Previous flight, great danger, reeducation camp	LR
Karlehagen et al., 1993	Train driver N = 101	Few hours/days, 1 month, 12 months	Previous accidents, IES, risk expectancy	
Koopman et al., 1993	Oakland/Berkeley firestorm N = 187	1 week, 7 months	Dissociation, recent life events	MR
Lee et al., 1995	World War II vets N = 979	Pre-World War II every 5 years to 1988	Combat exposure, less mature defenses	
Nolen-Hoeksema & Morrow, 1991	Earthquake victims N = 137	14 days pretrauma, 10 days, 7 months post	Depression and stress pretrauma, danger during trauma, ruminations 10 days post-trauma	
Perry et al., 1992	Burn patients N = 51	1 weeks, 2, 6, 12 months	Less burns, less social support, > POMS[a]	LR
Rothbaum et al., 1992	Rape victims N = 95	Weekly from 12 to 94 days	RAST and intrusion symptoms	DFA
Southwick et al., 1995	Desert Storm veterans N = 62	1, 6, 12 months	Symptoms increase over 2 years, greatest changes 1–6 months	
Shalev et al., 1996	Civilian trauma survivors N = 51	1 week, 6 months	Peritraumatic dissociation, intrusion, avoidance	MR Path analysis

[a]GHQ—General Health Questionnaire; POMS—Profile of Mental States.
[b]MR—multiple regression; LR—logistic regression; DFA—discriminant functional analysis.

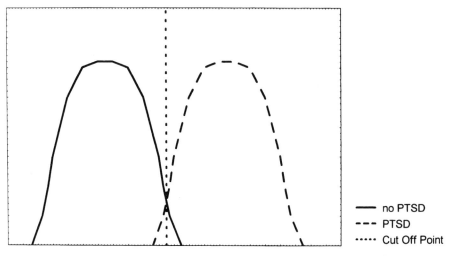

FIGURE 1. Two overlapping, normal distribution curves with cutoff points.

The best known statistical analysis for arriving at a critical amount is *discriminant functional analysis*. This model assumes that the two groups, PTSD and non-PTSD, are essentially "different," and that for any variable, two distinct normal distribution curves will be found (Figure 1). If this variable is a "good" predictor of PTSD status, then the two curves will be far apart; if it is not, there will be considerable overlap. Clearly, in most cases, something between the two extremes is found, and there is some overlap between the groups. Discriminant functional analysis measures the distance between the means of each group as a way of measuring the relative power of the variable in question to discriminate between the two groups. Discriminant analysis generally takes the midpoint between the two means (i.e., the mean of the means) as the "cutoff point," although this can be changed to reflect factors such as prior probabilities or the importance of eliminating false positives. Then this single cutoff point can be used in subsequent analyses to test predictive ability.

This approach will clearly help in obtaining critical amounts of a variable, but this may not be appropriate for each setting, and the degree to which the results of one research study apply to another event are uncertain.

A second general problem concerning both multiple regression and dicriminant functional analyses is that they are based on the *mean value* of the variables. Although this underlies many statistical techniques, there is a potential problem with it. For example, PTSD subjects are shown to have higher intrusion scores than non-PTSD subjects—in other words, the mean intrusion score of the PTSD group is higher than that of the non-PTSD group. It is possible, however, that a high degree of overlap exists between these two groups, such that some individuals in the PTSD group actually have lower intrusion scores than some of the non-PTSD group (and vice versa). Although this overlap will reduce the significance level of the difference between the mean intrusion scores, it is still possible to obtain a statistically significant difference which is, in practical terms, very misleading. A recent paper by Putnam et al. (1996) examined dissociation in PTSD and illustrated precisely this point.

The final methodological issue to be considered is less directly concerned with the statistics but more with the choice of *assessment instruments.* Two major issues have affected the knowledge gap in PTSD: one that the same assessment instruments have not been used in all studies and the second that different systems of diagnosing PTSD status are utilized. The first problem, although inherent to any "group" of studies not undertaken "together," is a serious issue when attempting to find general conclusions from studies because in multiple regression the addition of one more factor to the equation can seriously alter the results. Also, if several studies find that social support is a good predictor of PTSD and another group of studies does not, then it is important to know whether these studies even examined social support. If not, then any conclusions about the importance of it in predicting PTSD are tentative at best.

Despite the proliferation of validated and reliable instruments for assessing PTSD, it is remarkable how few studies use them. Many studies use instruments designed to assess levels of symptomatology as indicators of PTSD status (e.g., Dalgleish et al., 1996), and others use nonstandardized assessment tools (Malt, 1988; Basoglu et al., 1994). This makes replication of results almost impossible and again means that generalizing between studies is difficult.

A combination of all of the factors presented has led to the results that longitudinal studies are less useful in nonresearch settings than would be expected.

Choosing Between Instruments and Using Cutoff Points

In a recent paper (Shalev et al., 1997), we presented results of a study that in its design and analysis was able to answer some of these limitations. The study examined consecutive patients arriving at the Emergency Room of a large teaching hospital; most were traffic accident victims, although other types of trauma were seen. Subjects were seen 1 week, 1 month, and 6 months after their trauma. PTSD was assessed twice, at the 1 month and 6 month assessments, and questionnaires completed at 1 week and 1 month were examined for their predictive ability.

In attempting to provide data useful to clinicians, the study used commonly used assessment tools and instead of analyzing the data using multiple regression or discriminant functional analysis, used a statistical technique relatively new to psychiatry, *receiver operator characteristics* (ROC). This was considered more appropriate because it evaluates a full range of cutoff points for each questionnaire and may, therefore, be more useful than discriminant functional analysis in addressing clinician needs.

The assumption underlying ROC analysis is that every questionnaire has a range of scores and that it is theoretically possible to use *any* of these scores as a cutoff point, that is, the score below which subjects do not have PTSD and above which they do. The ability of a given cutoff point to correctly classify subjects can be explained by examining the rates of true and false positives and true and false negatives. The rate of true positives is the sensitivity, and the rate of true negatives is the specificity.

ROC analysis further uses the sensitivity and specificity scores of *all* possible values of a questionnaire to examine its ability to predict the correct diagnosis. This is related to discriminant functional analysis, outlined previously—in the latter, the midpoint cutoff point is usually used, whereas in ROC analysis, all possible cut off points are examined. ROC curves are constructed by plotting the false and true positive rates. They evaluate and express the global yield of all cutoff points of an instrument or a test. If the test is a good one, the ROC curve will be near the upper left-hand side of the graph, and the area between the curve and the diagonal line (the line of no informa-

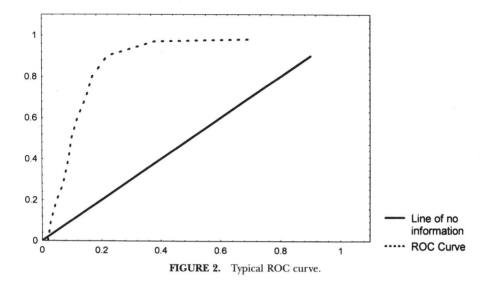

FIGURE 2. Typical ROC curve.

tion) will be maximal. A poor instrument, on the other hand, may not differ from chance, and its ROC curve will coalesce with the line of no information (Figure 2).

Several important results emerged from using ROC curves in a prospective study. The first was that although all the questionnaires were better than chance at predicting PTSD status, none was particularly efficient. Importantly, there were no significant differences between specific PTSD questionnaires (i.e., Impact of Event Scale, Horowitz et al., 1979, and Mississippi Scale—Civilian version, Keane et al., 1988) and other more general questionnaires (Spielberger Anxiety Scale, Spielberger, 1983; PDEQ, Marmar et al., 1994). Second, there was no difference in predictive ability between assessments carried out at 1 week and at 1 month. This implies that the course of PTSD is stable enough that assessing predictors of chronic PTSD 1 week after trauma is as efficient as assessing the patient at 1 month.

In attempting to "choose" appropriate cutoff points and thus help make sensible clinical decisions in the ER scenario presented, the problem outlined with discriminant functional analysis was very clearly demonstrated: there was never one obvious cutoff point, but appropriate cutoff points could be chosen on the basis of needs. For example, in a clinical setting where only potential PTSD cases are likely to receive preventative treatment, the initial assessment could be used to identify the very few cases who are almost certainly likely to develop it (a high cutoff point). However, where it is imperative to identify any potential case (e.g., in situations or professions that involve repeated exposure), then a lower cutoff point would be chosen. Table 2 illustrates the choice that one has to make between cutoff points in terms of predicting chronic PTSD from psychometric instruments administered 1 week and 1 month following trauma. These data are based on studying 211 trauma survivors, 39 of whom developed PTSD. The use of more than one cutoff point allows greater flexibility and is more closely related to the specific needs of the clinician. Thus, the clinician is invited to use cutoff points according to needs and resources.

There are obvious advantages to the data resulting from ROC analysis. First, it allows informed decisions to be made, based on circumstances and need, and cutoff

TABLE 2. Selected Cutoff Points with Related Sensitivity and Specificity

	Cutoff Point	Sensitivity (%)	Specificity (%)	Positive Predictive Value (%)	Negative Predictive Value (%)	N (PTSD)
IES total 1 week						
High sensitivity	11	100	7.68	19.9	99	32/32
High specificity	71	0	99.4	0	0.6	0/32
High sensitivity and specificity	30	75	60.98	28.2	43	24/32
IES total 1 month						
High sensitivity	13	100	47.3	23.8	78.7	31/31
High specificity	55	19.4	97.8	66.9	2	6/31
High sensitivity and specificity	28	80.6	77.4	33.6	37.2	25/31
STAI 1 month						
High sensitivity	37	100	27.3	21.9	87.5	33/33
High specificity	72	15	96	45.4	3.8	5/33
High sensitivity and specificity	54	66.7	65.2	28.2	37.9	22/33
Mississippi 1 month						
High sensitivity	60	100	19.6	20.3	96.8	32/32
High specificity	144	12.5	100	100	0	4/32
High sensitivity and specificity	94	71.8	82.9	46.2	19.2	23/32

points can be chosen accordingly. Second, because it was solely based on commonly used questionnaires, it provides results that are of potential use to clinicians who may wish to use these instruments. Third, ROC analysis is not mean-based and thus takes into account the wide range of scores obtained from the whole sample and the subsequent overlap between PTSD and non-PTSD groups.

Conclusions

Longitudinal studies have provided invaluable information regarding the course and predictors of PTSD, and our ideas and conceptualization of the disorder have, consequently, changed dramatically (Yehuda & McFarlane, 1995). There are, however, many things still not known about the disorder, and this is due in part to the way in which these studies have been carried out and their results analyzed. Although most studies were focused on causes and pathogenesis of PTSD and hence evaluated contributory factors for even small affect, clinicians have largely remained without practical ways of predicting the disorder in individual cases. We have presented an approach, which although not necessarily practical or realistic in all research settings, may help provide some of the missing information if utilized with other populations in the future. Perhaps the most salient point is that the needs and reality of the clinician should be addressed more closely in the theoretical research being carried out in the future.

References

American Psychiatric Association (1980). *Diagnostic and statistical manual of mental disorders*, 3rd ed. Washington, DC: American Psychiatric Press.

American Psychiatric Association (1987). *Diagnostic and statistical manual of mental disorders*, 3rd ed., rev. Washington, DC: American Psychiatric Press.

American Psychiatric Association (1994). *Diagnostic and statistical manual of mental disorders*, 4th ed. Washington, DC: American Psychiatric Press.

Basoglu, M., Paker, M., Ozmen, E., Tasdemir, O., & Sahin, D. (1994). Factors related to long-term traumatic stress responses in survivors of torture in Turkey [see comments]. *Journal of the American Medical Association, 272*(5), 357–363.

Blanchard, E. B., Hickling, E. J., Barton, K. A., Taylor, A. E., Loos, W. R., & Jones-Alexander, J. (1996). One-year prospective follow-up of motor vehicle accident victims. *Behaviour Research and Therapy, 34*(10), 775–786.

Bremner, J. D., Southwick, S. M., Darnell, A., & Charney, D. S. (1996a). Chronic PTSD in Vietnam combat veterans: Course of illness and substance abuse. *American Journal of Psychiatry, 153*(3), 369–375.

Bremner, J. D., Krystal, J. H., Charney, D. S., & Southwick, S. M. (1996b). Neural mechanisms in dissociative amnesia for childhood abuse: Relevance to the current controversy surrounding the "false memory syndrome." *American Journal of Psychiatry, 153*(7 Suppl.), 71–82.

Breslau, N., Davis, G. C., & Andeski, P. (1995). Risk factors for PTSD-related traumatic events: A prospective analysis. *American Journal of Psychiatry, 152*(4), 529–535.

Burstein, A. (1989) Posttraumatic stress disorder in victims of motor vehicle accidents. *Hospital and Community Psychiatry, 40*(3), 295–297.

Carlier, I. V., Lamberts, R. D., Fouwels, A. J., & Gersons, B. P. (1996). PTSD in relation to dissociation in traumatized police officers. *American Journal of Psychiatry, 153*(10), 1325–1328.

Carlier, I. V., Lamberts, R. D., & Gersons, B. P. (1997). Risk factors for posttraumatic stress symptomatology in police officers: A prospective. *Journal of Nervous and Mental Disease, 185*(8), 498–506.

Dalgleish, T., Joseph, S., Thrasher, S., Trannah, T., & Yule, W. (1996). Crisis support following the Herald of Free Enterprise disaster: A longitudinal perspective. *Journal of Traumatic Stress, 9*(4), 833–845.

Davidson, L. M., & Baum, A. (1993). Predictors of chronic stress among Vietnam veterans: Stress exposure and intrusive recall. *Journal of Traumatic Stress, 6*(2), 195–212.

Donovan, B. S., Padin-Rivera, E., Dowd, T., & Blake, D. D. (1996) Childhood factors and war zone stress in chronic PTSD. *Journal of Traumatic Stress, 9*(2), 361–368.

Eich, E. (1995). Searching for mood dependent memory. *Psychological Science, 6*(2) 67–75.

Feinstein, A., & Dolan, R. (1991). Predictors of post-traumatic stress disorder following physical trauma: An examination of the stressor criterion. *Psychological Medicine, 21*, 85–91.

Fisher, N., & Jacoby, R. (1992). Psychiatric morbidity in bus crews following violent assault: A follow-up study. *Psychological Medicine, 22*, 685–693.

Foy, D. W., Sipprelle, R. C., Rueger, D. B., & Carroll, E. M. (1984). Etiology of posttraumatic stress disorder in Vietnam veterans: Analysis of premilitary, military, and combat exposure influences. *Journal of Consulting and Clinical Psychology, 52*, 79–87.

Fraser, F., & Wilson, R. M. (1918). The sympathetic nervous system and the "irritable heart of soldiers." *British Medical Journal, II*, 27–31.

Green, B. L., Grace, M. C., & Gleser, G. C. (1985) Identifying survivors at risk: Long term impairment following the Beverly Hills Supper Club fire. *Journal of Consulting and Clinical Psychology, 53*(5), 672–678.

Green, B. L., Lindy, J. D., Grace, M. C., Gleser, G. C., Leonard, A. C., Korol, M., & Wurget, C. (1990). Buffalo Creek survivors in the second decade: Stability of stress symptoms. *American Journal of Orthopsychiatry, 60*(1), 43–54.

Green, B. L., & Lindy, J. D. (1994) Post-traumatic stress disorder in victims of disasters. *Psychiatric Clinics of North America, 17*(2), 301–309.

Grinker, R. R., Willerman, B., Bradley, A. D., & Fastowsky, A. (1946). A study of psychological predisposition to the development of operational fatigue. *American Journal of Orthopsychiatry, 16*, 191–214.

Hauff, E., & Vaglum, P. (1994). Chronic posttraumatic stress disorder in Vietnamese refugees. A prospective community study of prevalence, course, psychopathology, and stressors. *Journal of Nervous & Mental Disorders, 182*(2), 85–90.

Horowitz, M. J. (1986). Stress-response syndromes: A review of posttraumatic and adjustment disorders. *Hospital and Community Psychiatry, 37*(3), 241–249.

Horowitz, M., Wilner, N., & Alvarez, W. (1979). Impact of event scale: A measure of subjective stress. *Psychosomatic Medicine*, *41*(3), 209–218.

Joseph, S., Yule, W., Williams, R., & Hodgkinson, P. (1994). Correlates of post-traumatic stress at 30 months: The Herald of Free Enterprise disaster. *Behaviour Research and Therapy*, *32*(5), 521–524.

Karlehagen, S., Malt, U. F., Hoff, H., Tibell, E., Herrstromer, U., Hildingsa, K., & Leymann, H. J. (1993). The effect of major railway accidents on the psychological health of train drivers II. A longitudinal study of the first year outcome after the accident. *Psychosomatic Research*, *37*(8), 807–817.

Keane, T. M., Caddell, J. M., & Taylor, K. L. (1988). Mississippi Scale for combat-related posttraumatic stress disorder: Three studies in reliability and validity. *Journal of Consulting and Clinical Psychology*, *56*, 85–90.

Kemp, A., Green, B., Hovanitz, C., & Rawlings, E. (1995). Incidence and correlates of posttraumatic stress disorder in battered women: Shelter and community samples. *Journal of Interpersonal Violence*, *10*(1), 43–55.

Kessler, R. C., Sonega, A., Bromet, E., Hughes, M., & Nelson, C. B. (1995). Posttraumatic stress disorder in the National Comorbidity Survey. *Archives of General Psychiatry*, *52*, 1048–1060.

Kilpatrick D. G., Best, C. L., Veronen, L. J., Amick, A. E., Villeponteaux L. A., & Ruff, G. A. (1985). Mental health correlates of criminal victimization: A random community survey. *Journal of Consulting and Clinical Psychology*, *53*(6), 866–873.

Koopman, C., Classen, C., & Spiegel, D. A. (1994) Predictors of posttraumatic stress symptoms among survivors of the Oakland/Berkeley, Calif. firestorm. *American Journal of Psychiatry*, *151*(6), 888–894.

Lee, K. A., Vaillant, G. E., Torrey, W. C., & Elder, G. H. (1995). A 50 year prospective study of the psychological sequelae of World War II combat. *American Journal of Psychiatry*, *152*(4), 516–522.

Malt, U. (1988). The long term psychiatric consequences of accidental injury: A longitudinal study of 107 adults. *British Journal of Psychiatry*, *153*, 810–818.

Marmar, C. R., Weiss, D. S., Schlenger, W. E., Fairbank, J. A., Jordan, B. K., Kulka, R. A., & Hough, R. L. (1994). Peritraumatic dissociation and posttraumatic stress in male Vietnam theater veterans. *American Journal of Psychiatry*, *151*, 902–907.

McFarlane, A. C. (1992). Avoidance and intrusion in posttraumatic stress disorder. *Journal of Nervous and Mental Disease*, *180*(7), 439–445.

McNally, R. J., & Shin, L. M. (1995). Association of intelligence with severity of posttraumatic stress disorder symptoms in Vietnam combat veterans. *American Journal of Psychiatry*, *152*(6), 936–938.

Nolen-Hoeksema, S., & Morrow, J. (1991). A prospective study of depression and posttraumatic stress symptoms after a natural disaster: The 1989 Loma Prieta earthquake. *Journal of Personality and Social Psychology*, *61*(1) 116–121.

Norman E. M., Getek, D. M., & Griffin, C. C. (1991). Post-traumatic stress disorder in an urban trauma population. *Applied Nursing Research*, *4*(4), 171–176.

Orr, S. P., Pitman, R. K., Lasko, N. B., & Herz, L. R. (1993). Psychophysiological assessment of posttraumatic stress disorder imagery in World War II and Korean combat veterans. *Journal of Abnormal Psychology*, *102*(1), 152–159.

Perry, S., Difede, J., Musgni, G., Frances, A. J., & Jacobsberg, L. (1992). Prediction of post-traumatic stress disorder after burn injury. *American Journal of Psychiatry*, *149*(7), 931–935.

Putnam, F. W., Carlson, E. B., Ross, C. A., Anderson, G., Clark, P., Torem, M., Bowman, E. S., Coons, P., Chu, J. A., Dill, D. L., Loewenstein, R. J., & Braun, B. G. (1996). Patterns of dissociation in clinical and nonclinical samples. *Journal of Nervous and Mental Disease*, *184*(11), 673–679.

Rachman, S. (1980). Emotional processing. *Behaviour Research and Therapy*, *18*(1), 51–60.

Resnick, H. S., Kilpatrick, D. G., Best, C. L., & Kramer, T. L. (1992). Vulnerability-stress factors on development of posttraumatic stress disorder. *Journal of Nervous and Mental Disease*, *180*(7), 424–430.

Rivers, W. H. F. (1918). The repression of war experiences. *Lancet*, February 2, 1918.

Rothbaum, B. O., Foa, E. B., Riggs, D. S., & Murdock, T. (1992). A prospective examination of post-traumatic stress disorder in rape victims. *Journal of Traumatic Stress*, *5*(3) 455–475.

Shalev, A. Y. (1992). Posttraumatic stress disorder among injured survivors of a terrorist attack: Predictive value of early intrusion and avoidance symptoms. *Journal of Nervous and Mental Disease*, *180*(8), 505–509.

Shalev, A. Y., Orr, S. P., & Pitman, R. K. (1993). Psychophysiologic assessment of traumatic imagery in Israeli civilian patients with posttraumatic stress disorder. *American Journal of Psychiatry*, *150*(4), 620–624.

Shalev, A. Y., Peri, T., Canetti, L., & Schreiber, S. (1996). Predictors of PTSD in injured trauma survivors: A prospective study. *American Journal of Psychiatry*, *153*(2), 219–225.

Shalev, A. Y., Freedman, S., Peri, T., Brandes, D., & Sahar, T. (1997). Predicting PTSD in civilian trauma survivors: Prospective evaluation of self-report and clinician administered instrument. *British Journal of Psychiatry*, *170*, 558–564.

Solomon, Z. (1989). Psychological sequelae of war. A 3 year prospective study of Israeli combat stress reaction casualties. *Journal of Nervous and Mental Disease, 177*(6), 342–346.

Southwick, S. M., Morgan, A., Darnell, A., Bremner, D., Nicolaov, A. C., Nagy, L. M., & Charney, D. S. (1995). Trauma related symptoms in veterans of Operation Desert Storm: A 2 year follow-up. *American Journal of Psychiatry, 152*(8), 1150–1155.

Spielberger, C.D. (1983). *Manual for state trait anxiety inventory.* Palo Alto: Consulting Psychologists Press.

Sutker, P. B., Bugg, F., & Allain, A. N. (1990). Person and situation correlates of post-traumatic stress disorder among POW survivors. *Psychological Reports, 66*(3, Pt 1), 912–914.

Sutker, P. B., Davis, J. M., Uddo, M., & Ditta, S. R. (1995). War zone stress, personal resources, and PTSD in Persian Gulf War returnees. *Journal of Abnormal Psychology, 104*(3), 444–452.

Ursano, R. J., Fullerton, C. S., Kao, T. C., & Bhartiga, V. R. (1995). Longitudinal assessment of post-traumatic stress disorder and depression after exposure to traumatic death. *Journal of Nervous and Mental Disease, 183*(1), 36–42.

Wilson, J. P., & Kraus, G. E. (1982). Predicting post-traumatic stress disorders among Vietnam veterans. In W. E. Kelly (Ed.), *PTSD and the war veteran patient.* New York: Brunner/Mazel.

Yehuda, R., & McFarlane, A. C. (1995). Conflict between current knowledge about posttraumatic stress disorder and its original conceptual basis. *American Journal of Psychiatry, 152*(12), 1705–1713.

V

Neurobiology of Human Response to Trauma

In the past decade, it has become clear that distinct neurobiological alterations can be identified in symptomatic trauma survivors. These studies have had an enormous impact from political, clinical, and scientific perspectives. The idea of a specific biology for post-traumatic disorders certainly provides ammunition for those who feel that these disorders are posthoc rationalizations based on sociopolitical ideologies. The fact of these alterations attests to the longevity and severity of these events on the neurocircuitry and neurochemistry of the brain. The transition of traumatic stress reactions from the psychosocial into the biological arena has also opened up new horizons for treating post-traumatic reactions. Finally, the idea that traumatic stress responses are biologically mediated and that some of these biological mediators may become irreversible may ultimately link this construct across cultures, as suggested in previous sections.

Clinicians usually skip biological chapters. However, as the findings and their clinical implications become increasingly salient, their relevance to clinical work becomes too difficult to ignore. The changes produced following stressful exposure relate to elementary biological survival systems of the human body, whose physiology is widely understood. Clinicians need information beyond medicating patients. They need to know why their patients cannot sleep, cannot concentrate, have difficulty performing usual tasks without interference, are overly vigilant, and often become violent, detached, or depressed.

Now there are several major reviews that summarize the neurobiological systems that are thought to be altered in PTSD. We have chosen to focus on four particularly relevant parameters. In the first chapter Rachel Yehuda summarizes results of what has been the most surprising of the biological data thus far, that individuals who have PTSD appear to have a very different profile of stress hormone alterations compared to patients with other psychiatric disorders, and more, importantly, compared to the kinds of alterations that have been described as part of the neuroendocrine stress response. These differences are present in the chronic traumatic aftermath and also immediately following exposure. Yehuda's data suggest that the neurobiological circuitry controlling the hormonal stress response actually becomes more sensitized as a result of traumatic stress and the repeated reexperiencing of the trauma. The findings help explain why low-magnitude environmental events produce exaggerated behavioral responses in trauma survivors.

The hormonal differences observed in PTSD have certainly suggested that there may be important brain changes that either explain or occur as secondary consequences of neuroendocrine alterations. Israel Liberzon and Stephan Taylor provide a summary of neuroanatomical findings in PTSD that have evaluated both the morphology and functional chemistry of different brain regions. They mention the provocative observations of hippocampal atrophy in PTSD patients and describe several studies showing that the brain responds exaggeratedly to both reminders of traumatic stress and pharmacological challenges of alarm systems, as captured by PET technology. Indeed, Liberzon and Taylor make the point that it is important to distinguish between the way the brain looks under basal or resting conditions and the way it may respond to provocation. It has been exciting that these sophisticated tools are available to probe the brain. However, the subtle interaction of these brain mechanisms with meaningful psychological constructs still needs to be analyzed.

One of the prime symptoms of PTSD is difficulty in sleep. Trauma survivors most often complain about insomnia and traumatic nightmares. Thomas Mellman provides a comprehensive summary of studies of sleep in PTSD. Sleep has been one of the easier symptoms to study because it can be easily quantified by objective and relatively non-intrusive measures. However, contrasting with the apparently ubiquitous clinical complaints of sleep disturbances, empirical observations have failed to observe a consistent pattern of sleep abnormalities in PTSD. It may be that the laboratory condition inadvertently provides a therapeutic and safe environment that lacks the normal cues that trigger disturbed sleep. Certainly, the discrepancy between the empirical and clinical observations reminds us of the complexity of accurately characterizing PTSD. Nonetheless, the gains made in this important area have direct relevance to the clinical treatment of sleep disorders associated with PTSD.

It is so tempting to apply the burgeoning knowledge about neurobiology to clinical constructs, even in the absence of direct empirical data. The field of dissociation has suffered greatly because of the elusive nature of this clinical phenomenon, as well as sharp ideological differences in ways to view and define dissociation. John Krystal and his colleagues provide a scholarly review of the brain systems that are likely to be associated with dissociation and related phenomena. He begins by summarizing some of the interesting results of pharmacological challenges that have successfully demonstrated that certain PTSD symptoms can be induced in the laboratory. Interestingly, dissociative symptoms such as flashbacks and intrusive thoughts, have been particularly easy to induce in this manner. Pharmacological challenges offer a wonderful opportunity to ferret out the biological systems that may be involved in expressing diseases and particular symptoms because it is clear which systems may be affected during such an experimental manipulation. However, as Krystal et al. point out, similar symptoms can be provoked by activating very different neurotransmitter systems. Moving from these empirical studies, Krystal et al. hypothesize alterations in one of the most widely distributed neurotransmitter systems in the brain—glutamate. Such theories advance the field by offering concrete models that are empirically testable.

19

Cortisol Alterations in PTSD

RACHEL YEHUDA

Introduction

When post-traumatic stress disorder (PTSD) became a diagnosis in 1980, many psychiatrists felt that this disorder was redundant with current biopsychosocial formulations of mental illness. Given the acknowledged importance of stress in precipitating the development of any psychiatric disorder—but primarily of mood and anxiety disorders (Bidzinska, 1984; Ghaziuddin et al., 1990; McFarlane, 1990; Pitman et al., 1987; Post et al., 1986; Swann et al., 1990)— many felt that there was little to gain by having a discrete psychiatric disorder that specifically focused on targeting the effects of traumatic stressors. This feeling was further bolstered by the similarities between the proposed symptoms of PTSD and those seen in other mood and anxiety disorders (Friedman & Yehuda, 1995). Thus, many mental health practitioners in the early 1980s felt that the formulation of PTSD did not particularly add much to the psychiatric nosology in describing a novel syndrome. Rather, these practitioners considered PTSD to be a concession to social and political agendas of trauma survivors (Yehuda & McFarlane, 1995). Although this, in and of itself, did not particularly prompt antagonism within the field of mental health, it did generate some skepticism about whether PTSD was a "real" (i.e., legitimate and discrete) psychiatric disorder. This skepticism was reminiscent of past feelings that led to earlier descriptions of traumatic stress disorders as a "compensation neurosis."

When investigators began to address the possible biological underpinnings of PTSD, the more skeptical among them might have anticipated no biological changes at all in these trauma survivors (because they felt that there was no "real" disorder). More optimistic investigators predicted that biological alterations in PTSD would be similar to those that had already been well described in other mood and anxiety disorders. The latter hypothesis was quite reasonable, given the link between the biology of mood and anxiety disorders and the biology of stress responses in general.

Indeed, the acknowledgment of a link between stressful life events and the development of mood and anxiety disorders in the 1970s had been critical in generating hypotheses about the biological underpinnings of these disorders. After about two

RACHEL YEHUDA • Mount Sinai School of Medicine, Posttraumatic Stress Disorder Program, Bronx Veterans Affairs Medical Center, Bronx, New York 10468.

International Handbook of Human Response to Trauma, edited by Shalev, Yehuda, and McFarlane. Kluwer Academic / Plenum Publishers, New York, 2000.

decades of research, investigators had clearly concluded that the biology of mood disorders and to a lesser extent, of anxiety disorders was remarkably similar to the biological alterations described as part of the classic stress response (Chrousos & Gold, 1992). In particular, investigators were fascinated by the observation that about half of patients with major depressive disorder showed evidence of hypercortisolism (i.e., high cortisol levels) and also showed other abnormalities that were consistent with a chronic, biological stress response. So, too, it was predicted that PTSD patients would show evidence of hypercortisolism. However, the empirical findings that emerged from neuroendocrine investigation of PTSD suggested quite a different biological profile from the one that had been described in major depression and stress.

Indeed, rather than showing evidence of hypercortisolism, as initially predicted, trauma survivors with PTSD actually had lower cortisol levels than healthy control subjects. The low cortisol levels in PTSD were accompanied by a series of other abnormalities that further clarified the nature of the stress response in this disorder. Ironically, however, the very fact that cortisol levels are different in PTSD from those in normal patients or in other psychiatric disorders has done much more to validate the idea of PTSD as a distinct disorder than if cortisol levels would have simply been high as initially predicted. The fact that cortisol levels are low helps underscore that PTSD does describe a rather circumscribed set of symptoms and helps differentiate this syndrome from seemingly similar disorders with overlapping symptoms. As will be extensively reviewed in this chapter, the results from neuroendocrine studies have also helped clarify the nature of the stress response represented by PTSD.

Providing a Context for the Biological Findings: A Brief Review of the Prevalence and Course of PTSD

As mentioned, it seemed surprising initially that many of the neuroendocrine alterations in PTSD do not resemble those described in classic descriptions of stress because PTSD is precipitated by a stressor. However, as epidemiological studies emerged and clarified the prevalence and course of PTSD, the apparent paradox became more easy to understood. Less than half of those exposed to traumatic events develop this disorder (Breslau et al., 1991; Kessler et al., 1995), and less than half of those fail to show remission within a few years (Kessler et al., 1995). Thus, from a biological perspective, PTSD, particularly chronic PTSD, represents a particular type of stress response, which may not necessarily have the characteristics of the "classic" stress response (Yehuda & McFarlane, 1995; Yehuda et al., 1994). By emphasizing the limited prevalence of PTSD compared with the prevalence of traumatic events, it is easier to place into context the fact that there may be multiple biological and psychological responses to traumatic events and multiple determinants of those responses. Indeed, many trauma-exposed individuals develop other psychiatric disorders, such as major depression, dissociative disorders, eating disorders, substance abuse, anxiety disorders, and physical disorders. Some individuals develop "physical" rather than "psychological" symptoms, whereas others may seem impervious or resistant to the effects of particular types of life events (Shalev & Yehuda, 1998). Because PTSD is only one type of response to trauma, it may be that some aspects of the biological alterations in PTSD reflect risk for the development of this disorder rather than consequences of trauma exposure. This possibility is reasonable considering the contrast between the hypothalamic–

pituitary–adrenal (HPA) alterations in PTSD and those described in the stress literature. A brief description of the HPA axis and its role in stress is provided now.

The Hypothalamic–Pituitary–Adrenal Axis

According to classic descriptions, stress results in stimulating a cascade of events.
One of the most immediate responses to stress is the release of neurochemicals such as
norepinephrine (NE), dopamine (DA), acetylcholine (ACH) and serotonin (5-HT) in
the brain. These neurochemicals stimulate the release of a peptide called corticotrophin-
releasing factor (CRF) from the hypothalamus (Rivier & Plotsky, 1986). CRF (with the
help of other neurochemicals and neuropeptides) stimulates the release of a hormone
called adrenocorticotrophic hormone (ACTH) from the pituitary gland, which in turn,
stimulates the release of the hormone cortisol from the adrenal glands (Figure 1). This
response has generally been thought to be dose-dependent, that is, the more severe the
stressor, the higher the cortisol level (for reviews, see Mason, 1968, 1975; Selye, 1980). In
fact, Selye believed that it was possible to infer the severity of a stressor and its impact on
the individual from the concentration of cortisol levels. This implied that the objective
characteristics of stressors were far less important in determining the effect of events on

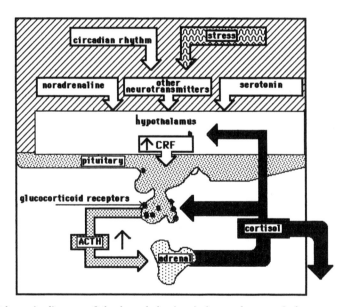

FIGURE 1. Schematic diagram of the hypothalamic–pituitary–adrenocortical stress response cascade.
Stress activates higher brain centers to release several neurotransmitters that stimulate the release of CRF
from the hypothalamus. CRF stimulates the release of ACTH from the pituitary, and ACTH stimulates the
release of cortisol from the adrenal glands. Cortisol exerts a negative feedback inhibition at the level of the
pituitary and the hypothalamus but more importantly, attends to the inhibition of myriad biological reactions
that are activated during stress. Importantly, according to classic descriptions, CRF, ACTH, and cortisol levels
are increased in response to stress. In PTSD, stress activates neurotransmitters to release CRF from the
hypothalamus. However, because of an increased number of glucocorticoid receptors on the pituitary, the
normal stress response cascade is disrupted. Although ACTH stimulates the adrenal to release cortisol,
cortisol acts at the level of the pituitary to shut off ACTH release from the pituitary, and ultimately less cortisol
is made and released from the adrenal glands.

organisms than the cortisol response (Selye, 1956). It is interesting to point out that
Selye's position was quite different from that taken in the DSM-IV, which tries to focus
primarily on the importance of the objective nature of the event (i.e., as involving life
threat) in determining subsequent emotional responses.

For decades after Selye's initial description in 1956, the release of cortisol during
stress was considered potentially harmful. Selye and numerous investigators who followed him described many detrimental consequences that were a direct or indirect
result of cortisol secretion following stress (Selye, 1956, 1980). One of the worst consequences of cortisol release, according to Selye, is that it causes a shrinkage of the thymus
gland and reductions in the number of lymphocytes in the blood, which leads to a
subsequent weakening of the immune system and increased susceptibility to a myriad of
other illnesses. It was also thought that many negative coping behaviors such as smoking, drinking, overeating, and undereating were a result of increased cortisol release
following stress (Lazarus et al., 1980). These behaviors, in turn, were thought to increase
the risk for hypertension, coronary disease, and other stress-related illnesses. Selye's
work led to the idea that stress has a negative effect on organisms, primarily via the
release of cortisol. More recently, stress (i.e., increased cortisol levels) has been implicated in causing brain changes. Indeed, Sapolsky (1996) hypothesized that sustained
stress and resultant increases in cortisol result in hippocampal atrophy and cell death.

It was not until relatively recently and about 50 years after Selye's initial descriptions of the pituitary-adrenocortical response to stress that investigators began to
question whether, indeed, cortisol was really the dangerous direct culprit of stress-
related disease. In 1984, a remarkable paper emerged which asserted that the function
of cortisol in stress was actually reparative, not destructive (Munck et al., 1984). Indeed,
it was postulated that perhaps the most important function of cortisol is to help shut
down the other biological reactions that were activated by stress (i.e., for example, the
release of adrenaline). Munck et al. correctly pointed out that the stress response is
ultimately contained by the negative feedback inhibition of cortisol on the pituitary,
hypothalamus, and other sites. Thus, cortisol was identified as the hormone necessary
for terminating the stress response—almost like an "antistress" hormone—by shutting
down the reactions that really could do long-term damage to organisms. From this it
stood to reason that not having enough cortisol might be detrimental to organisms that
are trying to cope with the initial demands of a stressor. On the other hand, however, the
truism that there can be too much of a good thing, also seemed to be true about cortisol.
Munck et al. also pointed out that when cortisol levels remain too high for too long, this
could also result in negative consequences, including medical illness (Ling et al., 1981)
neuronal death (Sapolsky et al., 1985), and impaired mood and cognitive alterations
(Wolkowitz et al., 1990).

Another important concept was introduced into our understanding of the way
hormones affect behavior as investigators began to identify the presence of hormone
receptors and study their mechanism of action. Selye formulated his ideas about
cortisol's actions in the absence of knowledge about steroid receptors and the way they
work. Now it is widely appreciated that cortisol exerts its actions by binding to glucocorticoid receptors (Svec, 1985). It is also known now that changes in the number and/or
sensitivity of glucocorticoid receptors can influence the body's response to stress (Lowy
et al., 1989), that is, although two individuals might have the same cortisol levels, if their
receptors differ in their ability to bind to cortisol and synthesize proteins, these

individuals might have very different biological and behavioral reactions to stress, and might function very differently, even under conditions where there is no active stressor. Because of this, simply knowing the concentration of circulating cortisol levels does not provide complete information about the neuroendocrine or behavioral effects of this hormone. To properly understand the nature of the HPA axis responses during tonic phases and in response to stress, it is necessary to know about the nature of the hormone receptors along the HPA axis, and it is also important to evaluate the effects of neuro-hormones on target tissue above the level of the adrenal (i.e., the pituitary, the hypothalamus, and other areas of the brain such as the hippocampus). As will be more comprehensively reviewed below, our group has made the observation that glucocorticoid receptors may actually be more sensitive in trauma survivors with PTSD. This has led to several plausible hypotheses about the nature of HPA axis alterations in PTSD. Primarily, now it is thought that although cortisol levels in PTSD are lower than normal in PTSD, this actually reflects a more sensitive HPA system, as further described following.

Hypothalamic–Pituitary–Adrenal Alterations in PTSD

Cortisol Levels.   The majority of the studies performed to date demonstrate that cortisol levels in PTSD are lower compared to those of other psychiatric groups and normal controls. In an initial investigation, lower means that 24-hour urinary cortisol excretion was observed in nine hospitalized combat Vietnam veterans with PTSD compared to patients with major depression, bipolar mania, undifferentiated schizophrenia, and schizoaffective disorder (Mason et al., 1986). A second study also found low urinary cortisol in combat veterans with PTSD compared to major depression, bipolar mania, panic disorder, and schizophrenia (Yehuda et al., 1993b). Urinary cortisol excretion was found to be lower in inpatient and outpatient combat veterans with PTSD compared to nonpsychiatric, healthy controls (Yehuda et al., 1990). A more recent study demonstrated that urinary cortisol levels were significantly lower in Holocaust survivors with PTSD compared with Holocaust survivors without PTSD and demographically comparable comparison subjects (Yehuda et al., 1995). The mean urinary cortisol levels in the PTSD and normal control groups in these four studies have been remarkably consistent (Figure 2). In contrast to these studies, Pitman and Orr reported that the 24-hour urinary cortisol excretion of cortisol in combat veterans with PTSD was elevated compared to cortisol levels of combat veterans without PTSD. These investigators did not use a nontraumatized comparison group. Lemieux and Coe (1995) also failed to demonstrate low cortisol in PTSD. In fact, their study showed increased urinary cortisol excretion in adult women with PTSD arising from sexual abuse.

One possible reason for the high cortisol levels in the study of sexually abused women may have been the inclusion of obese women in the sample (i.e., the weight range in the sample was 102–400 lbs). In trying to evaluate the reasons for the discrepancies across these studies, it is also important to consider that the established normal range of urinary cortisol excretion over a 24-hour period in man is estimated to be between 20–90 μg/day. Values at either extremes of this range may suggest endocrinologic abnormality. In both the Pitman and Orr (1990) and Lemieux and Coe (1995) studies, the mean cortisol excretions for the normal control groups were at the high end of the normal range (Figure 2). Because it is unlikely that the normal controls had endocrinologic disorder, it might be more reasonable to consider that differences

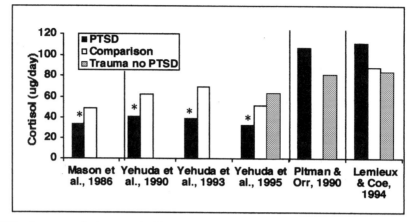

FIGURE 2. Summary of urinary cortisol levels across all PTSD studies to date. Comparison subjects were nonpsychiatric healthy age and gender comparable persons in Yehuda et al., 1990, 1995; and Lemiux & Coe, 1994. Comparison subjects in Mason et al., 1986, and Yehuda et al., 1993, were psychiatric patients. In Mason et al., 1986, subjects in this group consisted of major depression disorder ($N = 8$), mania ($N = 8$), schizophrenia ($N = 7$), and paranoid schizophrenia ($N = 12$). In Yehuda et al., 1993, subjects in the psychiatric comparison group were those with major depression disorder ($N = 10$), mania ($N = 7$), psychotic disorder ($N = 9$), and panic disorder ($N = 6$). The asterisk indicates that mean cortisol levels in PTSD subjects were significantly lower than those in other groups. In the Lemiex & Coe study, PTSD subjects had significantly higher mean cortisol levels than in the other groups. In the Pitman & Orr study, there were no significant differences in cortisol levels between PTSD and combat control subjects.

in the method of storage, collection, or assay of the urine may have led to artificially high or spurious cortisol values. For example, when acid preservative is added to the urine collection bottle (to prevent degradation of catecholamines), this may interfere with the antibody–antigen reaction in the radioimmunoassay procedure and yield artificially high or spurious cortisol values (Mason et al., 1986; Meikle et al., 1969).

Studies of 24-hour urinary cortisol excretion provide an overall assessment of cortisol output during the diurnal cycle. However, they do not provide information about the patterning of cortisol levels over the course of the cycle. This can be particularly important because what may be critical in evaluating the regulation of the HPA axis under tonic conditions is the dynamic range of hormonal release and not simply the ultimate amount of cortisol secreted.

In a recent investigation examining the circadian release of cortisol at 30-minute intervals over the 24-hour diurnal cycle, our group confirmed the finding of overall lower cortisol levels in combat veterans with PTSD compared to patients with major depression and normal controls. However, we also demonstrated that the patterning of cortisol release was substantially different in the three groups (Yehuda et al., 1996c). In PTSD, cortisol levels were found to be significantly lower only in the late evening and early morning hours, but comparable to normals from 7:00 A.M. until 7:00 P.M. Furthermore, the peak hormone release of cortisol was comparable to that of normal (Figure 3). Because cortisol levels were lower only at the nadir of the cycle, but not at the peak, this resulted in a greater range of cortisol release during the diurnal cycle that was reflected by a higher amplitude/mean ratio (Figure 4). Although the full significance of these findings awaits further clarification, the results suggest that there are important

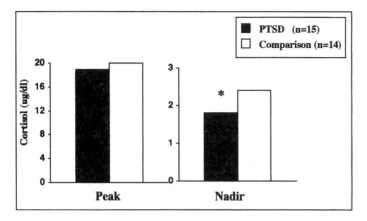

FIGURE 3.   Cortisol levels and the peak and nadir of the diurnal cycle in PTSD and nonpsychiatric healthy comparison subjects. These data are redrawn from Yehuda et al., 1996c, and demonstrate the mean peak cortisol levels and mean nadir levels in PTSD and nonpsychiatric healthy comparison subjects. There were no differences in peak cortisol levels (which occurred at approximately 7 A.M.) but PTSD subjects showed significantly lower levels at the nadir of the cycle (approximately 1 A.M.).

differences in the patterning of cortisol release, as well as the regulatory influences controlling cortisol release, that may have implications for the way the HPA axis might differentially respond to stress in PTSD and major depression.

Although this study did not demonstrate significant differences in cortisol levels at all times, it is interesting to note that a recent epidemiologic study conducted on a sample of almost 2500 Vietnam veterans demonstrated that veterans with current PTSD had lower plasma cortisol levels than veterans without PTSD (Boscarino, 1996). Although the actual effect size was quite small, which is consistent with the previously

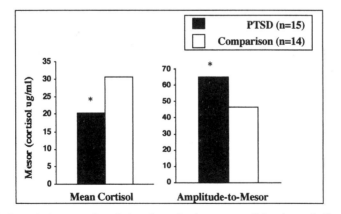

FIGURE 4.   Mathematical mean of cortisol and amplitude-to-mesor ("signal-to-noise") ratio of cortisol during the 24-hour diurnal cycle in PTSD and nonpsychiatric comparison subjects. These data are redrawn from Yehuda et al., 1996c, and demonstrate that mean cortisol levels during the 24-hour cycle in PTSD subjects were significantly lower than in comparison subjects. However, the amplitude-to-mesor ratio was significantly higher, indicating that the range of cortisol release reflects a larger peak-to-nadir difference in PTSD.

mentioned study, the significance of the finding may be a result of the very large sample size used. Other studies have similarly demonstrated low basal cortisol levels from single plasma or salivary estimates in subjects with PTSD (Goenjian et al., 1996; Heim et al., 1997; Jensen et al., 1997; Kellner et al., 1997).

There have also been reports of low cortisol in other chronically stressed or traumatized individuals. However, these studies did not evaluate subjects for the presence or absence of PTSD. Nonetheless, it is interesting to note that lower than normal cortisol levels have been observed in parents of chronically, fatally ill children (Friedman et al., 1963), and in persons exposed to highly chronically stressful jobs (Hellhammer & Wade, 1993; Vernikos Danellis et al., 1975). Low cortisol levels were observed in soldiers who were studied in Vietnam while under the threat of enemy attack (Bourne et al., 1967, 1968). A recent report also reported low cortisol levels in a group of detainees in a Bosnian prisoner of war camp (Dekaris et al., 1993). Low cortisol was also observed in a group of refugees who fled from East to West Germany shortly after their arrival in West Berlin (Bauer et al., 1994). These findings further support the idea that cortisol levels can be low in symptomatic individuals who have been exposed to traumatic stress.

Lymphocyte Glucocorticoid Receptors.   Because hormones, like cortisol, cannot exert their biological effects unless they are bound to steroid receptors (DeKloet et al., 1991; Svec, 1985), the examination of steroid receptors can provide information to help assess the biological activity of hormones. It is for this reason that our group examined glucocorticoid receptor number and sensitivity following the initial observations of lower cortisol levels.

Four studies have been performed to date, and all show that PTSD subjects have a larger number of lymphocyte glucocorticoid receptors compared with other groups. In contrast, major depression (Gormley et al., 1985; Lowy et al., 1989; Veith & Murburg, 1994; Yehuda et al., 1993) and stress (Sapolsky et al., 1985) have been associated with a decreased number of glucocorticoid receptors.

Studies of combat veterans with PTSD have consistently demonstrated significantly larger numbers of glucocorticoid receptors compared to nonpsychiatric (Yehuda et al., 1991, 1996) and psychiatric comparison groups of major depression, panic disorder, bipolar mania, and schizophrenia (Yehuda et al., 1993b). A more recent study demonstrated that adult women with PTSD from childhood physical or sexual abuse have an increased number of lymphocyte glucocorticoid receptors (Stein et al., 1997).

The finding of a larger number of glucocorticoid receptors is consistent with observations of low cortisol in PTSD because low circulating levels of a hormone or neurotransmitter are usually associated with an "upregulation" or increased number of receptors. However, in the case of PTSD, the direction of causality of the relationship between glucocorticoid receptors and low cortisol is not known. In more classic models of receptor–ligand interactions, changes in glucocorticoid receptor number are thought to be compensatory responses to the concentration of ligand (Rabkin & Struening, 1976; McEwen et al., 1986; Schlecte et al., 1982; Tornello et al., 1982). Therefore, an increased number of glucocorticoid receptors is usually considered to be a secondary consequence of low cortisol. However, it is possible that glucocorticoid receptors actually serve to regulate hormonal release by modifying the strength of negative feedback (Lowy et al., 1989).

Several years ago our group hypothesized that an increased sensitivity of glucocorticoid receptors might constitute a primary alteration in PTSD (Yehuda et al., 1995). However, to truly prove this hypothesis, it is necessary to perform a careful, prospective, and longitudinal characterization of glucocorticoid receptor changes beginning either before or in the immediate aftermath of trauma in exposed individuals who do and do not develop PTSD.

Cortisol Response to Dexamethasone.   Dexamethasone is a synthetic glucocorticoid that mimics the effect of cortisol and can act to substantially inhibit the release of ACTH from the pituitary (and possibly CRF from the hypothalamus). The dexamethasone suppression test (DST) involves administering 1 mg dexamethasone at 11:00 P.M. when normal cortisol secretion is at its lowest point in the diurnal cycle. In individuals with an intact negative feedback inhibition, this manipulation suppresses the normal morning rise in cortisol. In normals a dose of 1 mg usually suppresses plasma cortisol to a level below 5 μg/dl at 8:00 A.M. and remains at that level at 4:00 P.M.

Studies that examine the cortisol response to dexamethasone in major depressive disorder have repeatedly shown a "nonsuppression" of cortisol in about half of depressed patients (Carroll et al., 1981). The cortisol response to 1 mg dexamethasone has been investigated in five studies of PTSD. These studies all reported that PTSD patients without major depression show "normal" suppression to dexamethasone (Dinan et al., 1990; Halbreich et al., 1989; Kosten et al., 1990; Kudler et al., 1987; Olivera & Fero, 1990). However, closer examination reveals that PTSD patients as a group show an exaggerated suppression to dexamethasone—which is opposite of the nonsuppression observed in major depression.

The findings of cortisol suppression following dexamethasone in PTSD patients with major depression are less clear. In an initial study, Kudler et al., (1987) reported that PTSD patients with major depressive disorder showed a rate of nonsuppression comparable with that observed in major depressive disorder, whereas Halbreich et al. (1989) and Kosten et al. (1990) found normal responses to dexamethasone, even in depressed combat veterans with PTSD. Olivera and Fero (1990) reported a 32% rate of nonsuppression in 65 combat veterans with PTSD who met comorbid criteria for major depressive disorder. However, these individuals showed normal suppression after their major depression had remitted. A study that examined the cortisol response to dexamethasone in eight civilian woman with PTSD (Dinan et al., 1990) also showed normal responses to dexamethasone. It is possible that some of the differences between studies may be due to differences across laboratories in the way major depression is diagnosed in the PTSD patients. Some investigators may consider that patients who meet the diagnostic criteria for depression due to symptoms that overlap with PTSD (e.g., symptoms such as insomnia, impaired concentration) are patients with major depression, whereas other investigators might not consider that PTSD patients have a comorbid depression unless they meet criteria for major depression using symptoms that cannot be considered part of the PTSD syndrome. However, regardless of whether a more stringent or liberal interpretation of comorbidity is used, when the 4:00 P.M. postdexamethasone cortisol values of the 83 PTSD patients with comorbid depression are averaged across all studies, the overall mean was somewhat higher than that reported for PTSD patients without major depression but still well below the cutoff of 5.0 μg/dl commonly used as a threshold for major depression.

Studies Using the Low-Dose DST. DST studies using a 1.0 mg dose of dexamethasone in PTSD were conducted before it was known that cortisol levels in these patients were lower and the number of glucocorticoid receptors larger, than in comparison subjects. These earlier studies were designed to test for "nonsuppression" in PTSD and did not consider the possibility of an exaggerated cortisol response or hypersuppression to dexamethasone. Because of the failure to observe the classic nonsuppression response to cortisol and our own observations of low cortisol and an increased number of glucocorticoid receptors, we utilized lower doses of dexamethasone to explore the possibility of enhanced negative feedback sensitivity.

Hyperresponsiveness to low doses (0.50 and 0.25 mg) of dexamethasone in PTSD compared to controls, as reflected by significantly lower postdexamethasone cortisol levels, has been observed now in all studies published to date. In one study, the enhanced suppression of cortisol was accompanied by a decreased number, or downregulation, of cytosolic lymphocyte glucocorticoid receptors (Yehuda et al., 1996a). Interestingly, the hyperresponsiveness to dexamethasone was also present in trauma survivors with PTSD who met the diagnostic criteria for major depressive disorder (Stein et al., 1997; Yehuda et al., 1993a).

Although initial studies were performed on combat veterans, enhanced suppression to dexamethasone has been observed in adult survivors of childhood sexual abuse (Stein et al., 1997) and among women who have chronic pelvic pain and a history of sexual abuse and PTSD (Heim et al., 1997). Hypersuppression of salivary cortisol to 0.50 mg dexamethasone was also observed in Armenian children with PTSD following exposure to the great earthquake of 1988 (Goenjian et al., 1996) and in Persian Gulf War soldiers who were evaluated approximately 1 year after their return from the war theater (Kellner et al., 1997). Table 1 summarizes the results from studies using the low-dose DST.

When the DST was initially applied to the study of psychiatric disorder, many investigators felt hopeful that the DST could be used to aid in diagnosing and classifying major depressive disorder (Carroll et al., 1981). The original idea was to use a cutoff of 5 μg/dl at 4:00 P.M. to differentiate between "normal" cortisol suppression and "nonsuppression" typical of a major depressive disorder. As stated before, however, decades of research demonstrated that only about half of depressed patients exhibit this nonsuppression, and therefore, this test did not provide the sensitivity and specificity needed for diagnostic purposes. It is certainly interesting to note that none of the DST studies in major depression considered the possibility that any of their subjects might have experienced psychological trauma. Furthermore, the presence of current or lifetime PTSD was not an exclusion for any of these studies. Given the fact that about half of the normal population has experienced traumatic events, it may be that the failure to observe "nonsuppression" in all depressed patients can be attributed to the presence of a substantial trauma history or post-traumatic symptomatology in these individuals. This hypothesis has not yet been tested. Nonetheless, the extraordinary distinction between the "hypersuppression" of PTSD and the "nonsuppression" of major depressive disorder makes the low-dose DST an attractive tool to aid in the differential diagnosis of PTSD and major depressive disorder.

Suprapituitary Activation of the HPA Axis. Thus far we have discussed primarily measuring cortisol from the adrenals under basal conditions and in response to dexamethasone. However, because the stress response is actually best thought of as a

TABLE 1. DST Studies in PTSD

1A. Studies Using 1.0 mg DEX

Study/Year	Trauma Survivors with PTSD (µg/dl CORT)	N	Trauma Survivors with PTSD and MDD (µg/dl CORT)	N
Kudler et al., 1987	1.86 ± 1.87	18	3.83 ± 3.15	10
Kosten et al., 1990	2.38 ± 2.58	7	0.90 ± 0.53	4
Olivera and Fero, 1990	1.00 ± 0.10	44	2.70 ± 2.78	65
Halbreich et al., 1990			0.96 ± 1.63	14
Dinan et al., 1990	3.6 ± 0.28	8		

1B. Studies Using Low Dose (0.50 and 0.25) DEX

Study/Year	Trauma with PTSD X ± SD	N	Trauma without PTSD X ± SD	N	Normal Subjects X ± SD	N
0.5 mg						
Yehuda et al., 1993	1.4 ± 0.6[a]	21			4.8 ± 2.9	12
Stein et al., 1995	1.5 ± 1.4[a]	12	2.0 ± 1.2	6	3.2 ± 3.2	21
Yehuda et al., 1995	1.1 ± 0.6[a]	14	3.9 ± 3.5	12	3.9 ± 2.9	14
0.25 mg						
Yehuda et al., 1995	4.5 ± 2.5[a]	14	10 ± 3.6	12	9.0 ± 3.7	14

[a]Significantly different from other groups.

cascade that begins in the brain, it has been imperative to obtain information whether brain centers are activated in PTSD, and if so, how neurochemical activation in brain results in the lower cortisol levels observed in PTSD. Thus, it has been important to evaluate hypothalamic CRF release in PTSD.

As previously mentioned, CRF plays a critical role in modulating pituitary-adrenocortical activity. Furthermore, this peptide is also localized in extrahypothalamic areas that regulate emotionality, such as the amygdala (Fellman et al., 1982; Merchanthaler, 1984; Sawchenko & Swanson, 1985; Swanson et al., 1983) and locus coeruleus (Chappell et al., 1986; Sawchenko et al., 1985). Therefore, investigators hypothesized that there would be overproduction of CRF release in both major depression, and later, PTSD (Yehuda & Nemeroff, 1994).

Interestingly, both major depressive disorder (Arato et al., 1989; Banki et al., 1987; Nemeroff et al., 1984) and PTSD appear to be characterized by CRF hypersecretion. However, rather than showing the classic stress response cascade where increased CRF levels lead to increased cortisol release and ultimately to a pituitary hyporesponsivity and decreased negative feedback inhibition, the HPA system appears to be more sensitized in PTSD (Yehuda, 1998). This increased sensitivity is manifested by decreased cortisol release and an increased negative feedback inhibition.

Indirect evidence of an increase in CRF was recently obtained in a study that demonstrated increased concentrations of CRF in cerebrospinal fluid (CSF) of combat veterans with PTSD compared to healthy controls (Bremner et al., 1997). Because CSF provides an overall estimate of the CRF activity in the brain and spinal cord, it cannot be concluded from this study that hypothalamic CRF is also increased.

Rather, estimations of hypothalamic release of CRF have been made using neuroendocrine challenge strategies. The most popular of these tests has been the CRF stimulation test. The CRF challenge test measures the pituitary adrenocorticotropic hormone (ACTH) and adrenal cortisol response to exogenous infusion of the neuropeptide CRF and therefore provides an indirect estimate of CRF activity by examining the effects of this peptide on pituitary sensitivity. The "blunted" ACTH response to CRF observed in major depression (Nemeroff & Evans, 1989) is thought to reflect a downregulation of pituitary CRF receptors caused by the presumed state of chronic hypothalamic CRF hypersecretion (Krishnan et al., 1991).

Studies examining the ACTH response to CRF in trauma survivors have also reported blunting of the ACTH response to CRF. One study showed that the ACTH response to CRF was blunted in combat veterans with PTSD compared to normal controls (Smith et al., 1989). A second study demonstrated a blunted ACTH response to CRF in sexually abused girls (DeBellis et al., 1994). In the latter study, PTSD was not diagnosed. However, a third study found a blunted salivary cortisol response to CRF infusion in women with chronic pelvic pain and sexual abuse who also had PTSD (Heim et al., 1997).

Although the finding of a blunted ACTH to CRF may seem similar to that observed in patients with major depression, it seems likely that the mechanisms underlying the blunted ACTH response in PTSD are different from the mechanism described previously for major depression. This possibility was initially considered because the attenuated ACTH response in PTSD patients occurred in the presence of normal, not elevated, evening plasma cortisol levels (Smith et al., 1989). Thus, it seemed plausible that the ACTH blunting in response to CRF may have occurred as a result of hyperresponsivity of the pituitary gland to cortisol resulting directly from an increased number of glucocorticoid receptors on the pituitary gland (Yehuda et al., 1991).

A more direct way of assessing CRF hypersecretion is to utilize the metyrapone stimulation test. Metyrapone is a drug that prevents adrenal steroidogenesis by blocking the conversion of 11-deoxycortisol to cortisol and virtually eliminates the influences of negative feedback inhibition on the pituitary gland. Thus, metyrapone administration allows direct examination of pituitary release of ACTH without the potentially confounding effects of differing ambient cortisol levels or glucocorticoid receptor responsiveness (Lisansky et al., 1989).

The abrupt disruption of cortisol synthesis following metyrapone administration results in a sudden and significant increase in the release of ACTH. The normal response to metyrapone results in a two- to fourfold increase in plasma levels of ACTH within 2 to 8 hours of metyrapone administration. Under these conditions, it is possible to use the concentration of ACTH or even 11-deoxycortisol as index of hypothalamic CRF activity (Tepperman, 1981). If levels of ACTH or 11-deoxycortisol are substantially higher (i.e., greater than a fourfold increase in response to metyrapone), this provides direct evidence that the pituitary is receiving greater stimulation by CRF. Interestingly, this test has not been utilized as extensively as other challenge strategies in major depression. However, some studies have demonstrated that the ACTH response to metyrapone is increased (Ur et al., 1992; Young et al., 1994).

One published study examined the ACTH and 11-deoxycortisol response to metyrapone in PTSD. In that study metyrapone resulted in a significantly greater increase of ACTH and 11-deoxycortisol in combat veterans with PTSD ($N = 11$) compared with normal male volunteers ($N = 8$) (Yehuda et al., 1996b). These data are consistent with the results of the CRF challenge test in suggesting an increased sensitivity of the pituitary gland that may arise as a result of CRF hypersecretion.

One of the challenges that has arisen in trying to make sense out of the HPA axis alterations in PTSD has been to explain how there could be suprapituitary activation (i.e., increased CRF release) that does not necessarily result in hypercortisolism. To date, the theoretical model that best accounts for all the data obtained is the enhanced negative feedback model described here.

Enhanced Negative Feedback Model. If PTSD were characterized by an enhanced negative feedback sensitivity of cortisol (see Figure 1), this would nicely account for the alterations that have been observed. According to this model, PTSD is characterized by chronic or transient increases in the release of hypothalamic CRF, likely resulting from differences in neuropeptide modulation. The high levels of CRF lead to an altered responsivity of the pituitary, as evidenced by the blunted ACTH response to CRF challenge and increased ACTH levels following metyrapone in PTSD. However, because of primary alteration in glucocorticoid receptor responsivity, there would be a stronger negative feedback inhibition resulting in attenuated baseline ACTH and cortisol levels, as well as enhanced responsivity to dexamethasone. To date, the etiology of the proposed alteration in glucocorticoid receptor responsiveness is unknown.

Biological Studies in the Acute Aftermath of Traumatic Events: Relationship to the Biology of PTSD

The previous discussion demonstrates that the neuroendocrine alterations in PTSD are different from those associated with other types of stress responses and other psychiatric disorders. However, several questions have arisen in attempting to understand these findings. First, because the findings summarized before were performed on subjects with chronic PTSD (i.e., trauma survivors who have been symptomatic for years and even decades), it was possible that the alterations observed represented a biological adaptation to chronic symptoms of PTSD over time and not necessarily the neurobiological response to a traumatic event. Furthermore, as it became increasingly clear that individuals without PTSD did not show the biological alterations despite their comparable exposure to trauma, it became important to consider the possibility that prior and subsequent stressors, in addition to the focal trauma, contributed to the neuroendocrine alterations in PTSD. Additionally, the possibility of a preexisting biological diathesis to stress could also be a contributing factor to the observed findings.

Figure 5 presents a schematic diagram that provides a "road map" for future biological studies. This diagram underscores the necessity of elucidating the relationships among pretraumatic, acute (peritraumatic), and post-traumatic stress responses in all trauma survivors. Furthermore, the diagram demonstrates that trauma survivors should be studied in terms of the current PTSD status and also in terms of whether or not they may have developed PTSD in the first place. Currently, there is no information describing biological alterations in trauma survivors who recover from PTSD, as differentiated from trauma survivors who never developed this disorder. However, to the extent that some of the biological alterations in PTSD predate the development of

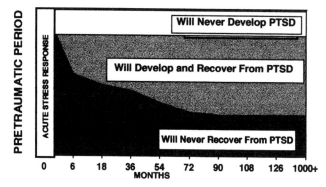

FIGURE 5. A schematic "road map" for future biological studies in PTSD. This hypothetical schematic is loosely based on data summarized from Kessler et al., 1995, which demonstrated that a majority of individuals who develop PTSD recover from this disorder over time (shaded grey), whereas a substantial minority of individuals appear to develop a chronic and unremitting form of PTSD (shaded black). Kessler et al.'s study also demonstrates that some individuals never develop PTSD following exposure to trauma (white area). Although neuroendocrine studies have demonstrated differences between trauma survivors with and without PTSD, several questions remain concerning the relationship of these changes to the pretraumatic state of individuals, as well to their neuroendocrine response during the acute phase. Ultimately it will be important to determine the extent to which trauma survivors in the different shaded areas differ from one another in biological measures when these differences are first manifest.

symptoms, or even trauma exposure, such information may become quite useful in predicting risk for, or remission from, PTSD.

Recent longitudinal studies have begun to explore some of these questions by examining the acute biological response to trauma in those who subsequently do and do not develop PTSD (see Figure 6). One study demonstrated that women who are most likely to develop PTSD had lower cortisol levels at the time of the trauma. Low cortisol levels at the time of rape was associated with a prior history of rape, which was the strongest predictor of the subsequent development of PTSD (Resnick et al., 1995). Interestingly, the severity of the rape did not predict either cortisol levels or the subsequent development of PTSD.

In a second study (Figure 6), the cortisol response to motor vehicle accidents was examined in individuals who appeared at the Emergency Room in the immediate aftermath of the trauma. Six months later subjects were evaluated for the presence or absence of psychiatric disorder. In subjects who had developed PTSD, the cortisol response in the immediate aftermath of the motor vehicle was substantially lower, and the cortisol response in those who developed major depression was substantially higher than in individuals who did not develop psychiatric disorder. In the aggregate, the two longitudinal studies demonstrate that acute cortisol responses to trauma in individuals who develop PTSD may be different from those of individuals who do not develop PTSD in response to a similar trauma. Furthermore, the data raise the possibility that the low cortisol levels observed in chronic PTSD reflect more than simply the state of having a chronic illness.

Unfortunately, the two longitudinal studies do not directly address whether individuals may have had low cortisol levels before the traumatic event. Thus, it would be premature to conclude that the neuroendocrine findings in PTSD manifest an under-

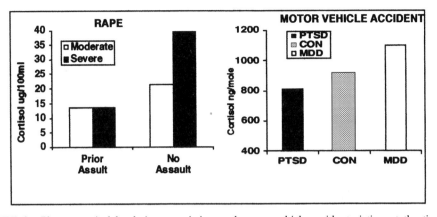

FIGURE 6. Plasma cortisol levels in rape victims and motor vehicle accident victims at the time of presentation to the emergency room in the acute aftermath of the trauma. The first panel contains data redrawn from Resnick et al., 1995, indicating that cortisol levels in the acute aftermath of rape were lower in victims with a prior history of rape, regardless of the severity of rape. The second panel contains preliminary data from a sample of 35 motor vehicle accident victims redrawn from Yehuda et al., 1998, demonstrating that lower cortisol following a motor vehicle accident was more likely to be associated with the subsequent development of PTSD, whereas higher cortisol levels were more likely to be associated with the subsequent development of major depressive disorder.

lying risk for this disorder rather than describe the consequences of chronic symptoms following trauma exposure. The resolution of this question necessitates prospective studies that assess cortisol levels in subjects before and after they experience traumatic events, which for obvious reasons, are difficult to perform.

What remains increasingly clear is that it is difficult to ascribe neuroendocrine alterations in PTSD solely to exposure to traumatic events. It is even possible that some features of the atypical neuroendocrine response to trauma in those who develop chronic PTSD might be present at the time of the trauma, or even before the traumatic event occurs (and would therefore predispose the individual to responding). This study does not directly address the question whether the enhanced negative feedback response may be a more "adaptive" stress response, but it does suggest that there are important individual differences that may contribute to the reason some people respond to stress by becoming more hypervigilant (e.g., similar to PTSD) versus more withdrawn and disengaged (e.g., similar to major depression).

Conclusion

Although most initial hypotheses about the biology of PTSD proposed very similar alterations in PTSD compared to those observed in major depression and other anxiety disorders, a review of the neuroendocrine findings in PTSD to date indicates very specific and qualitatively different abnormalities in this disorder. The most prominent of these differences appear to be in the hypothalamic–pituitary–adrenal axis. PTSD patients show evidence of enhanced negative feedback inhibition characterized by an exaggerated cortisol response to dexamethasone, an increased number of glucocorticoid receptors, and lower basal cortisol levels. These findings contrast with the blunted cortisol response to dexamethasone, the decreased number of glucocorticoid receptors, and the increased basal cortisol levels described in major depression. Most studies also suggest increased activation of the catecholamine system in PTSD. Now the task is to determine the extent to which findings in chronic PTSD represent the same types of changes as those seen in the early aftermath of trauma and to determine whether any long-term consequences can be predicted on the basis of the nature of the changes observed.

Acknowledgments.   Supported by NIMH grant-49536 and 49555 and Merit Review Funds (awarded to Dr. Yehuda).

References

APA Task Force on Laboratory Tests in Psychiatry. (1987). The dexamethasone suppression test: An overview of its current status in psychiatry. *American Journal of Psychiatry, 144*, 1253–1262.

Arato, M., Banki, C. M., Bissette, G., & Nemeroff, C. B. (1989). Elevated CSF CRF in suicide victims. *Biological Psychiatry, 25*, 355–359.

Banki, C. M., Bissette, G., Arato, M., O'Connor, L., & Nemeroff, C. B. (1987). CSF corticotropin-releasing factor-like immunoreactivity in depression and schizophrenia. *American Journal of Psychiatry, 144*, 873–877.

Bauer M., Priebe, S., Graf, K. J., et al. (1994). Psychological and endocrine abnormalities in refugees from East Germany: Part II. Serum levels of cortisol, prolactin, luteinizing hormone, follicle stimulating hormone and testosterone. *Psychiatry Research, 51*(1), 75–85.

Bidzinska, E. J. (1984). Stress factors in affective diseases. *British Journal of Psychiatry, 144*, 161–166.

Bourne, P. B., Rose, R. M., & Mason, J. W. (1967). Urinary 17-OHCA levels. Data on seven helicopter ambulance medics in combat. *Archives of General Psychiatry, 17*, 104–110.

Bourne, P. B., Rose, R. M., & Mason, J. W. (1968). 17-OHCS levels in combat: Special forces "A" team under threat of attack. *Archives of General Psychiatry, 19*, 135–140.

Boscarino, J. A. (1996). Posttraumatic stress disorder, exposure to combat, and lower plasma cortisol among Vietnam veterans: Findings and clinical implications. *Journal of Consulting and Clinical Psychology, 64*(1), 191–201.

Bremner, J. D., Southwick, S. M., Johnson, D. R., Yehuda, R., & Charney, D. S. (1993). Childhood physical abuse and combat-related posttraumatic stress disorder. *American Journal of Psychiatry, 150*, 234–239.

Bremner, J., Licinio, J., Darnell, A., Krystal, J. H., Owens, M. J., Southwick, S. M., Nemeroff, C. B., & Charney, D. S. (1997). Elevated CSF corticotropin-releasing factor concentrations in posttraumatic stress disorder. *American Journal of Psychiatry, 154*(5), 624–629.

Breslau, N., Davis, G. C., Andreski, P., & Peterson E. (1991). Traumatic events and posttraumatic stress disorder in an urban population of young adults. *Archives of General Psychiatry, 48*, 216–222.

Caroll, B. J., Feinberg, M., Greden, J. F., Tarika, J., Albala, A. A., Haskett, R. F., James, N. M., Kronfolz, S., Lohr, N., Steiner, M., deVigne, J. P., & Young, E. (1981). A specific laboratory test for the diagnosis of melancholia. *Archives of General Psychiatry, 38*, 15–22.

Chappell, P. B., Smithe, M. A., Kilts, C. D., Bissette, G., Ritchie, J., Anderson, C., & Nemeroff, C. B. (1986). Alterations in corticotropin-releasing factor-like immunoreactivity in discrete rat brain regions after acute and chronic stress. *Journal of Neuroscience, 6*, 2908.

Chrousos, G. P., & Gold, P. W. (1992). The concepts of stress and stress system disorders. Overview of physical and behavioral homeostasis. *Journal of the American Medical Association, 267*, 1244–1252.

DeBellis, M., Chrousos, G. P., Dorn, L. D., Burke, L., Helmers, K., Kling, M. A., Trickett, P. K., & Putnam, F. W. (1994). Hypothalamic-pituitary-adrenal axis dysregulation in sexually abused girls. *Journal of Clinical Endocrinology and Metabolism, 78*, 249–255.

Dekaris, D., Sabioncello, A., Mazuran, R., et al. (1993). Multiple changes of immunologic parameters in prisoners of war. *Journal of the American Medical Association, 270*, 595–599.

DeKloet, R., Joels, M., Oitzl, M., & Sutanto, W. (1991). Implication of brain corticosteroid receptor diversity for the adaptation syndrome concept. *Methods Achieve Experimental Pathology, 14*, 104–132.

Dinan, T. G., Barry, S., Yatham, L. N., Moyabed, M., & Brown, I. (1990). A pilot study of a neuroendocrine test battery in posttraumatic stress disorder. *Biological Psychiatry, 28,* 665–672.

Fellman, D., Bugnon, C., & Gouger, A. (1982). An immunocytochemical demonstration of corticoliberin-like immunoreactivity (CLI) in neurons of the rat amygdala central nucleus (ACN). *Neuroscience Letters, 34,* 253.

Friedman, M. J., & Yehuda, R. (1995). PTSD and comorbidity: Psychobiological approaches to differential diagnosis. In M. J. Friedman, D. S. Charney, & A. Y. Deutch (Eds.), *Neurobiological and clinical consequences of stress: From normal adaptation to PTSD.* New York: Raven Press.

Ghaziuddin, M., Ghaziuddin, N., & Stein, G. S. (1990). Life events and the recurrence of depression. *Canadian Journal of Psychiatry, 35,* 239–242.

Goenjian, A. K., Yehuda, R., Pynoos, R. S., Steinberg, A. M., Tashjian, M., Yang, R. K., Najarian, L. M., & Fairbanks, L. A. (1996). Basal cortisol and dexamethasone suppression of cortisol among adolescents after the 1988 earthquake in Armenia. *American Journal of Psychiatry, 153*(7), 929–934.

Gormley, G. J., Lowy, M. T., Reder, A. T., Hospelhorn, V. D., Antel, J. P., & Meltzer, H. Y. (1985). Glucocorticoid receptors in depression: Relationship to the dexamethasone suppression test. *American Journal of Psychiatry, 142,* 1278–1284.

Green, B. (1993). Identifying survivors at risk: Trauma and stressors across events. In J. Wilson & B. Raphael (Eds.), *International handbook of traumatic stress syndromes.* New York: Plenum.

Halbreich, U., Olympia, J., Carson, S., Glogowski, J., Yeh, C., Axelrod, S., & Desu, M.M. (1989). Hypothalamic-pituitary-adrenal activity in indigenously depressed post-traumatic stress disorder patients. *Psychoneuroendocrinology, 14,* 365–370.

Heim, C., Ehlert, U., Rexhausen, J., Hanker, J. P., & Hellhammer, D. H. (1997). Psychoendocrinological observations in women with chronic pelvic pain. In R. Yehuda & A. C. McFarlane (Eds.), *Psychobiology of posttraumatic stress disorder,* Vol. 821 (pp. 456–458). New York: New York Academy of Sciences.

Hellhammer, D. H., & Wade, S. (1993). Endocrine correlates of stress vulnerability. *Psychother-Psychosom, 60*(1), 8–17.

Jensen, C. F., Keller, T. W., Peskind, E. R., McFall, M. E., Veith, R. C., Martin, D., Wilkinson, C. W., & Raskind, M. (1997). Behavioral and plasma cortisol responses to sodium lactate infusion in posttraumatic stress disorder. In R. Yehuda & A. C. McFarlance (Eds.), *Psychobiology of posttraumatic stress disorder* (pp. 444–447). New York: New York Academy of Sciences.

Kellner, M., Baker, D. G., & Yehuda, R. (1997). Salivary cortisol in Operation Desert Storm returnees. *Biological Psychiatry, 42,* 849–850.

Kessler, R. C., Sonnega, A., Bromet, E., Hughes, M., & Nelson, C. B. (1995). Posttraumatic stress disorder in the national comorbidity survey. *Archives of General Psychiatry, 52,* 1048–1060.

Kosten, T. R., Mason, J. W., Giller, E. L., Harkness, L., & Ostroff, R. (1987). Sustained urinary norepinephrine and epinephrine levels in post-traumatic stress disorder. *Psychoneuroendocrinology, 12,* 13–20.

Kosten, T. R., Wahby, V., Giller, E., & Mason, J. (1990). The dexamethasone suppression test and thyrotropin-releasing hormone stimulation test in post-traumatic stress disorder. *Biological Psychiatry, 28,* 657.

Krishnan, R. R., Ritchie, J. C., Reed, D., et al. (1991). CRF stimulation test results before and after dexamethasone in depressed patients and normal controls. *Journal of Neuropsychiatry and Clinical Neuroscience.*

Kudler, H., Davidson, J., Meador, K., Lipper, S., & Ely, T. (1987). The DST and post-traumatic stress disorder. *American Journal of Psychiatry, 144,* 1068–1071.

Lazarus, R. S., Cohen, J. B., Folkman S., Kanner, A., & Schaefer, C. (1980). Psychological stress and adaptation: Some unresolved issues. In H. Selye (Ed.), *Selye's guide to stress research,* Vol. 1 (pp. 90–117). New York: Van Nostrand Reinhold.

Lemieux, A. M., & Coe, C. L. (1995). Abuse-related posttraumatic stress disorder: Evidence for chronic neuroendocrine activation in women. *Psychosomatic Medicine, 57,* 105–115.

Ling, M. H. M., Perry, P. J., & Tsuang, M. T. (1981). Side effects of corticosteroid therapy. *Archives of General Psychiatry, 38,* 471–477.

Lisansky, J., Peake, G. T., Strassman, R. J., Kualls, C., Meikle, A. W., Risch, S. C., Fava, G. A., Zownir-Brazis, M., Hochla, P., & Britton, D. (1989). Augmented pituitary corticotropin response to a threshold dosage of human corticotropin-releasing hormone in depressive pretreated with metyrapone. *Archives of General Psychiatry, 46,* 641–649.

Lowy, M. T., Gormley, G. J., & Reder, A. T. (1989). Immune function, glucocorticoid receptor regulation and depression. In *Depressive disorders and immunity* (pp. 105–134). Washington DC: American Psychiatric Press.

March, J. S. (1993). What constitutes a stressor: the "criterion A" issue. In J. R. T. Davidson & E. B. Foa (Eds.), *Posttraumatic stress disorder: DSM-IV and beyond.* Washington, DC: American Psychiatric Press.

Mason, J. W. (1968). A review of psychoendocrine research on the sympathetic-adrenal-medullary system. *Psychosomatic Medicine, 30,* 631–653.

Mason, J. W. (1975). A historical view of the stress field, part I. *Journal of Human Stress, 1,* 6–12.

Mason, J. W., Giller, E. L., Kosten, T. R., Ostroff, R. B., & Podd, L. (1986). Urinary-free cortisol levels in posttraumatic stress disorder patients. *Journal of Nervous and Mental Disorders, 174,* 145–159.

Mason, J. W., Giller, E. L., Kosten, T. R., & Yehuda R. (1990b). Psychoendocrine approaches to the diagnosis and pathogenesis of PTSD. In *Biological assessment and treatment of PTSD* (pp. 65–86). Washington, DC: American Psychiatric Press.

McEwen, B. S., DeKloet, E. R., & Rostene, W. H. (1986). Adrenal steroid receptors and actions in the nervous system. *Physiological Reviews, 66,* 1121–1188.

McFarlane, A. C. (1990). Vulnerability to posttraumatic stress disorder. In M. E. Wolf & A. D. Mosnaim (Eds.), *Posttraumatic stress disorder: Etiology, phenomenology and treatment.* Washington, DC: American Psychiatric Press.

Meikle, A. W., Jubiz, W., Hutchings, M. P., West, C. D., & Tyler, F. H. (1969). A simplified metyrapone test with determination of plasma 11-deoxycortisol. *Journal of Clinical Endocrinology, 29,* 985–987.

Merchanthaler, I. (1984). Corticotropin-releasing factor (CFR)-like immunoreactivity in the rat central nervous system. Extrahypothalamic distribution. *Peptides, 5,* 53.

Munck, A., Guyre, P. M., & Holbrook, N. J. (1984). Physiological functions of glucocorticoids in stress and their relation to pharmacological actions. *Endocrinology Reviews, 93,* 9779–9783.

Nemeroff, C. B., Widerlov, E., Bissette, G., Walleus, H., Karlsson, I., Eklund, K., Kilts, C. D., Loosen, P. T., & Vale, W. (1984). Elevated concentrations of CSF corticotropin-releasing factor-like immunoreactivity in depressed patients. *Science, 226,* 1342–1344.

Olivera, A. A., & Fero, D. (1990). Affective disorders, DST, and treatment in PTSD patients: Clinical observations. *Journal of Traumatic Stress, 3,* 407–414.

Pitman, R. K., & Orr, S. (1990). Twenty-four hour urinary cortisol and catecholamine excretion in combat-related posttraumatic stress disorder. *Biological Psychiatry, 27,* 245–247.

Pitman, R. K., Orr, S. P., Forgue, D. F., DeJong, J. B., & Clairborn, J. M. (1987). Psychophysiologic assessment of posttraumatic stress disorder imagery in Vietnam combat veterans. *Archives of General Psychiatry, 44,* 970–975.

Post, R. M., Rubinow, D. R., & Ballenger, J. C. (1986). Conditioning and sensitization in the longitudinal course of affective illness. *British Journal of Psychiatry, 149,* 191–201.

Rabkin, J. G., & Struening, E. L. (1976). Life events, stress and illness. *Science, 194,* 1013–1020.

Resnick, H. S., Yehuda, R., Pitman, R., et al. (1995). Effect of previous trauma on acute plasma cortisol level following rape. *American Journal of Psychiatry, 152,* 1675–1677.

Rivier, C. L., & Plotsky, P. M. (1986). Mediation by corticotropin releasing factor (CRF) of adenohypophysial hormone secretion. *Annual Review of Physiology, 48,* 475–494.

Sapolsky, R. M. (1996). Does stress damage the brain? *Science, 273,* 749–750.

Sapolsky, R. M., Krey, L. C., & McEwen, B. S. (1985). Prolonged glucocorticoid exposure reduces hippocampal neuron number. Implications for aging. *Journal of Neuroscience, 5,* 1221–1226.

Sawchenko, P. E., & Swanson, L. W. (1985). Localization, colocalization and plasticity of corticotropin-releasing factor immunoreactivity in rat brain. *Fed Proceedings, 44,* 221.

Schlecte, J. A., Ginsburg, B. H., & Sherman, B. M. L. (1982). Regulation of the glucocorticoid receptor in human lymphocytes. *Journal of Steroid Biochemistry, 16,* 69–74.

Selyle, H. (Ed.). (1980). *Selye's guide to stress research,* Vol. 1. New York: Van Nostrand Reinhold.

Selye, H. (1956). *The stress of life.* New York: McGraw-Hill.

Shalev, A. Y., & Yehuda R. (1998). Longitudinal development of posttraumatic disorders. In *Psychological trauma: Annual review of psychiatry,* Vol. 17, Section 5. Washington, DC: American Psychiatric Association Press.

Smith, M. A., Davidson, J., Ritchie, J. C., Kudler, H., Lipper, S., Chappell, P., & Nemeroff, C. B. (1989). The corticotropin releasing hormone test in patients with posttraumatic stress disorder. *Biological Psychiatry, 26,* 349–355.

Stein, M. B., Yehuda, R., Koverola, C., & Hanna, C. (1997). Enhanced dexamethasone suppression of plasma cortisol in adult women traumatized by childhood sexual abuse. *Biological Psychiatry, 42,* 680–686.

Svec, F. (1985). Minireview: Glucocorticoid receptor regulation. *Life Sciences, 35,* 2359–2366.

Swann, A. C., Secunda, S. K., Stokes, P. E., Croughan, J., Davis, J. M., Koslow, S. H., & Maas, J. W. (1990). Stress, depression, and mania: Relationship between perceived role of stressful events and clinical and biological characteristics. *Acta Psychiatrica Scandinavica, 81,* 389–397.

Swanson, L. W., Sawchenko, P. E., Rivier, J., & Vale, W. W. (1983). Organization of ovine corticotropin-releasing factor immunoreactive cells and fibers in the rat brain: An immunohistochemical study. *Neuroendocrinology, 36,* 165.

Tepperman, J. (1981). *Metabolic and endocrine physiology*, 4th ed. New York: Year Book Medical.

Tornello, S., Orti, E., DeNicola, A. F., Rainbow, T. C., & McEwen, B. S. (1982). Regulation of glucocorticoid receptor in brain corticosterone treatment of adrenalectomized rats. *Neuroendocrinology, 35*, 411–417.

Ur, E., Dinan, T. G., O'Keane, M., Clare, A., McLoughline, L., Reese, L., Turner, T., Grossman, M., & Besser, M. (1992). Effect of metyrapone on the pituitary adrenal axis in depression: Relation to dexamethasone suppressor status. *Neuroendocrinology, 56*, 533–538.

Veith, R. C., & Murburg, M. M. (1994). Assessment of sympathetic nervous system functioning in PTSD: A critique of methodology. In *Catecholamine function in post-traumatic stress disorder: Emerging concepts* (pp. 309–334). Washington, DC: American Psychiatric Press.

Vernikos Danellis, J., Goldenrath, W. L., & Dolas C. B. (1975). The physiological cost of flight stress and flight fatigue. *US Navy Medical Journal, 66*, 12–16.

Wolkowitz, O. M., Reus V. I., Weingartner, H., et al. (1990). Cognitive effects of corticosteroids. *American Journal of Psychiatry, 147*, 1297–1303.

Yehuda, R. (1998). Neuroendocrinology of trauma and PTSD. In *Psychological trauma: Annual review of psychiatry*, Vol. 17, Section 5 (pp. 97–125). Washington, DC: American Psychiatric Press.

Yehuda, R., & McFarlane, A. C. (1995). Conflict between current knowledge about posttraumatic stress disorder and its original conceptual basis. *American Journal of Psychiatry, 152*, 1705–1713.

Yehuda, R., & Nemeroff, C. B. (1994). Neuropeptide alterations in affective and anxiety disorders. In J. A. DenBoer & A. Sitsen (Eds.), *Handbook on depression and anxiety: A biological approach* (pp. 543–571). New York: Dekker.

Yehuda, R., Southwick, S. M., Nussbaum, G., Giller, E. L., & Mason, J. W. (1990). Low urinary cortisol excretion in PTSD. *Journal of Nervous and Mental Disorders, 178*, 366–369.

Yehuda, R., Giller, E. L., Southwick, S. M., Lowy, M. T., & Mason, J. W. (1991). Hypothalamic-pituitary-adrenal dysfunction in posttraumatic stress disorder. *Biological Psychiatry, 30*, 1031–1048.

Yehuda, R., Lowy, M. T., Southwick, S. M., Shaffer, S., & Giller, E. L. (1991). Increased lymphocyte glucocorticoid receptor number in posttraumatic stress disorder. *American Journal of Psychiatry, 149*, 499–504.

Yehuda, R., Southwick, S. M., Krystal, J. M., Charney, D. S., & Mason, J. W. (1993a). Enhanced suppression of cortisol following dexamethasone administration in combat veterans with posttraumatic stress disorder and major depressive disorder. *American Journal of Psychiatry, 150*, 83–86.

Yehuda, R., Boisoneau, D., Mason, J. W., & Giller, E. L. (1993b). Relationship between lymphocyte glucocorticoid receptor number and urinary-free cortisol excretion in mood, anxiety, and psychotic disorder. *Biological Psychiatry, 34*, 18–25.

Yehuda, R., Teicher, M. H., Levengood, R. A., Trestman, R. L., & Siever, L. J. (1994). Circadian regulation of basal cortisol levels in posttraumatic stress disorder. In *Corticosteroid receptors and function*. New York: Academy of Sciences.

Yehuda, R., Giller, E. L., Levengood, R. A., Southwick, S. M., & Siever, L. (1995). Hypothalamic-pituitary-adrenal alterations in PTSD: Expanding the stress-response spectrum. In M. J. Friedman, D. S. Charney, & A. Y. Deutch (Eds.), *Neurobiological and clinical consequences of stress: From normal adaptation to PTSD*. New York: Raven Press.

Yehuda, R., Kahana, B., Binder-Brynes, K., Southwick, S., Zemelman, S., Mason, J. W., & Giller, E. L. (1995). Low urinary cortisol excretion in Holocaust survivors with posttraumatic stress disorder. *American Journal of Psychiatry, 152*, 7–12.

Yehuda, R., Boisoneau, D., Lowy, M. T., & Giller, E. L. (1996a). Dose-response changes in plasma cortisol and lymphocyte glucocorticoid receptors following dexamethasone administration in combat veterans with and without posttraumatic stress disorder. *Archives of General Psychiatry, 52*, 583–593.

Yehuda, R., Levengood, R., Schmeidler, J., Wilson, S., Guo, L. S., & Gerber, D. (1996b). Increased pituitary activation following metyrapone administration in post-traumatic stress disorder. *Psychoneuroendocrinology, 21*, 1–16.

Yehuda, R., Teicher, M. H., Trestman, R. L., Levengood, R. A., & Siever, L. J. (1996c). Cortisol regulation in post-traumatic stress disorder and major depression: A chronobiological analysis. *Biological Psychiatry, 40*, 79–88.

Yehuda, R., McFarlane, A. C., & Shalev, A. Y. (1998). Predicting the development of posttraumatic stress disorder from the acute response to a traumatic event. *Biological Psychiatry, 44*, 1305–1313.

Young, E. A., Haskett, R. F., Grunhaus, L., Pande, A., Murphy-Weinberg, V., & Watson, S. J. (1994). Increased evening activation of the hypothalamic-pituitary-adrenal axis in depressed patients. *Archives of General Psychiatry, 51*, 701–707.

20

Brain Imaging Studies of PTSD

ISRAEL LIBERZON AND STEPHAN F. TAYLOR

The last decade has witnessed a major transformation in the concepts of mental function and behavior. Dualistic models, such as mental versus physical or psychological versus biological, are giving way to more integrative views of the functional organism, where function and structure are interrelated and affect each other. New concepts of neuroplasticity and improved tools of visualization have both provided a conceptual frame and demonstrated this structure–function interaction. These developments also offer a new conceptualization of psychiatric disorders, which were traditionally seen as psychological or functional in nature. In traditional dualistic terms, post-traumatic stress disorder has been considered a preeminently functional disorder. However, in 1987 Lawrence Kolb (1987) proposed a neuropsychological hypothesis for PTSD, suggesting that neuroanatomical changes as a result of stress and stress-related neuro-endocrine changes might underlie symptoms of PTSD. Since then, multiple lines of evidence have demonstrated stress-related neurobiological changes and neuroanatomical sequelae of traumatic exposure. Accordingly, an increasing number of investigators are actively pursuing possible structural or functional neuroanatomical abnormalities that are associated with PTSD or that underlie PTSD symptomatology.

Structural Neuroimaging in PTSD

With the advent of magnetic resonance imaging (MRI), neuroscientists have been able to examine the neuroanatomy of small CNS structures, previously inaccessible with computerized tomography (CT). In particular, MRI reveals structural details of medial temporal lobe areas relevant to PTSD, anxiety, and other psychiatric disorders, including the hippocampal formation, the parahippocampal gyrus, and amygdaloid nuclei.

Bremner and colleagues (1995) first reported neuroanatomical abnormalities by MRI in a sample of 26 PTSD patients. They found that the right hippocampus of PTSD patients was approximately 8% smaller than that of a matched control group. This was a unilateral finding with no significant difference in hippocampus size on the left. There was also an association between deficits in short-term memory and smaller hippocampal

ISRAEL LIBERZON AND STEPHAN F. TAYLOR • Department of Psychiatry, University of Michigan, Ann Arbor VAMC, Ann Arbor, Michigan 48105.

International Handbook of Human Response to Trauma, edited by Shalev, Yehuda, and McFarlane. Kluwer Academic / Plenum Publishers, New York, 2000.

size in PTSD patients. In a follow-up study of a new cohort of 17 PTSD patients with histories of childhood sexual abuse, this group replicated their finding of reduced hippocampal size, except that the significant finding occurred in the left and not right hippocampus (Bremner et al. 1997b). Gurvitz and colleagues (1996) reported on a small sample of 7 PTSD subjects, in which hippocampal size was reduced on both the right and left compared to two control groups. Overall, their effect size was larger than the study by Bremner and co-workers, and the PTSD group's hippocampal size was as much as 30% smaller than that of the controls. The patients in these studies had significant alcohol histories, although they were matched to their control group on life-long alcohol consumption. Gurvitz and co-workers found good correlation between combat exposure and hippocampal volume loss, leading them to propose that combat exposure plays an etiologic role in the loss of hippocampal tissue. In all three studies, there were no other regional differences in the temporal lobes, amygdalae or other limbic regions.

The reduced volume of the medial temporal lobe in PTSD patients suggests a potentially important link between environmental stress and structural changes underlying PTSD. In the last decade, Sapolsky (Sapolsky, 1996; Sapolsky et al., 1984, 1990) and others have shown in animal studies that high cortisol levels can be neurotoxic and cause specific damage to hippocampal neurons. Support for this idea in humans comes from work by Starkman and colleagues, who found smaller hippocampal volumes in patients with Cushing's disorder, whose very high plasma cortisol levels result from abnormal cortisol secretion (Starkman et al., 1992). Arguing from this data, Bremner and colleagues have suggested that the smaller hippocampal volume in PTSD could result from excessive cortisol secretion and subsequent neurotoxicity. Although this interpretation has intuitive appeal, it does fail to integrate Yehuda et al.'s data suggesting that PTSD patients have low 24-hour cortisol secretion (Yehuda et al., 1990, 1995). Another possibility is that the hippocampal abnormalities in PTSD are unrelated to cortisol secretion and actually predate the development of a clinical syndrome. If this is true, then they might reflect a preexisting neurobiological abnormality that predisposes individuals to develop PTSD. Thus, although fascinating, the MRI work is preliminary, and many more questions, such as the question of asymmetrical volume loss, longitudinal course, effect of treatment, etc., remain to be answered by subsequent studies.

High-resolution structural neuroimaging will continue to contribute valuable neuroanatomical data in future studies. In addition to the questions outlined, prospective longitudinal studies can address questions of structural changes in time and treatment effects. For example, does hippocampal size increase as symptoms abate? New techniques like magnetic resonance spectroscopy (MRS) might be used to assess cellular integrity, and new warping analytic techniques will explore the relative spatial relationships of different CNS structures. These will make a valuable contribution to the understanding of PTSD and stress responses in general.

Functional Neuroimaging

Overview of Functional Neuroimaging

In contrast to structural neuroimaging, functional neuroimaging depicts the brain as it carries out a particular activity, such as neuronal metabolism, blood flow, or neurotransmission. Compared to structural images, images of brain function sacrifice resolution, but they provide considerably greater information about the way neurons carry out their jobs. Current technologies include positron emission tomography (PET) and single photon emission computed tomography (SPECT), both of which use radionuclide-labeled, tracer molecules. Functional magnetic resonance imaging (fMRI), which typically uses the paramagnetic properties of deoxyhemoglobin to mark blood flow changes, is a newer application of standard magnetic resonance scanners. PET, which uses short-lived, positron-emitting radionuclides of carbon, oxygen, and fluorine, and SPECT, which uses slightly longer lived, gamma-emitting radionuclides, are the principal techniques for mapping radioligand binding in specific cortical structures, e.g., dopamine receptor binding in the striatum. However, investigators have only recently begun to apply these technically challenging neurochemical approaches to PTSD, and we will not discuss them further.

The most common application of PET or SPECT in a modern nuclear medicine facility is in measuring either cerebral blood flow or cerebral metabolism. Neurons require glucose for metabolism, and by measuring the uptake of deoxyglucose, PET scans can generate a quantitative map of metabolism throughout the brain. This has diagnostic utility in several diseases of the central nervous system. For instance, in Alzheimer's disease, a distinctive pattern of reduced metabolism in the temporoparietal regions of the brain often shows up before significant structural changes appear on MRI scans (Jagust, 1994). Cerebral blood flow also varies with neuronal activity, closely matching the pattern of metabolism. It can be measured either by SPECT, using compounds usually labeled with technetium-99m, or by PET, usually using water labeled with oxygen-15 (^{15}O). Although PET provides greater flexibility, including better quantitation and better spatial resolution, these studies require considerably more resources, such as an on-site cyclotron.

Activation Studies

Neuroimaging studies of metabolism and blood flow are sensitive to change, and in the past decade, investigators have exploited this sensitivity in *activation paradigms*. For example, an [^{15}O]water PET scan measuring regional CBF is done while a subject performs a particular task that recruits or "activates" brain regions that carry out this task. Tasks, usually two or more, are designed to elicit particular functions, and a comparison between the images obtained during each condition provides a map of the anatomical structures that subserve a particular function. Such a scan can be repeated up to 12–15 times during the session because of the short half-life of the radiotracer. Providing a relatively noninvasive means of doing functional neuroanatomy *in vivo*, this approach has generated significant excitement in recent years. Once principally the domain of PET, activation paradigms are more often performed with the newer technique of fMRI. Unlike PET, fMRI does not expose subjects to ionizing radiation, permitting more data collection in individual subjects and superior anatomical resolution. In general, the activation approach provides a natural marriage between neuroimaging and symptom provocation paradigms in PTSD, as well as a methodology for studying the functional neuroanatomy of the normal emotional processing that becomes pathological in PTSD.

Functional Neuroimaging of Emotions

Recent work has begun to identify brain regions involved in regulating emotions. Animal experiments and neuropsychological studies in humans have pointed to so-called "limbic" regions, such as the anterior cingulate cortex and amygdaloid complex, as well as the nearby inferior orbital and ventromedial cortex, that have roles in regulating emotion. Direct stimulation of the amygdala in animals elicits dramatic behavioral responses, including fear, rage, and aggression (Kling & Brothers, 1992), and electrophysiological experiments show that it performs a mediating role in the fear-conditioning response (Davis, 1992). In humans viewing pictures of aversive visual stimuli, such as facial mutilation, cerebral perfusion increases in the amygdala, particularly on the left side (Breiter et al., 1996; Irwin et al., 1996; Taylor et al., 1998), but other investigators have not found this effect (Kosslyn et al., 1996). Interestingly, this may reflect desensitization (or falling off in the blood flow signal) in this region with repeated presentation of the aversive stimuli, observed by the groups that have found activation in the amygdala (Breiter et al., 1996; Taylor et al., 1998).

Emotional processing is frequently described as "coloring" specific perceptions, which captures the idea that emotions can enhance the salience of an object but are not required to perceive the object. The amygdala appears to play this "coloring" role. McGaugh and co-workers have demonstrated in animals how the amygdaloid complex can modulate memory for aversively motivated learning, but it is not indispensable for this learning (McGaugh et al., 1996). Cahill et al. found that recall for films with emotional content correlates with blood flow in the right amygdala (1996). Thus, the functional neuroimaging data show that the amygdala responds to salient stimuli, perhaps to increase the strength of memory. Of course, this data supports the idea that dysfunction in the amygdala might be involved in the symptoms of PTSD.

Emotions include both the way salient stimuli are processed and the type of response elicited by stimuli, and a particular set of brain regions appears to code emotional behaviors or responses. The recall of a sad experience can cause a change in brain blood flow relative to the recollection of an emotionally neutral experience, causing activation in the inferior orbital cortex (Pardo et al., 1993) or the medial frontal and anterior cingulate cortex (George et al., 1995). The role of these cortical regions is less well understood than that of the amygdala, which may reflect the fact they appear to mediate emotional dimensions of complex social behavior, for which animal models are not readily available. Lesions to these brain regions cause notable difficulties in impulse control and a loss of the ability to ascertain the appropriate social context for behavior (Damasio et al., 1990; Reitman, 1946; Stuss & Benson, 1986). Although findings to date are very preliminary, one readily appreciates that the "limbic brain," which really denotes the "emotional" brain, implicates a significant proportion of the neocortex.

Functional Neuroimaging in Other Anxiety Disorders

Symptom provocation studies during blood flow activation have been employed in the study of anxiety disorders to illustrate the role of these limbic brain regions. For example, a patient with obsessive compulsive disorder with fears of contamination is exposed to stimuli that elicit compulsive behavior, such as a glove dropped in the toilet. CBF changes by PET and by fMRI show activation in the orbitofrontal cortex, anterior cingulate, basal ganglia, thalamus, and lateral frontal cortex (Baxter et al., 1987; Breiter et al., 1996; Rauch et al., 1994). Patients with simple phobias to small animals, such as spiders, show blood flow increases in similar regions, including the anterior cingulate, left orbitofrontal cortex, left thalamus and right temporal pole (Rauch et al. 1995).

Although these preliminary studies suffer from some shortcomings, such as possible confounding by order effects (because the provocative stimuli could not be given at the beginning of the scanning session), they do provide support for an emerging functional neuroanatomy of anxiety disorders.

Functional Neuroimaging in PTSD

We will discuss how PET and SPECT have been applied to PTSD in studying cerebral metabolism and blood flow, where research findings are uncovering some clues to the pathophysiology of PTSD. Although metabolism and blood flow, closely coupled in normal physiological states, are often considered roughly similar indexes of brain activity, it is important to keep in mind that these parameters are indirect measurements and subject to multiple confounds. For instance, the mechanisms whereby local changes in blood flow track local changes in neuronal activity are imperfectly understood. Some evidence shows that oxygen extraction tends to fall when glucose metabolism and blood flow increase. Effects of medications on these measurements are also poorly understood, so that findings that involve pharmacological manipulation need to be considered with caution. In spite of these caveats, the techniques of functional neuroimaging provide tremendous opportunity in the study of PTSD—in the provocation of symptoms and in the response of local metabolism to medication and pharmacological challenge. We will begin by reviewing the work looking for potential differences in nonspecific brain activity between PTSD and comparison groups and then move on to the studies that examine how PTSD patients exhibit differential responses to environmental and pharmacological challenges.

Baseline Activity in PTSD

One of the major unanswered questions in PTSD is whether various reported physiological abnormalities are present only during response to specific, trauma-related triggers or also during "nonspecific" or "baseline" conditions. One obvious place to start with functional neuroimaging studies of PTSD is by searching for an abnormal pattern of activity during a baseline state. Semple and colleagues examined the regional cerebral blood flow (rCBF) of eight PTSD patients and nine controls with ^{15}O water PET scans. Subjects performed an auditory continuous performance test (CPT) that consisted of listening to auditory tones and discriminating them with the press of a button. The baseline (or "rest") state presents a challenge for scans sensitive to brain activity because the brain is never truly "at rest." The CPT, as a nonspecific task for PTSD patients not related to traumatic stimuli, served to stabilize the brain state and establish a relatively unchanging baseline.

Overall, PTSD patients performed more poorly on CPT than the control subjects, in large part due to a more liberal response threshold (more false positives). The authors found lower blood flow (8–11%) in the right angular gyrus of PTSD patients. There were no differences between the PTSD and the control groups in other regions examined or in whole brain blood flow. Several factors make the interpretation of these findings quite difficult. First, the CPT showed no effects on rCBF, suggesting that all experimental conditions might have similar effects on rCBF and that the differences found stem from baseline variability. Similarly, the absence of any diagnosis by region by task interactions suggests that there was no response specific to PTSD. In addition, all PTSD subjects had an active substance abuse problem (alcohol, marijuana and cocaine) whereas control subjects did not. Therefore, the reported finding could reflect the effects of recent substance use, the effects of substance dependence, or the direct vascular effect of the substance on rCBF (especially in six cocaine users). Future studies corroborating these results will be critical to ascertain baseline rCBF in PTSD.

Symptom Provocation in PTSD

It is, perhaps, surprising that marrying symptom provocation studies in PTSD to the activation paradigms of functional neuroimaging has not occurred until recently. Investigators have reliably demonstrated specific psychophysiological changes in PTSD patients by exposing them to cues that derive from the traumatic experience. Both "generic" reminders of traumatic experience, such as battle footage from movies and imagery induced by personalized "scripts" of the traumatic event, elicit a specific set of physiological responses in PTSD patients, such as exaggerated skin conductance and heart rate responses or enhanced plasma catecholamine secretion. However, better understanding of the underlying neuroanatomical circuitry of normal emotions was first needed to identify potential neuroanatomical correlates of the abnormal responses of PTSD patients. With recent progress in the functional neuroanatomy of emotions, the exploration of rCBF changes associated with the specific psychophysiological responses in PTSD patients has begun.

The first study to combine these approaches was performed by Rauch and colleagues in 1996. They used PET to examined eight PTSD subjects with the ^{15}O water method (Rauch et al., 1996). They contrasted cerebral blood flow during three different conditions: (1) while imagining the traumatic experience, (2) while imagining a neutral experience, and (3) while clenching teeth together. There was significant variability in gender, age, and type of trauma that required the use of individualized trauma scripts (Pitman, 1987; Pitman et al., 1990) to structure the imagery process. Conditions that provoke anxiety and lead to jaw contraction show increased blood flow in the region of the temporalis muscle, which can appear to come from the adjacent temporal pole. By having subjects clench their teeth and measuring CBF, the experimenters could identify where extracerebral activity occurred during this condition.

A number of limbic and paralimbic regions were activated by traumatic imagery in this study. Four regions had activation peaks during traumatic imagery compared to both neutral imagery and teeth clenching conditions: the medial (posterior) orbitofrontal cortex, the insular cortex, the anterior temporal pole, and the medial temporal cortex—all on the right. One area, the secondary visual cortex, showed activation in the traumatic minus neutral subtraction but not in the traumatic minus teeth clenching subtraction. Two other areas, the amygdala and the anterior cingulate cortex, showed peaks in the traumatic minus teeth clenching subtraction but not in the traumatic minus neutral condition. The left inferior frontal cortex (Broca's area) showed deactivation (decrease in the rCBF) in traumatic minus neutral conditions.

These findings were interpreted as evidence of right-sided limbic and paralimbic activation associated with PTSD symptom production. Right-side activation is compelling because these regions are implicated in mediating negative emotions. However, in the absence of control subjects, it is difficult to assess whether this activation pattern is a "physiological" response to negatively valenced imagery or phenomena specific to PTSD. Although activations in the amygdala and anterior cingulate cortex are intriguing, given links of amygdala to negative emotions (LeDoux, 1986) and of anterior cingulate to memory processes (Devinsky et al., 1995), the absence of significant activation in the negative minus neutral subtraction precludes one from deriving definitive conclusions from these data.

Shin and colleagues (1997) also conducted a PET activation study in more homogeneous groups of combat veterans and combat controls (seven subjects each). Psychological challenge was induced using combat-related, neutral, and emotionally negative (but combat-unrelated) pictures, with verbal descriptions. Subjects underwent separate conditions in which they viewed the image and in which they imagined the image without the picture before their eyes. Thus, the authors aimed to distinguish separate CBF patterns for trauma-specific images from the flow patterns for negative images, as well as a network for visual perception from a network for visual imagery.

Out of six limbic regions predicted from previous studies, the authors demonstrated activation in two, the anterior cingulate and the right amygdala. Activation in the anterior cingulate was present in PTSD patients during combat imagery compared with perception of combat images. Because a relative decrease, sometimes called "deactivation," occurred in the same region while viewing combat images relative to neutral images, the authors suggested that this activation was associated with the cognitive process of imagery, rather than an emotional response. Activation in the right amygdaloid regions in PTSD patients was found in the comparison of combat imagery to the combat perception condition. Although the amygdala was among the predicted results, interpretation was not straightforward because a relative deactivation also occurred for normal controls when the combat perception condition was compared to the negative perception condition.

In summary, the studies described suggest involvement of several limbic and paralimbic structures in PTSD. Orbitofrontal cortex, insular cortex, medial temporal lobe, and temporal pole findings are interesting but represent findings clearly in need of replication. Activity in the amygdala and anterior cingulate regions support roles for these structures in the disorder, but inconsistent results across various provocation conditions preclude one from suggesting specific roles for these regions.

To address some of these questions and to identify rCBF patterns that are specific to PTSD patients, we have studied PTSD patients, normal controls, and combat controls in our laboratory, using SPECT imaging to measure rCBF. To identify specific brain regions associated with PTSD, rCBF was measured during the time interval indicated by psychophysiological studies to show the greatest discrimination between PTSD and control groups—the imagery period immediately following exposure to traumatic stimuli (Pitman 1987). We recruited 14 Vietnam veterans with post-traumatic stress disorder, 11 Vietnam veterans without PTSD, but with combat exposure, and 14 age- and sex-matched nonveteran controls. Subjects were diagnosed according to DSM-III-R criteria, using the SCID (Structured Clinical Interview for Diagnosis (Spitzer et al., 1990)) for PTSD patients and SCID-NP for control groups. All subjects were medication-free, and those with histories of substance abuse had to have been in remission for at least six months.

The study consisted of two sessions on separate days, 48 hours apart, in randomized order. During one session, subjects were exposed to nonspecific arousing stimuli (white noise) and during another to trauma-related stimuli (combat sounds). Traumatic stimuli consisted of a three-minute audio tape of combat sounds (e.g., helicopter sounds, explosions, small arms fire) at gradually increasing volume (up to 75 dB). The control condition consisted of nonspecific stimuli in the form of white noise, with the same frequency spectrum at the identical ramped intensity. Subjects were instructed to imagine whatever came to their mind, with their eyes closed for approximately five minutes immediately following the termination of the auditory stimuli. To minimize differences in brain activity due to the characteristics of the different sounds, CBF was measured at the beginning of the imagining phase after the sounds finished.

Activation within the left amygdaloid region of the PTSD patients confirmed our hypothesis (see Figure 1). We found no activation foci in this region in control subjects, and there was no activation in the right amygdala of any group. This activation appeared to be specific to subjects with PTSD, consistent with an exaggerated emotional response to trauma-related stimuli. Whether this amygdaloid region activation merely reflected an exaggerated emotional response of PTSD patients or whether it generated the abnormal emotional response will have to be addressed in future studies.

All three groups did show a common site of activation in the rostral anterior cingulate cortex/medial prefrontal cortex. This site was very near a focus of activity reported in association with anxiety symptoms after yohimbine infusion in both healthy controls and in panic disorder patients (Woods et al., 1988). If activation of the medial prefrontal cortex is associated with PTSD/anxiety symptom generation, these findings might also implicate noradrenergic mechanisms in PTSD symptomatology. This area of the brain is also associated with emotional regulation, including the recall of emotional experiences (Lane et al., 1997; Reiman et al., 1997) and processing of emotional responses (George et al., 1995). Therefore, it appears that this medial frontal cortex activation may be associated with the processing of meaningful stimuli in general, regardless of its content (whether positive or negative). Because the medial prefrontal cortex appears to be activated in PTSD and is selectively modulated by noradrenergic transmission, it is possible that activation of this region is specifically associated with the arousal component of emotional response.

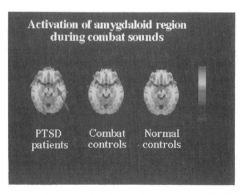

FIGURE 1. Activation peaks (combat sounds minus white noise) in PTSD patients and controls are superimposed on a reference MRI image in stereotactic space and in radiological orientation (left/right reversed). Color bar indicates T scores magnitude.

Symptom Correlation

In addition to examining rCBF activity at the baseline or during a particular psychological or pharmacological challenge, imaging techniques can be used in correlation with the appearance of a specific symptom. Finding a specific pattern of cerebral blood flow associated with a particular symptom identifies potential areas of the brain that originate specific symptoms. Because very few psychiatric symptoms are disorder-specific, this type of finding provides information that might be relevant to a number of different clinical conditions. Among the most intriguing and poorly understood psychiatric symptoms are the dissociative states. These symptoms appear frequently in PTSD (Amdur & Liberzon, 1997; Bremner et al., 1992), and the intrusive, sudden sense of reliving the traumatic experience, commonly known as a "flashback," has been accepted as one of the characteristic diagnostic criteria of PTSD.

While performing a traumatic challenge study in PTSD patients, we induced an actual flashback in one of the patients during CBF measurement. Behaviorally, the patient was visibly distressed, tearful, diaphoretic, and agitated. In debriefing, he stated "I had a flashback; I forgot were I was; I saw the black pajamas right in front of me, I was back in Vietnam." No other subject in the comparison group experienced an actual flashback during the study. Analysis of this patient's rCBF patterns showed an altered pattern of rCBF that was dramatically different from all other subjects, including patients and control subjects (see Figure 2). Greater uptake in subcortical regions, particularly the thalamus, was evident compared with cortical regions. In contrast, the pattern of relative rCBF during the control scan in the same patient looked normal.

To our knowledge, this represents the first time that rCBF has been visualized during a PTSD flashback (Liberzon et al., 1997). Although generalization from a single case requires caution, the unusual pattern of blood flow in this case is noteworthy because clinical conditions, such as flashbacks, are very difficult to study experimentally. The state of agitation, accompanied by hyperventilation, would have reduced the concentration of carbon dioxide in the subject's circulation, inducing a decrease in cerebral circulation. However, when this occurs, the CBF in all regions of the brain decreases uniformly; one does not observe a change in the ratio of cortical to subcorti-

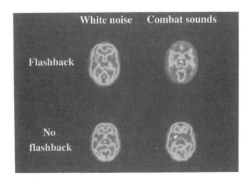

FIGURE 2. The images depict the relative perfusion pattern of a PTSD subject who experienced a flashback during the presentation of traumatic stimuli (battle sounds) and showed an altered perfusion pattern during the flashback, compared with the presentation of white noise. Transverse image planes from another PTSD subject who did not experience a flashback show the grossly normal perfusion pattern in this subject for both conditions.

cal(thalamic) flow which we observed. The altered cortical/thalamic rCBF pattern may have represented the shift of attention away from external stimuli and toward the internal stimuli of the flashback, consistent with a hypothesized role of the thalamus in regulating the conscious state and the generation of dissociative symptoms in PTSD (Krystal et al., 1995).

Clearly, additional data are needed to determine whether changes in cortico/thalamic activity actually cause flashback phenomena. The literature is still divided regarding the nature of a "flashback," and suggestions have been made that memory processes, panic attacks, perceptual distortions, fantasy, and dream-like states contribute to its development (Burstein, 1985; Frankel, 1994; Mellman & Davis, 1985).

Pharmacological Challenge

In addition to psychological challenge paradigms, pharmacological challenge procedures have also been used with PET imaging. Here, pharmacological agents are used to activate a specific neurotransmitter system or elicit a set of psychiatric symptoms that the investigator wants to study. As with psychological challenge procedures, rCBF or glucose update can be studied to assess the activity of specific brain regions following administration of a pharmacological probe. Yohimbine, a CNS alpha adrenergic agonist that increases central catecholamine secretion, elicits anxiety and trauma-related symptoms in PTSD patients (Morgan et al., 1995; Southwick et al., 1993, 1997). Bremner and colleagues (Bremner et al., 1997a) used PET FDG to assess the effects of yohimbine on the cerebral metabolism in a group of 10 PTSD patients and 10 normal controls. CNS catecholamine secretion can differentially affect brain metabolism, initially increasing it, and then causing a decrease in metabolism if large increases in catecholamine secretion occur. Based on the hypothesis that PTSD patients hypersecrete central catecholamines (Aston-Jones et al., 1991, 1994), Bremner predicted that administration of 0.4 mg/kg of yohimbine would result in a mild increase in catecholamines and an increase in brain metabolism in controls and a larger increase in catecholamines and subsequent decrease in brain metabolism in PTSD subjects.

Yohimbine administration produced more anxiety, panic, and flashbacks in PTSD subjects, and the authors also noted a differential effect of yohimbine on brain metabolism in three out of seven hypothesized regions (orbitofrontal cortex, temporal cortex, and postcentral gyrus) and one out of eleven in a nonhypothesized region (globus pallidus). These findings supported the *a priori* hypothesis of a hypersensitive response to catecholamine secretion in some regions in PTSD. However, there was no association between anxiety symptoms and changes in brain metabolism.

One of the major challenges in pharmacological studies is interpreting the results. A pharmacological probe is merely a tool to elicit a specific set of symptoms; however, agents might exert a direct effect on rCBF or brain metabolism, mechanistically unrelated to symptoms elicited by the drug. In addition, pharmacological probes are seldom symptom-specific, and they elicit a set of different symptoms, making a connection between a specific symptom and rCBF change problematic. On the other hand, the pharmacological specificity of these probes provides additional information regarding the possible neurochemical processes underlying the observed blood flow changes. Although many promises exist in combining selective pharmacological agents and neuroimaging technologies, many problems must be carefully dealt with to produce meaningful and interpretable results.

Comment

Today, the structural and functional neuroanatomy of human emotional responses and the response to trauma are clearly in their early stages of development. The exciting findings of the last decade delineate a set of neuroanatomical regions such as medial temporal lobe structures, the medial prefrontal and orbitofrontal cortex, the thalamus, and the anterior cingulate that are involved in human emotions. The careful study of these regions and their function should elucidate the functional neuroanatomy of normal emotional responses and the pathophysiology of various conditions where this response is altered. Our findings suggest that at least in the left amygdaloid region, disorder-specific findings might be present in PTSD. Future studies that examine the specificity and neurochemical substrates underlying these abnormalities—with fMRI, PET receptor imaging, and MRS—should prove very helpful in clarifying the patho-physiology of abnormal responses to stress and trauma.

References

Amdur, R., & Liberzon, I. (1996). Factor structure of the dissociative experiences survey in PTSD patients. *Dissociation, 9*, 118–124.

Aston-Jones, G., Chiang, C., & Alexinsky, T. (1991). Discharge of noradrenergic locus coeruleus neurons in behaving rats and monkeys suggests a role in vigilance. *Progress in Brain Research, 88*, 501–520.

Aston-Jones, G., Valentino, R. J., Van Bockstaele, E. J., & Meyerson, A. T. (1994). Locus coeruleus, stress, and PTSD: Neurobiological and clinical parallels. In M. M. Murburg (Ed.), *Catecholamine function in post-traumatic stress disorder: Emerging concepts* (pp. 17–62). Washington, DC: American Psychiatric Press.

Baxter L., Jr., Phelps, M. E., Mazziotta, J. C., Guze, B. H., Schwartz, J. M., & Selin, C. E. (1987). Local cerebral glucose metabolic rates in obsessive-compulsive disorder. A comparison with rates in unipolar depression and in normal controls. *Archives of General Psychiatry, 44*, 211–218.

Breiter, H. C., Etcoff, N. L., Whalen, P. J., Kennedy, W. A., Rauch, S. L., Buckner, R. L., Strauss, M. M., Hyman, S. E., & Rosen, B. R. (1996). Response and habituation of the human amygdala during visual processing of facial expression. *Neuron, 17*, 875–887.

Bremner, J. D., Innis, R. B., Ng, C. K., Staib, L. H., Salomon, R. M., Bronen, R. A., Duncan, J., Southwick, S. M., Krystal, J. H., Rich, D., Zubal, G., Dey, H., Soufer, R., & Charney, D. S. (1997a). Positron emission tomography measurement of cerebral metabolic correlates of yohimbine administration in combat-related posttraumatic stress disorder. *Archives of General Psychiatry, 54*, 246–254.

Bremner, J. D., Randall, P., Scott, T. M., Bronen, R. A., Seibyl, J. P., Southwick, S. M., Delaney, R. C., McCarthy, G., Charney, D. S., & Innis, R. B. (1995). MRI-based measurement of hippocampal volume in patients with combat-related posttraumatic stress disorder. *American Journal of Psychiatry, 152*, 973–981.

Bremner, J. D., Randall, P., Vermetten, E., Staib, L., Bronen, R. A., Mazure, C., Capelli, S., McCarthy, G., Innis, R. B., & Charney, D. S. (1997b). Magnetic resonance imaging-based measurement of hippocampal volume in posttraumatic stress disorder related to childhood physical and sexual abuse—a preliminary report. *Biological Psychiatry, 41*, 23–32.

Bremner, J. D., Southwick, S., Brett, E., Fontana, A., Rosenheck, R., & Charney, D. S. (1992). Dissociation and posttraumatic stress disorder in Vietnam combat veterans. *American Journal of Psychiatry, 149*, 328–232.

Burstein, A. (1985). Posttraumatic flashbacks, dream disturbances, and mental imagery. *Journal of Clinical Psychiatry, 46*, 374–378.

Cahill, L., Haier, R. J., Fallon, J., Alkire, M. T., Tang, C., Keator, D., Wu, J., & McGaugh, J. L. (1996). Amygdala activity at encoding correlated with long-term, free recall of emotional information. *Proceedings of the National Academy of Sciences USA, 93*, 8016–8021.

Damasio, A. R., Tranel, D., & Damasio, H. (1990). Individuals with sociopathic behavior caused by frontal damage fail to respond autonomically to social stimuli. *Behavioral Brain Research, 41*, 81–94.

Davis, M. (1992). The role of the amygdala in conditioned fear. In J. P. Aggleton (Ed.), *The amygdala: Neurobiological aspects of emotion, memory and mental dysfunction* (pp. 255–395). New York: Wiley-Liss.

Devinsky, O., Morrell, M. J., & Vogt, B. A. (1995). Contributions of anterior cingulate cortex to behaviour. *Brain, 118,* 279–306.

Frankel, F. H. (1994). The concept of flashbacks in historical perspective. *International Journal of Clinical and Experimental Hypnosis, 42,* 321–336.

George, M. S., Ketter, T. A., Parekh, P. I., Horwitz, B., Herscovitch, P., & Post, R. M. (1995). Brain activity during transient sadness and happiness in healthy women. *American Journal of Psychiatry, 152,* 341–351.

Gurvits, T. V., Shenton, M. E., Hokama, H., Ohta, H., Lasko, N. B., Gilbertson, M. W., Orr, S. P., Kikinis, R., Jolesz, F. A., McCarley, R. W., & Pitman, R. K. (1996). Magnetic resonance imaging study of hippocampal volume in chronic, combat-related posttraumatic stress disorder. *Biological Psychiatry, 40,* 1091–1099.

Irwin, W., Davidson, R. J., Lowe, M. J., Mock, B. J., Sorenson, J. A., & Turski, P. A. (1996) Human amygdala activation detected with echo-planar functional magnetic resonance imaging. *Neuroreport, 7,* 1765–1769.

Jagust, W. J. (1994). Functional imaging in dementia: An overview. *Journal of Clinical Psychiatry, 55*(Suppl.), 5–11.

Kling, A. S., & Brothers, L. (1992). The amygdala and social behavior. In J. P. Aggleton (Ed.), *The amygdala: Neurobiological aspects of emotion, memory and mental dysfunction* (pp. 353–377). New York: Wiley-Liss.

Kolb, L. C. (1987). A neuropsychological hypothesis explaining posttraumatic stress disorders. *American Journal of Psychiatry, 144,* 989–995.

Kosslyn, S. M., Shin, L. M., Thompson, W. L., McNally, R. J., Rauch, S. L., Pitman, R. K., & Alpert, N. M. (1996). Neural effects of visualizing and perceiving aversive stimuli: A PET investigation. *Neuroreport, 7,* 1569–1576.

Krystal, J. H., Bennett, A., Bremner, J. D., & Southwick, S. S. (1995). Toward a cognitive neuroscience of dissociation and altered memory functions in post-traumatic stress disorder. In M. J. Friedman, D. S. Charney, & Y. A. Deutsch (Eds.), *Neurobiological and clinical consequences of stress: From normal adaptation to PTSD* (pp. 239–269). New York: Raven Press.

Lane, R. D., Reiman, E. M., Ahern, G. L., Schwartz, G. E., & Davidson, R. J. (1997). Neuroanatomical correlates of happiness, sadness, and disgust. *American Journal of Psychiatry, 154,* 926–933.

LeDoux, J. E. (1986). The neurobiology of emotion. In J. E. LeDoux & W. Hirst (Eds.), *Mind and brain* (pp. 301–354). Cambridge: Cambridge University Press.

Liberzon, I., Taylor, S. F., Fig, M. F., & Koeppe, R. A. (1997). Alteration of thalamo cortical perfusion ratio during PTSD flashback. *Depression and Anxiety, 4,* 146–150.

McGaugh, J. L., Cahill, L., & Roozendaal, B. (1996). Involvement of the amygdala in memory storage: Interaction with other brain systems. *Proceedings of the National Academy of Sciences USA, 93,* 13508–13514.

Mellman, T. A., & Davis, G. C. (1985). Combat-related flashbacks in posttraumatic stress disorder: phenomenology and similarity to panic attacks. *Journal of Clinical Psychiatry, 46,* 379–382.

Morgan, C. A., Grillon, C., Southwick, S. M., Nagy, L. M., Davis, M., Krystal, J. H., & Charney, D. S. (1995). Yohimbine facilitated acoustic startle in combat veterans with post-traumatic stress disorder. *Psychopharmacology (Berlin), 117,* 466–471.

Pardo, J. V., Pardo, P. J., & Raichle, M. E. (1993). Neural correlates of self-induced dysphoria. *American Journal of Psychiatry, 150,* 713–719.

Pitman, R. K. (1987). Psychophysiologic assessment of posttraumatic stress disorder imagery in Vietnam combat veterans. *Archives of General Psychiatry, 44,* 970–975.

Pitman, R. K., Orr, S. P., Forgue, D. F., Altman, B., de Jong, J. B., & Herz, L. R. (1990). Psychophysiologic responses to combat imagery of Vietnam veterans with posttraumatic stress disorder versus other anxiety disorders. *Journal of Abnormal Psychology, 99,* 49–54.

Rauch, S. L., Jenike, M. A., Alpert, N. M., Baer, L., Breiter, H. C., Savage, C. R., & Fischman, A. J. (1994). Regional cerebral blood flow measured during symptom provocation in obsessive-compulsive disorder using oxygen 15-labeled carbon dioxide and positron emission tomography. *Archives of General Psychiatry, 51,* 62–70.

Rauch, S. L., Savage, C. R., Alpert, N. M., Miguel, E. C., Baer, L., Breiter, H. C., Fischman, A. J., Manzo, P. A., Moretti, C., & Jenike, M. A. (1995). A positron emission tomographic study of simple phobic symptom provocation. *Archives of General Psychiatry, 52,* 20–28.

Rauch, S. L., van der Kolk, B. A., Fisler, R. E., Alpert, N. M., Orr, S. P., Savage, C. R., Fischman, A. J., Jenike, M. A., & Pitman, R. K. (1996). A symptom provocation study of posttraumatic stress disorder using positron emission tomography and script-driven imagery. *Archives of General Psychiatry, 53,* 380–387.

Reiman, E. M., Lane, R. D., Ahern, G. L., Schwartz, G. E., Davidson, R. J., Friston, K. J., Yun, L. S., & Chen, K. (1997). Neuroanatomical correlates of externally and internally generated human emotion. *American Journal of Psychiatry, 154,* 918–925.

Reitman, F. (1946). Orbital cortex syndrome following leucotomy. *American Journal of Psychiatry, 103,* 238–241.

Sapolsky, R. M. (1996). Why stress is bad for your brain [see comments]. *Science, 273*, 749–750.

Sapolsky, R. M., Armanini, M. P., Packan, D. R., Sutton, S. W., & Plotsky, P. M. (1990). Glucocorticoid feedback inhibition of adrenocorticotropic hormone secretagogue release. Relationship to corticosteroid receptor occupancy in various limbic sites. *Neuroendocrinology, 51*, 328–336.

Sapolsky, R. M., Krey, L. C., & McEwen, B. S. (1984). Glucocorticoid-sensitive hippocampal neurons are involved in terminating the adrenocortical stress response. *Proceedings of the National Academy of Sciences USA, 81*, 6174–6177.

Semple, W. E., Goyer, P. F., McCormick, R., Compton-Toth, B., Morris, E., Donovan, B., Muswick, G., Nelson, D., Garnett, M. L., Sharkoff, J., Leisure, G., Miraldi, F., & Schultz, S. C. (1996, May 31). Attention and regional cerebral blood flow in posttraumatic stress disorder patients with substance abuse histories. *Psychiatry Research, 67*(1), 17–28.

Shin, L. M., Kosslyn, S. M., McNally, R. J., Alpert, N. M., Thompson, W. L., Rauch, S. L., Macklin, M. L., & Pitman, R. K. (1997). Visual imagery and perception in posttraumatic stress disorder. A positron emission tomographic investigation. *Archives of General Psychiatry, 54*, 233–241.

Southwick, S. M., Krystal, J. H., Morgan, C. A., Johnson, D., Nagy, L. M., Nicolaou, A., Heninger, G. R., & Charney, D. S. (1993). Abnormal noradrenergic function in posttraumatic stress disorder [see comments]. *Archives of General Psychiatry, 50*, 266–274.

Southwick, S. M., Morgan, C. A., Bremner, A. D., Grillon, C. G., Krystal, J. H., Nagy, L. M., & Charney, D. S. (1997). Noradrenergic alterations in posttraumatic stress disorder. *Annals of the New York Academy of Sciences, 821*, 125–141.

Spitzer, R. L., Williams, J. B. W., Gibbon, M., & First, M. B. (1990). *Structured clinical interview for DSM-III-R, patient edition (SCID-P)*. Washington, DC: American Psychiatric Association.

Starkman, M. N., Gebarski, S. S., Berent, S., & Schteingart, D. E. (1992). Hippocampal formation volume, memory dysfunction, and cortisol levels in patients with Cushing's syndrome. *Biological Psychiatry, 32*, 756–765.

Stuss, D. T., & Benson, D. F. (1986). *The frontal lobes*. New York: Raven Press.

Taylor, S. F., Liberzon, I., Fig, L. M., Minoshima, S., & Koeppe, R. A. (1998). The effect of emotional content on visual recognition memory: A PET activation study. *NeuroImage, 8*, 188–197.

Woods, S. W., Koster, K., Krystal, J. K., Smith, E. O., Zubal, I. G., Hoffer, P. B., & Charney, D. S. (1988). Yohimbine alters regional cerebral blood flow in panic disorder. *Lancet, 2*, 678.

Yehuda, R., Kahana, B., Binder-Brynes, K., Southwick, S. M., Mason, J. W., & Giller, E. L. (1995). Low urinary cortisol excretion in Holocaust survivors with posttraumatic stress disorder. *American Journal of Psychiatry, 152*, 982–986.

Yehuda, R., Southwick, S. M., Nussbaum, G., Wahby, V., Giller, E. L., Jr., & Mason, J. W. (1990). Low urinary cortisol excretion in patients with posttraumatic stress disorder. *Journal of Nervous and Mental Disease, 178*, 366–369.

21

Sleep and the Pathogenesis of PTSD

THOMAS ALAN MELLMAN

Most, if not all, clinicians in the field of traumatic stress would agree that sleep disturbances are among the most prominent and distressing complaints associated with post-traumatic stress disorder or PTSD. This recognition is formalized in the *Diagnostic and Statistic Manual of Mental Disorders IV* by the inclusion of nightmares and difficulty initiating and maintaining sleep as symptom criteria. Overall, a pathogenic role for sleep disturbance in PTSD is supported by the prominence of sleep-related symptoms, the association of traumatic incidents with sleep disruption, and the overlap of the effects of sleep deprivation and PTSD symptoms. Although the importance of sleep disturbance in PTSD may seem self evident, there has been uncertainty regarding the objective nature of sleep abnormalities in PTSD. Historically, the deficiency of data allowed for speculative hypotheses. Although uncertainty regarding the role of sleep in PTSD remains, the topic has been the subject of a number of recent investigations by an international group of investigators. Therefore, it seemed timely with the convening of the meeting that inspired this volume, the *Second World Conference of the International Society for Traumatic Stress Studies* that met in June 1996 in Israel, to address investigations of sleep and PTSD. Researchers who are actively investigating the topic were invited to participate. They included Ehud Klien of Israel who presented a longitudinal study of recent accident victims that included actigraphic and polysomnographic sleep assessments. Thomas Hurwitz of the United States presented sleep laboratory evaluations of Vietnam combat veterans. Wybrand Op den Weld and J. M. H. de Groen of the Netherlands presented sleep and circadian studies of aging World War II Resistance fighters. Peretz Lavie of Israel presented a study of awakening thresholds from rapid eye movement or REM sleep in PTSD subjects, and this author (Thomas Mellman of the United States) reviewed sleep studies of combat veterans and more acutely affected subjects who had PTSD related to a natural disaster. Richard Ross of the United States could not attend but was involved in conceiving and planning the symposium.

THOMAS ALAN MELLMAN   Dartmouth Hitchcock Medical Center, Department of Psychiatry, Lebanon, New Hampshire 03756-0001.

International Handbook of Human Response to Trauma, edited by Shalev, Yehuda, and McFarlane. Kluwer Academic / Plenum Publishers, New York, 2000.

Findings from international and otherwise diverse study populations were presented, and there were opportunities to examine commonalities, as well as discrepancies in the data and their possible reconciliation. With these discussions in mind, this chapter reviews research on sleep aspects of PTSD. Specific subtopics include the nature and prevalence of sleep complaints in PTSD, a review of studies that objectively assess sleep disturbances via polysomnographic methods, the status of REM sleep in PTSD, treatment implications, thoughts regarding divergent findings, and potential future directions for research.

Sleep Symptoms

A review of studies that was utilized for considering revisions of diagnostic criteria for PTSD in the DMS-IV indicates that sleep disturbances are the most highly endorsed category of symptoms across a range of traumatized populations who have PTSD (Green, 1993). The 4th edition of the *Diagnostic and Statistics Manual of Mental Disorders* (DSM-IV) includes nightmares that replicate traumatic events and impairment in initiating and maintaining sleep among PTSD symptom criteria.

The more specific nature of sleep complaints in PTSD has been addressed by several studies using survey methodologies. We found that, among Vietnam combat veterans with and without PTSD, disturbing dreams about topics other than combat were common in both groups. The findings, however, supported previous observations that dreams referring to military combat were specifically associated with having PTSD (Mellman, et al., 1995a). In a study of subjects exposed to Hurricane Andrew, we found that endorsement of dreams referring to the disaster was relatively infrequent approximately 6 to 8 months after the hurricane struck. All of the subjects who endorsed nightmares about the hurricane had PTSD (David & Mellman, 1997). Our study, another that surveyed combat veterans (Inman et al., 1990), and a survey of survivors of the Nazi Holocaust (Rosen et al., 1990) are consistent in reporting body movement during sleep and awakenings with increased psychophysiological arousal as frequently endorsed symptoms.

In summary, complaints of general sleep disturbances such as insomnia are quite common in PTSD. However, it appears that they are more sensitive than specific to having the disorder. Replicative nightmares are characteristic of the more severe end of PTSD and are relatively specific to PTSD. Sleep complaints associated with PTSD also include body movement during sleep and nondream awakenings with somatic anxiety.

Polysomnographic Studies Evaluating Sleep Disturbance

Polysomnography (PSG) is a laboratory procedure for evaluating sleep that features the recording of electroencephalographic and other physiological data through the sleep period. PSG provides objective indexes of the initiation, duration, and maintenance of sleep, as well as the distribution and timing of sleep stages and the presence of sleep-related pathology. Most PSG studies of PTSD subjects have used small to moderately sized samples of chronically affected combat veterans from the United States or Israel. Many of the published results at least partially support the occurrence of disrupted sleep in terms of reduced sleep time or efficiency or increased awakenings or arousals in the PTSD patients (Dow et al., 1996; Glaubman et al., 1990; Hefez et al., 1987; Mellman et al., 1995a). Findings from our laboratory (Mellman et al., 1995), as well as those of Brown & Boudewyns (1996), have also corroborated the subjective complaints in terms of documenting frequent limb or gross body movements during sleep.

In one of the studies with American veterans (Ross et al., 1994a), as well as in a study of Israeli veterans (Dagan et al., 1991), these measures of sleep maintenance did not differ between PTSD patients and controls. Similarly, new findings presented by Hurwitz at the conference were striking for the absence of objective sleep abnormalities in a group of combat veterans with PTSD who had sleep complaints. In the aforementioned study by Dagan et al. (1991) conducted in Lavie's laboratory, the PTSD patients were additionally found to have an increased threshold of arousal by white noise from slowwave sleep. Replication of this paradoxical finding with respect to REM sleep was presented by Lavie at the conference. The higher threshold of arousal from REM sleep in these Israeli PTSD subjects was greater among those with more disrupted sleep and higher aggression ratings from dream reports. Thus, compensatory mechanisms may contribute to the variability within sleep findings among subjects with PTSD.

More generally, the findings from studies of chronic PTSD likely reflect progression over time and an unknown number of secondary factors. Information regarding the sleep aspects of acute traumatic reactions is scant. Schlossberg and Benjamin (1978) reported PSG findings in three acute combat fatigue cases that included marked fragmentation of sleep. We evaluated 10 subjects with PTSD symptoms related to Hurricane Andrew 6 to 8 months after the hurricane struck and during a stressful period of recovery. These subjects exhibited increased tendencies to arousal within sleep compared to the controls (Mellman et al., 1995b). In the symposium, Klein presented preliminary findings from an acute and longitudinal study of motor vehicle accident victims. Subjects who developed PTSD did have evidence of objective sleep disturbance, however, greater subjective complaints more substantially distinguished the group with PTSD. These types of studies are important because a greater understanding of acute changes in sleep patterns that precede the consolidation of PTSD could have implications for secondary preventive strategies.

REM Sleep and Dreaming

Polysomnographic studies in PTSD are also of interest for documenting the status of rapid eye movement or REM sleep activity. REM sleep activity can be applied to evaluating the biological relationship of PTSD and major depression (Mellman et al., 1997). Major depression overlaps PTSD clinically but has been found to be divergent with respect to certain biological markers. Reduced REM latency is a well-established marker of severe depression (Kupfer, 1976).

The other reasons for focusing on REM activity in PTSD are the status of dreams in PTSD and the relationship of dreaming and REM sleep. Abnormal dream patterns, in which repetitive nightmares replicate traumatic events, have been considered a hallmark symptom of PTSD (Ross et al., 1989). Although not all mentation during sleep is associated with REM, REM is the sleep stage where the most elaborate and affectively laden dreaming occurs (Foulkes, 1962). The literature reports that nightmares in PTSD are associated with both REM and non-REM sleep stages. Non-REM nightmares have been inferred on the basis of body movement that occurs during stage II sleep when nightmares were reported in the morning (van der Kolk et al., 1984). Kramer and Kinney (1988) also identified subgroups of combat veterans with nightmares that predominantly arise from stage II sleep. In other studies, spontaneous awakenings with nightmares in PTSD subjects during PSG recordings have arisen from REM sleep (Ross et al., 1994a; Mellman et al., 1995a; Hefez et al., 1987). Thus REM sleep appears to be associated with, albeit not the exclusive province of PTSD nightmares. Perhaps the more salient issue is the tendency for dreams reported by PTSD patients not to feature contemporaneous references and distortions that normally characterize dreams associated with REM sleep (Dow et al., 1996; Foulkes, 1962).

Overall, there is variability between and within studies regarding standard measures of the timing and amount of REM sleep in PTSD. The amount of REM sleep has been found to be reduced (Hefez et al., 1987), increased (Ross et al., 1994a), or not significantly different (Dow et al., 1996; Glaubman et al., 1990; Mellman et al., 1997) from controls. In contrast to the finding associated with severe depression, shortened REM latency has not been consistently reported in PTSD. In fact, a wide range of REM latency values has been found in the aforementioned PTSD studies. We have recently noted early REM sleep onsets during daytime sleep in 5 out of 10 chronic PTSD patients who slept during evaluation by the multiple sleep latency test. In these evaluations, short REM latency, which can be considered indicative of "REM pressure," was more characteristic of daytime than nighttime sleep. The presentation of de Groen and Op den Velde included 24-hour monitoring of sleeping and waking in aging subjects with PTSD related to Dutch Resistance activity during World War II. In these subjects, nightmare complaints were associated with phase advance phenomena that also included recordings of daytime REM sleep. The significance of variable patterns of REM timing and duration, as well as the preliminary evidence for early REM onsets in subsets of PTSD patients, remains to be clarified.

The frequency of eye movements within REM periods (REM density) was found to be increased in combat veterans with chronic PTSD by Ross et al. (1994a) and our laboratory (Mellman et al., 1997). REM density correlated with self-ratings of PTSD severity in our more acutely affected subjects with PTSD related to Hurricane Andrew (Mellman et al., 1995b). In our study of combat veterans, the increase in REM density was similar to that of a comparison group with primary depression. However, the amount of REM sleep was significantly lower in the PTSD group compared to the depressed group. Thus, mechanisms that underlie increased REM density in PTSD may diverge from mechanisms that occur in major depression where overall REM activity overall is increased. The etiology and significance of increased REM density in PTSD is unresolved at present. A possible relationship to an enhanced wake function in the disorder is suggested by a neurophysiological overlap of REM phasic activity and the alerting or startle responses in animal models (Morrison et al., 1995). REM density has been found to be elevated in association with nonpathological adaptations to life stressors (Reynolds et al, 1993), to periods of intense learning (Smith & Lapp, 1991), and to recovery sleep following REM deprivation (Reynolds et al., 1993) and following periods of suppression of tonic REM activity with antidepressant medication (Kupfer et al., 1994).

Ross et al. (1994b) also reported increased phasic muscle activation during REM sleep with PTSD. We have noted that a trend for symptomatic awakenings arises from REM (Mellman et al., 1995a). The observations of increased phasic eye movement activity and movement arousals during REM and symptomatic awakenings arising from

REM sleep suggest an increased level of arousal in relation to REM sleep with PTSD. In some circumstances, increased REM activity associated with active dreaming appears to be facilitating a positive adaptation to distressing events (Cartwright et al., 1991). The propensity to replay threatening events, disrupted REM sleep continuity due to symptomatic awakenings, and phasic muscle intrusion may be factors that impair REM sleep from facilitating emotional adaptation in individuals with PTSD.

Treatment Considerations

Chronic PTSD presents a difficult treatment challenge and has not been shown to be robustly responsive to either psychological or pharmacological interventions. The PTSD treatment literature is not very specific with regard to the effects of interventions on sleep disturbances. Because of the association with dreaming, there has been speculation regarding the therapeutic implications of pharmacologically altering REM sleep. In the review article by Ross et al. (1989), it was noted that monoamine oxidase inhibitors (MAOIs) that are potent REM sleep suppressants have sometimes ameliorated PTSD reexperiencing symptoms. However, intensification of daytime intrusive symptoms has also been observed with phenelzine treatment. In a PTSD treatment study from Israel phenelzine was reported to improve sleep and nightmares. However, there was no benefit to daytime intrusive symptoms for which ratings worsened, albeit not at a statistically significant level (Lerer et al., 1987). Pharmacological reduction of central noradrenergic activity via clonidine has also been preliminarily observed to ameliorate nightmares and improve sleep with PTSD (Kinzie & Leung, 1989). Relevant mechanisms could include suppression of REM sleep and/or the more general effect of reducing arousal during sleep.

With regard to the possibility of worsening daytime intrusive symptoms within phenelzine treatment, it is noteworthy that a subset of individuals will respond to REM deprivation with intrusive dream-like mentation during wake states (Cartwright et al., 1967). Another consideration that challenges the desirability of suppressing REM pharmacologically is the potentially adaptive relationship of REM sleep and emotional adaptation (Cartwright et al., 1991). With these considerations in mind, we recently conducted a pilot evaluation of the recently released antidepressant medication nefazodone in a relatively treatment-refractive, chronic group of PTSD patients. Unlike other serotonergically active antidepressants, nefazodone has been found to preserve or modestly enhance REM sleep and also reduces arousals in depressed patients (Armitage et al., 1994). In our preliminary observations of open label treatment, PTSD symptoms were significantly reduced at 6 weeks of treatment and subjective, diary-based ratings of sleep time were increased at a trend level during the first week of treatment. Ratings from the morning diary of the degree to which recalled dreams replicated traumatic experiences became reduced. Thus, treatment with an agent that potentially enhances REM sleep and improves sleep maintenance was associated with similar rates of dream recall overall, but with seemingly fewer PTSD-like characteristics.

In addition to pharmacological approaches, psychotherapeutic interventions can target disturbed dreaming. Although an interest of psychoanalytic treatment is the symbolic nature of dream content, the repetitive, replicative nightmare would not seem amenable to this type of approach. "Nightmare rehearsal" is a cognitive-behavioral technique applied to the content of a target dream that has been effective in treating subjects with recurrent nightmares and has shown preliminary promise in being applied to nightmares that occur with chronic PTSD (Krakow et al., 1997). We have found that this technique effects improvements in reported nightmares and sleep quality. However, it is sometimes resisted, particularly among patients who view their dreams as historical truth.

The disturbances in arousal that appear to characterize sleep disturbances in PTSD could also be an important target for therapeutic intervention. One of the few medication trials that demonstrated improvement in veterans with chronic PTSD used amitriptyline (Davidson et al., 1990). Among antidepressant medications, amitriptyline is often prescribed specifically for its benefit in maintaining sleep.

The difficulty in reversing processes that have gained momentum over periods of years speaks to the potential value of intervening early in disrupted sleep in the wake of trauma exposure. To this end, we recruited three patients from a surgical trauma service and one who had sought treatment in a psychiatric setting. All were within 1 to 3 weeks of trauma exposure and had acute PTSD symptoms that included disturbed sleep. Temazepam, a benzodiazepine hypnotic, was administered for 5 nights, tapered for 2 nights, and then discontinued. Evaluations 1 week after the medication had been discontinued revealed improved sleep and reduced PTSD severity. These observations are quite preliminary and the strategy is currently being evaluated by our group with placebo-controlled, double-blinded conditions. In addition to medication, environmental modifications and patient education regarding healthy sleep behaviors could be useful and efficient interventions. It further seems that querying regarding sleep disturbance would be a sensitive and efficient means of screening and monitoring recently traumatized populations.

Conclusions and Future Directions

As stated earlier, sleep complaints are prominent among individuals presenting with a diagnosis of PTSD. Disrupted sleep can have a substantial impact on vitality and mood. These rather straightforward observations justify the effort to form a better understanding of the role of sleep and sleep disturbance in the pathogenesis and treatment of PTSD. The absence of consistent objective corroboration of disturbed sleep from sleep laboratory recordings is a problem. As previously noted, although findings are mixed, there is a need to understand discrepancies in the degree of subjective and objective sleep disturbances, at least in some of the patient populations. One consideration is the effect of the sleep laboratory, which paradoxically can be considered a relatively safe environment by the patient subject. To address this limitation, there have been recent developments to monitor sleep in habitual environments utilizing ambulatory techniques. Selection bias may also be a factor because there is a need to record subjects in medication-free states which could lead to recruitment of less severe subgroups. Longitudinal effects also merit consideration because periods of sleep disruption may lead to subsequent apprehension regarding sleep and sleep state misperception.

Measures regarding the timing and duration of REM sleep, which have garnered much interest in depression research, have not distinguished PTSD populations. Therefore, an open question is whether these aspects of REM activity are normal in PTSD or reflect abnormal processes that vary within populations and possibly within individuals over time. Increased phasic activity, such as eye movements, has been more consistently found in PTSD but is not entirely specific to the disorder. Its significance remains to be fully clarified. REM density could represent heightened arousal stimulated by cholinergic brain stem centers, a correlate of affective processing and a primary pathogenic versus compensatory mechanism. Longitudinal PSG studies across different clinical states and treatment conditions would be ideal for addressing these considerations.

Dreams are associated with REM sleep and normally feature a hyperassociative form of mentation that often bridges past and present and does not typically follow logical narrative. Dreams in PTSD tend to replay threat and do not appear to effectively serve the adaptive function that some attribute to normal dreams. The malleability of dream patterns in PTSD as a function of treatment conditions is another matter for future research.

Interventions that target sleep disturbance appear to have a role in treating PTSD. Hypnotics merit consideration as early, time-limited and/or adjunctive approaches. Antidepressants and mood stabilizers that are applied to treating chronic PTSD can benefit sleep maintenance. The significance of the differential impact of these agents on REM sleep requires further elucidation. Cognitive-behavioral interventions can also effectively target sleep symptoms. Possible interventions include education and reinforcement of adaptive sleep hygiene, as well as desensitization to and cognitive restructuring of dream content. All of these approaches merit further systematic evaluation. It is recommended that future treatment studies evaluate sleep phenomena more systematically.

Like other psychobiological dimensions of a complex and likely heterogeneous disorder, uncertainties and controversy remain. In-depth presentations from an international group of investigators impressed this author that apparent discrepancies are likely to be a function of variability among study populations. Hopefully, the next generation of research will bring greater clarity and knowledge that will translate into more effective interventions.

References

Armitage, R., Rush, J. A., Trivedi, M., Cain, J., & Roffwarg, H. (1994). The effects of nefazodone on sleep architecture in depression. *Neuropsychopharmacology, 10,* 123–127.

Brown, T. M., & Boudewyns, P. A. (1996). Periodic limb movements of sleep in combat veterans with posttraumatic stress disorder. *Journal of Traumatic Stress, 9,* 129–136.

Cartwright, R. D., Kravitz, H., Eastman, C. I., & Wood, E. (1991). REM latency and the recovery from depression. Getting over divorce. *American Journal of Psychiatry, 148,* 1530–1535.

Cartwright, R. D., Monroe, L. J., & Palmer, C. (1967). Individual differences in response to REM deprivation. *Archives of General Psychiatry, 16,* 297–303.

Dagan, Y., Lavie, P., & Bleich, A. (1991). Elevated awakening thresholds in sleep stage 3–4 in war-related posttraumatic stress disorder. *Biological Psychiatry, 30,* 618– 622.

David, D., & Mellman, T. A. (1997). Dreams following Hurricane Andrew. *Dreaming, 7,* 209–214.

Davidson, J. R. T., Kudler, H., Smith, R., Mahorney, S. L., Lipper, S., Hammett, E., Saunders, W. B., & Cavenar, J. O. (1990). Treatment of posttraumatic stress disorder with amitriptyline and placebo. *Archives of General Psychiatry, 47,* 259–266.

Dow, B. M., Kelsoe, J. R., & Gillin, J. C. (1996). Sleep and dreams in Vietnam PTSD and depression. *Biological Psychiatry, 39,* 42–50.

Foulkes, W. D. (1962). Dream reports from different stages of sleep. *Journal of Abnormal Social Psychology, 65,* 14–25.

Glaubman, H., Mikulincer, M., Porat, A., Wasserman, O., & Birger, M. (1990). Sleep of chronic posttraumatic patients. *Journal of Traumatic Stress, 3,* 255–263.

Green, B. L. (1993). Disasters and posttraumatic stress disorder. J. R. T. Davidson & E. B. Foa, (Eds.), *Posttraumatic stress disorder DSM-IV and beyond.* Washington, DC: American Psychiatric Press.

Hefez, A., Metz, L., & Lavie, P. (1987). Long-term effects of extreme situational stress on sleep and dreaming. *American Journal of Psychiatry, 144,* 344–347.

Inman, D. J., Silver, S. M., & Doghramji, K. (1990). Sleep disturbance in post-traumatic stress disorder: A comparison with non-PTSD insomnia. *Journal of Traumatic Stress, 3,* 429–437.

Kinzie, J. D., & Leung, P. (1989). Clonidine in Cambodian patients with posttraumatic stress disorder. *Journal of Nervous and Mental Disorders, 177,* 546–550.

Krakow, B., Tandberg, D., Cutchen, L., McBride, L., Hollifield, M., Lauriello, J., Schrader, R., Yau, C. L., & Chang, D. T. (1997). *Sleep Research, 26,* 245.

Kramer, M., & Kinney, L. (1988). Sleep patterns in trauma victims with disturbed dreaming. *Psychiatric Journal University of Ottawa, 13,* 12–16.

Kupfer, D. J. (1976). REM latency—a psychobiological marker for primary depressive disease. *Biological Psychiatry, 11,* 159–174.

Kupfer, D. J., Ehlers, C. L., Frank, E., Grochocinski, V. J., McEarchran, A. B., & Buhari, A. (1994). Persistent effects of antidepressants: EEG sleep studies in depressed patients during maintenance treatment. *Biological Psychiatry, 35,* 781–793.

Lerer, B., Bleich, A., Kotler, M., Garb, R., Hertzberg, M., & Levin, B. (1987). Posttraumatic stress disorder in Israeli combat veterans. Effect of phenelzine treatment. *Archives of General Psychiatry, 44,* 976–981.

Mellman, T. A., Kulick-Bell, R., Ashlock, L. E., & Nolan, B. (1995a). Sleep events in combat-related post-traumatic stress disorder. *American Journal of Psychiatry, 152,* 110–115.

Mellman, T. A., David, D., Kulick-Bell, R., Hebding, J., & Nolan, B. (1995b). Sleep disturbance and its relationship to psychiatric morbidity following Hurricane Andrew. *American Journal of Psychiatry, 152,* 1659–1663.

Mellman, T. A., Nolan, B., Hebding, J., Kulick-Bell, R., & Dominguez, R. (1997). A polysomnographic comparison of veterans with combat-related PTSD, depressed men, and non-ill controls. *Sleep, 20,* 46–51.

Morrison, A. R., Sanford, L. D., Ball, W. A., Mann, G. L., & Ross, R. J. (1995). Stimulus-elicited behavior in rapid eye movement sleep without atonia. *Behavioral Neuroscience, 109,* 972–979.

Reynolds, C. F., Buysse, D. J., Kupfer, D. J., Hoch, C. C., Houch, P. R., Matzzie, J., & George, C. J. (1990). Rapid eye movement sleep deprivation as probe in elderly subjects. *Archives of General Psychiatry, 47,* 1128–1136.

Reynolds, C. F., Hoch, C. C., Buysse, D. J., Houch, P. R., Schlernitzauer, M., Pasternack, R. E., Frank, E., Mazumdar, S., & Kupfer, D. J. (1993). Sleep after spousal bereavement: A study of recovery from stress. *Biological Psychiatry, 34,* 791–797.

Rosen, J., Reynolds, C. F., Yeaer, A. L., Houck, P. R., & Hurwitz, L. F. (1990). Sleep disturbances in survivors of the Nazi holocaust. *American Journal of Psychiatry, 148,* 62–66.

Ross, R. J., Ball, W. A., Dinges, D. F., Kribbs, N. B., Morrison, A. R., Silver, S. M., & Mulvaney, F. D. (1994a). Rapid eye movement sleep disturbance in posttraumatic stress disorder. *Biological Psychiatry, 35,* 195–202.

Ross, R. J., Ball, W. A., Dinges, D. F., Kribbs, N. B., Morrison, A. R., Silver, S. M. & Mulvaney, F. D. (1994b). Motor dysfunction during sleep in posttraumatic stress disorder. *Sleep, 17,* 723–732.

Ross, R. J., Ball, W. A., Sullivan, K. A., & Caroff, S. N. (1989). Sleep disturbance as the hallmark of post-traumatic stress disorder. *American Journal of Psychiatry, 146,* 697–707.

Schlosberg, A., & Benjamin, M. (1978). Sleep patterns in three acute combat fatigue cases. *Journal of Clinical Psychiatry, 39,* 546–549.

Smith, C., & Lapp, L. (1991). Increases in number of REMs and REM density in humans following an intensive learning period. *Sleep, 14,* 325–330.

van der Kolk, B. A., Blitz, R., Burr, W. A., Sheery, S., & Hartmann, E. (1984). Nightmares and trauma: A comparison of nightmares after combat with lifelong nightmares in veterans. *American Journal of Psychiatry, 141,* 187–190.

22

The Emerging Neurobiology of Dissociative States

Relevance to PTSD

JOHN H. KRYSTAL, J. DOUGLAS BREMNER,
D. CYRIL D'SOUZA, AMIT ANAND,
STEVEN M. SOUTHWICK, AND DENNIS S. CHARNEY

Sensory perception often appears to be a fixed process that produces an exact transcription of the world. This view conflicts with the increasingly well-characterized distortions in perception, identity, and memory that are commonplace in everyday life (Krystal et al., 1995; Ray 1996). Generally, modest levels of stress distort perception in a manner that optimizes information processing. For example, stress may enhance the focusing of attention and the efficiency of several cognitive processes at the expense of reduced processing of peripheral stimuli in the environment. As stress becomes extreme, gross perceptual distortions emerge, including illusions and hallucinations. These perceptual alterations may occur in association with identity-related disturbances such as derealization and depersonalization. Equally profound perceptual alterations take place as people fall asleep or undergo prolonged sensory deprivation.

The term dissociation was coined by Janet (1920) to describe states where the integration of consciousness is disrupted. This concept has been employed to describe a spectrum of subjective experiences in which perceptual, affective, memory, and identity functions are altered. Particular symptoms or syndromes associated with dissociative states include distorted sensory perceptions, altered time perception, amnesia, derealization, depersonalization, conversion symptoms, fugue states, and multiple personality (Spiegel & Cardena, 1991; Bremner et al., 1992). As suggested before, dissociation may occur during traumatization (Krystal, 1968; Spiegel & Cardena, 1991; Bremner et al., 1992; Griffin et al., 1997). Clinicians have long debated whether dissociation is an adverse or adaptive consequence of traumatic stress response. Both clinical experience

JOHN H. KRYSTAL, J. DOUGLAS BREMNER, D. CYRIL D'SOUZA, AMIT ANAND, STEVEN M. SOUTHWICK, AND DENNIS S. CHARNEY   Department of Psychiatry, VA Medical Center, Yale University School of Medicine, West Haven, Connecticut 06516.
International Handbook of Human Response to Trauma, edited by Shalev, Yehuda, and McFarlane. Kluwer Academic / Plenum Publishers, New York, 2000.

(Freud and Breuer, 1953) and laboratory data (Griffin et al., 1997) suggest that peritraumatic dissociation may reduce both the initial impact of traumatization and the degree of subsequent physiological hyperactivity. However, these studies cannot untangle the genetic and environmental factors that might have influenced the vulnerability to dissociation and the pattern of post-traumatic response (Krystal et al., 1998b).

Dissociative states and increased vulnerability to hypnotic states may also develop as ongoing sequelae of traumatization (Spiegel et al., 1988; Bremner et al., 1992). Although dissociated, acutely traumatized individuals may appear confused, emotionally dulled, or even catatonic (Kardiner, 1941; Grinker & Spiegel, 1945; Krystal, 1968). Decades following traumatization, while recalling their traumatic experiences, individuals may experience time as being slow, have altered sensory perceptions, and have feelings of unreality (Bremner et al., 1998). Less frequently, adult traumatization may produce fugue states, conversion reactions, or multiple personality as ongoing symptoms of post-traumatic stress disorder (PTSD) (Grinker & Spiegel, 1945; McDougle & Southwick, 1990).

Flashbacks, perhaps the most distinctive PTSD symptom, link dissociative, memory-related, and arousal regulatory processes pertinent to this disorder. During flashbacks, patients vividly reexperience aspects of the traumatic response while feeling detached from their surrounding environment. Ongoing sensory processing may be altered or disrupted, and patients may report that they are in a fog or that they blacked out (Bremner et al., 1993). Flashbacks involving the recollection of traumatic experiences are frequently associated with intense emotional responses and panic-like states (Mellman & Davis, 1985). Most flashbacks are brief and last only a few minutes. However, some flashbacks may last several hours or several days. Some flashbacks are accurate depictions of a traumatic situation, and others have unreal or distorted qualities, similar to dreams. Out-of-body experiences may also be associated with flashbacks (Rainey et al., 1987; Spiegel & Cardena, 1991).

Despite progress in identifying, characterizing, and quantitatively assessing dissociative states, there has been surprisingly little study of their neurobiology and few pharmacological trials specifically aimed at reducing dissociation. This chapter reviews a series of studies in PTSD patients and healthy subjects that have utilized psychopharmacological processes to evoke or suppress dissociative states in patients or perceptual alterations resembling dissociation in healthy individuals. The implications of these studies for the evaluation of novel pharmacotherapies for dissociative states in PTSD patients is considered.

Pharmacological Challenge Studies in PTSD Patients

Flashbacks have been precipitated in Vietnam veterans who have chronic PTSD by the intravenous administration of sodium lactate (Rainey et al., 1987), yohimbine (Southwick et al., 1993), and m-chlorophenylpiperazine (MCPP; Southwick et al., 1997). Administration of each of these substances produces panic attacks in a significant proportion of patients with either panic disorder (Pitts & McClure, 1967; Charney et al., 1984, 1987) or PTSD (Rainey et al., 1987; Southwick et al., 1993, 1997), but not in other patient groups. However, PTSD patients are the first group studied who experience flashbacks after administration of these substances.

Rainey and his associates (1987) compared the response to intravenous sodium lactate, isoproterenol, and a dextrose placebo in seven Vietnam combat veterans, six of whom also met criteria for panic disorder. All seven patients experienced flashbacks following lactate, two patients also experienced flashbacks after isoproterenol infusion, and one patient experienced a flashback during placebo infusion. The authors described these flashbacks as similar to those that occur naturally as part of PTSD. Six of the seven lactate-induced flashbacks, both isoproterenol flashbacks, and the dextrose flashback were followed by panic-like states. However, the absence of reported anxiety ratings makes it impossible to determine whether subpanic increases in anxiety preceded the flashbacks. The overlap of panic disorder and PTSD in the patients in this study was another limitation of this study because it raised concerns that lactate-induced flashbacks were a property of panic disorder and not independently associated with PTSD. Little is known about the mechanisms through which lactate produces panic attacks and flashbacks in PTSD patients.

The precipitation of flashbacks and panic attacks in PTSD patients by yohimbine, linked noradrenergic systems are implicated in fear and arousal regulation with the symptoms of PTSD (Southwick et al., 1993). Yohimbine activates central noradrenergic neurons through a blockade of alpha-2 receptors located on noradrenergic neurons. These alpha-2 receptors mediate, in part, feedback inhibition of noradrenergic neurons (Starke et al., 1975). Following yohimbine, 40% (8/20) of the patients experienced flashbacks and 70% (14/20) of the patients experienced panic attacks. No panic attacks and only one flashback emerged following placebo administration. Although 45% of the patients in this study also met DSM-III-R criteria for panic disorder, 43% of the yohimbine-induced panic attacks occurred in individuals without panic disorder. The risk of a yohimbine-induced panic attack was increased in patients with panic disorder relative to those without comorbid panic disorder (89% vs. 43%). However, a history of panic disorder did not appear to influence the likelihood of experiencing a yohimbine-induced flashback. The following vignette illustrates the features of yohimbine-induced flashback:

10:00 A.M.: Initiation of yohimbine infusion
10:05 A.M.: Subject reports hot and cold flashes, goose bumps, palpitations.
10:10 A.M.: Subject reports clammy hands, he asked the nurse to move away from him … in case he felt like running. "I feel like I'm picking up dead bodies the centrifuge sounds like a helicopter …. A chopper is shooting at us, we're trying to shoot back at it! One of the guys' head is shot off! Brains are coming at me! I smell burnt flesh … I feel scared, I can't hear what's going on …."

The operational definition for flashback employed in this study led to the exclusion of many dissociative states produced by yohimbine in the PTSD patients. The following criteria were employed to define a drug-induced flashback: (1) reexperiencing a past traumatic event during drug infusion, (2) the reexperiencing must involve one or more sensory modalities, and (3) the drug-induced state must be similar to naturally occurring flashbacks. Despite the expedient characterization of flashbacks as being present or absent, yohimbine actually produced a continuum of dissociative phenomena. Patients experienced varying degrees of derealization and depersonalization that were often accompanied by other dissociative symptoms. Yohimbine also elicited a rang of altered perceptual experiences, some of which were fragmentary or vague. For example, one patient perceived the shadow produced by a sink in the testing facility to be the shadow made by a tank turret. In addition to stimulating flashbacks, yohimbine significantly increased the recall of traumatic memories. Although yohimbine produced symptoms of autonomic arousal in many patients, these symptoms were not the sole predictors of flashbacks within a session. Yohimbine also significantly increased the recall of traumatic memories. In some cases, symptoms of autonomic arousal followed or were coincident with the reported retrieval of traumatic memories (S. M. Southwick, personal communication). Thus, it appeared that noradrenergic systems might be involved in eliciting dissociative symptoms as a direct consequence of their central pharmacological actions on neural circuitry that contribute to dissociation and memory retrieval. These data contrasted with models in which noradrenergic contributions of PTSD symptoms were entirely mediated by peripheral autonomic systems.

A subsequent study evaluated the cortical localization of yohimbine effects in PTSD patients and in controls by studying its effects on cortical metabolism using fluorodeoxyglucose and PET (Bremner et al., 1997). This study found that yohimbine increased orbital frontal cortical metabolism in healthy subjects, perhaps by blocking the inhibitory effects of postsynaptic alpha-2 adrenergic receptors. In PTSD patients, however, yohimbine reduced orbital frontal cortex metabolism. Because locus coeruleus stimulation inhibits frontal cortical metabolism, it is possible that the finding in PTSD patients reflects enhanced norepinephrine release after yohimbine administration. This study also linked yohimbine-stimulated PTSD symptoms to modulation of the orbital frontal cortex, a brain region implicated in both emotion and cognitive functions.

One question raised by the initial yohimbine study was whether the elicitation of flashbacks by yohimbine reflected a specific response to alpha-2 receptor blockade or whether all anxiogenic drugs produce flashbacks in PTSD patients. To investigate this question, yohimbine and MCPP effects were compared in 26 PTSD patients and 14 healthy controls (Southwick et al., 1997). This study found that flashback occurred in 8 (31%) patients following yohimbine, 7 (27%) after mCPP, and 2 (8%) following placebo. Four patients (16%) had flashbacks on both the yohimbine and mCPP test days. No flashbacks occurred in control subjects. These observations do not allow one to determine whether common or distinct mechanisms mediated the drug-induced evocation of flashbacks.

Although yohimbine and mCPP produce panic attacks and flashbacks in subgroups of PTSD patients, they do not appear to have these effects when administered in comparable doses to healthy subjects. The source of the differential sensitivity of patients and healthy subjects to these medications is not yet clear. One hypothesis suggests that an adaptive reduction in alpha-2 adrenergic receptor function contributes to increased yohimbine sensitivity. This hypothesis is supported by the finding that yohimbine produced greater noradrenergic activation, as suggested by increased accumulation of the norepinephrine metabolite 3-methoxy-4-hydroxy phenethyleneglycol (MHPG) in plasma in patients with panic attacks relative to patients who did not experience panic attacks or controls (Southwick et al., 1993). To date, there is not clear evidence to support the hypothesis that alterations in the sensitivity of 5-HT receptor targets for mCPP account for the differential vulnerability to flashbacks in patients.

The vulnerability to yohimbine- and mCPP-induced flashbacks in PTSD patients may also occur as a consequence of inhibitory deficits within brain networks involving serotonin and noradrenergic systems. Deficits in endogenous opiate systems may have contributed to the PTSD-related vulnerability to yohimbine-evoked flashbacks. Opiate antagonist-induced withdrawal has stimulated flashbacks in opiate-dependent PTSD patients (Kosten & Krystal, 1988). The association between endogenous opiate systems and noradrenergic systems is also suggested by the potentiation of the panicogenic and MHPG-increasing effects of yohimbine by naloxone in healthy subjects (Charney et al., 1986). Although this study did not directly measure dissociative states, yohimbine-precipitated panic has been previously linked to symptoms including derealization and depersonalization (Krystal et al., 1988).

Deficits in gamma aminobutyric acid-A (GABA-A) receptor function may also contribute to a vulnerability to mCPP-induced dissociation. In a clinical laboratory-based model, deficits in GABA function may be produced by the benzodiazepine partial inverse agonist, iomazenil. This drug created a vulnerability to mild dissociation-like perceptual changes in healthy subjects administered mCPP (Gil et al., 1996). Alterations in GABA function have been studied in PTSD patients. The failure of the benzo-diazepine antagonist, flumazenil, to produce flashbacks in PTSD patients suggests that this disorder is not associated with significant constriction of their field of attention that results in the sensation of tunnel vision or the feeling that they were surrounded by fog. Ketamine also produced learning and memory impairments. Its effects increased proportionately to the dose administered and the duration of delay between stimulus presentation and testing. In addition, ketamine interfered with executive functions, such as abstraction, assessed by proverb interpretation, and problem solving, evaluated by the Wisconsin Card Sorting Test. Ketamine also produced emotional responses. At low doses, it had mild anxiolytic properties, whereas larger doses produced euphoria and anxiety. Anxiety stimulated by ketamine appeared to follow perceptual alterations and thought disorganization and to be related to their degree of comfort with ketamine effects on perception and thought processes.

To date, a series of studies has attempted to block the perceptual alterations produced by ketamine (summarized in Table 1). Several studies conducted in the anesthesiology field suggested that lorazepam reduced the perceptual effects of ket-amine, particularly at high lorazepam doses. To evaluate this possibility, the effects of lorazepam pretreatment upon ketamine response was studied. Lorazepam (2 mg) administered orally two hours before ketamine administration tended to reduce altered environmental perceptions produced by ketamine. However, it had no effects on other dissociative symptoms or psychotic states produced by ketamine (Krystal et al., 1998a).

TABLE 1. Pharmacological Modulation of Perceptual Changes Resembling Dissociation Produced by the NMDA Antagonist, Ketamine, in Healthy Subjects[a]

Pretreatment	Degree of reduction[b]	N
Lorazepam, 2 mg, p.o.	+	23
Haloperidol, 5 mg, p.o.	0	20
Clozapine, 25 mg, p.o.	0	8
Glycine, 0.1 or 0.2 g/kg, i.v.		7
Lamotrigine, 300 mg, p.o.	++	10

[a]Krystal et al., 1999; Krystal et al 1998a; Lipschitz et al., 1997; D'Souza et al., 1997; Anand et al., 1997.
[b]Degree of reduction: 0 = no change to ++ = significant reduction.

Haloperidol (5 mg) and clozapine (25 mg) failed to reduce dissociative symptoms or amnesic effects produced by ketamine (Krystal et al., 1998a; Lipschitz et al., 1997). These data are consistent with the literature suggesting that neuroleptics have limited efficacy in treating dissociative symptoms (Kluft, 1987). Haloperidol reduced other ketamine-induced cognitive impairments, such as concrete ideation or poor performance on the Wisconsin Card Sorting Test (Krystal et al., 1999b).

To date, there have not been formal evaluations of ketamine effects in PTSD patients or patients with other dissociative disorders. However, anecdotal data from Russian studies suggest that ketamine induces dissociative states and may promote guided recollection of traumatic material in Russian-Afghanistan war veterans with PTSD (E. Krupitsky, personal communication).

Dissociative states have also been produced by psychoactive cannabinoids, such as tetrahydrocannabinol, the principal psychoactive component of marijuana and hashish. Cannabinoids bind to a specific G-protein-coupled receptor (Herkenham et al., 1990) through which they alter cellular functions, including blockade of N-type calcium channels, inhibition of cyclic AMP accumulation, and stimulation of arachidonic acid and intracellular calcium release (Felder et al., 1993). Some cannabinoid effects may be mediated by stimulation of glucocorticoid receptors (Eldridge & Landfield, 1990) and blockade of N-methyl-D-aspartate receptors (Feigenbaum et al., 1989). At high doses, cannabinoid intoxication produces depersonalization, derealization, temporal disorientation, perceptual alterations, and insight impairments (Melges et al., 1970; Dittrich et al., 1973). Depersonalization and temporal disorientation produced by marijuana smoking were associated with increased cortical regional cerebral blood flow assessed with the [133]xenon inhalation technique (Mathew et al., 1992). Cannabis has been reported to produce flashbacks in the drug-free state that resemble cannabis intoxication (Hollister, 1986). In one study (Stanton et al., 1976), 3% (1/31) of habitual marijuana users and 1% (3/348) of nonhabitual users reported flashbacks when drug-free, suggesting that flashbacks were not a frequent consequence of cannabis use. However, this study suggested that marijuana use also enhanced the likelihood of experiencing flashbacks following ingestion of serotonergic hallucinogens.

Serotonergic hallucinogens, such as lysergic acid diethylamide (LSD), mescaline, and dimethyltryptamine (DMT), also produce dissociative symptoms. These agents stimulate serotonin-2 ($5\text{-}HT_2$) receptors (Rasmussen et al., 1986). Serotonergic hallucinogens produce pronounced visual hallucinations, illusions, synesthesia, and expansive or portentous emotional responses (Freedman, 1968; Strassman et al., 1994). Following ingestion of psychedelics, feelings of derealization or depersonalization are prominent. Environmental stimuli may be experienced in a fragmented manner, body image distortion is common, and feelings of emotional detachment may arise (Savage, 1955; Freedman, 1968). Some clinicians have also reported that LSD may facilitate the recall of repressed memories (Freedman, 1968), although this capacity has never been rigorously evaluated. Relative to the phencyclidine or ketamine experience, psychedelic hallucinogens tend to produce perceptual effects that predominate over dissociative effects and impairments in higher cognitive functions (Rosenbaum et al., 1959).

Flashbacks have been reported in healthy individuals following serotonergic hallucinogen use. Freedman (1968) and Horowitz et al. (1969) suggested that LSD intoxication was traumatic for some users because it diminished control over awareness, resulting in intense emotional states experienced as beyond their control. In such cases, LSD flashbacks might have a traumatic etiology. However, some LSD-like experiences, such as synesthesia, may be reexperienced long after drug ingestion by individuals who find such experiences pleasant. These effects do not easily fit a trauma model, suggesting that sensitization, conditioning, or state-dependent learning might also apply (Freedman, 1968, 1984; Horowitz et al., 1969; McGee, 1984). Subject expectancy may also play a role in drug-like flashbacks. One study found that flashbacks may be produced in healthy subjects following placebo administration, if subjects are coached to anticipate that a placebo will produce flashbacks (Heaton, 1975). Heaton suggested that the expectancy of flashbacks led subjects to mislabel and selectively attend to aspects of normal experience that are consistent with a flashback-like experience.

Synthesis and Clinical Implications

The studies reviewed in this chapter chart the slow but steady progress made in characterizing the psychopharmacology of dissociative states in PTSD patients and dissociation-like perceptual changes in healthy individuals. The studies reviewed in this chapter suggest that one fundamental insight into the neurobiology of dissociation may come from the observation that some drugs given at specific doses produce dissociative symptoms in traumatized individuals, but not in healthy controls. Yohimbine and mCPP fit into this class. Other drugs, such as ketamine, cannabis, and hallucinogens, produce dissociation-like responses in individuals without histories of traumatization or dissociative disorders.

Dissociative States and the Activation of Cortical Glutamatergic Neurons

The significance of these distinctions is not yet clear but may be linked to the intrinsic organization of the cerebral cortex or the pharmacology of cortical function, as illustrated in Figure 1 (reviewed in Lewis, 1992; Krystal et al., 1999a). The cerebral cortex contains both pyramidal and nonpyramidal neurons. Pyramidal neurons release excitatory amino acids, primarily glutamate. Cortical pyramidal neurons are primarily responsible for cortico–cortical and cortico–subcortical communication. The nonpyramidal neurons predominantly release GABA and inhibit the activity of pyramidal neurons. One class of GABAergic interneurons is the chandelier cells. These cells provide feedback inhibition to cortical pyramidal neurons. Cortical pyramidal neurons and interneurons receive innervation from noradrenergic, serotonergic, and opiatergic neurons. These monoamine and peptide systems provide important modulation of the release of both amino acid neurotransmitters.

Stress has important modulatory effects on the release of many neurotransmitters, including monoamines, endogenous opiates, GABA, and serotonin (Charney et al., 1993). More recently, research has begun to characterize stresss-related stimulation of cortical glutamate release in the prefrontal cortex (Moghaddam, 1993). A series of studies suggested that stress-related glutamate release in conjunction with parallel enhancements in the levels of circulating glucocorticoids promoted the death of hippocampal neurons in the CA3 region of the hippocampus (Sapolsky, 1992). However, the release of glutamate may have important implications in evoking stress-related perceptual changes.

Some insights into the importance of alterations in cortical glutamate function for dissociation may be derived from studies of NMDA antagonists, including ketamine.

NEUROTRANSMITTERS IMPLICATED IN DISSOCIATION:
RELATION TO CORTICAL AND LIMBIC CIRCUITRY

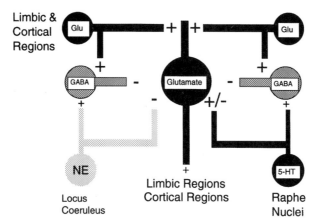

FIGURE 1. This figure provides a schematic representation of interactions that are predicted to contribute to dissociative states on the basis of human psychopharmacological studies and preclinical studies reviewed in the text. This schematic depicts the convergence of cortical GABAergic and glutamatergic inputs on a prototypical glutamatergic pyramidal neuron. This neuron, in turn, provides glutamatergic input to both cortical and limbic regions. Extrinsic inputs to the cortex from the noradrenergic locus coeruleus and serotonergic raphe nuclei appear to modulate the activity of intrinsic cortical populations. Activation of these inputs or direct stimulation or blockade of postsynaptic receptors, as reviewed in the text, appears to precipitate dissociative symptoms in vulnerable traumatized patients. In contrast, blockade of NMDA receptors by ketamine or stimulation of 5-HT$_2$A receptors by serotonergic hallucinogens appears to activate glutamatergic activity and to evoke dissociation-like perceptual changes in healthy subjects. Abbreviations: Glu: glutamate-containing; NE: norepinephrine-containing; 5-HT: serotonergic. All other abbreviations are defined in the text.

Components of ketamine response may mimic the impact of stress upon glutamate release. For example, ketamine and other NMDA antagonists increase the release of glutamate within the frontal cortex (Moghaddam et al., 1997). Although the mechanism underlying the glutamate-releasing effect of NMDA antagonists is not fully clear, some preclinical research suggests that these drugs may inhibit the activity of chandelier cells in the cortex or GABAergic cells that play similar roles in the hippocampus (see Krystal et al., in press c). Glutamate that is released during NMDA antagonist administration primarily stimulates non-NMDA receptors (AMPA/kainate and metabotropic glutamate receptors) because the NMDA receptors are blocked by the antagonist (Figure 2). Thus, NMDA antagonists effects might reflect the direct postsynaptic effects of NMDA receptor blockade, the excessive stimulation of non-NMDA glutamate receptors, and possibly shifts in the relative degree of stimulation of NMDA and non-NMDA receptors.

Recent clinical data support the hypothesis that cognitive and perceptual changes produced by NMDA antagonists reflect a hyperglutamatergic state combined with a deficit in NMDA receptor function. Consistent with the preclinical literature, ketamine increases cortical metabolism, as assessed by the FDG-PET technique (Breier et al., 1997). Further, two ongoing studies suggest that the effects of ketamine on perception may be reduced by enhancing NMDA receptor function or by reducing ketamine-

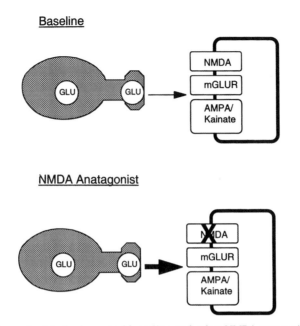

FIGURE 2. This figure depicts the impact of ketamine and other NMDA antagonists upon glutamate neuronal activity. The neuronal release of glutamate stimulates postsynaptic NMDA, AMPA, kainate, and metabotropic glutamate receptors. NMDA antagonists, such as ketamine, active glutamate neuronal activity causing increased stimulation of non-NMDA receptors. Abbreviations not defined in the text: GLU: glutamate; AMPA: alpha-amino-3-hydroxy-5-methyl-4-isoxazoleproprionic acid.

stimulating glutamate release. The first of these studies evaluated the effects of large intravenous glycine doses on ketamine response (D'Souza et al., 1997). Glycine binds to a strychnine-insensitive site on the NMDA receptor complex where it acts as a coagonist (D'Souza et al., 1995). In the initial seven patients studied, both glycine 0.1 g/kg and glycine 0.2 g/kg reduced CADSS (Clinician-Administered Dissociative States Scale) scores in healthy subjects administered ketamine. Another study evaluated the effects of lamotrigine pretreatment upon ketamine response. Lamotrigine reduces glutamate release through several mechanisms, including blockade of sodium channels and antagonism of N-type calcium channels (Rataud et al., 1994; Wang et al., 1996).

Cortical Networks, Dissociation, and PTSD

As suggested by Figure 1, one consequence of activation of cortical glutamate neurone by stress, ketamine, or 5-HT$_2$A receptors is enhancing glutamate release within key limbic and cortical projection areas. Kctamine, for example, has activated frontal cortex and cingulate gyrus metabolism and blood flow in healthy humans and schizophrenic patients (Breier et al., 1997; Lahti et al., 1995). NMDA antagonists have also shown evidence of activating a cortical network involving the striatum, globus pallidus, subthalamic nucleus, and thalamus (Carlsson and Carlsson, 1990). Recent neuroimaging studies have suggested that the cingulate gyrus and thalamus may be activated in PTSD patients by exposure to reminder s of their traumas (Rausch et al., 1996; Liberzon et al., 1996/1997). In contrast, the orbital frontal gyrus may be inhibited during worsening of PTSD symptoms produced by reminders of the trauma or yohimbine (Rausch et al., 1996; Bremner et al., 1997). The involvement of the thalamus and cingulate gyrus in evoking PTSD is interesting in the light of other data implicating these regions in the control of attention and sensory processing (Krystal et al., 1995). The overlap among the neuroimaging studies reviewed in this paragraph raise the possibility that cortico–striato–thalamic circuitry modulated by ketamine also contributes to evoking the reexperiencing cluster of PTSD symptoms, including flashbacks.

Therapeutic Implications

The introduction of benzodiazepines and antidepressants into the pharmaco-therapeutic armamentarium advanced the treatment of post-traumatic stress disorder significantly (Friedman and Southwick, 1995). The efficacy of these medications in treating PTSD is quite consistent with the yohimbine and mCPP testing performed in PTSD patients. Thus, the efficacies of benzodiazepines and antidepressants are consistent with the view that activation of monamine is intimately involved in the interplay of neurobiological processes that give rise to PTSD symptoms, including dissociation. Further, the impact of monoaminergic activation may be reduced by facilitation of GABA-A receptor function (reviewed in Gil et al., 1996). However, several promising treatments based on preclinical models have remained peripheral in treating PTSD. For example, clonidine and propranolol were evaluated in PTSD to prevent or reduce the consequences of central noradrenergic systems based on promising clinical and pre-clinical evidence that implicated central noradrenergic systems in the symptoms of PTSD (Kolb et al., 1984). The anticonvulsants carbamazepine and valproic acid were evaluated in PTSD based on the hypothesis that repeated exposure to stress sensitizes or "kindles" cortical networks (Lipper et al., 1986). Similarly, naltrexone was evaluated in PTSD based on the hypothesis that traumatic stress and subsequent stressful experience causes a rewarding release of endogenous opiates (Friedman and Southwick, 1995). Despite their limited use in treating PTSD, the precise role of each of these novel treatments remains to be precisely characterized. Generally, the pharmacotherapeutic approaches to PTSD referred to in this paragraph are now more than 10 years old. Given the limited, but important, efficacy of these approaches, it appears that there is a need for novel approaches to the neurobiology of clusters of PTSD symptoms to drive the next generation of medication development for this disorder.

The central question of this chapter is whether the effects of NMDA antagonists in healthy humans have pharmacotherapeutic implications for dissociative symptoms in PTSD patients or patients with other dissociative disorders. It may be that the perceptual effects of ketamine do not provide an accurate model for dissociative symptoms associated with PTSD or other dissociative disorders beyond the level of phenomenological similarity. Bearing this concern in mind, one might attempt to build on a glutamatergic model by testing the efficacy of drugs that block the perceptual effects of ketamine in humans. Based on this criterion, one would endorse the efficacy of benzodiazepines and the relative lack of efficacy of neuroleptics in PTSD. This laboratory-based model also suggests two novel pharmacological approaches to the treatment of PTSD: (1) agonists of the strychnine-insensitive glycine site of the NMDA receptor complex and (2) drugs, such as lamotrigine, that reduce ketamine effects on glutamate release. One might also evaluate drugs that block the postsynaptic consequences of enhanced glutamate release by studying the effects of antagonists of non-NMDA glutamate receptors. The caveat here, though, is that a subclass of metabotropic glutamate receptors inhibit glutamate, the mGLUR II/III receptors (Schoepp and Conn, 1993). Agonists, rather than antagonists of these receptors would be predicted to be helpful in PTSD.

Implications

This chapter continues a line of discourse that began almost 15 years ago (van der Kolk et al., 1985) that attempts to integrate animal research and human laboratory-based paradigms in developing models for the neurobiology and pharmacotherapy of PTSD. The utility of these models is ultimately determined by the definitive evaluation of the effectiveness of rationally developed pharmacotherapies. In advance of the clinical data, the laboratory-based paradigms continue to be a source of creative approaches to the pathophysiology and pharmacotherapy of PTSD.

Acknowledgments.   The work described in this paper was supported by the U.S. Department of Veterans Affairs through its clinical research centers (Clinical Neurosciences Division of the National Center for PTSD, VA-Yale Alcoholism Research Center, and VA Schizophrenia Biological Research Center) and the Merit Review Program.

References

Anand, A., Charney, D. S., Berman, R. M., Oren, D. A., Cappiello, A., & Krystal, J. H. (1997). Reduction in ketamine effects in humans by lamotrigine. *Social Neuroscience Abstracts, 23*, (#686.3).

Breier A., Malhotra A. K., Pinals D. A., Weisenfeld, N. I., & Pickar, D. (1997). Association of ketamine-induced psychosis with focal activation of the prefrontal cortex in healthy volunteers. *American Journal of Psychiatry, 154*, 805–811.

Bremner, J. D., Southwick, S., Brett, E., Fontana, A., Rosenheck, R., & Charney, D. S. (1992). Dissociation and posttraumatic stress disorder in Vietnam combat veterans. *American Journal of Psychiatry, 149*, 328–332.

Bremner, J. D., Steinberg, M., Southwick, S. M., Johnson, D. R., & Charney, D. S. (1993). Use of the structured clinical interview for DSM-IV dissociative disorders for systematic assessment of dissociative symptoms in posttraumatic stress disorder. *American Journal of Psychiatry, 150*, 1011–1014.

Bremner, J. D., Innis, R. B., Ng, C. K., Staib, L., Salomon, R., Bronen, R. A., Markey, J., Duncan, J., Krystal, J. H., Rich, D., Zubal, G., Dey, H., Soufer, R., & Charney, D. S. (1997). PET measurement of cerebral metabolic correlates of yohimbine administration in combat-related posttraumatic stress disorder. *Archives of General Psychiatry, 54*, 246–256.

Bremner, J. D., Mazure, C. M., Putnam, F. W., Southwick, S. M., Marmar, C., Hansen, C., Lubin, H., Roach, L., Freeman, G., Krystal, J. H., & Charney, D. S. (1998). Measurement of dissociative states with the Clinician-Administered Dissociative States Scale (CADSS). *Journal of Traumatic Stress, 11*, 125–136.

Carlsson, M., & Carlsson, A. (1990). Schizophrenia: A subcortical neurotransmitter imbalance syndrome? *Schizophrenia Bulletin, 16*, 425–432.

Charney, D. S., Heninger, G. R., & Breier, A. (1984). Noradrenergic function in panic anxiety: Effects of yohimbine in healthy subjects and patients with agoraphobia and panic disorder. *Archives of General Psychiatry, 41*, 751–763.

Charney, D. S., & Heninger, G. R. (1986). α-2 Adrenergic and opiate receptor blockade: Synergistic effects on anxiety in healthy subjects. *Archives of General Psychiatry, 43*, 1037–1041.

Charney, D. S., Woods, S. W., Goodman, W. K., & Heninger, G. R. (1987). Serotonin function in anxiety. II. Effects of the serotonin agonist MCPP in panic disorder patients and healthy subjects. *Psychopharmacology, 92*, 14–24.

Charney, D. S., Deutch, A. Y., Krystal, J. H., Southwick, S. M., & Davis, M. (1993). Psychobiologic mechanisms of posttraumatic stress disorder. *Archives of General Psychiatry, 50,* 294–305.

Dittrich, A., Battig, K., & von Zeppelin, I. (1973). Effects of $(-)\Delta^9$-trans-tetrahydrocannabinol (Δ^9-THC) on memory, attention and subjective state: A double blind study. *Psychopharmacologia (Berlin), 33,* 369–376.

Domino, E. F., Chodoff, P., & Corssen, G. (1965). Pharmacologic effects of CI-581, a new dissociative anesthetic, in man. *Clinical Pharmacology Therapy, 6,* 279–291.

D'Souza, D. C., Gil, R., Zuzarte, E., Abi-Saab, D., Damon, D., White, J., Zimmerman, L., & Krystal, J. H. (1997). Glycine ketamine interactions in healthy humans. *Schizophrenia Research, 24,* 213.

Eldridge, J. C., & Landfield, P. W. (1990). Cannabinoid interactions with glucocorticoid receptors in rat hippocampus. *Brain Research, 534,* 135–141.

Feigenbaum, J. J., Bergmann, F., Richmond, S. A., Mechoulam, R., Nadler, V., Kloog, Y., & Sokolovsky, M. (1989). Nonpsychotropic cannabinoid acts as a functional *N*-methyl-D-aspartate receptor blocker. *Proceedings of the National Academy of Sciences of the USA, 86,* 9584–9587.

Felder, C. C., Briley, E. M., Axelrod, J., Simpson, J. T., Mackie, K., & Devane, W. A. (1993). Anandamide, an endogenous cannabimmetic eicosanoid, binds to the cloned human cannabinoid receptor and stimulates receptor-mediated signal transduction. *Proceedings of the National Academy of Sciences of the USA, 90,* 7656–7660.

Freedman, D. X. (1968). On the use and abuse of LSD. *Archives of General Psychiatry, 18,* 330–347.

Freedman, D. (1984). LSD: The bridge from human to animal. In B. L. Jacobs (Ed.), *Hallucinogens: Neurochemical, behavioral, and clinical perspectives* (pp. 203–226). New York: Raven Press.

Friedman, M. J., & Southwick, S. M. (1995). Towards pharmacotherapy for post-traumatic stress disorder. In M. J. Friedman, D. S. Charney, & A. Y. Deutch (Eds.), *Neurobiological and clinical consequences of stress: From normal adaptation to post-traumatic stress disorder,* pp. 465–482. Philadephia: Lippincott-Raven.

Freud, S., & Breuer, J. (1953). On the psychical mechanism of hysterical phenomena. In E. Jones (Ed.), *Sigmund Freud, M.D., LL.D. Collected papers,* Vol. 1, pp. 24–41. London: Hogarth Press.

Gil, R., D'Souza, D. C., Zuzarte, E., Damon, D., White, J., Boutros, N., Abi-Dargham, A., Seibyl, J., Innis, R., Charney, D. S., & Krystal, J. (1996). Serotonergic and GABAergic contributions to psychosis: Psychotogenic interactions of MCPP and iomazenil in healthy subjects. Presented to the American College of Neuropsychopharmacology. *Scientific Abstracts, 35th Annual Meeting.* December 9–13, p. 192.

Griffin, M. G., Resick, P. A., & Mechanic, M. B. (1997). Objective assessment of peritraumatic dissociation: Psychophysiological indicators. *American Journal of Psychiatry, 154,* 1081–1088.

Grinker, R. R., & Spiegel, J. P. (1945). *War neuroses.* Philadelphia: Blakiston.

Heaton, R. K. (1975). Subject expectancy and environmental factors as determinants of psychedelic flashback experiences. *Journal of Nervous and Mental Disorders, 161,* 157–165.

Herkenham, M., Lynn, A. B., Little, M. D., Johnson, M. R., Melvin, L. S., De Costa, B. R., & Rice, K. C. (1990). Cannabinoid receptor localization in brain. *Proceedings of the National Academy of Sciences of the USA, 87,* 1932–1936.

Hollister, L. E. (1986). Health aspects of cannabis. *Pharmacology Review, 38,* 2–20.

Horowitz, M. J. (1969). Flashbacks: Recurrent intrusive images after the use of LSD *American Journal of Psychiatry, 126,* 565–569.

Janet, P. (1920). *The major symptoms of hysteria.* New York: Macmillan.

Kardiner, A. (1941). The traumatic neuroses of war. Psychosomatic Monograph II-III, Washington, DC: National Research Council.

Kluft, R. F. (1987). An update on multiple personality disorder. *Hospital and Community Psychiatry, 38,* 363–373.

Kolb, L. C., Burris, B. C., & Griffiths, S. (1984). Propranolol and clonidine in the treatment of the chronic post traumatic stress disorders of war. In B. A. van der Kolk (Ed.), *Post traumatic stress disorder: Psychological and biological sequelae* (pp. 97–107). Washington DC: American Psychiatric Press.

Kosten, T. R., & Krystal, J. H. (1988). Biological mechanisms in post traumatic stress disorder: Relevance for substance abuse. In M. Galenter (Ed.), Recent developments in alcoholism. Vol. VI, pp. 49–68. New York: Plenum.

Krupitsky, E. [personal communication].

Krystal, H. (1968). *Massive psychic trauma.* New York: International Universities Press.

Krystal, J. H., Woods, S. W., Hill, C. L., & Charney, D. S. (1988). Characteristics of self-defined panic attacks. New Research Program & Abstracts, *American Psychiatric Association, 141st Annual Meeting,* Montreal, Quebec, Canada, May 7–12, NR 263.

Krystal, J. H., Kosten, T. R., Perry, B. D., Southwick, S., Mason, J. W., & Giller, E. L., Jr. (1989). Neurobiological aspects of PTSD: Review of clinical and preclinical studies. *Behavioral Therapy, 20,* 177–198.

Krystal, J. H., Karper, L. P., Seibyl, J. P., Freeman, G. K., Delaney, R., Bremner, J. D., Heninger, G. R., Bowers,

M. B., Jr., & Charney, D. S. (1994). Subanesthetic effects of the NMDA antagonist, ketamine, in humans: Psychotomimetic, perceptual, cognitive, and neuroendocrine effects. *Archives of General Psychiatry, 51,* 199–214.

Krystal, J. H., Bennett A., Bremner J. D., Southwick, S., & Charney, D. S. (1995). Toward a cognitive neuroscience of dissociation and altered memory functions in post-traumatic stress disorder. In M. J. Friedman, D. S. Charney, & A. Y. Deutch (Eds.), *Neurobiological and clinical consequences of stress: From normal adaptation to PTSD* (pp. 239–269). New York: Raven Press.

Krystal, J. H., Karper, L. P., Bennett, A., D'Souza, D. C., Abi-Dargham, A., Morrissey, K. A., Abi-Saab, D., Bremner, J. D., Bowers, M. B., Jr., Suckow, R. F., Stetson, P., Heninger, G. R., & Charney, D. S. (1998a). Interactive effects of subanesthetic ketamine and subhypnotic lorazepam in humans. *Psychopharmacology, 135,* 213–229.

Krystal, J. H., Nagy, L. M. Southwick, S. M., & Charney D. S. (1998b). Initial clinical evidence of genetic contributions to post-traumatic stress disorder. In Y. Danieli (Ed.), *An international handbook of multigenerational legacies of trauma* (pp. 657–667). New York: Plenum.

Krystal, J. H., Abi-Dargham, A., Laruelle, M., Moghaddam, B. (1999a). Pharmacologic model psychoses. In D. S. Charney, E. Nestler, & B. S. Bunney (Eds.), *Neurobiology of mental illness* (pp. 214–224). New York: Oxford University Press.

Krystal, J. H., D'Souza, D. C., Karper, L. P., Bennett, A., Abi-Dargham, A., Abi-Saab, D., Cassello, K., Bowers, M. B., Jr., Vegso, S., Heninger, G. R., & Charney, D. S. (1999b). Interactive effects of subanesthetic ketamine and haloperidol in healthy human subjects. *Psychopharmacology, 145,* 193–204.

Lahti, A. C., Holcomb, H. H., Medoff, D. R., & Tamminga, C. A. (1995). Ketamine activates psychosis and alters limbic blood flow in schizophrenia. *Neuroreports, 6,* 869–872.

Lewis, D. A. (1992). The catecholaminergic innervation of primate prefrontal cortex. *Journal of Neural Transmission, 36* (suppl), 179–200.

Liberzon, I., Taylor, S. F., Fig, L. M., & Koeppe, R. A. (1997). Alteration of corticothalamic perfusion ratios during a PTSD flashback. *Depression and Anxiety, 4,* 146–150.

Lipper, S., Davidson, J. R. T., Grady, T. A., Edinger, J., Hammett, E. B., Mahorney, S. L., & Cavenar, J. O. (1986). Preliminary study of carbamazepine in post traumatic stress disorder. *Psychosomatics, 27,* 849–854.

Lipschitz, D. S., D'Souza, D. C., White, J. A., Charney, D. S., & Krystal, J. H. (1997). Clozapine blockade of ketamine effects in healthy subjects. *Biological Psychiatry, 41*(S):23S (abstract #76).

Luby, E. D., Cohen, B. D., Rosenbaum, G., Gottlieb, J. S. & Kelley, R. (1959). Study of a new schizophreno-mimetic drug-sernyl. *AMA Archives of Neurology and Psychiatry, 81,* 363–369.

Mathew, R. J., Wilson, W. H., Humphreys, D. F., Lowe, J. V., & Wiethe, K. E. (1992). Regional cerebral blood flow after marijuana smoking. *Journal Cerebral Blood Flow and Metabolism, 12,* 750–758.

McDougle, C. J., & Southwick, S. M. (1990). Emergence of an alternate personality in combat-related posttraumatic stress disorder. *Hospital and Community Psychiatry, 41,* 554–556.

McGee, R. (1984). Flashbacks and memory phenomena: A comment on flashback phenomena-clinical and diagnostic dilemmas. *Journal of Nervous and Mental Disorders, 172,* 273–278.

Melges, F. T., Tinklenberg, J. R., Hollister, L. E., Gillespie, H. K. (1970). Temporal disintegration and depersonalization during marihuana intoxication. *Archives of General Psychiatry, 23,* 204–210.

Mellman, T. A., & Davis, G. C. (1985). Combat-related flashbacks in post-traumatic stress disorder: Phenomenology and similarity to panic attacks. *Journal of Clinical Psychiatry, 46,* 379–382.

Moghaddam, B. (1993). Stress preferentially activates extraneuronal levels of excitatory amino acids in the prefrontal cortex: A comparison to hippocampus and basal ganglia. *Journal of Neurochemistry, 60,* 1650–1657.

Moghaddam, B., Adams, B., Verma, A., & Daly, D. (1997). Activation of glutamatergic neurotransmission by ketamine: A novel step in the pathway from NMDA receptor blockage to dopaminergic and cognitive disruptions associated with the prefrontal cortex. *Journal of Neuroscience, 17,* 2921–2927.

Pitts, F. N., & McClure, J. N. (1967). Lactate metabolism in anxiety neurosis. *New England Journal of Medicine, 277,* 1329–1336.

Rainey, J. M., Jr., Aleem, A., Ortiz, A., Yeragani, V., Pohl, R., & Berchou, R. (1987). A laboratory procedure for the induction of flashbacks. *American Journal of Psychiatry, 144,* 1317–1319.

Randall, P. K., Bremner, J. D., Krystal, J. H., Heninger, G. R., Nicolaou, A. L., & Charney, D. S. (1995). Effects of the benzodiazepine antagonist, flumazenil, in PTSD. *Biological Psychiatry, 38,* 319–324.

Rasmussen, K., Glennon, R. A., & Aghajanian, G. K. (1986). Phenethylamine hallucinogens in the locus coeruleus: Potency of action correlates with rank order of 5-HT_2 binding affinity. *European Journal of Pharmacology, 132,* 79–82.

Rataud, J., Debarnot, F., Mary, V., Pratt, J., & Stutzmann, J. M. (1994). Comparative study of voltage-sensitive sodium channel blockers in focal ischemia and electric convulsions in rodents. *Neuoscience Letters, 172,* 19–23.

Rausch, S. L., van der Kolk, B. A., Fisler, R. E., Alpert, N. M., Orr, S. P., Savage, C. R., Fischman, A. J., Jenicke, M. A., & Pitman, R. K. (1996). A symptom provocation study of posttraumatic stress disorder using positron emission tomography and script-driven imagery. *Archives of General Psychiatry, 53,* 380–387.

Ray, W. J. Dissociation in normal populations. (1996). In L. K. Michelson, & W. J. Ray (Eds.), *Handbook of dissociation: Theoretical, empirical, and clinical perspectives* (pp. 51–68). New York: Plenum.

Rosenbaum, G., Cohen, B. D., Luby, E. D., Gottlieb, J. S., & Yelen, D. (1959). Comparison of sernyl with other drugs. *AMA Archives of General Psychiatry, 1,* 651–656.

Sapolsky, R. M. (1992). *Stress, the aging brain, and the mechanisms of neuron death.* Cambridge, MA: MIT Press.

Savage, C. (1995). Variations in ego feeling induced by D-lysergic acid diethylamide (LSD-25). *Psychoanalytic Review, 42,* 1–16.

Schoepp, D. D., & Conn, P. J. (1993). Metabotropic glutamate receptors in brain function and pathology. *Trends in Pharmacologic Science, 14,* 13–25.

Southwick, S. M. [personal communication].

Southwick, S. M., Krystal, J. H., Morgan, C. A., Johnson, D. R., Nagy, L. M., Nicolaou, A., Heninger, G. R., & Charney, D. S. (1993). Abnormal noradrenergic function in post traumatic stress disorder. *Archives of General Psychiatry, 50,* 266–274.

Southwick, S. M., Krystal, J. H., Bremner, J. D., Morgan , C. A. III, Nicolaou, A., Nagy, L. M., Johnson, D. R ., Heninger, G. R., & Charney, D. S. (1997). Noradrenergic and serotonergic function in post-traumatic stress disorder. *Archives of General Psychiatry, 54,* 246–254.

Spiegel, D., Hunt, T., & Dondershine, H. E. (1988). Dissociation and hypnotizability in posttraumatic stress disorder. *American Journal of Psychiatry, 145,* 301–305.

Spiegel, D., & Cardena, E. (1991). Disintegrated experience: The dissociative disorders revisited. *Journal of Abnormal Psychology, 100,* 366–378.

Stanton, M. D., Mintz, J., & Franklin, R. M. (1976). Drug flashbacks. II. Some additional findings. *International Journal of Addictions, 11,* 53–69.

Starke, K., Borowski, E., & Endo, T. (1975). Preferential blockade of presynaptic α-adrenoceptors by yohimbine. *European Journal of Pharmacology, 34,* 385–388.

Strassman, R., Qualls, C., Uhlenhuth, E., & Kellner, R. (1994). Dose-response study of N, N-dimethyltryptimine in humans, II. Subjective effects and preliminary results of a new rating scale. *Archives of General Psychiatry, 51,* 98–108.

van der Kolk, B., Greenberg, M., Boyd, H., & Krystal, J. (1985). Inescapable shock, neurotransmitters, and addiction to trauma: Toward a psychobiology of post traumatic stress. *Biological Psychiatry, 20,* 314–325.

Wang, S. J., Huang, C. C., Hsu, K. S., Tsai, J. J., & Gean, P. W. (1996). Inhibition of N-type calcium currents by lamotrigine in rat amygdalar neurons. *Neuroreports, 7,* 3037–3040.

VI

Treating the Survivor
in the Acute and Chronic
Aftermath of an Adverse Event

The impact of defining PTSD via the medical-psychological model is ultimately measured by the effects of subsequent therapies. Hence, evaluating the efficacy of different treatments for PTSD is essential for the practical task of clinical work and also for heuristic purposes. Many forms of therapy have been offered to PTSD patients, some based on approaches that predated the definition of stress-related disorders. The enlightened clinician may find the plethora of divergent solutions daunting, particularly given the limited efficacy of each. Overestimating human power to reverse the effect of severe traumatization and idealizing or expecting too much from the clinician may lead to unnecessary frustration or despair. On the other hand, clearly, certain kinds of symptoms can be substantially improved by current therapies, and indeed, even partial improvement may be of great benefit to those who are suffering.

This section summarizes the current knowledge concerning theory, implementation, and efficacy of the major treatment approaches to PTSD. It can be clearly seen that most treatment modalities, when properly applied, are somewhat efficacious. What still must be done in the field is to properly match trauma survivors to the type of therapeutic modality that is likely to work best for that person. Indeed, although it has not yet been explicitly demonstrated, different treatments may work better depending on the stage of illness, type of traumatization, type of comorbid problems, and other variables, not the least of which are cultural and social. Although each chapter focuses on a particular treatment, we actually advocate the use of multimodal treatments and hope that clinicians will synthesize many different approaches in their treatment of patients.

As a prelude to discussing treatment options, Jeannine Monnier and Stevan Hobfoll cogently express what is being lost during trauma. As such, the authors offer an alternative way of viewing trauma exposure in terms of loss of resources. It follows that treatment strategies would be aimed at assessing the magnitude of loss, as well as evaluating the particular impact of these losses on the individual's well-being, integrity, and chances for recovery. Grounded in empirical studies, the theory of resource loss is introduced here as a paradigm for clinical reflection relevant to the treatment of individuals and groups alike.

Elizabeth Meadows and Edna Foa present a review of cognitive behavioral therapy as applied to trauma-related disorders. These treatments have been widely studied and found to be among the most efficacious in alleviating symptoms. Particularly impressive about the approach suggested by the authors is that it has been formulated to parallel conceptual understanding of the effects of trauma. If what is traumatic to individuals is a consequence of either learned responses or erroneous assumptions about the way the event could have been prevented or otherwise controlled, then directly addressing such learned behaviors and related cognitions constitutes a direct avenue for achieving treatment gains. Although often viewed as mechanistic and avoiding deeper layers of psychic experience, this approach in fact addresses emotions, thoughts, behaviors, and imagination in a way that is often difficult to address using other modalities. It also offers the advantage of dealing directly with the traumatic event and seeing exposure as the true cause of subsequent psychological distress. In so doing, it avoids the pitfalls that have led to the notion that trauma survivors must have had a preexisting weakness that dictated the traumatic stress response.

Randall Marshall, Rachel Yehuda, and Stanley Bone try to link the traditional, time-honored psychodynamic approach to the current needs of trauma survivors. Rather than offering a narrow interpretation of traumatization, its antecedents, and its consequences, they cover a large area of expertise gathered through years of tackling the resistant trauma survivor. Indeed, insights gained by applying disciplined psychodynamic psychotherapy are reflected in this thoughtful synthesis. For example, the intent of psychodynamic psychotherapy is shifted from exploring the event to exploring the meaning of the event, and its goal in the severely traumatized becomes a stabilization, rather than "cure." The treatment of trauma-related disorders is a major challenge for psychodynamically oriented psychotherapists as many shorter and seemingly more efficacious therapies are advertised. However, if one does not address the profound layers of meaning that traumas may pervert—as psychodynamic therapy does— then the cognitive dimension of the response to trauma is likely to be ignored in the long run.

As with all other therapies, the pharmacotherapy of PTSD does not offer uniquely effective solutions to either the complex neurobiology of PTSD or its clinical presentation. Arieh Shalev and Omer Bonne provide an updated review of empirical studies of the pharmacotherapy of PTSD. Although clearly aware of the gaps between neurobiological theories and current implementation of pharmacological agents, nonetheless, the authors provide a framework for the clinician to assess and implement a sound pharmacological approach to PTSD, including the implementation of newly available agents.

Given how long-lasting and treatment-resistant chronic PTSD may be, it has certainly been understandable that clinicians have searched for ways to treat trauma survivors in the immediate aftermath of an event. The hope of such treatments is to intervene when the traumatic response is still incubating, so as to disrupt this process and prevent the development of this disorder. One such attempt was in the development of Critical Incidence Stress Debriefing (CISD). Despite the seductive promise offered by being present at the time of the trauma to offer such help, Ingrid Carlier reveals that long-term studies have failed to show a preventative effect of CISD on trauma-related disorder. The reason for these unfulfilled promises may in fact have to do with the biological observations noted in the previous section. A careful documentation of heterogeneity in the acute aftermath of trauma may in the future delineate the subgroups of patients for whom immediate interventions might be most useful.

Back to community resources, Shmuel Lahad, Yehuda Shacham, and Shulamit Niv report experience addressing traumatized children within their immediate social environment, Lahad et al. describe a model for community interventions in which individual strengths and coping resources are primarily addressed and present data from two studies in which this model has been applied. Their observation of children evacuated during a disaster highlights the role of family support in mediating the effect of stressful events. They also show that successful psychological intervention in a school disaster could reduce the effect of subsequent traumatization.

23

Conservation of Resources in Individual and Community Reactions to Traumatic Stress

JEANNINE MONNIER AND STEVAN E. HOBFOLL

Community stressors, such as natural and man-made disasters, major epidemics, famine, war, and political upheaval, are powerful events that impact individuals, families, and communities alike (Weisaeth, 1992). The number of community stressors that occur yearly is staggering. For example, Solomon and Green (1992) reported that approximately 2 million U.S. households experience injuries and physical damage each year from fire, floods, hurricanes, and the like. Freedy et al. (1993) reported that between 1974 and 1980 there were 37 major catastrophes in the United States alone. Furthermore, Vogel and Vernberg (1993) remind us that dozens of countries are at war or suffer violent internal strife at any one time. An individual's reaction to extreme stress can lead to the development of individual psychopathology, family and relationship turmoil, substance abuse, and loss of employment (Kilpatrick et al., 1989; McFarlane, 1987; Resnick et al., 1993; Solomon et al., 1987). On the community level, such stress may mean the breakdown of social codes and networks, as well as increased disease and violence (Wallace, 1990; Wallace et al., 1992; Wardak, 1992). Additionally, the manner in which communities cope with such stressors has both short-term and long-term implications for individual community members, families, social institutions, and the community as a whole. Interventions have been developed for the previously mentioned individual reactions to trauma (e.g., Foa et al., 1989; Resick & Schnicke, 1993). However, little is known about the way communities manage such stressors and about the best ways to intervene communitywide after such events.

de Jong (1995) states that the impact of trauma following a man-made disaster or natural disaster is often too great to manage by current models of psychology or psychiatry, which are based on individuals and crisis intervention or brief individual

JEANNINE MONNIER • National Crime Victims Research and Treatment Center, Medical University of South Carolina, Charleston, South Carolina 29425. STEVAN E. HOBFOLL • Department of Psychology, Kent State University, Kent, Ohio 44242.

International Handbook of Human Response to Trauma, edited by Shalev, Yehuda, and McFarlane. Kluwer Academic / Plenum Publishers, New York, 2000.

psychotherapy. An individualistic perspective may not be the most helpful perspective when examining the broader social context of community reactions to traumatic stress because it minimizes objective reality and fails to capture collective responding. Stepping beyond the individual and examining community issues can improve the functioning of a community as a whole. As a result, this can also improve the functioning of community members. Most mental health professionals have limited training or experience in working at broader community, national, or international levels and therefore are not well prepared to intervene on these levels. However, mental health professionals are important in both the short-term and long-term for victims of traumatic events (Punamaki, 1989; Westermeyer, 1987; Williams & Berry, 1991). New models of stress are needed to provide mental health professionals with a framework for intervention at the community level.

Conservation of Resources

Conservation of Resources (COR) theory is a general stress model that has been applied to both individuals (Hobfoll, 1988, 1989) and communities (Hobfoll et al., 1995) in an effort to best explain the impact of stress. COR theory posits that stress can be conceptualized in terms of resource loss and is based on the premise that individuals strive to obtain, retain, and protect their resources. Arguments have been made that this same process applies to communities, in that communities also work to acquire and maintain resources (Hobfoll et al., 1995). Stress occurs when individuals or communities are faced with significant loss of resources or a threat of significant loss. COR theory also holds that stress occurs when resources are invested without a significant gain of resources, resulting in an overall loss of resources. However, if resources are invested and additional resources are gained, the occurrence of stress can be eliminated or its duration reduced. In sum, loss of resources can cause significant distress, and resources can be used to limit the impact of stressful events on psychological well-being (Freedy et al., 1993; Hobfoll, 1991). Following this premise, COR theory allows predictions about the social context of community stressors and thus seems to be especially germane to prevention and intervention efforts for communities in the face of major stressors. It provides a framework for understanding how traumatic stress acts immediately on individuals and on communities through loss experienced due to the initial event (e.g., a home during a fire, loss of health during a motor vehicle accident, the loss of roads and bridges during an earthquake) and over time through the further loss of resources (e.g., time off from work, lifelong injuries, draining of financial reserves).

The resources that are integral to the underlying principles of this theory fall into one of four categories: personal characteristics, objects, conditions, and energies. These same categories of resources can be employed when considering both individuals and communities. Personal characteristics are attributes that are valued in and of themselves or that facilitate the acquisition or protection of other resources. Personal characteristics of the individual include occupational skills and sense of self-esteem. When considering these same types of resources for the community, personal characteristics extend to such concepts as community pride and community cohesion. Object resources for an individual can include tangible material goods such as one's car, home, and clothing, and object resources for the community can include roads, bridges, and industry. Condition resources are social structures and circumstances that apply to both individuals and larger groups. For individuals, tenure or seniority at work and a good marriage are included in condition resources. For a community, conditions resources can include availability of employment and the level of emergency services. Energy resources are important because they can be exchanged or used to obtain and retain other resources. On an individual level, such resources include money, credit, and insurance. On a community level, energy resources include money, credit, and heating and transportation fuel reserves. The above-mentioned resources highlight the importance of their consideration as key components of everyday life, and indeed, it has been shown that the loss of such resources elicits significant distress (Freedy et al., 1993; Kaniasty & Norris, 1993).

Existing theories of stress tend to focus on individual perceptions of stressful events, suggesting that events are stressful only if an individual perceives them as such. However, it may be too simplistic to assume that events are stressful only to the extent that they are perceived as such. COR theory frames stress in the context of loss of resources and suggests that people's actual loss of resources and their perception of the loss of resources are what influence their reactions to stress. Additionally, COR theory posits that these perceptions of loss are not idiographic, but are realistic interpretations of one's environment, and that others in that same environment would make similar interpretations, especially in the face of major community stressors. Lazarus and Folkman (1984) concurred with this point and argued that perception plays a lesser role in major stressors because such events would cause stress for nearly everyone. Additionally, existing resources can offer a buffer against the negative impact of resource loss. Therefore, the impact of different stressors depends in part on how extensive the loss was, how critical the lost resources were, and how many other resources are available to protect against further resource loss.

Principles of COR Theory

COR theory is based on a number of principles and corollaries that can aid in predicting and developing interventions for individuals and communities after major stressors.

Principle 1: The Primacy of Loss

COR theory proposes that a resource loss is more powerful than an equivalent resource gain. The power of loss has been well documented across individuals and communities. McFarlane (1992) demonstrated that major fires, which occurred in the Australian bush, did not produce severe, prolonged psychological distress. Only the individuals who were part of communities that were severely damaged by the fire, experienced long-term distress. Similar findings resulted from a study of cyclone survivors. Only those who experienced continued losses, such as loss of a home and dislocation from support systems, experienced serious, long-term psychological impairment (Parker, 1977). Moreover, longitudinal studies of Buffalo Creek flood survivors showed that loss of community support, loss of support from neighbors and friends, and length of dislocation were powerful predictors of outcome (Green & Gleser, 1983). Additionally, it was found that the level of resource loss is strongly related to distress, and is more important than demographic or coping variables in psychological outcome for people after a hurricane and an earthquake (Freedy et al., 1994; Freedy et al., 1992).

An equal, yet opposite, impact of resource gain has not been found; it has been shown that resource loss is strongly related to individual psychological distress, but resource gains alone are not related to distress, unless they occur in the wake of loss (Hobfoll & Lerman, 1988; Hobfoll & Lilly, 1993). Gains that are equivalent in magnitude to losses (i.e., gain versus loss of the same object) may have less of an impact for several reasons. For example, consider the amount of time and energy required to acquire a house, car, or other similar resources compared with the time in which these resources can be lost in a natural disaster. With this illustration, it can be seen that in one day a person and/or community can lose what has taken years to gain. However, resource gains do become important in the face of resource loss because they can be used to stop or curtail losses (see Figure 1; Hobfoll et al., 1988). For example, a small gain in mastery may be critical in withstanding threats to the self, and having insurance becomes critical in the face of the losses that result from disaster.

Principle 2: Resource Investment

Because resource loss can have such devastating effects on individuals and communities, efforts must be made to obtain new resources and to retain and protect existing resources. Investment of resources can offset current loss, protect against future loss, or contribute to resource gain. In turn, investment can improve well-being and thus be viewed as a key part of the coping process (Schönpflug, 1985). Because resources are employed to reduce stress, the more stress one experiences, the more resources are invested to reduce the existing stress. This investment of resources leads to a depletion of resource reservoirs and, if resources are not actively replenished, can reduce de-

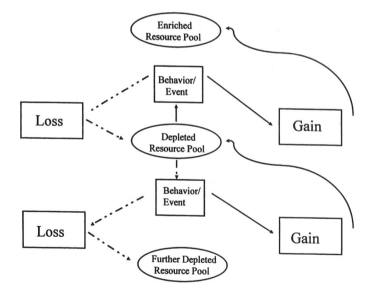

FIGURE 1.   Loss and gain spirals can result from a behavior or event. Loss after a behavior or event depletes one's resource pool, and additional action must be taken to replenish the resource pool. Gains enable one to replenish resources.

fenses against future stress. Additionally, if resources are invested and gains are not made, distress will occur or increase (Wells et al., 1997).

Many examples of the way resource investment enhances coping ability can be found on both the individual and community level. For instance, on an individual level, people invest energy in developing and maintaining social support networks so that they are intact in a time of need (Cohen & Wills, 1985). Additionally, Holahan and Moos (1986) found that personal and social resources act together to buffer against the negative impact of stress. This same process is at work on the community level. For example, money, energy, and time are just a few resources that are invested in the maintenance of emergency services such as a fire service and police force, so that the community will be protected during times of crisis. Without the initial and continued investment of resources, the ability of an individual or community to cope with stressors would be greatly impaired.

Once invested, a resource is lost (Schönpflug, 1985). The cost or loss of this resource is often weighed against the potential benefit or gain that results from the investment. Those who invest wisely will increase their resource reservoir; those who invest poorly will reduce their resource reservoir. Wise investments can act to offset future loss because they will add to the potential for coping with future stressors. Schönpflug's (1985) work in this area of resource investment has provided both theory and laboratory analogs explaining how resource investment options are considered and evaluated by individuals. There is an existing bias toward action in the face of a stressor. However, when coping is viewed as a resource investment process and the risks involved in resource investment are considered, the choice not to act becomes a viable option. This is especially true for those with low resources, to whom loss of any existing resources would be extremely detrimental. Consider, for example, the plight of a woman with three children who is the victim of domestic violence and has not been permitted to work outside the home by her abusive spouse. Does she risk losing the benefits of shelter, food, and clothing for her and her children for the potential gain of her own physical safety? Many women decide that the potential for loss far outweighs the uncertainty of any gains and remain in abusive relationships (Rusbult & Martz, 1995).

The Cycle of Loss and Gain

A number of corollaries emerge from the principles of loss salience and resource investment. These more finely tuned points involving the impact of stress and the consequences of resource loss and gain that can provide additional information for designing and implementing individual community itnervention programs after a traumatic event.

Corollary 1: Greater Resources Reduce Vulnerability to Resource Loss

To counteract resource loss after a stressful event, one must have resources. Additionally, to gain resources, one must have resources above and beyond those necessary for everyday existence and must be able to invest these resources to ensure resource gain.

Following from this, the first corollary of COR theory posits that individuals who have greater resources are less vulnerable to resource loss and more capable of resource gain. This premise also holds true for communities. Those communities that have more resources to start with will be better able to cope with stress than those that have fewer resources. Such resource-endowed communities will be better able to invest resources to aid the community in the face of a stressful event and will be more likely to have resources that fit the demand of a crisis. As a result, they will be more prepared to cope with the crisis at hand. Furthermore, in wealthy communities, reserves will be greater and therefore last longer in the face of a crisis.

Corollary 2: Initial Loss Begets Future Loss

The second corollary of COR theory states that initial loss begets future loss. As stated earlier, initial resource loss increases one's vulnerability to further resource loss (see Figure 1). After an initial resource loss, communities and individuals have fewer or less powerful resources to cope with any additional stressors that occur after the first loss event (Hobfoll, 1991). A community or individual left with fewer resources is more vulnerable to further resource loss. This cycle of loss has been labeled a loss spiral. COR theory predicts that such loss cycles have advancing momentum and strength. When losses are contained, distress and impairment will be limited. However, if this spiral cannot be contained, the resulting distress and impairment will be great (Freedy et al., 1994; Green, 1995). Following from this, individuals who have minimal resources are more likely to experience loss spirals in the wake of major crises (Hobfoll, 1988, 1989).

This same loss spiral can occur on the community level. Resources exist within a community because they are needed and helpful for the development and prosperity of the community and its members. When these resources are disrupted, the natural progress of the community is also disrupted. This interrelationship among resources suggests that resource loss in one domain will reverberate into other domains, such that one loss event (e.g., fire) will lead to further loss of resources (e.g., unemployment, homelessness, and draining of financial reserves) and propel a community into a loss spiral. The longer resources are strained and the more resources expended, the more difficulty a community will have in meeting its usual obligations (Trickett, 1984).

Corollary 3: Gain Cycles

As loss spirals occur, so do gain spirals. Unlike resource loss, however, resource gain is thought to be a slow process, and gain cycles are far less powerful than loss cycles. Resource gain usually involves risking of resources to meet goals and aspirations. The motivation behind resource gain is either a product of desiring to better one's self or the social system within which one exists (e.g., family, organization) or is intended to offset potential future loss (Aspinwall & Taylor, 1997). Positive outcomes of resource investment increase the number of available resources to protect against future loss and add to resource reservoirs. In this context, resource gain is not as immediate as the need to reduce loss.

Corollary 4: Guarding Resources

Individuals are likely to take a defensive stance to guard against the loss of their resources. Such a defensive posture enables one to hold resources in reserve so they can be used to forestall the impact of a possible major loss sequence. Guarding resources in this manner may at first appear to be a poor coping strategy because it prevents resource investment. However, such an approach does have benefits; it holds resource reservoirs intact, which will ensure that resources are ready and accessible in the event of a crisis. This is particularly true for individuals and communities that have few resources.

For example, Jerusalem et al. (1995) found that individuals who experienced personal loss were less likely to invest in helping others in their community who were more severely impacted by a community stressor. Having themselves lost resources, they may have felt that this further resource expenditure would have placed them at undue risk.

Intervention

Clearly, disasters impact mental health in both the short-term and long-term (Bravo et al., 1990; Green, 1995; Norris et al., 1994; Palinkas et al., 1993). Researchers have suggested that the implementation of interventions that limit resource loss immediately after disasters might be particularly beneficial for individuals and communities (Ørner & Thompson, 1993; Solomon, 1986; Weisaeth, 1992). Additionally, at least in some populations interventions can aid in the acquisition of resources, leading to reductions of long-term mental health risks (Freedy & Hobfoll, 1994). COR theory provides a possible framework for such interventions and indicates that intervention should be based on resource investment and conservation. A series of recommendations stemming from the principles of COR theory was developed by Hobfoll and Lilly (1993) for interventions with individuals. These recommendations were broadened to encompass the needs of communities and to explain reaction to and recovery from community stress (see Hobfoll et al., 1995). Integrating these recommendations would provide a comprehensive approach to intervention after a large-scale disaster. Such an integrated approach is discussed below.

COR theory stipulates that limiting and preventing resource loss will best minimize the negative outcome after a stressor. To ensure that appropriate resources are targeted for intervention, the structure and needs of that community must be assessed before intervention begins. Interventionists should first assess the extent of loss or damage to both people and property. Next, resource reservoirs must be assessed to evaluate which resources are available for interventionists to employ. Finally, expectations about the long-term consequences of these stressful events must be assessed to inform the interventionist how to best direct their energies.

During and after the assessment process, mental health professionals should limit interference with more immediate services, such as emergency services workers, and enable them to perform their duties in entirety. The primacy of emergency services exists because emergency personnel have the ability to limit devastation (e.g., limit the death toll by rescuing individuals), whereas other professionals, including mental health professionals, are better suited to help individuals cope with their losses and limit further losses after the stressor. Additionally, immediate efforts should be made to eliminate the risk of further injury to community members and emergency workers alike.

The next step for interventionists is to identify community and subcommunity leaders who can educate interventionists about the character and the scope of the problems they will be confronting due to the disaster (de Jong, 1995; Trickett, 1995), and to provide information regarding the consequences of a traumatic event as perceived by the community. Community leaders can also provide information about the communities' coping strategies (including religious and political coping behaviors) and the help-seeking behavior of community members (e.g., willingness to travel to community centers for assistance). Finally, information about community resources such as health-care facilities, relief organizations, and other formal and cultural aids can be provided by community leaders.

Initiation of gain cycles can help to increase resources, which, in turn, can help to limit future loss. It follows that resource gain can be used in two ways which will greatly benefit communities. First, gain cycles can be initiated to build reserves before disasters occur. Prevention efforts should firmly establish gain cycles, so that future loss can be limited and better managed when and if it does occur (de Jong, 1995; Freedy et al., 1992). Second, after a disaster, gain cycles can be initiated to counteract loss. For example, if homes are destroyed by an earthquake, important initial areas for gains would include helping people take initial steps to clear debris, obtain midterm shelter, and navigate insurance processes.

When acute traumas cause severe loss to individuals or communities, people are typically handicapped in dealing with normal life (Kaniasty & Norris, 1993; Pearlin et al., 1981) and thus more vulnerable to future physical and emotional stress. In the case of more chronic stressors, such as wars and chemical disasters, the draining of resources is even more salient (Baum, 1987). The long-term demands of these stressors compete with new demands for the same diminishing set of resources. Thus, interventionists must work with community leaders to develop a plan of action that will best ensure that key community resources are targeted for intervention first and foremost (Green et al., 1990). Additionally, plans must be set in place that begin gain cycles, so that resource reservoirs can be naturally replenished over the course of time.

Communities that have limited resources may not have the resources to adequately meet additional demands placed on their systems by a disaster. Communities with strong and plentiful resources may also begin to falter if they must expend too many of their coping resources. Interventionists should be cognizant of the secondary losses that may occur as a result of resource depletion. When secondary losses begin, low coping reserves will reduce a community's ability to manage usual demands, as well as new demands. For example, a community that had the means to protect its members against crime may lose these abilities following a political upheaval. Individuals who are forced into refugee camps often become the victims of robbery, rape, and kidnapping (de Jong, 1995). Providing a means to secure refugee camps would limit the likelihood of these secondary resource losses after a traumatic stressor.

COR theory suggests that because loss cycles occur more rapidly and impact more severely than do gain cycles, interventions should target resource loss and the slowing or cessation of such loss. This point becomes even more poignant when interventionists are dealing with resource-poor communities, because their resource reservoirs are likely to be drained quickly. Social services such as public health care, low-cost housing, or social welfare systems are often important components of resource-poor communities and are likely to be the first impacted by a communitywide traumatic event. As a result, communities that are highly dependent on these services will be severely impacted (Jerusalem et al., 1995). Therefore, in addition to any new difficulties caused by the traumatic event, intervention should be targeted at reinforcing such social services so that they are not interrupted or so that the interruption is minimal.

Interventionists must approach communities following a traumatic stressor to reduce the likelihood of barriers to successful interventions. COR theory can be utilized to predict potential barriers and to provide a means of overcoming these barriers. Because community stressors often enter the political arena and are used by agencies, department administrators, politicians, and community leaders to make gains with their constituents, subcommunity leaders will act to limit the loss to their subcommunity members. This will place subcommunities in competition with each other for the same resources. Identifying and working with the leaders of subcommunities will allow interventionists to best assess community strengths and weaknesses and to access resources for all community members (Norris et al., 1995). Additionally, because actions are often considered for their potential negative side effects and not necessarily for their benefits, some leaders will be slow to act for fear that they will experience negative repercussions if the intervention does not proceed successfully. COR theory offers clear pathways for intervention that will minimize danger while maximizing return for all community members and thus should minimize the reluctance to act.

Another potential barrier to successful intervention involves poor communication of information within a community after a stressor. Social interaction, in part, may exacerbate stress, especially through the spread of unfavorable news or untruths (Hobfoll & London, 1986; Kessler et al., 1985; Riley & Eckenrode, 1986). Thus, a means of communicating with community members should be quickly developed. One voice or a unified group should convey accurate information to the community members and keep them informed of any changes or news, which can help them regain control over their environment and help them make informed choices of how best to proceed.

Conclusions

Community stressors can have severe and long-lasting effects on individuals and communities as a whole. Interventions must be designed and implemented that can act to reasonably reduce the impact of such stressors. To date, most research in the area of stress and coping has focused on individual response to stress and ways to reduce the individual's negative response to stress. However, community perspectives may be more helpful in assisting both the individual community member and the community as a whole following traumatic events. COR theory provides an avenue for community intervention which is focused on reducing resource loss and initiating resource gain for both the individual and the community.

If we are correct in our thesis that the stress literature is biased toward a perception-based view of stress and the impact of perceptions of stress on well-being, then it is natural that most interventions work to change perceptions of stressors and stress. The difficulty with this approach can be seen no more clearly than when examining community stressors, where large groups of people have perceived one event as overwhelming, disrupting, exhausting, and the like. How can perceptions of earthquakes, tornadoes, and plane crashes, or the undeniable trauma, carnage, and losses that result from these events be changed? COR theory suggests that these events are traumatic and that intervention cannot simply target changing perceptions but must work to change the real-life circumstances of victims of such trauma. COR theory specifically targets resources as the mechanism for this change. Although perceptions do play a part in stress reactions, it may be most helpful to see those perceptions as a result of resource loss. Thus, if initial resource loss could be limited or further resource loss prevented, the formation of negative perceptions could be prevented and/or eliminated.

It has been shown that resources have important implications for individuals under both normal stress and extreme traumatic stress (Butcher & Dunn, 1989; Freedy et al., 1992, 1993; Green & Gleser, 1983; Hobfoll, 1991). For a community facing a major stressor, we also suggest that the presence or absence of resources will best predict outcome. If resources are depleted over time and cannot be replenished, the consequences for a community and its individual members will be severe and long-lasting. As with individuals, communities may require some outside assistance and intervention to help overcome the trauma and start gain cycles.

Researchers and clinicians can also help limit the impact of extreme stress on communities and community members by conducting more research on decision making, communication, and organizational breakdowns in the face of extreme loss. Such information can aid in designing and implementing more effective community interventions after traumatic events. The power of a successful intervention should not be ignored. It can have lasting impact on a community and make the same community more likely to accept intervention in the future. In sum, COR theory emphasizes the importance of limiting initial losses because it is these losses that will lead to future losses and have a cascading effect on individuals and communities.

References

Aspinwall, L. G., & Taylor, S. E. (1997). A stitch in time: Self-regulation and proactive coping. *Psychological Bulletin, 121*, 417–436.

Baum, A. (1987). Toxins, technology, and natural disasters. In G. R. Vanderbos & B. K. Bryant (Eds.), *Cataclysms, crises, and catastrophes: Psychology in action.* Washington, DC: American Psychological Association.

Bravo, M., Rubio-Stipec, M., Canino, G., Woodbury, M. A., & Ribera, J. C. (1990). The psychological sequelae of disaster stress prospectively and retrospectively evaluated. *American Journal of Community Psychology, 18*, 661–680.

Butcher, J. N., & Dunn, L. A. (1989). Human responses and treatment needs in airline disasters. In R. Gist & B. Lubin (Eds.), *Psychological aspects of disasters* (pp. 86–119). New York: John Wiley & Sons.

Cohen, S., & Wills, T. A. (1985). Stress, social support and the buffering hypothesis of life change. *Psychological Bulletin, 98*, 310–357.

de Jong, J. T. V. M. (1995). Prevention of the consequences of man-made or natural disaster at the (inter)national, the community, the family, and the individual level. In S. E. Hobfoll & M. V. de Vries (Eds.), *Extreme stress and communities: Impact and intervention* (pp. 207–228). Dordrecht, The Netherlands: Kluwer Academic.

Foa, E. B., Steketee, G., & Olasov-Rothbaum, B. (1989). Behavioral/cognitive conceptualizations of post-traumatic stress disorder. *Behavioral Therapy, 20*, 155–176.

Freedy, J. R., & Hobfoll, S. E. (1994). Stress inoculation for reduction of burnout: A conservation of resources approach. *Anxiety, Stress, and Coping, 6*, 311–325.

Freedy, J. R., Hobfoll, S. E., & Ribbe, D. P. (1994). Life events, war and adjustment: Lessons for the Middle East. *Anxiety, Stress, and Coping, 7*, 191–203.

Freedy, J. R., Kilpatrick, D. G., Resnick, H. S. (1993). Natural disasters and mental health: Theory, assessment, and intervention. In R. Allen (Ed.), Handbook of post-disaster interventions. [Special Issue]. *Journal of Social Behavior and Personality, 8*(5), 49–103.

Freedy, J. R., Resnick, H. S., & Kilpatrick, D. G. (1992). A conceptual framework for evaluating disaster impact: Implications for clinical intervention. In L. S. Austin (Ed.), *Clinical response to trauma in the community* (pp. 3–23). Washington, DC: American Psychiatric Press.

Freedy, J. R., Saladin, M. E., Kilpatrick, D. G., Resnick, H. S., & Saunders, B. E. (1994). Understanding acute psychological distress following natural disaster. *Journal of Traumatic Stress, 7*(2), 257–273.

Freedy, J. R., Shaw, D. L., Jarrell, M. P., & Masters, C. R. (1992). Toward an understanding of the psychological impact of disasters. *Journal of Traumatic Stress, 5,* 441–454.

Green, B. L. (1995). Long-term consequences of disasters. In S. E. Hobfoll & M. W. deVries (Eds.), *Extreme stress and communities: Impact and intervention* (pp. 307–324). Dordrecht, The Netherlands: Kluwer Academic.

Green, B. L., & Gleser, G. C. (1983). Stress and long term psychopathology in survivors of the Buffalo Creek disaster. In D. Ricks & B. S. Dohrenwend (Eds.), *Origins of psychopathology* (pp. 73–90). New York: Cambridge University Press.

Green, B. L., Grace, M. C., Lindy, J. D., Gleser, G. C., Leonard, A. C., & Kramer, T. L. (1990). Buffalo Creek survivors in the second decade: Comparison with unexposed and nonlitigant groups. *Journal of Applied Social Psychology, 20,* 1033–1050.

Hobfoll, S. E. (1988). *The ecology of stress.* Washington, DC: Hemisphere Publishing.

Hobfoll, S. E. (1989). Conservation of resources: A new attempt at conceptualizing stress. *American Psychologist, 44*(3), 513–524.

Hobfoll, S. E. (1991). Traumatic stress: A theory based on rapid loss of resources. *Anxiety Research, 4,* 187–197.

Hobfoll, S. E., Briggs, S., & Wells, J. D. (1995). Community stress and resources: Actions and reactions. In S. E. Hobfoll and M. V. de Vries (Eds.), *Extreme stress and communities: Impact and intervention* (pp. 137–158). Dordrecht, The Netherlands: Kluwer Academic.

Hobfoll, S. E., & Lerman, M. (1988). Personal relationships, persona attributes, and stress resistance: Mothers' reactions to their child's illness. *American Journal of Community Psychology, 16,* 565–589.

Hobfoll, S. E., & Lilly, R. S. (1993). Resource conservation as a strategy for community psychology. *Journal of Community Psychology, 21,* 128–148.

Hobfoll, S. E., & London, P. (1986). The relationship of self-concept and social support to emotional distress among women during war. *Journal of Social and Clinical Psychology, 12,* 87–100.

Hobfoll, S. E., London, P., & Orr, E. (1988). Mastery, intimacy, and stress resistance during war. *Journal of Community Psychology, 16,* 317–331.

Holahan, C. J., & Moos, R. H. (1986). Personality, coping, and family resources in stress resistance: A longitudinal analysis. *Journal of Personality and Social Psychology, 51,* 389–395.

Jerusalem, M., Kaniasty, K., Lehman, D. R., Ritter, C., & Turnbull, G. J. (1995). Individual and community stress: Integration of approaches at different levels. In S. E. Hobfoll and M. V. de Vries (Eds.), *Extreme stress and communities: Impact and intervention* (pp. 105–130). Dordrecht, The Netherlands: Kluwer Academic.

Kaniasty, K., & Norris, F. H. (1993). A test of social support deterioration models in the context of natural disaster. *Journal of Personality and Social Psychology, 64,* 395–408.

Kessler, R. C., McLeod, J. D., & Wethington, E. (1985). The costs of caring: A perspective on the relationship between sex and psychological distress. In I. G. Sarason & B. R. Sarason (Eds.), *Social support: Theory, research, and applications* (pp. 491–506). The Hague, The Netherlands: Martinus Nijhoff.

Kilpatrick, D. G., Saunders, B. E., Amick-McMullan, A., Best, C. L. Veronen, L. J., & Resnick, H. S. (1989). Victim and crime factors associated with the development of crime-related post-traumatic stress disorder. *Behavioral Therapy, 20,* 199–214.

Lazarus, R. S., & Folkman, S. (1984). *Stress, appraisal, and coping.* New York: Springer.

McFarlane, A. H. (1987). Family functioning and overprotection following a natural disaster: The longitudinal effects of post-traumatic morbidity. *Australian and New Zealand Journal of Psychiatry, 21,* 210–218.

McFarlane, A. H. (1992). Avoidance and intrusion in posttraumatic stress disorder. *Journal of Nervous and Mental Disorders, 180*(7), 439–445.

Norris, F. H., Freedy, J. R., DeLongis, A., Sibilia, L., & Schönpflug, W. (1995). Research methods and directions: Establishing the community context. In S. E. Hobfoll and M. V. de Vries (Eds.), *Extreme stress and communities: Impact and intervention* (pp. 283–300). Dordrecht, The Netherlands: Kluwer Academic.

Norris, F. H., Phifer, J. F., & Kaniasty, K. Z. (1994). Individual and community reactions to the Kentucky floods: Findings from a longitudinal study of older adults. In R. Ursanom, B. McCaughey, & C. Fullerton (Eds.), *Individual and community responses to trauma and disaster* (pp. 378–400). Cambridge, Great Britain: Cambridge University Press.

Ørner, R. J., & Thompson, M. (1993). Current provision for traumatic stress reactions in N. H. S. personnel: A survey of critical incident stress management services (CISMS) in England, Scotland, and Wales. Unpublished manuscript.

Palinkas, L., Downs, M., Patterson, J., & Russell, J. (1993). Social, cultural, and psychological impacts of the Exxon Valdez oil spill. *Human Organization, 52,* 1–13.

Parker, G. (1977). Cyclone Tracy and Darwin evacuees: On restoration of the species. *British Journal of Psychiatry, 130,* 548–555.

Pearlin, C. I., Menaghan, E. G., Lieberman, M. A., & Mullan, J. T. (1981). The stress process. *Journal of Health and Social Behavior, 22,* 337–356.

Punamaki, R. (1989). Political violence and mental health. *International Journal of Mental Health, 17,* 3–15.

Resick, P. A., & Schnicke, M. K. (1993). *Cognitive processing therapy for rape victims.* Newbury Park, Calif.: Sage.

Resnick, H., Kilpatrick, D. G., Dansky, B. S., Saunders, B. E., & Best, C. L. (1993). Prevalence of civilian trauma and posttraumatic stress disorder in a representative national sample of women. *Journal of Consulting and Clinical Psychology, 61,* 984–991.

Riley, D., & Eckenrode, J. (1986). Social ties: Subgroup differences in costs and benefits. *Journal of Personality and Social Psychology, 51,* 770–778.

Rusbult, C. E., & Martz, J. M. (1995). Remaining in abusive relationships: An investment model of non-voluntary dependence. *Personality & Social Psychology Bulletin, 21,* 558–571.

Schönpflug, W. (1985). Goal-directed behavior as a source of stress: Psychological origins and the consequences of inefficiency. In M. Frese and J. Sabini (Eds.), *The concept of action in psychology* (pp. 172–188). Hillsdale, NJ: Laurence Erlbaum.

Solomon, S. D. (1986). Mobilizing social support networks in times of disaster. In C. R. Figley (Ed.), *Trauma and its wake, Volume II: Traumatic stress, theory, research, and intervention* (pp. 232–263). New York: Brunner/Mazel.

Solomon, S. D., & Green, B. L. (1992). Mental health effects of natural and human made disasters. *PTSD Research Quarterly, 3,* 1–8.

Solomon, Z., Mikulincer, M., & Hobfoll, S. E. (1987). Objective versus subjective measurement of stress and social support: The case of combat related reactions. *Journal of Consulting and Clinical Psychology, 55,* 577–583.

Trickett, E. J. (1984). Toward a distinctive community psychology: An ecological metaphor for the conduct of community research and the nature of training. *American Journal of Community Psychology, 12,* 261–279.

Trickett, E. J. (1995). The community context of disaster and traumatic stress: An ecological perspective from community psychology. In S. E. Hobfoll and M. V. de Vries (Eds.), *Extreme stress and communities: Impact and intervention* (pp. 11–26). Dordrecht, The Netherlands: Kluwer Academic.

Vogel, J. M., & Vernberg, E. M. (1993). Psychological responses of children to natural and human-made disasters: I. Children's psychological responses to disasters. *Journal of Clinical Child Psychology, 22,* 464–484.

Wallace, R. (1990). Urban desertification, public health, and public order: Planned shrinkage, violent death, substance abuse and AIDS in the Bronx. *Social Science, 31,* 801–813.

Wallace, R., Fullilove, M. T., & Wallace, D. (1992). Family systems and deurbanization: Implications for substance abuse. In J. H. Lowinson, P. Rueiz, & R. Millman (Eds.), *Substance abuse: A comprehensive textbook,* 2nd ed. (pp. 944–955). Baltimore: Williams and Wilkins.

Wardak, A. W. H. (1992). The psychiatric effects of war stress on Afghanistan society. In J. P. Wilson & B. Raphael (Eds.), *International handbook of traumatic stress syndromes* (pp. 349–364) New York: Plenum.

Weisaeth, L. (1991). The information and support center: Preventing the after-effects of disaster trauma. In T. Sorensen, P. Abrahamsen, & S. Torgersen (Eds.), *Psychiatric disorders in the social domain* (pp. 50–58). Oslo: Norwegian University Press.

Weisaeth, L. (1992). Prepare and repair: Some principles in prevention of psychiatric consequences of traumatic stress. *Psychiatria Fennica, 23,* 11–18.

Wells, J. D., Hobfoll, S. E., & Lavin, J. (1997). Resource loss, resource gain, and communal coping during pregnancy among women with mulltiple roles. *Psychology of Women Quarterly, 21,* 645–662.

Westermeyer, J. (1987). Prevention of mental disorders among Hmong refugees in the US: Lessons from the period 1976–1986. *Social Science and Medicine, 25,* 941–947.

Williams, C. L., & Berry, J. W. (1991). Primary prevention of acculturative stress among refugees. *American Psychologist, 6,* 632–641.

24

Cognitive Behavioral Treatment for PTSD

ELIZABETH A. MEADOWS AND EDNA B. FOA

Cognitive behavioral therapies encompass a range of procedures, a number of which have been found efficacious in treating PTSD. These include variations of exposure, cognitive restructuring, and anxiety management training, as well as combinations of methods. In this chapter, we review the cognitive behavioral treatments that have been studied in PTSD populations and describe the theories underlying the treatments and the research literature examining their efficacy.

Exposure Therapy

The treatment that has been most studied with different trauma populations is exposure therapy. This therapy consists of confronting one's fears systematically. In PTSD, these fears include thoughts and memories about the traumatic event, as well as external stimuli that remind one of the trauma, such as the site where it happened. Exposure therapy is rooted in learning tradition; the largest influence is Mowrer's two-factor theory (1960). In this theory, fear is acquired via classical conditioning during pairing of a neutral stimulus with an aversive stimulus (unconditioned stimulus, or UCS), and then this fear is maintained via operant conditioning as the feared stimuli are avoided to circumvent anxiety. Higher order conditioning and generalization may also occur, so that related stimuli also begin to evoke fear and thus avoidance. The avoidance, however, prevents the individual from learning that the CS (i.e., the site of the trauma) is no longer followed by the UCS (the trauma), and thus fear is maintained.

According to this theory, exposure works by breaking the associations between the CS and the UCS by repeatedly presenting the CS, either imaginally or *in vivo*. Because the UCS does not reoccur during the exposure, the client's conditioned responses to

ELIZABETH A. MEADOWS • Department of Psychology, Central Michigan University, Mt. Pleasant, Michigan 48859.   **EDNA B. FOA** • University of Pennsylvania Health System, Center for the Treatment and Study of Anxiety, Philadelphia, Pennsylvania 19104.

International Handbook of Human Response to Trauma, edited by Shalev, Yehuda, and McFarlane. Kluwer Academic / Plenum Publishers, New York, 2000.

the CS are weakened. This process is referred to as extinction (Stampfl & Levis, 1967) or habituation (Watts, 1979).

Recent theories of the mechanism of action for exposure have gone beyond simple conditioning processes. Foa and Kozak (1986) suggested that exposure works because it promotes emotional processing, in which corrective information is introduced to counter the pathological elements of the client's fear structure. The corrective information includes the fact that the reminders of the trauma do not in fact signal a return of the trauma, that remembering the trauma is not the same as reexperiencing it, that anxiety decreases in the presence of feared situations and memories even without avoidance, and that experiencing PTSD symptoms does not lead to a loss of control (Foa & Rothbaum, 1998).

Systematic Desensitization

Exposure methods vary in several dimensions, including level of arousal, length of exposure, and medium of exposure (Foa et al., 1989). The earliest form of exposure examined in treating PTSD was systematic desensitization (SD; Wolpe, 1958). SD falls on one extreme of these dimensions, and exposure is conducted imaginally, briefly, and in a minimally arousing fashion. The exposures to trauma memories are interrupted by relaxation exercises when the client becomes anxious, followed by a return to the memory once the anxiety has diminished.

Early case reports and uncontrolled studies (e.g., Frank & Stewart, 1983, 1984; Schindler, 1980; Turner, 1979; Wolff, 1977) indicated that SD was effective in reducing post-trauma symptoms. Although these studies indicated promise for the procedure, definitive conclusions cannot be drawn from them because of the lack of methodological rigor.

In a larger and somewhat more controlled study, Frank et al. (1988) found SD efficacious in decreasing symptoms in female rape victims. SD was compared with cognitive restructuring, and outcomes of both treatments were compared with those in a group of untreated women. Although this study also included methodological problems (i.e., a less than ideal control group derived from other studies and the inclusion of recent victims who might be expected to improve via natural recovery), it does provide additional support for the use of SD for treating post-trauma reactions.

Additional support comes from a controlled study of 112 victims of various traumas (Brom et al., 1989). In this study, SD was compared with hypnotherapy, psychodynamic therapy, and a wait-list control group. Unlike the earlier studies reviewed, the Brom et al. study specifically assessed and targeted symptoms of PTSD, rather than "trauma symptoms," although it should also be noted that several of the earlier studies predated the DSM diagnosis of PTSD. Clients in all three treatments evidenced PTSD symptom reduction relative to the control group.

Prolonged Exposure

Recent studies of exposure in treating PTSD have focused more on prolonged rather than brief exposure, thus decreasing the emphasis on SD in favor of prolonged exposure therapy. Prolonged exposure can include both imaginal exposure, in which frightening memories are confronted, and *in vivo* exposure, in which trauma-related situations or activities are confronted. Prolonged exposure (also called flooding or implosive therapy) was also examined in early case reports and uncontrolled studies (Fairbank & Keane, 1982; Johnson et al., 1982; Keane & Kaloupek, 1982) with promising results. The earliest controlled studies of prolonged exposure were conducted with combat veterans, often as an adjunct to standard VA hospital treatment. Cooper and Clum (1989) compared standard treatment (pharmacological and psychosocial) with and without the adjunct of imaginal flooding (IF). Patients who received IF showed greater reduction of some symptoms such as nightmares, as well as less anxiety during a behavioral avoidance test, relative to those who received only standard treatment.

Similarly, Boudewyns and his colleagues (Boudewyns & Hyer, 1990; Boudewyns et al., 1990) compared direct therapeutic exposure (DTE) with a control condition of individual traditional counseling, both as adjuncts to standard inpatient milieu treatment in a special PTSD unit. Patients in the DTE condition showed greater improvement than control group patients in self-report measures of general psychological functioning, but no differences were observed in physiological responding. Thus, it appears that DTE may have some benefit for general distress. However, data was not presented on specific symptoms of PTSD other than physiological responding. This omission, combined with other methodological issues such as inclusion of some DTE elements in the standard treatment and a lack of blind independent assessment makes it impossible to determine the efficacy of DTE for PTSD in these studies.

A more rigorously controlled study of exposure for combat-related PTSD compared flooding and a wait-list control group (Keane et al., 1989). Flooding significantly reduced a number of PTSD symptoms, as well as fear and depression, although some PTSD symptoms (those of numbing/avoidance) were unaffected.

Two well-controlled studies examined exposure for assault-related PTSD in women. In the first (Foa et al., 1991), prolonged exposure (PE) was compared with stress inoculation training (SIT) and supportive counseling (SC). The second study compared PE, SIT, and a combination of PE and SIT (Foa, Dancu, Hembree, Jaycox, Meadows, & Street, 1999). Both studies also included a wait-list control group. In both studies, women who received PE improved significantly in PTSD symptoms relative to those in the wait-list group, both at post-test and at follow-up. In the first study, SIT also produced improvement in all PTSD symptoms at post-test, but SC produced improvement only in PTSD arousal symptoms. At follow-up, PE generally appeared superior to the other two treatments. In the second study, the three treatments performed similarly well. However, patients who received PE improved significantly more than patients who did not, whereas no differences were found between patients who received SIT and those who did not.

Another controlled study supporting the use of exposure compared exposure, cognitive restructuring, and their combination, compared with a relaxation control group (Marks et al., 1998). The exposure, cognitive, and combination groups all showed greater improvement in PTSD symptoms than the relaxation group, although relaxation produced some improvement as well.

Two studies examined exposure in open trials with samples of mixed trauma victims. Richards et al. (1994) compared imaginal and *in vivo* exposure in a crossover design and found both types of exposure effective in reducing PTSD symptoms. No differences between them were observed except that for avoidance symptoms, *in vivo* exposure appeared more effective regardless of whether conducted before or after imaginal exposure. The second study (Thompson et al., 1995) indicated that trauma victims treated with imaginal and *in vivo* exposure improved in measures of PTSD, general psychological symptoms, and general health symptoms.

Finally, exposure has also been studied as a component of several combination treatment programs (e.g., Echeburua, de Corral, Sarasua, & Zubizarreta, 1997; Echeburua, de Corral, Zubizarreta, & Sarasua, 1997; Frueh, Turner, Beidel, Mirabella, & Jones, 1996; Hickling & Blanchard, 1997) that have also been shown to effectively reduce symptoms of PTSD.

Thus, both controlled and uncontrolled studies attest to the efficacy of prolonged exposure in ameliorating the severity of PTSD and related symptoms.

EMDR

Eye movement desensitization and reprocessing (EMDR; Shapiro, 1995) is another form of exposure therapy, in which elements such as saccadic eye movements are added to the sessions of imaginal exposure. Considerable controversy surrounds the use of EMDR, both due to claims by its originator as to large improvement very quickly and to differing opinions as to whether EMDR is efficacious only because of its exposure component. For a review of this controversy, see Tolin et al. (1996).

Some studies of EMDR compared the treatment with alternative treatments such as exposure alone, whereas others compared it with a variation of the procedure. Most studies of EMDR as a treatment for PTSD suffered from significant methodological flaws (i.e., lack of control groups, random assignment, clearly defined diagnostic criteria, and/or standardized and independent outcome measures), making it impossible to evaluate their results.

Both Rothbaum (1997) and Pitman et al. (1996) conducted well-controlled studies of EMDR. Rothbaum compared EMDR with a wait-list control group in 21 female rape victims; EMDR produced significant improvement both post-treatment and at follow-up. The extent to which the exposure component of EMDR is responsible for this improvement, however, cannot be addressed in this study. This issue was addressed by Pitman et al., who compared EMDR with and without the eye movements in a crossover design with 17 male veterans. Results showed no improvement in independent assessment and mild improvement in both conditions (with slightly higher improvement in the non-eye-movement condition) in self-report, suggesting that the eye movements that are the feature that most distinguishes EMDR from exposure are not relevant to outcome.

Anxiety Management Training

Anxiety management techniques were developed to teach clients specific skills to use when anxious, taking the view that pathological anxiety results from skills deficits (e.g., Suinn, 1974). A number of strategies have been used to reduce anxiety, including self-instruction, biofeedback, and relaxation training. Relaxation training served as a control group in several studies (Silver, 1995; Vaughan et al., 1994), including the Marks et al. (1999) study reviewed earlier, but only the Vaughan et al. study showed positive results for this method. Biofeedback has also been examined in treating clients with PTSD (Blanchard & Abel, 1976; Hickling et al., 1986; Peniston, 1986). These reports consisted of case reports and small studies, and although they suggest that biofeedback may be helpful in reducing trauma-related symptoms, there is not yet sufficient data to adequately evaluate the use of biofeedback for treating PTSD.

The anxiety management program that has been studied the most in treating PTSD is stress inoculation training (SIT). SIT was developed by Meichenbaum (1974) as an anxiety treatment and was modified by Kilpatrick et al. (1982) for use with rape victims. Skills included in the modified SIT program are muscle relaxation training, breathing retraining, role playing, covert modeling, guided self-dialogue, and thought stopping.

The use of SIT in treating rape victims was examined in several case reports and uncontrolled studies (Kilpatrick & Amick, 1985; Kilpatrick et al., 1982; Pearson et al., 1983; Veronen & Kilpatrick, 1982) with promising results. The first controlled study of SIT in treating rape victims was conducted by Resick et al., (1988). In this study, SIT was compared with assertion training and supportive counseling, all conducted in a group format and compared with a naturally occurring wait list in a quasi-experimental design. Clients in all three treatments showed improvement in rape-related fear and anxiety relative to those on the wait list. These improvements were generally modest, and the largest effect of SIT was observed in self-reported symptoms of intrusion and avoidance.

The two Foa et al. studies (Foa et al., 1991, 1997) described in the earlier section on exposure treatment also examined the efficacy of SIT in reducing assault-related PTSD. In the first study, SIT and PE were equally effective in reducing PTSD symptoms relative to wait list at post-treatment, although there was a tendency for PE to show superiority to SIT at follow-up. The 1997 study showed similar findings. PE, SIT, and the PE/SIT combination all proved effective relative to wait list at both post-treatment and follow-up. Although it did not always reach statistical significance, PE outperformed the other two treatments in all measures in this study.

Thus, SIT has proven efficacious in treating assault-related PTSD. Its efficacy in reducing PTSD symptoms that stem from other types of trauma, or in men, has yet to be tested.

Cognitive Therapy

Cognitive theories argue that the interpretation of an event, rather than the event itself, determines emotional states. Accordingly, pathological emotions stem from dysfunctional interpretations of events, e.g., overestimation of danger leads to pathological fear. Cognitive therapy, initially developed by Beck (1972; Beck et al., 1979) to treat depression and further developed by others (Beck et al., 1985; Clark, 1986) to treat anxiety disorders, aims to modify those dysfunctional thoughts, thus alleviating the pathological emotional response.

Cognitive therapy includes several steps. First, clients identify their dysfunctional thoughts, typically by self-monitoring their thoughts in a diary. Then, they gather evidence to evaluate the validity of these thoughts. Thoughts found to be erroneous or unhelpful are then challenged, using the evidence gathered in the previous step, and are replaced with thoughts that are more accurate or helpful.

Cognitive restructuring (CR) is one component of SIT, and to the extent that this program is effective, it lends indirect support for the efficacy of this treatment. Stronger support comes from two studies that examined the efficacy of CR alone. Frank et al. (1988) found that CR (as well as SD) was effective in reducing post-rape symptoms. As discussed previously, methodological flaws such as lack of an adequate control group and the inclusion of recent victims make it difficult to draw strong conclusions regarding the efficacy of CR in this study.

In their comparison of CR, PE, and a CR/PE combination, Marks et al. (1997) found that all three treatments were effective in reducing PTSD, providing support for the use of CR in PTSD treatment. An inspection of the means suggests that the two conditions that included PE were somewhat superior to the CR alone condition at follow-up.

Thus, there is some evidence that CR is effective in treating chronic PTSD, although this treatment has clearly not yet been studied extensively.

Combination Programs

Combination programs include therapies that combine existing procedures, such as the SIT/PE and CR/PE programs described earlier, as well as new therapies that incorporate aspects of different treatments. Cognitive processing therapy (CPT) developed by Resick and Schnicke (1992a) to treat rape-related PTSD, is an example of the latter type of program.

The theories that underlie CPT include cognitive and information processing models. Several theorists (Epstein, 1989; Janoff-Bulman, 1992; McCann & Pearlman, 1990) have suggested that schema changes result from traumatization. McCann and her colleagues (McCann & Pearlman, 1990; McCann et al., 1988) suggested that the trauma of rape leads to schema disruptions in the specific areas of safety, trust, power, esteem, and intimacy. The cognitive component of CPT targets each of these areas, and each theme is slated for cognitive restructuring at designated sessions. In addition to this cognitive restructuring, CPT includes an exposure component in which the client writes a detailed description of her rape and then reads this account. Thus, both exposure and cognitive therapy are conducted somewhat differently in CPT than in traditional exposure or cognitive therapies. Two reports have indicated that CPT, conducted in a group format, is an efficacious treatment for rape-related PTSD. Resick and Schnicke (1992a) compared CPT in 19 rape victims with a naturally occurring wait list; women in the CPT group showed significant improvement in symptoms of PTSD and depression as measured by a standardized self-report. Other standardized measures and interviews were conducted as well, but as these changed over time, the authors reported findings only for a measure completed by all clients.

The second report (Resick & Schnicke, 1992b) was a follow-up of the first. The results from a larger sample of 54 women, including the 19 from the first report, continued to support the use of CPT. This report included interview data as well, indicating that CPT resulted in a loss of PTSD diagnosis in 88% of the clients who had met the diagnosis at pretreatment; the reduction in self-reported symptoms observed in the first study was replicated in the larger sample.

Although the lack of random assignment to a true control group is problematic, the Resick and Schnicke studies suggest that CPT is an efficacious treatment for rape-related PTSD. More rigorously controlled studies and studies conducted by research groups other than the one that developed the treatment will allow drawing stronger conclusions regarding the efficacy of CPT. Preliminary findings of such a controlled trial (Resick, Nishith, & Astin, 1998), in which sexual assault survivors were randomly assigned to either CPT, exposure, or a minimal attention waiting group, support the published findings, showing both exposure and CPT to have reduced PTSD.

The SIT/PE (Foa et al., 1999) and CR/PE (Marks et al., 1998) combination programs described earlier were developed with the hope of enhancing the efficacy of single-method treatments by combining them. As evident from the earlier review, the combination programs have not outperformed their individual components. In some measures the combination was somewhat inferior to the single treatments. However, both combination programs proved efficacious, and thus in certain circumstances that will be described shortly, they may be preferred. A modified version of Foa and colleagues' (1999) SIT/PE program was examined in a sample of motor vehicle accident (MVA) victims (Hickling & Blanchard, 1997). In addition to the components included in the original SIT/PE treatment, Hickling and Blanchard included activity scheduling and discussion of existential issues. Results indicated that the modified SIT/PE treatment produced significant improvement in PTSD symptoms. Although this study did not include a control group or blind assessments, the results replicate the positive findings observed in the Foa et al. study and thus provide further support for the use of SIT/PE in a different trauma population.

The failure of combination programs to outperform single treatments may result from decreased time allotted for each individual component in the combined treatment, although this has not yet been tested.

Summary

Of the cognitive-behavioral treatments (CBT) that have been evaluated in PTSD populations, exposure therapy currently has the largest number of well-controlled studies to support its efficacy. Cognitive therapy, SIT, and combination treatments such as CPT have also been found efficacious in treating PTSD. Further, recent studies examining these treatments have implemented more rigorous controls than did earlier studies, leading to firmer conclusions regarding their efficacy. For example, the majority of the studies reviewed here required as an inclusion criterion that patients have had PTSD symptoms for a minimum of three months. In this way, the chances of seeing improvement due to natural recovery following a trauma are considerably reduced, as such recovery tends to have leveled off by that time, at least in assault victims (see Rothbaum et al., 1992). Clearly, studies that show improvement in veterans with combat-related PTSD that has persisted for decades provide further evidence that change may be attributed to treatment rather than to natural recovery. In addition to refuting the idea that improvement following CBT may be attributed to natural recovery, these studies also demonstrate that CBT can be effective even for individuals with severe and chronic PTSD. In the studies reviewed in this chapter, there was a wide range of duration following the trauma, and in no case was duration of PTSD noted as a predictor of poor outcome. Thus, it is even clearer that cognitive-behavioral treatments can be quite effective in alleviating PTSD.

Considering the greater evidence behind exposure, the fact that several studies comparing PE to other treatments have suggested that PE is superior and that PE might be more easily learned because it has fewer components than the other treatments reviewed (see Foa & Meadows, 1997), we recommend the use of PE as a first choice in most cases of PTSD. However, there are circumstances in which PE may not be appropriate, such as for clients who exhibit anger rather than anxiety or those whose traumas relate to perpetration rather than victimization. In these cases, alternate treatments such as CPT, SIT, or CR might be preferable. Similarly, some patients, such as those who exhibit extreme levels of anxiety or who dissociate during exposure, may require modifications of the way in which exposure is conducted; with these modifications, PE may still be quite effective with such patients (for a detailed discussion of these issues, see Jaycox & Foa, 1996). Combination programs might be useful with clients who encounter difficulties in conducting PE but who still may benefit from it. For example, clients who have extreme levels of anxiety might be better able to tolerate PE following the acquisition of skills taught in SIT. Thus, there are a number of cognitive-behavioral treatment options with demonstrated efficacy available to clients with PTSD.

References

Beck, A. T. (1972). *Depression: Causes and treatment.* Philadelphia: University of Pennsylvania Press.

Beck, A. T., Emery, G., & Greenberg, R. L. (1985). *Anxiety disorders and phobias: A cognitive perspective.* New York: Basic Books.

Beck, A. T., Rush, A. J., Shaw, B. F., & Emery, G. (1979). *Cognitive therapy of depression.* New York: Guilford.

Blanchard, E. B., & Abel, G. G. (1976). An experimental case study of the biofeedback treatment of a rape induced psychophysiological cardiovascular disorder. *Behavior Therapy, 7,* 113–119.

Boudewyns, P. A., & Hyer, L. (1990). Physiological response to combat memories and preliminary treatment outcome in Vietnam veteran PTSD patients treated with direct therapeutic exposure. *Behavior Therapy, 21,* 63–87.

Boudewyns, P. A., Hyer, L., Woods, M. G., Harrison, W. R., & McCranie, E. (1990). PTSD among Vietnam veterans: An early look at treatment outcome using direct therapeutic exposure. *Journal of Traumatic Stress, 3,* 359–368.

Brom, D., Kleber, R. J., & Defares, P. B. (1989). Brief psychotherapy for posttraumatic stress disorders. *Journal of Consulting and Clinical Psychology, 57,* 607–612.

Clark, D. M. (1986). A cognitive approach to panic. *Behaviour Research and Therapy, 24,* 461–470.

Cooper, N. A., & Clum, G. A. (1989). Imaginal flooding as a supplementary treatment for PTSD in combat veterans: A controlled study. *Behavior Therapy, 20,* 381–391.

Echeburua, E., de Corral, P., Sarasua, B., & Zubizarreta, I. (1996). Treatment of acute posttraumatic stress disorder in rape victims: An experimental study. *Journal of Anxiety Disorders, 10,* 185–199.

Echeburua, E., de Corral, P. Zubizarreta, I., & Sarasua, B. (1997). Psychological treatment of chronic posttraumatic stress disorder in victims of sexual aggression. *Behavior Modification, 21,* 433–456.

Epstein, R. S. (1989). Posttraumatic stress disorder: A review of diagnostic and treatment issues. *Psychiatric Annals, 19,* 556–563.

Fairbank, J. A., & Keane, T. M. (1982). Flooding for combat-related stress disorders: Assessment of anxiety reduction across traumatic memories. *Behavior Therapy, 13,* 499–510.

Foa, E. B., & Kozak, M. J. (1986). Emotional processing of fear: Exposure to corrective information. *Psychological Bulletin, 99,* 20–35.

Foa, E. B., & Meadows, E. A. (1997). The psychosocial treatment of PTSD: A critical review. *Annual Review of Psychology, 48,* 449–480.

Foa, E. B., & Rothbaum, B. O. (1998). *Treating the trauma of rape.* New York: Guilford.

Foa, E. B., Dancu, C. V., Hembree, E., Jaycox, L. H., Meadows, E. A., & Street, G. (1999). A comparison of exposure therapy, stress inoculation training, and their combination for reducing posttraumatic stress disorder in female assault victims. *Journal of Consulting and Clinical Psychology, 67,* 194–200.

Foa, E. B., Rothbaum, B. O., & Kozak, M. J. (1989). Behavioral treatments of anxiety and depression. In P. Kendall & D. Watson (Eds.), *Anxiety and depression: Distinctive and overlapping features* (pp. 413–454). New York: Academic Press.

Foa, E. B., Rothbaum, B. O., Riggs, D. S., & Murdock, T. B. (1991). Treatment of posttraumatic stress disorder in rape victims: A comparison between cognitive-behavioral procedures and counseling. *Journal of Consulting and Clinical Psychology, 59,* 715–723.

Frank, E., & Stewart, B. D. (1983). Physical aggression: Treating the victims. In E. A. Bleckman (Ed.), *Behavior modification with women* (pp. 245–272). New York: Guilford.

Frank, E., & Stewart, B. D. (1984). Depressive symptoms in rape victims. *Journal of Affective Disorders, 1,* 269–277.

Frank, E., Anderson, B., Stewart, B. D., Dancu, C., Hughes, C., & West, D. (1988). Efficacy of cognitive behavior therapy and systematic desensitization in the treatment of rape trauma. *Behavior Therapy, 19,* 403–420.

Frueh, B. C., Turner, S. M., Beidel, D. C., Mirabella, R. F., & Jones, W. J. (1996). Trauma Management Therapy: A preliminary evaluation of a multicomponent behavioral treatment for chronic combat-related PTSD. *Behaviour Research and Therapy, 34,* 533–543.

Hickling, E. J., & Blanchard, E. B. (1997). The private practice psychologist and manual-based treatments: Post-traumatic stress disorder secondary to motor vehicle accidents. *Behaviour Research and Therapy, 35,* 191–203.

Hickling, E. J., Sison, G. F. P., & Vanderploeg, R. D. (1986). Treatment of posttraumatic stress disorder with relaxation and biofeedback training. *Biofeedback & Self-Regulation, 11,* 125–134.

Janoff-Bulman, R. (1992). *Shattered assumptions: Towards a new psychology of trauma,* New York: The Free Press.

Jaycox, L. H., & Foa, E. B. (1996). Obstacles in implementing exposure therapy for PTSD: Case discussions and practical solutions. *Clinical Psychology and Psychotherapy, 3,* 176–184.

Johnson, C. H., Gilmore, J. D., & Shenoy, R. Z. (1982). Use of a feeding procedure in the treatment of a stress-related anxiety disorder. *Journal of Behavior Therapy and Experimental Psychiatry, 13,* 235–237.

Keane, T. M., & Kaloupek, D. G. (1982). Imaginal flooding in the treatment of post-traumatic stress disorder. *Journal of Consulting and Clinical Psychology, 50,* 138–140.

Keane, T. M., Fairbank, J. A., Caddell, J. M., & Zimering, R. T. (1989). Implosive (flooding) therapy reduces symptoms of PTSD in Vietnam combat veterans. *Behavior Therapy, 20,* 245–260.

Kilpatrick, D. G., & Amick, A. E. (1985). Rape trauma. In M. Hersen & C. G. Last (Eds.), *Behavior therapy casebook.* New York: Springer.

Kilpatrick, D. G., Veronen, L. J., & Resick, P. A. (1982). Psychological sequelae to rape: Assessment and treatment strategies. In D. M. Doleys, R. L. Meredith, & A. R. Ciminero (Eds.), *Behavioral medicine: Assessment and treatment strategies* (pp. 473–497). New York: Plenum.

Marks, I., Lovell, K., Noshirvani, H., Livanou, M., & Thrasher, S. (1998). Treatment of post-traumatic stress disorder by exposure and/or cognitive restructuring: A controlled study. *Archives of General Psychiatry, 55,* 317–325.

McCann, I. L., & Pearlman, L. A. (1990). *Psychological trauma and the adult survivor: Theory, therapy, and transformation.* New York: Brunner/Mazel.

McCann, I. L., Sakheim, D. K., & Abrahamson, D. J. (1988). Trauma and victimization: A model of psychological adaptation. *The Counseling Psychologist, 16,* 531–594.

Meichenbaum, D. (1974). Self-instructional methods. In F. H. Kanfer & A. P. Goldstein (Eds.), *Helping people change.* New York: Pergamon.

Mowrer, O. A. (1960). *Learning theory and behavior.* New York: John Wiley & Sons.

Pearson, M. A., Poquette, B. M., & Wasen, R. E. (1983). Stress inoculation and the treatment of post-rape trauma: A case report. *The Behavior Therapist, 6,* 58–59.

Peniston, E. G. (1986). EMG biofeedback-assisted desensitization treatment for Vietnam combat veterans' post-traumatic stress disorder. *Clinical Biofeedback Health, 9,* 35–41.

Pitman, R. K., Orr, S. P., Altman, B., Longpre, R. E., Poire, R. E., & Macklin, M. L. (1996). Emotional processing during eye movement desensitization and reprocessing therapy of Vietnam veterans with chronic posttraumatic stress disorder. *Comprehensive Psychiatry, 37,* 419–429.

Resick, P. A., & Schnicke, M. K. (1992a). Cognitive processing therapy for sexual assault victims. *Journal of Consulting and Clinical Psychology, 60,* 748–756.

Resick, P. A., & Schnicke, M. K. (1992b). Cognitive processing therapy for sexual assault victims. In E. G. Foa (Chair), *Treatment of PTSD: An update.* Presented at the Eighth Annual Meeting of the International Society for Traumatic Stress Studies, Los Angeles, CA.

Resick, P. A., Jordan, C. G., Girelli, S. A., Hutter, C. K., & Marhoefer-Dvorak, S. (1988). A comparative outcome study of group behavioral therapy for sexual assault victims. *Behavior Therapy, 19,* 385–401.

Resick, P. A., Nishith, P., & Astin, M. (1998, March). *A controlled trial comparing cognitive processing therapy and prolonged exposure: Preliminary findings* Paper presented at the Lake George Research Conference on Posttraumatic Stress Disorder, Lake George, NY.

Richards, D. A., Lovell, K., & Marks, I. M. (1994). Post-traumatic stress disorder: Evaluation of a behavioral treatment program. *Journal of Traumatic Stress, 7*, 669–680.

Rothbaum, B. O. (1997). A controlled study of eye movement desensitization and reprocessing in the treatment of posttraumatic stress disordered sexual assault victims. *Bulletin of the Menninger Clinic, 6,* 317–334.

Rothbaum, B. O., Foa, E. B., Murdock, T., Riggs, D., & Walsh, W. (1992). A prospective examination of post-traumatic stress disorder in rape victims. *Journal of Traumatic Stress, 5*, 455–475.

Schindler, F. E. (1980). Treatment by systematic desensitization of a recurring nightmare of a real life trauma. *Journal of Behavior Therapy and Experimental Psychiatry, 11*, 53–54.

Shapiro, F. (1995). *Eye movement desensitization and reprocessing: Basic principles, protocols, and procedures.* New York: Guilford.

Silver, S. M., Brooks, A., & Obenchain, J. (1995). Treatment of Vietnam war veterans with PTSD: A comparison of eye movement desensitization and reprocessing, biofeedback, and relaxation training. *Journal of Traumatic Stress, 8*, 337–342.

Stampfl, T. G., & Levis, D. J. (1967). Essentials of implosive therapy: A learning-theory-based psychodynamic behavioral therapy. *Journal of Abnormal Psychology, 72*, 496–503.

Suinn, R. (1974). Anxiety management training for general anxiety. In R. Suinn & R. Weigel (Eds.), *The innovative therapy: Critical and creative contributions.* New York: Harper & Row.

Thompson, J. A., Charlton, P. F. C., Kerry, R., Lee, D., & Turner, S. W. (1995). An open trial of exposure therapy based on deconditioning for post-traumatic stress disorder. *British Journal of Clinical Psychiatry, 34*, 407–416.

Tolin, D. F., Montgomery, R. W., Kleinknecht, R. A., & Lohr, J. M. (1996). An evaluation of eye movement desensitization and reprocessing (EMDR). In T. Jackson (Ed.), *Innovations in clinical practice,* Vol. 15. Sarasota, FL: Professional Resources Press.

Turner, S. M. (1979). *Systematic desensitization of fears and anxiety in rape victims.* Presented at the Annual Meeting of the Association for Advancement of Behavior Therapy, San Francisco, CA.

Vaughan, K., Armstrong, M. S., Gold, R., O'Connor, N., Jenneke, W., & Tarrier, N. (1994). A trial of eye movement desensitization compared to image habituation training and applied muscle relaxation in post-traumatic stress disorder. *Journal of Behavior Therapy and Experimental Psychiatry, 25*(4), 283–291.

Veronen, L. J., & Kilpatrick, D. G. (1981). *Stress inoculation training for victims of rape: Efficacy and differential findings.* Presented at the 16th Annual Convention of the Association for Advancement of Behavior Therapy, Los Angeles, CA.

Watts, F. N. (1979). Habituation model of systematic desensitization. *Psychological Bulletin, 86*, 627–637.

Wolff, R. (1977). Systematic desensitization and negative practice to alter the after effects of a rape attempt. *Journal of Behavior Therapy and Experimental Psychiatry, 8*, 423–425.

Wolpe, J. (1958). *Psychotherapy by reciprocal inhibition.* Stanford: Stanford University Press.

25

Trauma-Focused Psychodynamic Psychotherapy for Individuals with Post-Traumatic Stress Symptoms

RANDALL D. MARSHALL, RACHEL YEHUDA, AND STANLEY BONE

This chapter discusses the empirical and anecdotal clinical literature on psycho-dynamically based psychotherapy for individuals who meet the criteria for post-traumatic stress disorder (PTSD), and includes a number of practical strategies and interventions based on the authors' clinical experience. The patient with PTSD presents with prominent intrusive reexperiencing of the traumatic experience through thoughts, images, and dreams, together with heightened anxiety, overt attempts to avoid reminders of the trauma, emotional numbing, and profound demoralization. Repetitive thoughts about the trauma may have a ruminative quality, may be completely unbidden, and/or triggered by environmental cues. Symptoms of depression and panic are also often present, and a subgroup of patients may also manifest problems with aggressive impulses and behavior.

In trauma-focused psychodynamic therapy for PTSD, the therapist's overarching objective is exploring the personal meaning of the traumatic event. Specific attention is devoted to examining the impact of the event on the self-concept and views of others, as well as to defensive maneuvers being used to ward off painful emotions and nihilistic, frightening, or hopeless meanings attributed to the trauma or its aftermath. Support, advice, active expressions of empathy, and education can also be crucial components of this kind of treatment.

It should be noted that, although traumatic experiences have been implicated in the development of a wide range of psychological disorders, treatment of individuals

RANDALL D. MARSHALL • Anxiety Disorders Clinic, New York State Psychiatric Institute, New York, New York 10032.   RACHEL YEHUDA • Mount Sinai School of Medicine, Posttraumatic Stress Disorder Program, Bronx Veterans Affairs Medical Center, Bronx, New York 10468.   STANLEY BONE • Columbia Center for Psychoanalytic Training and Research, New York Psychiatric Institute, New York, New York 10032.

International Handbook of Human Response to Trauma, edited by Shalev, Yehuda, and McFarlane. Kluwer Academic / Plenum Publishers, New York, 2000.

presenting with other primary trauma-related diagnoses such as dissociative disorders or personality disorders may differ substantially (Marshall et al., 1998).

Contemporary Views on Psychodynamic Psychotherapy

This chapter emphasizes universal psychological themes observed in responses to serious adverse events, and in individuals meeting criteria for PTSD. The range of types of trauma and diversity of individuals' reactions to trauma, however, poses a challenge to any attempt to prescribe a generic approach to psychodynamic treatment. In fact, psychodynamically informed treatments have traditionally emphasized individual dynamics over categorical, generic constructs such as diagnosis. This may account in part for the relative paucity of efficacy studies, although an increasing number of rigorous outcome studies use psychodynamically based treatment guidelines (Marshall et al., 1997). The individual life history and psychology may be said to be embedded in more universal forms of responses to trauma.

The clinical presentation of trauma survivors does in fact vary considerably. Many trauma survivors are individuals with no prominent preexisting psychopathology who can rapidly engage in exploration of the trauma and recover quickly. A significant proportion of individuals, however, presents with histories of multiple trauma and preexisting affective, anxiety, and/or personality disorders, whose therapy requires ongoing attention to the treatment alliance and careful titration of supportive and interpretive interventions while reconstructing the trauma narrative and its implications for the individual.

The term psychodynamic will be used here in a broad contemporary sense, to reflect treatment that considers the complexities of defense, motivation, internal representations of self and other, and other schema as major influences on perception and behavior, which therefore dictate emotional response. As such, the psychodynamic view differs from cognitive and behavioral approaches in that it incorporates a broader range of issues and encourages more individualized treatment. Cognitive and behavioral treatments, as the best researched and validated psychotherapies to date in PTSD, are reviewed in detail in chapter 24.

In actual application, there are important resemblances between the major treatment approaches recommended for trauma survivors by experts. For example, education about typical responses to trauma, persistent encouragement of the patient to verbalize the traumatic experience in detail, and exploration of themes of helplessness, guilt, rage, defectiveness, safety, and failure are recommended in both cognitive-behavioral and psychodynamic approaches. In the only study to compare psychodynamic, desensitization, and hypnotherapy treatments, all three appeared equivalent and superior to a wait-list control (Brom et al., 1989). Thus, knowledge of the basic principles of empathic psychotherapy, and the characteristic dynamic configurations observed in trauma survivors can be useful in all psychotherapeutic approaches.

Efficacy of Psychodynamic Therapy for Individuals with PTSD

There is only one controlled study of trauma-focused psychodynamic therapy in the literature, which was conducted in the Netherlands (Brom et al., 1989). The study also fortunately includes other well-validated treatments for comparison, allowing preliminary conclusions to be drawn regarding the relative efficacy of different treatments. Brom, Kleber, and Defares (1989) randomly assigned 112 persons to one of four treatment cells: psychodynamic treatment ($N = 29$, two therapists, mean number of sessions = 18.8), hypnotherapy ($N = 29$, two therapists, mean number of sessions = 14.4), trauma desensitization ($N = 31$, three therapists, mean number of sessions = 15), or a waiting list ($N = 23$, 4 months). The psychodynamic treatment used was based on manualized treatment guidelines developed by Horowitz that integrate principles from psychodynamic, information-processing, and cognitive theory (Horowitz, 1986). In application, this therapy is an active, supportive-interpretive treatment that aims to work through trauma-related themes, as they arise, using the usual techniques of supportive dynamic therapy (e.g., clarification and interpretation of defenses, motives, and responses to fears). The explicit goal is to restore function to preevent levels and to maintain a focus on the traumatic event wherever possible.

Patients met DSM-III criteria for PTSD with the restriction that no more than 5 years had elapsed since the incurring event. The majority were women (79%), with a mean age of 42 years (range 18 to 73) and 3–4 years of high school education. For most subjects, the traumatic event was loss of an immediate family member (74%). Other trauma included violent crime (17%), traffic accidents (3.6%), and other (5.4%). Therapists were highly experienced in the therapy provided (>10 years) and provided the treatment he or she preferred in practice. Supervision by senior advisors was provided, although the frequency of supervision was not reported. Measures were taken before and after treatment and after a 3 month follow-up period. The drop-out rate was unusually low ($N = 12$, 11% of the total) and was evenly distributed across treatments.

In the overall analysis, all treatments appeared equally effective and superior to wait-list control on multiple measures of post-traumatic symptoms, general psychopathology, and personality functioning. No differences emerged in direct comparisons of the different treatments. The authors noted that clinically significant improvement was observed in 60% of treated patients versus 26% of the untreated group.

There was some evidence of differences in the course of treatment response across the different treatments. With respect to PTSD symptoms, desensitization and hypnotherapy resulted in a more rapid decrease in intrusive symptoms (assessed immediately after treatment), although in the follow-up period, all treatments were equally effective for both intrusive and avoidance symptoms.

This subject population did report clinically significant symptomatology (range 47.4–51.1 total score, Impact of Event Scale). However, this study possesses a number of limitations, including an absence of structured diagnostic interviews, lack of direct monitoring of the treatments provided, absence of ratings to ensure adherence to treatment protocols and difference between treatments, and the study of a population of individuals mostly suffering from bereavement. Comorbid psychiatric diagnoses were also not reported. This limits the generalizability of the study because comorbidity in PTSD is common, and significant comorbidity may limit the outcome. Furthermore, the exclusion of individuals with more than 5 years' duration of symptoms limits generalizability to more chronic PTSD.

This study suggests that a trauma-focused therapy based on Horowitz' model may be as effective as cognitive and/or behavioral approaches. However, for the reasons cited, this conclusion must be considered tentative, primarily because there was no direct observation of the actual treatments provided. A recent complete review of the treatment outcome literature demonstrates that psychodynamic therapy is the least well-researched treatment for PTSD, despite the fact that psychodynamic principles are widely used in clinical practice (Shalev et al., 1996). More outcome studies of psychodynamic psychotherapy in PTSD are obviously needed, as well as studies of longer term treatment of patients who do not respond to brief treatment (Burton & Marshall, 1999).

Other comparative trials have reported similar results, in that credible therapies all appear beneficial and differences between treatments are small in comparison to overall effect sizes. If confirmed, the overall conclusion appears to support Jerome Frank's view that credible psychotherapies usually share common mechanisms, which in turn are largely responsible for benefit (Frank, 1982). That is, effective psychotherapy persuasively counters demoralization, which in turn explains a substantial proportion of the outcome. Preliminary research, however, suggests that therapy that focuses specifically on the trauma is most effective. Confronting the traumatic memory, experiencing the associated affects within a supportive relationship, and thereby processing the traumatic experience may be the common mechanism of efficacy across trauma therapies. A nondirective therapy that does not encourage confronting the traumatic memory may collude with emotional and behavioral avoidance. In support of this view, Foa et al. found that, although supportive counseling was significantly helpful for symptoms of general distress, trauma-focused cognitive behavioral treatment was superior specifically for PTSD symptoms (Foa et al., 1991).

Early and Contemporary Psychodynamic Models of Trauma

Freud noted that the compulsion to repeat aspects of the trauma in the play of traumatized children, and the repetition of traumatic material in recurring nightmares of adults contradicted his theory that the pleasure principle was the dominant motivating principle for humans (Freud, 1922/1950, pp. 9–11). His etiologic model of posttraumatic symptoms, based on neurophysiological models of his day, was that traumatic neuroses were due to "excitations from outside which are powerful enough to break through the protective shield (p. 35)" of the cortical layer of cells which receives internal stimuli (Freud, 1922/1950). Thus, the etiology of the syndrome was not entirely construed within his developmental model of neurosis formation. Similarly, Kardiner stressed the distinction of traumatic stress syndromes from hysteria and compulsion neurosis since the primary fear in war neurosis was danger to physical integrity (Kardiner & Spiegel, 1947, p. 336). Constitutional factors and pre-traumatic neuroses were viewed as vulnerability factors by Freud and later theorists (e.g., Fenichel, 1945, pp. 117–128). The contemporary view that vulnerability factors and the severity of the trauma interact in the etiology of PTSDD is in fact similar to early psychoanalytic views (Fenichel, 1945).

Clinicians have often noted the phenomenon of patients who become repeatedly involved in problematic situations or relationships. The repetition compulsion refers to the unconsciously experienced, motivated seeking of distressing circumstances or relationships, thereby repeating earlier familiar, distressing experiences. Early psychodynamic views, noting such behavioral patterns, developed the notion of masochism in which punishment was unconsciously sought, motivated by guilt feelings, and was a price paid for future pleasure. The primary motivation for such repetition has sometimes been construed as a wish to work through unresolved conflicts—i.e., a drive toward mastery. For example, traumatized children may become absorbed in play that dramatizes aspects of a traumatic experience. This has been viewed as attempts to master traumatic experiences and dispel their influence over the self. Attempts to work through may take many forms and of course may be repeatedly unsuccessful or a source of problems in themselves.

This concept has its limitations, however, and should not be misapplied to situations in which individuals do not have control. Often, victims of recurrent trauma simply cannot envision alternative approaches to relationships or life in general and therefore simply seek or remain involved with what is familiar. These issues may become more important in longer-term psychotherapy with trauma survivors, when, for example, an individual wants to become free of a pattern of forming risky or doomed unsatisfying relationships.

Care must be taken not to distort this concept that individuals seek mastery of past trauma into a form of "blaming the victim."

Contemporary psychodynamic theory is pluralistic and offers several theoretical perspectives on trauma. Object relations theory, drive theory, self-psychology, and interpersonal theory all may potentially contribute to the treatment of trauma survivors. In general, psychodynamic therapies for adults are based on the principle that many problems may be understood as repetitions of unfulfilled or unresolved strivings and conflicts rooted in earlier phases of development, particularly in relation to caretakers. Experiences of disappointment, neglect, or overt trauma are often seen as the reason for such fixation. Object relations theory holds that early parental figures, along with models of stereotypical interactions with others, are represented in the mind and exert a powerful influence on behavior by creating expectations about the self, others, and the world in general. Unacceptable wishes and fears related to earlier developmental periods (including the fear that earlier trauma or disappointment will be repeated) are seen as influencing judgment and behavior largely outside of awareness. The recognition of these unconscious influences, together with at least partial resolution, is the goal of therapy.

Perhaps the most important issue in the psychodynamic therapy of trauma survivors concerns the relative emphasis on the here and now versus emphasis on conflicts and deficits that derive from earlier developmental periods. Experts in the field generally recommend maintaining a focus on the traumatic event and its psychological ramifications and exploring associations with earlier developmental conflicts as they arise. The classical view that adult post-traumatic reactions can always be "explained" entirely as a reemergence of developmental conflicts is no longer tenable. In trauma-focused psychotherapy, earlier conflicts, losses, compromises, and trauma are used to explore conscious and unconscious associations with the current trauma wherever possible. Patterns of relating emerge in the transference that can be understood as derived both from the traumatic experience and the patient's inner world.

This is a crucial therapeutic principle with trauma survivors in psychodynamic treatment. If clinicians convey the impression that they believe that the patient's symptoms are entirely related to a reenactment of childhood conflicts and deficits, patients can feel that the traumatic experience itself is being minimized. If patients feel that their reactions to trauma are being invalidated in this way, an irreparable rupture in the alliance may result.

Horowitz has developed this more contemporary view (Horowitz, 1986) that acknowledges the importance of developmental and pretrauma experiences but also emphasizes the role of the traumatic event itself in the etiology of PTSD. Traumatic events that occur in adulthood are seen as activating earlier states of mind and producing new sources of unconscious influence. Thus, the symptoms of PTSD in adults are not seen as simply the result of reactivation of unresolved developmental conflicts.

Weiss and Sampson have advocated a model of dynamic therapy which views the process as marked by a series of unconscious tests of the therapist on the part of the patient (Weiss & Sampson, 1986). In this view, emotionally meaningful material emerges in successive stages as a condition of safety with the therapist. The patient seeks to establish and consolidate safety through largely unconscious behaviors designed to test and hopefully disconfirm pathogenic beliefs (Weiss & Sampson, 1986, p. 8).

In this model, the patient brings to therapy a constellation of pathogenic beliefs that reflect fearful, grim expectations about others' behavior and the natural course of things. For example, a patient may come to the initial session with a pathogenic belief (expectation) concerning the therapist's behavior: that the therapist will probably respond to her "complaining" about the trauma just as her family had—by being uninterested, overwhelmed, irritated, and intrusive. If the patient successfully disconfirms this belief by seeing that the therapist is genuinely concerned for her welfare and can tolerate hearing about the trauma, therapy can progress.

In the initial phase of treatment, patients test therapists to discover whether they will be judgmental or overwhelmed by the traumatic event. Later there may be tests of whether the therapist will maintain appropriate boundaries in treatment, will revictimize the patient, or will turn away with impatience and boredom from frequently repeating themes and images over the course of therapy. These beliefs are usually unarticulated and may predate the traumatic experience or be a consequence of it. For example, a woman with a history of sexual abuse may have already felt suspicious of any male attention and then have this pathogenic belief exacerbated or reinforced after a sexual assault in adulthood. The similarity between the pathogenic beliefs model and the cognitive theoretical model is noteworthy. In both, distorted, overgeneralized, overly judgmental, and catastrophic thoughts are seen as a primary source of symptomatology.

Personality and character structure are widely discussed in the anecdotal literature on trauma. The predominant use of primitive defenses and the presence of significant psychopathology before the traumatic event may limit the effectiveness of any brief psychosocial treatment. However, if the goal is a return to the previous level of functioning by addressing PTSD symptoms, a trauma-focused psychotherapy may still be immensely helpful.

The global impairment often seen in PTSD can promote regression to earlier periods of development and reactivate issues of dependency, competence, safety, and bodily or personal integrity. Clinicians who work with trauma survivors often caution against making premature assessments of character while the patient is in crisis. There may be prominent use of defenses traditionally considered primitive, such as splitting, projection, denial, and depersonalization. Often after a patient recovers, one sees that such defenses were an aspect of the crisis response only and not integral to character. Patients who have routinely used maladaptive defenses to manage affect will likely need more intensive treatment to promote further gains once PTSD symptoms have been addressed.

Feelings of shame and humiliation that surround the loss of adult coping abilities are often apparent in the initial presentation and link associatively to similar experiences in childhood. However, such feelings can often be effectively addressed by simply educating patients about normative responses to severe trauma. Procedurally, the therapist pursues an explicit goal (processing the traumatic events) and refrains from pursuing such association unless clearly relevant.

Conversely, younger patients who have experienced life-threatening trauma may be prematurely confronted with the fact of mortality and may become overwhelmed by an "acceleration" of adult development.

Addressing the Psychological Features of PTSD

Psychotherapy for individuals with PTSD is based on the premise that emotional and cognitive processing of the traumatic event has become inhibited by conscious and unconscious mechanisms, resulting in an arrest of the process of coping and recovery. The goal of treatment is to elicit these (often unconscious) meanings, sometimes challenge them, and ultimately facilitate resolution of the conflict surrounding the trauma. Although different theoretical models have been proposed, all have in common the view that problematic fears, beliefs, and mental schemas related to the trauma are the source of post-traumatic symptoms, together with the defensive response to those themes.

The DSM-IV and ICD-10 emphasize universal features of post-traumatic reactions, including overwhelming negative emotions (such as fear, anxiety, rage, and dissociative numbness), cognitive disorganization, intrusive reexperiencing of aspects of the event and thoughts of its implications, and psychological and behavioral attempts to avoid these dysphoric states. *Interpersonal* trauma (such as sudden loss, witnessed violence, torture, rape, physical assault) are associated with PTSD more frequently than natural disasters (such as fires, earthquakes, and accidents). For example, about 46% of women and 65% of men who had been raped reported developing PTSD in the National Comorbidity Survey (Kessler et al., 1995). By contrast, only about 4% of men and 5% of women identified being in a natural disaster with fire as the most upsetting trauma leading to PTSD.

In the course of treatment, one often observes a repetition of interpersonal responses to the trauma as a form of reexperiencing the trauma (such as withdrawal, avoidance of potentially problematic relationships, rage, suspiciousness). These can be interpreted as such. For example, a patient who was assaulted and developed fear of strangers may be told, "you seem to feel now as if no one can be trusted, and anyone you meet may be planning to hurt you."

Social withdrawal is a common symptom in PTSD even when the traumatic experience did not involve betrayal or failure on the part of another (Marmar et al., 1995). The person may withdraw socially due to feelings of loss of emotional control; to shame because of loss of previous abilities to function; may fear the harsh judgments of others (a fear that is unfortunately sometimes grounded in actual experiences); or may believe that no one can understand his or her predicament. Interpersonal avoidance is an especially important focus in therapy, because coping is more successful if available social support can be enhanced. The therapist can address this issue through interpretation (e.g., "you are turning away from your wife as if you believe she will think you are weak and unmasculine") as well as frank advice-giving ("it seems to me that this is precisely the time when you should rely on your friends and family for extra help").

The impact of the trauma on the individual's view of self and others has been emphasized by contemporary investigators (Marmar et al., 1995). If the personal meaning given to the trauma is discrepant with preexisting conscious and unconscious representations of the self, the result is anxiety, fear, and confusion. This view is particularly relevant to individuals with no overt psychopathology and adaptive defenses before the trauma. For example, beliefs (which may constitute unrealistic wishes) that the world is generally safe, that others can be trusted, and that the self is effective and in control may be disrupted. The patient may angrily portray the world as completely spoiled since the traumatic experience. In such instances, the therapist may consistently point out that the patient is reacting as if everything good since the trauma has been erased and no longer counts. Reminding patients of their strengths and successes and reframing responses to trauma more realistically can also help to counter unconscious overgeneralization of the meaning of a trauma.

Individuals with PTSD feel the natural inclination to ward off powerful, intensely painful emotions. Shame may be experienced over the failure to cope, the experience of being sexually violated, or feelings of weakness at being unable to control emotions. Tremendous fear is usually present: fears of repetition of the trauma, of reminders of the trauma, or of the responses of others. Rage may be experienced and expressed to varying degrees toward the self for some failure to act during or after the trauma, toward the perpetrator, toward others who might have helped, or toward others who do not help after the trauma. In particular, guilt may be felt over failure to assist others, over unrealistic self-blame for not preventing the trauma, or over acts of aggression during the trauma and its aftermath. There is usually a general heightening of narcissistic vulnerability to stress and adversity. This may be a consequence of damage to an unconscious wish for invulnerability and often improves as patients cultivate a more realistic view of the trauma. Sometimes, after severe and/or recurrent trauma or after a severe and protracted course of PTSD, however, the conviction that the self is weak and damaged is not easily interpreted away. In such cases, a succession of relatively gratifying and successful life experiences may be necessary to provide new evidence to counter the earlier nihilistic beliefs about the self. This underscores the importance of assessing the patient's out of session behavior to ensure that steps are being taken to resume the prior level of functioning.

Dissociative responses to negative emotions and emotional numbing may further complicate the clinical presentation and interfere with daily functioning, as well as with coming to terms with the meaning of the trauma (Jaycox & Foa, 1996). Addressing this defense using the triangle of conflict model may be important to further progress. This approach, developed by Malan (1979) and others, views conflict as represented by the three poles of defense, impulse-feeling, and anxiety. For example, a trauma patient may feel emotionally numb (defense) due to tremendous anxiety (anxiety) over allowing himself or herself to experience trauma-related emotions (impulse-feeling). The therapist can intervene by pointing out this defensive maneuver and by gently exploring the patient's fear of what would happen if emotions related to the trauma were fully experienced.

The search for an explanation, and thus the attribution of responsibility for the trauma, can be a predominant theme in psychotherapy. In particular, the wish to assign blame may dominate feelings both toward the self, and toward others who may or may not be realistically implicated. Rage may be displaced onto anonymous figures (e.g., authorities), groups (e.g., a particular race, gender, or type of person), or institutions (e.g., society, community, religious group). Finally, rage toward the self as unrealistically responsible for the trauma or for not preventing the trauma often brings guilt feelings. Clarifying such primary process mechanisms can relieve this guilt: "you seem to believe you really could have prevented the man from raping you. In fact, it looks like you did well to stay alive." This also helps a patient to develop a more realistic appreciation of events. Care must be taken, however, not to invalidate the patient's viewpoint because in many cases other individuals and institutions are legitimately blameworthy.

If the patient is in fact responsible in some way for the event (e.g., a veteran who committed atrocities in the field, the driver of a car involved in an accident), guilt feelings result from a realistic appreciation of actual errors in judgment or action. In these instances, the therapist must encourage compassion and forgiveness toward the self, because realistic guilt cannot be interpreted away as nonrational. Such treatments often touch upon profound philosophical issues such as the value of human life and the aggressive side of human nature.

The self-concept is often shaken or altered in PTSD patients. Views of the self as weak, defective, and vulnerable (deriving from difficulty overcoming the traumatic experience) may perpetuate symptoms of fear, guilt, anxiety, and depression. Ruminations about what may have been done differently (e.g., in fighting off an assailant or rescuing others at the scene) are often present. In such circumstances, an unarticulated view of the self as unrealistically powerful (and therefore to blame for not preventing the event) may generate guilt and emotional confusion (Marmar, 1991).

For example, after being sexually assaulted and injured, a woman with severe PTSD symptoms revealed the following fears and beliefs in the course of therapy. She felt a general distrust of sexual involvements (which was understood as a fear of repetition of the trauma) and experienced intense rage alternating with intense anxiety (wish to retaliate, fear of losing control), guilt associated with sexual feelings (unrealistic self-blame for the rape), and devaluation of the self as weak and fragile (unrealistic belief that she should be able to master any threat or assault). She withdrew from most of her available social supports over a period of several months (distrust of others, unwillingness to risk being hurt through emotional involvement with others). In addition, memories of being sexually abused as a girl by an uncle were activated. When the patient had informed her mother, she was accused of lying. Thus, the belief that others cannot be trusted in times of difficulty, and that attempts to seek help will be met with betrayal, was long-standing and reactivated by the adult trauma. This made forming an initial therapeutic alliance difficult because the patient presented herself initially as guarded, angry, and demanding.

The Course of Psychotherapy

The initial evaluation of the trauma patient can serve several therapeutic functions. First, the clinician acquires the necessary information to develop a diagnosis and treatment. Second, the process of forming a treatment alliance is initiated. The central themes of this phase of treatment often are whether the therapist can be trusted (whether the relationship is safe) and whether the therapist can help (whether there is hope). In communicating their histories, patients begin the process of overcoming avoidance of the traumatic material and constructing coherent narratives, often for the first time. Ideally, the patient will experience the therapist as sympathetic, nonjudgmental, competent, and able to comprehend and tolerate the hearing about the traumatic experience or experiences. This new relationship is then gradually internalized over the course of therapy. Internalization refers to a complex process of learning (both consciously and unconsciously) from the therapeutic relationship in a way that hopefully can replace or at least moderate symptoms or problems. This includes a synthesis of information (e.g., education about typical and understandable responses to severe trauma), as well as a more general approach to adversity and conflict. That is, benefit is gained from internalizing the supportive psychodynamic process—taking a sympathetic, reflective, relatively calm and optimistic approach to problem-solving and self-awareness.

The patient's initial behavior and experience of the assessment can vary considerably. Usually, intense affect is evoked by retelling the event or events. This may provoke dissociative symptoms in some patients, and the natural inclination to avoid talking about terrible experiences is usually an important clinical focus. Because the alternation of intrusive recollections with impulses to avoid these thoughts is a central problem in PTSD, the therapist must provide active support and encouragement throughout treatment to persist with a focus on the trauma and its personal implications. This is especially crucial in the beginning when a treatment formulation must be developed. If the patient's associations are attended to and followed, the personal meaning of the trauma often becomes apparent as links to pretraumatic character and circumstances are established.

Throughout treatment, the therapist's role is to facilitate the resumption of processing the traumatic event or events by constructing a verbal narrative of the experience and exploring its associated meanings. Psychotherapy consists of reconstructing the event, exploring the patient's associations, and encouraging him or her to identify and express these beliefs and emotions. The therapist provides support throughout, and also actively addresses the unrealistic distortions and overgeneralizations in these beliefs, while actively encouraging reengagement in gratifying relationships and activities and reversal of avoidance behavior.

Psychotherapy with trauma survivors can be particularly challenging because of the intensity of the emotions evoked. Patients and therapists alike will experience the desire to avoid discussing traumatic experiences. The therapist may experience this reaction in intellectualized form as the thought that the therapy is cruel and unnecessary, and feel a powerful desire to rescue or shelter the patient from further harm. The crucial distinction to keep in mind is that although the traumatic event itself may have been horrific, it is the *memory* of the trauma that is going to be explored and hopefully mastered in the therapy. As in pathological mourning, the normal process of resolution has been arrested through avoiding a full experience of the tragic event.

The therapist may need to assist the patient in managing impulses to avoid addressing the trauma by fleeing treatment or by using action-oriented defensive maneuvers such as using alcohol or illicit substances, rageful and impulsive outbursts, compulsive work, or sensation-seeking (McFarlane, 1994). Often such behaviors can be more destructive and cause more impairment than the primary symptoms. Empathic confrontation of such behavior is often necessary. In confronting such defenses, the therapist can offer the hope that addressing the traumatic experience directly, though painful, can eventually lead to release from the need to avoid.

Specific therapist interventions span the full range of psychodynamic therapy (Marmar et al., 1995). If patients are overwhelmed by the task of verbalizing the experience, the therapist can encourage a focus on reconstructing the actual sequence of events at a relatively slow pace. This also allows a fuller experiencing of the associated emotions and thoughts about the events and communicates the possibility of tolerating and eventually mastering the memories. For individuals whose predominant affect is numbness, interpretation of the fear that talking about the trauma will be intolerable often promotes further progress in the therapeutic process. Asking questions that help to fill in gaps in the narrative can also be helpful. For example, questions about the timing of events, thoughts going through the patient's mind, and sensory experiences— what was seen, smelled, and heard—can promote vivid reexperiencing. Care must be taken throughout the treatment to monitor the tolerability of emotional reexperiencing, and time should be allowed near the end of sessions for intense emotions to subside.

Weiss and Marmar state that the prototypical candidate for time-limited (12 session) psychodynamic psychotherapy is a relatively well-functioning individual with no remarkable premorbid psychiatric history, who has experienced a single traumatic event as an adult (Weiss & Marmar, 1993). Because a substantial proportion of patients who have PTSD do not fit this description, however, they also note that individuals who have a history of prior trauma and psychiatric disorder may require longer and more intensive treatment. Many individuals suffer multiple trauma through the course of childhood and adult development. The National Comorbidity Study found that the majority of adults surveyed had suffered more than two major traumatic events (Kessler et al., 1995).

Adult trauma may reactivate and exacerbate memories of prior trauma, and prior trauma is a risk factor for the development of PTSD after trauma in adulthood (Yehuda and McFarlane, 1996). Often there are intrusive symptoms related to both the current and past traumas, and both can be addressed in psychotherapy. Furthermore, if the patient experienced early, repeated trauma and manifested psychiatric disorder prior to being retraumatized in adulthood, the oft-cited goal of returning the patient to the previous level of functioning may be more modest. The impact of prior trauma and comorbid psychiatric disorder on treatment outcome is an important subject for empirical investigation in future psychotherapy studies.

Horowitz outlines three overarching goals for trauma-focused psychotherapy (Horowitz & Kaltreider, 1995).

1. *Retention of a sense of competence and self-worth after the trauma, if psychological functioning was relatively intact before the experience. This includes acceptance of the consequences and aftermath of the trauma.*
   Often, however, individuals who had multiple trauma throughout development and adulthood have lifelong histories of poor self-regard and impoverished and troubled relationships with others. In such cases, however, brief treatment may actually result in significant improvement over prior functioning.
2. *Continued realistic and adaptive action, including maintaining beneficial relationships and continuing to develop new ones.*
   Withdrawal from social and family support is often understandable as a wish to avoid further disappointment through emotional involvement with others. However, social withdrawal is a common, maladaptive response to a wide range of predicaments and symptom states, and is a common feature of both PTSD and depression. Furthermore, individuals with PTSD often show a global

decline in functioning because of impairment from symptoms or a hopeless "giving up" on activities and responsibilities. In fact, a supportive environment in the post-traumatic period appears to have a protective effect. For all of these reasons, the therapist should encourage resumption of activities, hobbies, and other pursuits as soon as possible. If important activities are being avoided because they function as traumatic reminders, education should be provided about the role of desensitization in the recovery process.

3. *Use of the experience for some type of growth.*
   Newly learned skills of self-reflection and coping and the new experience of a helpful and concerned clinician ideally constitute corrective experiences that can have enduring benefits. Individuals come to appreciate their ability to overcome serious problems.

Transference and the Patient with PTSD

Attending to and interpreting the ways in which the patient's problems appear in the relationship with the therapist is a hallmark of psychodynamic treatment. Transference may be defined as those aspects of the patient's experienced relationship with the therapist that constitute projected aspects of prior important relationships. Aspects of relationships with parental figures, siblings, spouses, close friends, and other influential persons, including persons related to the traumatic experience, may be activated in the therapeutic relationship. The characteristics and behavior of the therapist can significantly influence the quality of the transference. In trauma-focused therapy, an active, supportive, emotionally expressive style will frequently evoke a mild positive transference that can facilitate treatment.

The real (as opposed to projected) therapeutic relationship as the foundation for successful therapy has been recently emphasized. An effective working alliance may include a realistic response to the person of the therapist, and also recruit positive feelings from early nonconflictual trusting relationships (Freud 1912/1966, pp. 123–144).

Interpersonal fears and hopes that are direct consequences of the trauma may be reexperienced in the relationship with the therapist. For example, fears of being violated, dismissed as an object, humiliated, or forced are common in survivors of interpersonal trauma. Although the active, compassionate stance of a supportive therapist is often sufficient to counter a potential negative transference, transference distortions can and should be directly addressed, particularly if the treatment appears jeopardized. Often the most delicate problem, particularly with more severely troubled clients, involves getting them to talk about the trauma without feeling retraumatized, that is, reexperiencing the traumatic event without losing sight of the therapist's good intentions or the overall objective of processing the experience for purposes of recovery. Levine (1995) lists a range of possible negative transferences that can arise at these moments in therapy:

> ... they may believe the therapist is hurting them, intruding on their privacy, becoming voyeuristically invested in the gruesome or exciting details of their childhood sexual experiences, using them for his or her own pleasure, or failing to protect them from the pain of remembering.

The fact that there can be an element of truth in all of these negative views underscores the importance of self-awareness in the conduct of successful psychotherapy.

In trauma-focused psychotherapy, the therapist attempts to formulate transference interpretations that include aspects of the traumatic event whenever possible. When the therapy is going well, often there is no need for intensive focus on the transference, particularly if time and resources are limited. However, if a repetition of post-traumatic beliefs, fears, or reactions is observed and can be successfully appreciated by the patient, such moments can be immensely helpful.

Although these kinds of negative transference can also be observed in nontraumatized individuals, their intensity and level of conviction in trauma survivors can provoke especially difficult, parallel emotions in the therapist. Many authors have emphasized the importance of some form of supervision, support, or regular self-reflection for health professionals who work with trauma survivors. Grappling with countertransference is often an important focus of discussion.

The special role of transference interpretation in psychodynamic therapy for PTSD has also been described by Lindy (1989) based on a naturalistic treatment study of Vietnam veterans, and on survivors of the Beverly Hills Supper Club fire (May 1977) and the Buffalo Creek Dam (West Virginia) collapse of 1972. He describes several different types of transference that depart from the traditional view of transference as an unconscious projection of aspects of internalized parental figures. These include the following (Lindy, 1989):

1. manifestation of repressed or disavowed memories of traumatic events (such as experiences of betrayal);
2. recreation of the roles of an important figure within the traumatic circumstance (such as close friends in combat or victims not rescued in a fire);
3. projection of psychological functions distorted by the traumatic experience (such as the ability to regulate the intensity of emotion experienced in therapy); and
4. expectation of a depth of understanding (often idealized) that would allow finding personal meaning in the experience.

Termination and Follow-up

The goal of trauma-focused psychodynamic therapy, as in many time-limited treatments, is not necessarily to complete the process of recovery but rather to stabilize acute symptoms and initiate a process of recovery and personal growth that can be continued after termination (Vaillant, 1997, p. 3). Treatment studies examining both psychodynamic, cognitive-behavioral, and relaxation training therapies for PTSD have all observed continued gains on almost all symptom measures after termination (Brom et al., 1989; Foa et al., 1991; Marks et al., 1998). This is also consistent with naturalistic studies of the course of recovery after severe trauma, which can extend over a period of several months (Kessler et al., 1995; Rothbaum et al., 1992).

Anticipation of termination may evoke themes related to the trauma such as fear of being unable to function autonomously and anger at being abandoned or betrayed. This may lead to a transient reemergence of symptoms. This is also a difficult phase for the clinician because judgment must be exercised in distinguishing between feelings about termination which can resolve over time, and PTSD symptoms which need ongoing treatment. The clinician's countertransference may be that of a callous therapist who is abandoning a suffering patient. Communicating the treatment model as outlined above, as well as outcome research findings, can sometimes be helpful in this circumstance. Particularly if the treatment has been successful, ending treatment will constitute a real interpersonal loss that should be fully experienced rather than avoided or minimized.

Some patients will have become interested in further self-exploration and wish to continue in therapy, although many other individuals will be grateful and ready to end the relationship with a return to their previous level of functioning. As one patient wrote in a letter to our research clinic: "I am doing fine. Everyone was very helpful.... I miss all of you, and I also hope to never need to come back to the clinic again."

References

Brom, D., Kleber, R. J., & Defares, P. B. (1989). Brief psychotherapy for posttraumatic stress disorders. *Journal of Consulting and Clinical Psychology, 57,* 607–612.

Burton, J. K., & Marshall, R. D. (1999). Categorizing fear: The role of trauma in a clinical formulation. *American Journal of Psychiatry, 156,* 761–766.

Fenichel, O. (1945). Traumatic neuroses (Chapter 7). In *The psychoanalytic theory of neurosis.* New York: Norton.

Foa, E. B., Rothbaum, B. O., Riggs, D. S., et al. (1991). Treatment of posttraumatic stress disorder in rape victims: A comparison between cognitive-behavioral procedures and counseling. *Journal of Consulting and Clinical Psychology, 59,* 715–723.

Frank, J. D. (1982). Therapeutic components shared by all psychotherapies. In J. H. Harvey and M. M. Parks (Eds.), *Psychotherapy research and behavior change* (pp. 5–38). Washington, DC: American Psychological Association.

Freud, S. (1920/1950 edition used). *Beyond the pleasure principle* (pp. 9–11). New York: Liveright.

Freud, S. (1912/1966). *On beginning the treatment.* Standard Edition, Vol. 12 (pp. 123–144). London: Hogarth Press.

Horowitz, M. J. (1986). *Stress response syndromes* (2nd ed.). Northvale, NJ, London: Jason Aronson.

Horowitz, M. J., & Kaltreider, N. B. (1995). Brief therapy of the stress response syndrome. In G. S. Everly, Jr. & J. M. Lating (Eds.), *Psychotraumatology* (pp. 231–243). New York: Plenum.

Jaycox, L. H., & Foa, E. B. (1996). Obstacles in implementing exposure therapy for PTSD: Case discussions and practical solutions. *Clinical Psychology and Psychotherapy, 3,* 176–184.

Kardiner, A., & Spiegel, H. (1947). *War stress and neurotic illness.* 2nd edition. New York: Paul B. Hoeber, Inc.

Kessler, R. C., Sonnega, A., Bromet, E., Highes, M., & Nelson, C. B. (1995). Posttraumatic stress disorder in the National Comorbidity Survey. *Archives of General Psychiatry, 52,* 1048–1060.

Levine, H. B. (1995). The patient with a history of childhood sexual abuse or incest. In Schwartz et al. (Ed.), *Psychodynamic concepts in general psychiatry.* Washington, DC: American Psychiatric Press.

Lindy, J. D. (1989). Transference and Post-traumatic stress disorder. *Journal of the American Academy of Psychoanalysis, 17,* 397–413.

Malan, D. M. (1979). *Individual psychotherapy and the science of psychodynamics.* London: Butterworth.

Marks, I., Lovell, K., Noshirvani, H., Livanou, M., & Thrasher, S. (1998). Treatment of posttraumatic stress disorder by exposure and/or cognitive restructuring: A controlled study. *Archives of General Psychiatry, 55,* 317–325.

Marmar, C. R., Horowitz, M. J., Weiss, D., Wilner, N., & Kaltreider, N. (1988). A controlled trial of brief psychotherapy and mutual help treatment of conjugal bereavement. *American Journal of Psychiatry, 145,* 203–209.

Marmar, C. R. (1991). Brief dynamic psychotherapy of post-traumatic stress disorder. *Psychiatric Annals, 21,* 405–414.

Marmar, C. R., Weiss, D. S., & Pynoos, R. S. (1995). Dynamic therapy of post-traumatic stress disorder. In M. J. Friedman, D. S. Charney, & A. Y. Deutch (Eds.), *Neurobiological and clinical consequences of stress: From normal adaptation to PTSD.* Philadelphia: Lippincott-Raven.

Marshall, R. D., Davidson, J. R. T., & Yehuda, R. (1998). Pharmacotherapy in the treatment of posttraumatic stress disorder and other trauma-related syndromes. In R. Yehuda (Ed.), *Psychological Trauma.* Washington, DC: American Psychological Association.

Marshall, R. D., & Pierce, D. (in press). Posttraumatic stress disorder: Recent findings and implications for pharmacotherapy. *Harvard Review of Psychiatry.*

Marshall, R. D., Vaughan, S. C., Mackinnon, R. A., Mellman, L., & Roose, S. P. (1997). Assessing outcome in psychoanalysis and long-term psychodynamic psychotherapy. *Journal of the American Academy of Psychoanalysis, 24,* 575–604.

McFarlane, A. C. (1994). Individual psychotherapy for post-traumatic stress disorder. *Psychiatric Clinics of North America, 17,* 393–408.

Rothbaum, B. O., Foa, E. B., Riggs, D. S., Murdock, T., & Walsh, W. (1992). A prospective examination of post-traumatic stress disorder in rape victims. *Journal of Traumatic Stress, 5,* 455–475.

Shalev, A. Y., Bonne, O., & Spencer, E. (1996). Treatment of posttraumatic stress disorder: A review. *Psychosomatic Medicine, 58,* 165–182.

Vaillant, L. M. (1997). *Changing character: Short-term anxiety-regulating psychotherapy for restructuring defenses, affects, and attachment.* New York: Basic Books.

Van der Kolk, B. A., McFarlane, A. C., & van der Hart, O. (1996). A general approach to treatment of posttraumatic stress disorder. In B. A. van der Kolk, A. C. McFarlane, & L. Weisaeth (Eds.), *Traumatic Stress: The Effects of Overwhelming Experience on Mind, Body, and Society.* New York, London: Guilford Press.

Weiss, D. S., & Marmar, C. R. (1993). Teaching time-limited dynamic psychotherapy for post-traumatic stress disorder and pathological grief. *Psychotherapy, 30,* 587–591.

Weiss, J., & Sampson, H. (1986). *The psychoanalytic process: Theory, clinical observation, and empirical research.* New York, London: Guilford Press.

Yehuda, R. & McFarlane, A. C. (1995). Conflict between current knowledge about posttraumatic stress disorder and its original conceptual basis. *American Journal of Psychiatry, 152,* 1705–1713.

26

Pharmacological Treatment of Trauma-Related Disorders

ARIEH Y. SHALEV AND OMER BONNE

Traditionally, the etiology of PTSD has been construed in psychological terms, such as learned conditioning (Keane et al., 1985), shattered cognitive assumptions (Janoff Bullman, 1985), or impacted grief (Horowitz, 1974). Such understanding reflected an early belief about PTSD, according to which the disorder was an extension of a normal response to extreme events, and its persistence over time was mediated by "unresolved" psychological processes. The current trend of imputing all mental disorders to underlying brain pathology has not spared PTSD. Current biological formulations of PTSD emphasize the pathogenic effects of environmental "stressors" on (predisposed?) brain structures, and PTSD is the expression of the resulting neuropathology. Biological therapies attempt to redress, reduce, or balance such hypothetical dysfunction of the brain.

Notwithstanding the lacunar nature of its underlying proof (the psychobiology of PTSD is addressed in other parts of this book), the psychobiological model has become a powerful view of mankind and human tragedy and is so prevalent among professionals that most PTSD patients are likely to be "treated" by one neuroactive agent or another during the course of their illness. Fortunately, the endeavor of producing and prescribing psychotropics is subject to strict, "evidence-based" regulatory control. Substantial documentation has, therefore, been generated, by years of treating PTSD patients with psychotropics. This documentation points to some "successes" and other "failures" and these are addressed in this chapter.

Several reviews of the pharmacotherapy of PTSD have been published (Friedman, 1988, 1996; Solomon et al., 1992). Instead of repeating previously presented views, this chapter attempts to provide a conceptual framework within which the current knowledge may be better understood and its few insights properly implemented by clinicians.

ARIEH Y. SHALEV AND OMER BONNE • Center for Traumatic Stress, Department of Psychiatry, Hadassah University Hospital, Jerusalem, 91120, Israel.

International Handbook of Human Response to Trauma, edited by Shalev, Yehuda, and McFarlane. Kluwer Academic / Plenum Publishers, New York, 2000.

Review of the Literature

Before presenting the data, several points are worth mentioning. First, controlled pharmacological studies are often limited to evaluating overt and measurable expressions of the disorder (e.g., counting changes in symptoms). The effect of the treatment on other dimensions of behavior and experience (social life, morale, interpersonal violence, drinking habits; Johnson et al., 1996) may escape such a template (chapter 15). Improvements or worsening in these unmeasured areas cannot be simply inferred from information on symptomatic changes. For practicing clinicians and their patients, however, improvement in these "secondary" areas may have significant value. Therefore, we encourage clinicians to use their broader view and understanding of their patients in implementing pharmacotherapy in PTSD.

Second, none of the studies reviewed here has employed an agent which had been developed specifically for PTSD (i.e., developed on animal models of extreme stress, memory consolidation, overgeneralization of avoidance, etc.). Although the use of pharmacological agents across disorders is not uncommon and often successful (e.g., antidepressants in panic disorder and obsessive compulsive disorder, OCD), in a disorder as pervasive as PTSD, the lack of specifically developed agents should lower one's expectations.

Third, because PTSD tends to become chronic and tenacious (in contrast, for example, with major depression, which often involves a self-limited, episodic course), the achievement of full remission in PTSD is somewhat less plausible, regardless of treatment modality. In fact, total remission has not been claimed by any pharmacological study of PTSD (nor by controlled studies of other treatment approaches). Therefore, relief of symptoms may be as much as any therapy can offer to chronic PTSD patients. Such relief, however, can be of the greatest value for patients and their close relatives.

Finally, one may argue that because most pharmacological studies of PTSD have addressed chronic patients (this was primarily due to the amenability of this subgroup for research), the current literature is biased toward less favorable results. The extent to which lessons from studies of patients who have severe and chronic PTSD apply to the more recently traumatized, or less severely ill, is a matter of debate (Shalev, 1997). Common sense, epidemiological surveys (Kessler et al., 1995) and experience with other chronic disorders (e.g., early versus chronic schizophrenia) suggest that there are differences in drug responses between the chronic and the more acute forms of PTSD (van der Kolk et al., 1994).

Tricyclic Antidepressants

Most pharmacological studies of PTSD (Table 1) involved antidepressants. Among antidepressants, the tricyclic agents (TCAs) have been the main tool for treating depression for almost forty years. Moreover, TCAs have proven efficacy in treating other anxiety disorders and depression. Given the frequent occurrence of depressed mood and of phasic anxiety in PTSD, the rationale for using TCAs in this disorder is understandable.

Within the limits mentioned, most studies that employ TCAs report some relief in PTSD symptoms (e.g., sleep, intrusive symptoms and reexperiencing), as well as improvement of mood. Importantly, comparisons between TCAs and MAO inhibitors (see below), as well as an analysis of 15 such studies (Southwick et al., 1994), suggesting that MAOIs are superior to TCAs (Table 1a).

Monoamine Oxidase Inhibitors (MAOIs)

The clinical indications for prescribing MAOIs are similar to those for TCAs, yet these compounds may have distinctive efficacy in "atypical" depression. MAOIs are used sparingly because of life-threatening side effects (hypertensive crisis) that may occur when the patient does not observe the strict dietary restrictions that accompany the use of these agents (Table 1b). Trials of MAOIs in PTSD employed phenelzine, a frequently used "traditional" MAOI.

Results from phenelzine studies vary. Some reported significant improvement (Hogben & Cornfield, 1981; Davidson et al., 1987; Frank et al., 1988; Kosten et al., 1991), in others the drug was superior to a placebo (Frank et al., 1988; Kosten et al., 1991). Another study reported relatively minor effects (Lerer et al., 1987), whereas one study (Shestazki et al., 1988) found no advantage to phenelzine over a placebo. Improvement with MAOIs encompassed reexperiencing symptoms and insomnia. The latter may be attributed to the reduction in intrusive traumatic nightmares.

The use of traditional MAOIs in PTSD patients who have problems of illicit drug or alcohol use, or in those who are unlikely to adhere to a strict diet, is of obvious concern. However, new "reversible" MAOIs (e.g., moclobamide) are currently available, in which dietary-related side effects are of lesser concern. It would be of interest, therefore, to examine the effect of these reversible MAOIs on PTSD.

Serotonin-Specific Reuptake Inhibitors (SSRIs)

Because they combine equal efficacy, fewer side effects, ease of administration, and low toxicity, SSRIs have become a treatment of choice for depression, panic disorder, and OCD. Several recent studies have examined their effectiveness in PTSD (Table 1c). Symptoms that accompany PTSD, such as irritability, impulse dyscontrol, depressed mood, suicidality, and obsessional thinking, are thought to be mediated by serotonergic mechanisms—hence the rationale of trying these compounds.

As with other agents, success has been partial, at least in studies completed to date. Reduction in various symptom domains was reported, including depressed mood (van der Kolk et al., 1994, Shay, 1992; Kline et al., 1994), intrusive symptoms avoidance (Nagy et al., 1993; Brady et al., 1995; Marmar et al., 1996), explosiveness and irritability (Shay, 1993; Kline et al., 1994). A comparison of several drugs in PTSD (Dow & Kline, 1997) reported greater responses to SSRIs. Recently, results from an ongoing study (Davidson et al., 1997) showed reduction of 44–49% in PTSD symptom intensity with sertraline (compared to 35% reductions in placebo-treated patients).

Two recent studies of sertraline in PTSD have been reported. The first was a 12-week, double blind, flexible dose study of adult outpatients with PTSD (Davidson et al., 1997). Sertraline (50–200 mg/day) was administered to 100 PTSD patients and placebo to an additional 108 PTSD patients. Sertraline-treated patients showed significant improvements in symptom intrusion and avoidance, in the total severity of PTSD symptoms, and in occupational functioning. The second study (Brady et al., 1998) was equally a double blind, placebo controlled, flexible dose study ($N = 184$), and showed similar efficacy on PTSD symptoms, along with significant improvements in a measure of quality of life. Following these studies, sertraline may become the first SSRI to be formally indicated for treatment of PTSD.

TABLE 1a. Pharmacological Treatment of PTSD: Tricyclic Antidepressants (TCAs)

Tricyclic Antidepressants	Drug and Dose (mg/day)	Design,[a] Duration, Instruments[b]	Population	N	Results/Conclusion
Burstein, 1984 Falcon et al., 1985	Imipramine (50–350) Miscellaneous tricyclics (200)	OT OT Chart rev. and CGI	Road accidents Veterans	10 17	Improved sleep, decreased intrusions Marked improvement in 82% of subjects
Bleich et al., 1986	Amitriptyline (140) Doxepine (100) Maprotiline (150) Clomipramine (150)	OT Chart review	Veterans with recent (8–10 mo.) PTSD	25	Improved sleep, memory, concentration. Decreased frequency of nightmares
Kauffman et al., 1987	Desipramine (150–200)	OT 4 weeks BDI, HAM-D	Miscellaneous trauma	8	Significant decrease in depressive symptoms
Frank et al., 1988	Phenelzine (71) Imipramine (240) Placebo	CT, RA, PC 8 weeks SADS, SCID-PTSD, IES, DEPR	Veterans	34	Phenelzine and imipramine superior to placebo. IES intrusion improved, but no avoidance
Kinzie and Leung, 1989	Clonidine (0.2–6) and imipramine (50–100)	OT 12–19 mo. HAM-D	Refugees	9	Significant (16 pt.) decrease of HAM-D scores. Some improvement of intrusion, nightmares, startle
Reist et al., 1989	Desipramine (200)	DB, PC, CO 4 weeks BDI, HAM-D, IES	Veterans	18	Improvement in "some symptoms of depression," no change in anxiety and PTSD symptoms
Davidson et al., 1990	Amitriptyline (50–300) vs. Placebo	DB, PC 4 and 8 weeks HAM-A&D, CGI, IES	Miscellaneous PTSD	40	Significant effect on depression on week 4. Additional effet on anxiety, CGI, and IES on week 8
Kosten et al., 1991	Phenelzine (60–79) Imipramine (50–300) Placebo	RA, PC 8 weeks IES	Veterans	19 23 18	44% improvement with phenelzine and 25% with imipramine in week 5. Improved intrusion but not avoidance of depression
Davidson et al., 1993	Amitriptyline (160)	DB, PC 4 and 8 weeks CGI, HAM-D, IES	War veterans	55	Significant effect on depression and CGI, trend toward improvement in PTSD symptoms. Combat intensity predicts IES response

TABLE 1b. Pharmacological Treatment of PTSD: MAO Inhibitors (MAOIs)

MAOI Antidepressants	Drug and Dose (mg/day)	Design,[a] Duration,[b] Instruments	Population	N	Results/Conclusion
Hogben & Cornfield, 1981	Phenelzine (45–57)	OT	Veterans	5	Decreased frequency of nightmares, flashbacks, startle reactions, violence
Lerer et al., 1987	Phenelzine (60)	OT 4–18 weeks HAM-A&D PTSD	Army (Israeli) veterans	22	Minor improvement on most measures. Sleep significantly improved
Shestazki et al., 1987	Phenelzine (45–75) vs. Placebo	CT, RA, PC, CO 5 weeks CGI, HAM-A&D, IES	Miscellaneous trauma	13	No difference between the active drug and placebo (significant decrease in PTSD and anxiety in both)
Davidson et al., 1987	Phenelzine (45–60)	OT 4 weeks CGI, IES	Veterans	10	Improved PTSD symptoms

(For all tables)
[a]Design: CO = crossover; CR = case report; DB = double blind; OT = open trial; PC = placebo-controlled; RA = random assignment; TCAs = tricyclic antidepressants.
[b]Instruments: BDI = Beck Depression Inventory; BPRS = Brief Psychiatric Rating Scale; CAPS = Clinician Administered PTSD Scale; CGI = Clinical Global Impression; DEPR = Risking Depression Scale; DES = Dissociation Experience Scale; GAF = General Assessment of Functioning; HAM-A = Hamilton Anxiety Scale; HAM-D = Hamilton Depression Scale; Host. = Buss Durkee Hostility Inventory; IES = Impact of Events Scale; PMS = Profile of Mood States; SADS = Structured Interview for Affective Disorders and Schizophrenia; SANX = Spielberger Scale-Trail Anxiety Scale; SCL-90 = Derogatis' Symptoms Checklist 90.

TABLE 1c. Pharmacological Treatment of PTSD: SSRIs

SSRI Antidepressants and Others	Drug and Dose (mg/day)	Design,[a] Duration, Instruments[b]	Population	N	Results/Conclusion
Shay, 1992	Fluoxetine (20–80)	Clinical impression >12 mo.	Veterans	26	Reduced explosive behavior, improved mood and insomnia in 16 (61%) patients
Nagy et al., 1993	Fluoxetine (20–80)	OT 10 weeks CAPS	Veterans	19	Significant reduction in PTSD symptoms mostly after 6 weeks. 50% reduction in frequency of panic attacks. 30% drop-out due to side effects (anxiety)
van der Kolk et al., 1994	Fluoxetine (20) Placebo	DB, PC 5 weeks CAPS, HAM-D, DES, Hostility Scale	War veterans Civilian PTSD	23 24	Reduction in arousal, numbing, and depression. No significant effect on intrusion, dissociation, and hostility. Better results in civilians with recent PTSD
Kline et al., 1994	Sertaline (98.5)	OT 3 mo. BDI, IES, SANX, CGI	Veterans with PTSD and depression	19	Significant reduced dysphoria, irritability, and anger in 12 (63%)
Brady et al., 1995	Sertaline, up to 200, as tolerated	OT 12 weeks HAM-D, IES, PTSD Symptom Scale	PTSD with alcoholism	9	Decrease in avoidance, intrusion, hyperarousal, and alcohol after first 4 weeks
Marmar et al., 1996	Fluvoxamine (range 100–250)	OT 10 weeks SCID, SCID-II, IES, Stress Response Scale, SCL-90, BPRS, GAF	Vietnam veterans with chronic PTSD	11	Improvement in all measures by week 6 with marginal additional change by week 10. Effect on intrusion, avoidance, and arousal
Rothbaum et al., 1996	Sertraline (105)	OT 12 weeks CAPS, IES	Rape victims	7 (5)	5 completers. 4 of 5 participants—positive response, 53% reduction in CAPS

	Drug and Dose (mg/day)	Design,[a] Duration, Instruments[b]	Population	N	Results/Conclusion
Dow & Kline, 1997	SSRIs, TCAs, phenelzine, bupropion, lithium	OT 1–22 mo. CGI	Veterans with comorbid PTSD and major depression	72	Improvement in 50% of subjects after several trials; SSRIs seem better than NA specific TCAs
Hertzberg et al., 1996	Trazodone (300)	OT 16 weeks CAPS, Trauma Scale, Sleep Quality Index, BDI, SANX, CGI	Vietnam veterans	6	Improvement in PTSD symptoms (CAPS B-D) and sleep but not in depression and anxiety symptoms
Davidson et al., 1997	Sertraline (50–200) vs. placebo	BD, PC 12 weeks CAPS, IES, CGI, others	Adult PTSD patients	208	Significant decrease in PTSD severity, intrusion, avoidance symptoms; improved occupational functioning
Brady et al., 1998	Sertraline (50–200) vs. placebo	BD, PC 12 weeks CAPS, IES, CGI, others	Adult PTSD patients	184	Significant decrease in PTSD severity; improved quality of life

TABLE 1d. Pharmacological Treatment of PTSD: Benzodiazepines

Benzodiazepines	Drug and Dose (mg/day)	Design,[a] Duration, Instruments[b]	Population	N	Results/Conclusion
Feldman, 1987	Alprazolam (0.5–6; mostly 0.5–1.5)	Retrospective chart review 1 mo.–1 yr.	Veterans	20	Major improvement (16 of 20 subjects) in anxiety and function. Explosive behavior induced in non-responders???
Loewenstein et al., 1988	Clonazepam (1–6)	OT	PTSD + multiple personality disorder	5	Improved sleep, nightmares, flashbacks, and panic attacks
Braun et al., 1990	Alprazolam vs. Placebo (2.5–6)	DB, PC, CO 5 weeks PTSD Scale, IES, HAM-A, HAM-D	Miscellaneous PTSD	10	Significant improvement in anxiety. No effect on intrusion and avoidance. 41% drop-out (7 of 17)
Gelpin et al., 1996	Clonazepam, Alprazolam (2.5)	Prospective case control 6 mo. IES, SANX-state, CAPS	Recent trauma survivors	26	No effect of active treatment on the course of PTSD symptoms. More PTSD cases at 6 mo. in the active treatment group

TABLE 1e. Pharmacological Treatment of PTSD: Mood Stabilizers and Other Compounds

Mood Stabilizers and Other Compounds	Drug and Dose (mg/day)	Design,[a] Duration, Instruments[b]	Population	N	Results/Conclusion
Kitchner & Greenstein, 1985 (70)	Lithium (low doses; 300–600)	Clinical observation	Veterans	4	Reduced anger, irritability, anxiety, and insomnia
Lipper et al., 1986	Carbamazepine (577–780)	OT 6 weeks HAM-A, HAM-D, SCL-90, PMS, CGI	Veterans	10	Improved CGI scores. Reduced intensity and frequency of nightmares, flashbacks, and intrusion symptoms. No effects on avoidance
Wolf et al., 1987	Carbamazepine (dose not specified)	OT	Veterans	10	Improved impulse control, violent behavior, and anger
Brophy, 1991	Cyproheptadine (16–24) TCAs	CR Few days	Veterans	4	Stopped nightmares
Fesler, 1991	Valproate (250–2000)	OT 10.6 mo. PTSD scale	Veterans	14	Improved hyperarousal and hyperreactivity
Forster et al., 1995	Lithium 1200 (1200–1800)	CR 17 mo.; 11 mo. BPRS, GAF, clinical impression	Vietnam veterans	2	Decrease in irritability and anger outbursts

TABLE 1f. Pharmacological Treatment of PTSD: Miscellaneous Drugs

Miscellaneous Drugs	Drug and Dose (mg/day)	Design,[a] Duration, Instruments[b]	Population	N	Results/Conclusion
Katz et al., 1994–5	Brofaromine (50–150)	DB, PC, RA 14 weeks CAPS, CGI	Male > female, mostly noncombat	64	Improvement (CAPS and CGI) particularly in subjects with PTSD of less than 1 yr. Most of subjects remain symptomatic. 55% of treated patients and 26% of controls do not meet full PTSD criteria at end point.
Baker et al., 1995	Brofaromine (flexible dose titrated to 150)	DB, PC, RA 12 weeks CAPS, IES, PTSD scale, Global Evaluation	Male > female PTSD	113	Brofaromine = placebo. Higher than usual placebo response rate
Wells et al., 1991	Buspirone (35–90)	CR	Miscellaneous PTSD	3	Improved anxiety, insomnia, flashbacks, and depression
Duffy and Malloy, 1994	Buspirone (5–30)	OT 28 days Structured PTSD interview (SI-PTSD), IES, BDI	Vietnam veterans	8	Significant reduction in symptoms (7 of 8 subjects), particularly reexperiencing, avoidance, intrusion, and the BDI, less on the IES. Greatest change observed after 1 week

Brofaromine

Brofaromine is an investigational drug, which combines serotonin uptake inhibition and selective, reversible MAO-A inhibition. Two recent multicenter trials (Katz et al., 1995, Baker et al., 1995) have been conducted with the hope of deriving additional clinical benefit from the combined pharmacological effect of this compound. The results, however, were disappointing, and did not show any statistically significant advantage of brofaromine over a placebo. In both brofaromine studies, however, the placebo responses were unusually high, and perhaps obscured the efficacy of the active drug. Interestingly, post hoc analysis of Katz et al.'s study demonstrated greater improvement in a subgroup of PTSD patients whose disorder lasted for more than one year. Interestingly, 55% of the subjects treated with brofaromine did not meet the full diagnostic criteria for PTSD at the end of the study.

Benzodiazepines

Only few studies have assessed the efficacy of benzodiazepines in PTSD (Table 1d), and only one of those (Braun et al., 1990) was placebo-controlled. As expected, no major breakthrough in symptom reduction was achieved, although all studies reported improvement in anxiety and sleep symptoms. In a report on five patients with PTSD and multiple personality disorder, treatment with clonazepam seems to have reduced the occurrence of flashbacks, nightmares, and panic attacks (Loewenstein, 1988).

Importantly, Gelpin et al. (1996) compared 13 trauma survivors who received clonazepam or alprazolam within 18 days of their traumatic events with 13 trauma survivors, matched for symptoms severity one week after trauma, who did not receive any pharmacological treatment. The treatment had no effect on the course of PTSD symptoms, as measured 1 and 6 months following trauma. Moreover, the incidence of PTSD was higher in the group that received benzodiazepines. A weakness of this study, however, is the lack of random assignment to treatment groups and the relatively low doses of benzodiazepines administered (2.5–2.7 mg/day). It warns clinicians, however, of the possibility that some drug interventions may interfere with recovery from traumatic experiences and increase the risk for developing PTSD.

Mood Stabilizers

The administration of mood stabilizers in PTSD (Table 1e) has been construed as (1) an attempt to reduce the mood variations that are seen in PTSD and (2) a way to control a putative kindling phenomenon, which was thought to be involved in the genesis of the disorder. Although most studies were not placebo-controlled, improvement has been observed consistently, involving symptoms such as anger, irritability, violence, impulse control, as well as nightmares, flashbacks, intrusive recollections, and insomnia.

Other Agents

Attempts to treat PTSD with several other agents have been published, most as open, uncontrolled clinical trials or case reports (Table 1f). A study of trazodone, a $5HT_2$ receptor antagonist and weak 5HT reuptake inhibitor (Hertzberg et al., 1996), reported improvement in PTSD symptoms, as measured by clinician administered interviews. Buspirone, a $5HT_1$ partial agonist anxiolytic, has been administered in two open trials (Wells et al., 1991; Duffy & Malloy, 1994) and resulted in reduced reexperiencing symptoms, avoidance, and intrusion in most subjects. Inositol, a second-messenger precursor, was compared to a placebo in a study involving 13 subjects with PTSD (Kaplan et al., 1996) but was not found superior to a placebo. The beta adrenergic blocking agent, propranolol, was found useful in children who had acute PTSD (Famularo, 1988), whereas no improvement was noted after its administration to Cambodian refugees (Kinzie, 1989). The positive effect of propranolol in acute PTSD is of particular interest in the light of the recent report (Cahil et al., 1994) suggesting that this drug may reduce the amount of distressful information remembered after experimental exposure to a threatening story. Propranolol, as well as the so-called neuroprotective agents (i.e., those shown to prevent cortisol-induced cellular damage to the hippocampus, e.g., tianeptine, calcium channel blocking agents) and compounds that prevent the acquisition of kindled seizures (e.g., clonidine) may become candidates for the preventive treatment of PTSD.

Unexplored Agents and Treatment Modalities

Interestingly, antipsychotics, a most frequently used category of drugs, have not been studied in PTSD. Yet, some clinicians do administer neuroleptics to very chronic and agitated PTSD patients, when treatment with other agents fails or in conditions involving severe and prolonged dissociative states (A. Shalev, personal communication). The reason for not studying neuroleptics is unclear. It may be a reluctance to repeat past diagnostic errors, in which combat-related PTSD patients were misdiagnosed as suffering from psychoses and treated with neuroleptics. Another reason may be the presence of severe side effects (e.g., parkinsonism, dystonias, akathisia, tardive dyskinesia) which made the use of neuroleptics particularly unappealing for treating "neurotic" (that is, nonpsychotic) patients. Indeed, neuroleptics have not been tried in other anxiety disorders as well. However, the recent marketing of new antipsychotics that combine the classical dopamine receptor-blocking effect with activity on specific serotonin receptors and have fewer side effects might lead to increased interest in using these pharmacological agents to treat PTSD.

Discussion

Technical Limitations of Studies

Several important issues emerge from examining the literature on the pharmacological treatment of PTSD.

Unpublished Negative Studies.   Only a minority of the current studies is blind, randomized, and controlled. Aside from the frequently stated point about the shortcomings of uncontrolled trials, it is commonly acknowledged that the publication of open trials is facilitated by positive findings.

Expected Effect Size and Need for Larger Samples.   Given the chronic course of PTSD in some individuals, one should *a priori* expect a small treatment effect in those who remain with chronic PTSD (e.g., Kessler et al., 1995). For such a small effect to become statistically significant, larger studies are required because smaller changes may not be captured in small samples (Type II error).

Inclusion of Treatment Resistant PTSD Patients in Drug Trials.   The rule regarding the inclusion or exclusion of PTSD patients with resistance to prior pharmacotherapy has not been openly stated in any published treatment study of the disorder. Treatment resistance, however, is possibly the strongest predictor of another failure, particularly when similar compounds are used. For example, if many veterans who participated in currently published studies had prior histories of treatment failure, then the results of such studies are biased toward being smaller. Hence, we recommend that future studies openly consider and report on prior drug treatment and its effects. Indeed, the concept of treatment resistance should be borrowed from other disorders (e.g., depression, schizophrenia) and used in PTSD as a guideline for further treatment. Treatment of "drug-resistant" PTSD patients may include new agents as well as augmentation techniques, such as those used in treating depression.

Concurrent Psychosocial Stressors and Comorbid Disorders.   A similar case can be made for including information about extreme psychosocial conditions, in which many PTSD patients seem to be living (Johnson et al., 1996). The interference of ongoing stressors with the result of drug trials in PTSD has not been evaluated properly and may have a significant effect on outcome. The presence of comorbid disorders in up to 80% of PTSD patients is also a point to be considered in interpreting the current literature.

Boundaries of Underlying Assumptions   As pointed out in the introduction, several implicit assumptions underlie the practice of pharmacotherapy in PTSD. Some of those are shared by PTSD and other mental disorders (e.g., psychopathology is strongly compounded by neuropathology; current classification correctly identifies neurobiological entities). Other assumptions, however, are proper to PTSD. Among the latter is the idea that PTSD is the same disorder regardless of the triggering trauma. This idea leads to applying lessons learned in one group of survivors (e.g., war veterans) to other groups (e.g., rape victims). It also leads to including among the "triggering events" of PTSD both prolonged traumatizations (e.g., torture, concentration camp experiences, repeated abuse) and single short incidents such as motor vehicle accidents. The extent to which the results of these very different physiological and psychological events are equally amenable to pharmacotherapy is yet to be established. Traumatic events experienced during childhood may, similarly, affect the brain at a different developmental stage (or stages) and therefore require a specific treatment.

Another implicit idea is that pharmacotherapy alone should suffice to make a significant change in PTSD. It might be the case, however, that pharmacotherapy, at its best, only opens the way for individuals to start adapting themselves to living with the consequences of traumatic events. If such is the case, then pharmacotherapy is not sufficient—yet might be necessary because it opens a window of opportunity for psychosocial factors to operate. Rejecting pharmacotherapy for being partially successful in such a case is wrong. Pharmacological studies, therefore, may not reveal the full potential of pharmacotherapy in PTSD.

As stated before, successful pharmacotherapy does not lead to full remission in many chronic disorders, but rather to *stabilization and prevention of future exacerbations*.

TABLE 2. Pharmacotherapy at Different Stages of PTSD: Summary of Current Knowledge

Stage	Treatment Goals	Treatment Options	Documented Effect	Level of Certainty in Traumatic Stress
Impact phase (first hours)	• Reduce distress	Benzodiazepines, other tranquilizers	Anxiolytic effect	Anecdotal long-term effect uncertain. Many clinicians prefer to abstain from medication at this stage
	• Prevent primary neuronal "imprinting"	Propranolol	None	Theoretical
Immediate response (first days)	• Prevent "kindling" and memory consolidation	Clonidine, carbamazepine	None	Theoretical
	• Alleviate insomnia, agitation, dissociation	Clonidine, Bzs, other tranquilizers	Improved sleep, reduced distress	Preliminary. Bzs may increase the odds of developing PTSD
Short-term PTSD (first months)	• Prevent neuronal sensitization and chronic PTSD	Unknown	None	None
	• Prevent neuronal damage to hippocampi	Neuroprotective agents?	None	Theoretical
	• Alleviate symptoms of intrusion, avoidance	SSRIs, TCAs, MAOIs, others?	Anecdotal	Preliminary
	• Alleviate depression	SSRIs, TCAs	Favorable in depression	Preliminary
Chronic PTSD (>1 year)	• Reduce PTSD symptoms and associated anxiety and depression	SSRIs, TCAs, clonidine, MAOIs	Partial effect	Good
	• Reduce agitation, hyperarousal	Mood stabilizers	Partial effect	Fair

Many of our own patients, for example, continue to take the same drugs which, if one were to count their symptoms, have failed to produce a major change. Yet such treatment enables them a level of social adaptation and well-being that, in the absence of pharmacotherapy, might not have been possible.

Finally, the idea that similar neurobiological processes underlie each stage of the development of PTSD may obscure significant differences between stages of the disorder and consequently significant differences in treatment goals and potential responsivity. Table 2 presents a competing view of goals for pharmacotherapy at each stage of PTSD and shows areas to be explored in the future.

Guidelines for Treatment

The current literature indicates that pharmacotherapy can alleviate PTSD symptoms and associated depression and anxiety. Several agents identified are capable of producing such effects. The clinician, therefore, (1) can choose among different agents, (2) should anticipate partial effects, and (3) should often resolve to stabilize the patient's condition, and combine the treatment with psychosocial interventions or rehabilitation. Secondary features of the disorder (e.g., alcohol abuse, uncontrolled violence) should also be considered among the goals of pharmacotherapy.

The clinician's choice may be guided by the patient's most prominent symptoms, as follows: patients with severe reexperiencing, insomnia, and nightmares may be first treated with MAOIs or TCAs. In subjects whose depressed mood, explosiveness, and irritability are most prominent, SSRIs may be the logical first option. Hyperarousal and hyperactivity seem to respond well to mood stabilizers. The clinician should actively seek comorbidity, refrain from attributing all observed phenomena to PTSD, and monitor the effect of concurrent stressors. Future studies should show whether propranolol, clonidine, or other agents can effectively reduce the incidence of PTSD when administered immediately after exposure.

Finally, the treatment of PTSD is often experienced as frustrating and unrewarding. It would be advisable, therefore, to adopt a team approach in treating PTSD, to share responsibilities and to create multidisciplinary programs in which various treatment approaches are offered, according to individual needs.

References

Baker, D. G., Diamond, B. I., Gillette, G., Hamner, M., Katzelnick, D., Keller, T., Mellman, T. A., Pontius, E., Rosenthal, M., Tucker, P., van der Kolk, B. A., Katz, R. (1995). A double-blind, randomized, placebo controlled, multi-center study of brofaromine in the treatment of post traumatic stress disorder. *Psychopharmacology (Berlin)*, *122*(4), 386–389.

Bleich, A., Siegel, B., Garb, R., & Lerer, B. (1986). Post-traumatic stress disorder following combat exposure: Clinical features and psychopharmacological treatment. *British Journal of Psychiatry*, *149*, 354–369.

Brady K., Farfel, G., and the Sertraline PTSD Study Group (1998, December). Double blind mulitcenter comparison of sertraline and placebo in PTSD. ACNP annual meeting, Puerto Rico.

Brady, K. T., Sonne, S. C., & Roberts, J. M. (1995). Sertraline treatment of comorbid post traumatic stress disorder and alcohol dependence. *Journal of Clinical Psychiatry*, *56*(11), 502–505.

Braun, P., Greenberg, D., Dasberg, H., & Lerer, B. (1990). Core symptoms of posttraumatic stress disorder unimproved by alprazolam treatment. *Journal of Clinical Psychiatry*, *51*, 236–238.

Brophy, M. H. (1991). Cyproheptadine for combat nightmares in post-traumatic stress disorder and dream anxiety disorder. *Military Medicine*, *156*, 100–101.

Burstein, A. (1984). Treatment of post-traumatic stress disorder with imipramine. *Psychosomatics, 25,* 681–687.

Cahil, L., Prins, B., Weber, M., & McGaugh, J. L. (1994). Beta adrenergic activation and memory for emotional events. *Nature, 371,* 702–704.

Davidson, J., Kudler, H., Smith, R., Mahorney, S. L., Lipper, S., Hammett, E., Saunders, W. B., & Cavenar, J. O. J. (1990). Treatment of posttraumatic stress disorder with amitriptyline and placebo. *Archives of General Psychiatry, 47,* 259–266.

Davidson, J. R. T., Londborg, P. D., Pearlstein, T., Weisler, R. Sikes, C., Farfel, G. M. (1997, December). Double blind comparison of sertraline and placebo in patients with posttraumatic stress disorder. ACNP annual meeting, Hawaii.

Davidson, J., van der Kolk, B., Brady, K., Rothbaum, B., Sikes, C., & Farfe, G. (1997). Double-blind comparison of sertraline and placebo in patients with posttraumatic stress disorder. *Presented at the 36th Annual Meeting of the American College of NeuroPsychopharmacology,* Hawaii, December 8–12.

Davidson, J., Walker, J., & Kilts, C. (1987). A pilot study of phenelzine in the treatment of post-traumatic stress disorder. *British Journal of Psychiatry, 150,* 252–255.

Davidson, J. R., Kudler, H. S., Saunders, W. B., et al. (1993). Predicting response to amitriptyline in post-traumatic stress disorder. *American Journal of Psychiatry, 150,* 1024–1029.

Dow, B., & Kline, N. (1997). Antidepressant treatment of post traumatic stress disorder and major depression in veterans. *Annals of Clinical Psychiatry, 9*(1), 1–5.

Duffy, J. D., & Malloy, P. F. (1994). Efficacy of buspirone in the treatment of post traumatic stress disorder: An open trial. *Annals of Clinical Psychiatry, 6*(1), 33–37.

Falcon, S., Ryan, C., Chamberain, Y., & Curtis, G. (1985). Tricyclics: Possible treatment for posttraumatic stress disorder. *Journal of Clinical Psychiatry, 44,* 385–388.

Famularo, R., et al. (1988). Propranolol treatment for childhood post-traumatic stress disorder, acute type: A pilot study. *American Journal of Diseases of Childhood, 142,* 1244–1247.

Feldmann, T. B. (1987). Alprazolam in the treatment of posttraumatic stress disorder [letter]. *Journal of Clinical Psychiatry, 48,* 216–217.

Fesler, F. A. (1991). Valproate in combat-related posttraumatic stress disorder. *Journal of Clinical Psychiatry, 52,* 361–364.

Forster, P. L., Schoenfeld, F. B., Marmar, C. R., & Lang, A. J. (1995). Lithium for irritability in post traumatic stress disorder. *Journal of Traumatic Stress, 8*(1), 143–149.

Frank, J. B., Kosten, T. R., Giller, E. L., & Dan, E. (1988). A randomized clinical trial of phenelzine and imipramine for posttraumatic stress disorder. *American Journal of Psychiatry, 145,* 1289–1291.

Friedman, M. J. (1988). Toward rational pharmacotherapy for posttraumatic stress disorder: An interim report. *American Journal of Psychiatry, 145,* 281–285.

Friedman, M. J. (1996). Drug treatment for PTSD. Answers and questions. In R. Yehuda & A. C. McFarlane, (Eds.), *Annals of the New York Academy of Science,* Vol. 821, 358–371.

Gelpin, E., Bonne, O., Peri, T., Brandes, D., Pitman, R. K., & Shalev, A. Y. (1996). Treatment of recent trauma survivors with benzodiazepines: A prospective study. *Journal of Clinical Psychiatry, 57,* 390–394.

Hertzberg, M. A., Feldman, M. E., Beckham, J. C., & Davidson, J. R. T. (1996). Trial of trazodone for post traumatic stress disorder using a multiple baseline group design. *Journal of Clinical Psychopharmacology, 16*(4), 294–298.

Hogben, G. L., & Cornfield, R. B. (1981). Treatment of traumatic war neurosis with phenelzine. *Archives of General Psychiatry, 38*(4), 440–445.

Horowitz, M. J. (1974). Stress response syndromes: Character style and dynamic psychotherapy. *Archives of General Psychiatry, 31,* 768–781.

Janoff Bulman, R. (1985). The aftermath of victimization: Rebuilding shattered assumptions. In C. R. Figley (Ed.), *Trauma and its wake, the study and treatment of post-traumatic stress disorder* (pp. 15–36). New York: Brunner/Mazel.

Johnson, D. R., Rosenheck, R., Fontana, A., Lubin, H., Charney, D., & Southwick, S. (1996). Outcome of intensive inpatient treatment for combat-related posttraumatic stress disorder. *American Journal of Psychiatry, 153,* 771–777.

Kaplan, Z., et al. (1996). Inositol treatment of PTSD. *Anxiety, 2,* 51–52.

Katz, R. J., Lott, M. H., Arbus, P., Crocq, L., Herlobsen, P., Lingjaerde, O., Lopez, G., Loughrey, G. C., MacFarlan, D. J., McIvor, R., et al. (1994–1995). Pharmacotherapy of post-traumatic stress disorder with a novel psychotropic. *Anxiety, 1*(4), 169–174.

Kauffman, C. D., Reist, C., Djenderedjian, A., Nelson, J. N., et al. (1987). Biological markers of affective disorders and posttraumatic stress disorder: A pilot study with desipramine. *Journal of Clinical Psychiatry, 48,* 366–367.

Keane, T. M., Fairbank, J. A., Caddel, M. T., et al. (1985). A behavioral approach to assessing and treating post-traumatic stress disorders in Vietnam veterans. In C. R. Figley (Ed.), *Trauma and its wake, the study and treatment of post-traumatic stress disorder* (pp. 257–294). New York: Brunner/Mazel.

Kessler, R. C., Sonnega, A., Bromet, E. J., Hughes, M., & Nelson, C. B. (1995). Posttraumatic stress disorder in the National Comorbidity Survey. *Archives of General Psychiatry, 52,* 1048–1060.

Kinzie, J., & Leung, P. (1989). Clonidine in Cambodian patients with posttraumatic stress disorder. *Journal of Nervous and Mental Disorders, 177,* 546–550.

Kinzie, J. D. (1989). Therapeutic approaches to traumatized Cambodian refugees. *Journal of Traumatic Stress, 2,* 207–208.

Kitchner, I., & Greenstein, R. (1985). Low dose lithium carbonate in the treatment of post traumatic stress disorder: Brief communication. *Military Medicine, 150,* 378–381.

Kline, N. A., Dow, B. M., Brown, S. A., & Matloff, J. L. (1994). Sertraline efficacy in depressed combat veterans with posttraumatic stress disorder. *American Journal of Psychiatry, 151,* 621.

Kosten, T. R., Frank, J. B., Dan, E., et al. (1991). Pharmacotherapy for posttraumatic stress disorder using phenelzine or imipramine. *Journal of Nervous and Mental Disorders, 179,* 366–370.

Lerer, B., Bleich, A., Kotler, M., Garb, R., et al. (9187). Posttraumatic stress disorder Israeli combat veterans: Effect of phenelzine treatment. *Archives of General Psychiatry, 44,* 976–981.

Lipper, S., Davidson, J. R. T., Grady, T. A., et al. (1986). Preliminary study of carbammazepine in posttraumatic stress disorder. *Psychosomatics, 72,* 849–854.

Loewenstein, R. J., Hornstein, N., Farber, B. (1988). Open trial of clonazepam in the treatment of posttraumatic stress symptoms in MPD. *Dissociation, 1,* 3–12.

Marmar, C. R., Schoenfeld, F., Weiss, D. F., Metzler, T., Zatzick, D., Wu, R., Smiga, S., Tecott, L., & Neylan, T. (1996). Open trial of fluvoxamine for combat related post traumatic stress disorder. *Journal of Clinical Psychiatry, 57* (Suppl 8), 66–70; discussion 71–72.

Nagy, L., Southwick, S. M., & Charney, D . S. (1993). Open prospective trial of Fluoxetine for posttraumatic stress disorder. *Journal of Clinical Psychopharmacology, 13,* 107–113.

Riest, C., Kauffman, C. D., Haier, R. J. (1976). A controlled trial of desipramine in 81 men with post traumatic stress disorder. *American Journal of Psychiatry, 146,* 513–516.

Rothbaum, B. O., Ninan, P. T., & Thomas, L. (1996). Sertraline in the treatment of rape victims with post traumatic stress disorder. *Journal of Traumatic Stress, 9*(4), 865–871.

Shalev, A. (1997). Treatment of prolonged posttraumatic stress disorder—learning from experience. *Journal of Traumatic Stress, 10,* 415–422.

Shay, J. (1992). Fluoxetine reduces explosiveness and elevates mood of Vietnam combat vets with PTSD. *Journal of Traumatic Stress, 5,* 97–110.

Shestatzki, M., Greenberg, D., & Lerer, B. (1988). A controlled trial of phenelzine in posttraumatic stress disorder. *Psychiatry Research, 24,* 149–155.

Solomon, S. D., Gerrity, E. T., & Muff, A. M. (1992). Efficacy of treatment for posttraumatic stress disorder. *Journal of the American Medical Association, 268,* 633–638.

Southwick, S. M., et al. (1994). Use of tricyclics and monoamine oxidase inhibitors in the treatment of PTSD: A quantitative review. In M. M. Murburg (Ed.), *Catecholamine function in post-traumatic stress disorder: Emerging concepts* (pp. 293–305). Washington, DC: American Psychiatric Press.

van der Kolk, B. A., Dryfuss, D., Michaels, M., et al. (1994). Fluoxetine in post traumatic stress disorder. *Journal of Clinical Psychiatry, 55,* 517–522.

Wells, B. G., Chu, C. C., Johnson, R., Nasdahl, C., Ayubi, M. A., Sewell, E., & Statham, P. (1991). Buspirone in the treatment of posttraumatic stress disorder. *Pharmacotherapy, 11,* 340–343.

Wolf, M. E., Alavi , A., & Mosnaim, A. D. (1987). Pharmacological interventions in Vietnam veterans with post traumatic stress disorder. *Research communications in psychology, psychiatry and behavior, 12,* 169–176.

27

Critical Incident Stress Debriefing

INGRID V. E. CARLIER

Crisis theory has taught us that people who have been through a horrific event such as a plane crash, fire, or other disaster have a natural need to share their experiences and emotions with one another after it is over (see, for instance, Butcher & Maudal, 1976; Caplan, 1961, 1964). This natural process of social care and support is also known as the recoil phase (Tyhurst, 1951). It is thought that most crisis reactions are transitory and that a crisis is resolved within 6 to 8 weeks, either normally or into a pathological form (Bloom, 1963).

Besides this natural process of social care and support, we also know a professionalized form of trauma relief known as debriefing. Debriefing typically consists of a single group session, set up if possible within 48 or 72 hours of the traumatic event. It is meant to provide initial psychosocial relief to victims and rescue workers. A debriefing session is usually led by two debriefers and lasts an average of two to three hours. Debriefing should be just one component of a comprehensive Critical Incident Stress Management (CISM) program carried out by properly qualified and trained team members (Robinson & Mitchell, 1993). Although debriefing was originally developed to provide psychosocial relief to groups, the technique can also be employed for individuals, couples, or families.

The gradual professionalization of trauma relief in the form of debriefing is being stimulated by a number of factors. One factor is the supposition that certain trauma-sensitive occupations such as police work, fire fighting, and military service provide insufficient opportunities for the natural process of trauma relief, perhaps as a result of a "macho culture." It became clear that many victims of traumatic experiences, instead of finding support and understanding in their environment, are more likely to meet with reproaches ("you should have been paying more attention" or "you must have been asking for it"). A third stimulus was that large groups of war survivors have been found to be still suffering from chronic post-traumatic stress disorder (PTSD; APA, 1994) many years later. This has fostered a wish to develop prevention methods to counter these pernicious delayed effects. This wish was also inspired by the fact that PTSD, which was formerly called "traumatic neurosis," has achieved some notoriety

INGRID V.E. CARLIER • Department of Psychiatry, Academic Medical Center, University of Amsterdam, Amsterdam, 1101 BC, The Netherlands.

International Handbook of Human Response to Trauma, edited by Shalev, Yehuda, and McFarlane. Kluwer Academic / Plenum Publishers, New York, 2000.

due to the numerous financial claims made by victims of critical events. Governments and armies, police forces and fire brigades, and businesses whose employees are subject to risk, have all seized eagerly upon the idea that debriefing might avert the delayed effects of traumas.

The technique of debriefing is by no means new (see, for instance, Salmon, 1919), though it has been gaining popularity since the 1980s. The debriefing model created by Jeffrey Mitchell (1983) is the one most commonly applied worldwide, and others have developed more or less modified versions (see, for instance, Armstrong et al., 1991). Basically, differences among debriefing models are rather slight; all models include more or less the same key features: participants in a debriefing session are given the chance to talk about what they have gone through and to air their feelings; post-traumatic stress reactions are catalogued; and information is supplied about the post-traumatic stress syndrome, about coping techniques, and about further opportunities for aftercare should the condition persist.

A general assumption behind a method like debriefing is, for instance, that the group atmosphere will have a therapeutic effect on the individual. It is thought to counterbalance the fear and horror one experienced during the event in question. Black (1987) even speaks of a "libidinal cocoon." The idea is also that talking about the traumatic event can promote psychological recovery. Basically, this boils down to the psychoanalytic notion of catharsis. It is presumed that the individual is overwhelmed by emotions during the psychotrauma, and the hope is that the emotional ventilation ("abreaction") that occurs during debriefing will bring on relief of the inner psychological tensions and especially the recovery of emotional control, thus preventing post-traumatic stress symptomatology (Benyakar et al., 1989).

This brings us to the central question to be addressed here: Can professionalized trauma relief activities, such as debriefing, prevent post-traumatic stress symptoms? Even as the popularity of debriefing grows, manifest doubts have arisen among researchers as to the technique's effectiveness (see among others Raphael et al., 1995). This article first reviews research on debriefing and then goes on to consider whether the doubts raised about it must be taken seriously or can reasonably be dismissed.

Measuring Psychological Effectiveness After Debriefing

The point of departure for debriefing has always been that it has a preventive effect on psychological injury caused by psychotraumas. More specifically, it is presumed that debriefing discourages the development of PTSD (Mitchell, 1983; Dyregrov, 1989; Mitchell & Everly, 1994). PTSD is part of the DSM category Anxiety Disorders, and it may be regarded as the most common psychiatric disturbance after a psychotrauma, especially in trauma-sensitive occupations such as police work (Carlier & Gersons, 1992, 1994, 1995; Gersons & Carlier, 1993; Carlier et al., 1996).

How can we best measure the impact of debriefing? Controlled systematic studies are required that compare a group of debriefed subjects with a nondebriefed control group (Kazdin, 1992). Because debriefing is often made available standardly (e.g., the police), randomization of research samples is difficult to achieve due to ethical considerations. The minimum requirements in any case are that the nondebriefed control group should be formed by purely accidental circumstances and that the two subsamples (debriefed and nondebriefed) should be equivalent to each other in background variables, prior psychiatric history, and the nature of the traumatic experience.

Research on Debriefing

The first studies discussed are impact evaluation studies, which draw conclusions on the psychological efficacy of debriefing based on control group comparisons. Then exploratory studies are examined, which, due to the absence of a control group, do not allow definitive conclusions as to their effectiveness. And third, some related impact studies are discussed which evaluate not debriefing but other techniques of crisis intervention.

(a) Impact Evaluation Studies on Debriefing

McFarlane carried out a study in 1988 which today ranks as one of the classics. He studied a total of 469 firefighters after a series of Australian forest fires. His investigation pointed for the first time to the possibility of an alarming, long-term adverse impact of debriefing: subjects who were debriefed were significantly more likely to develop late-onset PTSD than those not debriefed (see also McFarlane, 1993). In 1989, Hytten and Hasle studied 58 volunteer firefighters who had performed rescue work at a large hotel fire in Norway. The researchers were unable to detect any preventive effect of debriefing on PTSD: both the debriefed and the nondebriefed developed post-traumatic stress symptomatology in the acute phase. Bohl (1991) studied the effects of debriefing in a group of 71 police officers three months after some of them underwent it. Contrary to her expectations, she found that debriefing failed to curb anxious feelings, though the debriefed did report less anger and fewer depressive feelings. Bohl's study, however, was complicated by the fact that the nondebriefed officers were from a police force which did not consider debriefing necessary. That meant that the two samples may have differed in organizational climate.

Following a civilian plane crash in the Netherlands, a rather unique situation arose in which one group of Amsterdam police officers underwent debriefing in accordance with the Mitchell model, whereas by chance a second group was not debriefed. The latter group was used as a control in a longitudinal research project. The two groups were equivalent in the principal background variables and in prior psychiatric history, trauma anamnesis, and the nature of the rescue work. PTSD and any other psychopathology were determined by structured diagnostic interviews. The results showed that in the short term, there were no significant differences between debriefed and nondebriefed participants. In the long term, the group of debriefed subjects developed significantly more PTSD symptomatology, in particular, hyperarousal symptoms. They also suffered more from depressive and agoraphobic symptoms and from more rage and distrust (Carlier et al., 1994, 1995; Gersons & Carlier, 1993).

Griffith and Watts (1994) followed a large group of 285 rescue workers after several large-scale road accidents. Here, too, a long-term adverse effect became evident as debriefing touched off psychological complaints in the workers. Doctor et al. (1994) investigated the impact of debriefing on a group of 171 police officers, and they came to the same troubling conclusion. It further emerged here for the first time that debriefing had no significant preventive effect on work absenteeism. Deahl and colleagues (1994) studied the effectiveness of debriefing on a group of 74 Gulf War soldiers. Both debriefed and nondebriefed soldiers developed post-traumatic stress complaints. In the studies by Vernberg (1995) and Hamada (1995), no significant difference could be found between debriefed and nondebriefed child disaster victims in their post-traumatic stress reactions.

Kenardy et al. (1996) studied 195 earthquake relief workers in a prospective, controlled design, and found that, over time, psychological complaints were slower to recede among debriefed than among nondebriefed workers. Lee et al. (1996) studied the influence of debriefing on emotional adaptation in women following early miscarriage. The results of this controlled study revealed that debriefing was perceived to be helpful but did not influence emotional adaptation. Also, a recent study by Bisson (1996) can be cited. He carried out a randomized, controlled trial on 113 victims of major fires, with follow-up measurements to over 13 months. He established that debriefing entails serious risks for traumatized people. In agreement with the study by Carlier and her colleagues (1994, 1995), Bisson showed that debriefing resulted in PTSD, as well as in anxiety and depression.

(b) Exploratory Studies on Debriefing

In addition to the impact evaluation studies just discussed, there are descriptive, noncontrolled studies. Sloan (1988) questioned 30 plane-crash survivors after debriefing, and discoved considerable symptomatology in all of them. Flannery et al. (1991) interviewed 62 psychiatric nurses who were debriefed after violent incidents involving patients. Some 69% of them indicated that they had experienced the debriefing as worthwhile. The remainder expressed varying degrees of criticism. Some 7% eventually needed professional treatment. Searle and Bisson (1992) described the condition of eight traumatized soldiers who were debriefed within five days of their Gulf War experiences. The results were distressing: six of them later qualified for the PTSD diagnosis and five underwent lengthy treatment. Scott and Jordan reported in 1993 on their study of 192 firefighters in the wake of the 1992 Los Angeles riots. This is an important study because it showed for the first time that satisfaction with debriefing varies widely among participants. Although 50% regarded it as more or less effective, the other 50% found it ineffective.

Stallard and Law (1993) studied a group of seven children after their involvement in a bus accident. After two debriefing sessions, held 4 months post-trauma, a significant decline in PTSD scores was recorded for some children. The best known satisfaction study is undoubtedly that by Robinson and Mitchell (1993). They studied 172 relief and care workers 2 weeks after they had undergone any of 31 debriefings. Most relief and care workers expressed that they were very happy with the debriefing. In 1994, Sutker and colleagues reported on the condition of 24 debriefed army reservists after Operation Desert Storm. Half of them were suffering from PTSD and also from depression and alcohol abuse.

(c) Related Crisis Intervention Studies

Some final studies can be cited which focus not on debriefing but on other types of crisis intervention, namely, preventive, brief trauma counselling. These are mostly individual rather than group interventions, which are often comprised of multiple sessions (for instance, two, three or four). Raphael's (1977) controlled study demonstrated the efficacy of "brief early intervention" in 30 widowed women. Because this involved a life event, it is uncertain how far the findings can be generalized to psychotraumas. Bunn and Clarke (1979) did a controlled study on the effects a "20-minute supportive interview" had on relatives of seriously ill or injured patients. Immediately after the interview, the relatives were found to be less fearful than noninterviewed subjects, but the lack of a follow-up measurement makes it hard to interpret the results any further. Bordow and Porritt (1979) studied 70 male road-accident victims in three groups: no intervention; intervention solely in the form of an "immediate review" (comparable to debriefing), and combined intervention in the form of "immediate review" and "2–10 hours of formal intervention." Some 3 months post-trauma, all three groups were suffering psychological complaints, but all in all the combined-intervention group proved best off. Interestingly, though, the group that underwent no intervention was the quickest to eventually resume work. Another complication was that significantly more of the men in the two intervention conditions turned out to be married. That makes it uncertain how much influence the interventions had. Clear in any case was that satisfying social support (relatives, friends, family) led to fewer psychological complaints by respondents (see also Joseph et al., 1992).

Another study is that by Kilpatrick and Veronen (1984). They evaluated a brief, preventive behavior program on the basis of a controlled study of 49 recent rape victims. They could detect no influence of the program on symptoms. Solomon and Benbenishty (1986) investigated all soldiers who had PTSD following the 1982 war in Lebanon. They found that early counseling served to reduce symptoms. Duckworth (1986) studied police officers after a major conflagration and offered them brief, individual counseling. Respondents reported a reduction of symptoms afterward, but given the lack of a control group, it is unclear whether that can be credited to the counseling. Steinmetz (1990) did a controlled study of the effects of crime-victim support and primary relief and came up with some remarkable findings. Although the ultimate "overall" effect of victim support was negligible, victims of less serious crimes (such as burglary or bag snatching) with crime-victim support did experience fewer short-term practical and coping problems than those who received no help. In contrast to this, however, the victims of very serious crimes (such as violent burglaries, assaults, or rapes) who had crime-victim support were more likely to suffer by reexperiencing symptoms in the long run compared to victims who had lacked help but who definitely would have accepted it.

Yule (1992) carried out a controlled study on the effectiveness of early interventions with child disaster survivors. Debriefing was held 10 days after the disaster in two small, open groups, making use of a problem-solving approach based on cognitive-behavioral methods. Debriefed children scored significantly lower than nondebriefed children on intrusions and on unrelated fears, but no significant differences were found in avoidance, depression, anxiety, or related fears. Ford et al. (1993) found tentative support for the efficacy of a proactive family psychosocial debriefing procedure with veterans and their families. The procedure was based on life-span developmental and self-psychology family systems theory and a communitarian social integration model. Brom and associates (1993) investigated the impact of an individual preventive counseling program on a group of 151 road-accident victims. They found no significant preventive effect whatsoever of this intervention in the acute phase: both the experimental and the control group developed PTSD. Satisfaction and symptoms were in no way linked. One final study by Foa and colleagues (1995) can be cited. They found evidence of a favorable effect of a brief preventive cognitive-behavioral program on 10 victims of sexual or other forms of violence.

Discussion

In the first place, quite a few studies have shown that the currently prevailing relief methodology of debriefing has failed to achieve its prophylactic aim of preventing post-traumatic stress problems in disaster victims. Even if the use of alternative outcome measures is considered for future research on the effects of debriefing (such as group cohesion; see Orner, 1995), assessing symptomatology remains imperative. After all, debriefing is quite a powerful influencing technique, and it can inadvertently disrupt the natural, fragile coping processes of traumatized people. Even allowing for possible methodological flaws that are inherent in field research (not all studies were randomized, prospective), we still have some evidence of possible hazards of debriefing from controlled impact evaluation studies. It would be prudent for care workers and policy makers to take such hazards into account.

A second point is that debriefing sessions are in themselves often valued by those who have taken part, and as such they appear compatible with the natural desire to meet with others who have had the same distressing experience, to talk about it, and to experience the emotions together. The latter observation is often used by the adherents of debriefing as an argument in favor of it.

The foregoing conclusions raise the question of how to go about providing the best professionalized trauma relief in the future. Professionalized trauma relief should avoid secondary traumatization and at the same time stimulate the recovery of emotional control (see also Turnbull, 1994). Regaining control over the emotions implies, for instance, that the traumatic event can be assimilated into the cognitive schemata or conceptions of the traumatized individual (see Lazarus & Folkman, 1984). Hence, if there is to be a place for professionalized trauma relief in the sense of debriefing, it must become effective, especially in this regard.

In this context, it is also important to note the more favorable findings obtained by impact evaluation studies on crisis intervention techniques other than debriefing. The methodology of these relevant techniques differs from debriefing in both form and content. Debriefing, according to the prevailing method, ordinarily consists of a single session within 2 or 3 days of the trauma. The other crisis intervention studies reviewed here, by contrast, show the operation of mostly individual and repeated interventions (two, three or four sessions). These interventions mostly commence later than debriefing, for instance, 1 or 2 weeks post-trauma or even later (see, for instance, Chemtob et al., 1997). Contrary to debriefing, these interventions are firmly structured, and they are founded on far more specific theoretical principles. Therefore, we can better speak of brief preventive trauma counselling, rather than debriefing. Such approaches may be based, for example, on the cognitive-behavioral model proposed by Foa et al. (1995), by Ellison and Genz (1983), or by Yule (1992). Further research is needed to see whether this alternative, more specific trauma relief method indeed produces better results than debriefing. Because the hazards of debriefing especially tend to emerge in the long term, longitudinal research is required.

Three other pertinent questions need to be included in future research. To begin with, one might wonder whether different traumatic events (hostage-takings, rapes, disasters, etc.) might require different relief methods. No conclusions can be drawn on this from the research now available. A second question pertains to the care providers themselves. Because trauma relief can be regarded as crisis intervention, it is often taken for granted that such relief can be carried out by paraprofessionals (Auerbach & Kilmann, 1977). In the trauma context, paraprofessionals are key figures (clergy, teachers, police, community workers, etc.), volunteers (Salvation Army, Red Cross, Victim Support, or, in the case of occupational traumas, co-workers), or primary care workers (such as family doctors, district nurses, and social workers). They have their professional counterparts, in this case psychologists and psychiatrists (secondary care workers, that is, specialized mental health workers). It has yet to be determined whether the effectiveness of preventive trauma care is linked to the care providers' level of training (paraprofessionals versus professionals). In the third place one might wonder whether it is necessary and indeed wise to administer professionalized trauma relief to all disaster victims or rather than just to the high-risk cases. This suggestion is in line with Bisson and Deahl's (1994) proposition that healthy traumatized people who have adequate social networks will ordinarily need no professionalized trauma relief. In this light, the most important task for public authorities after a disaster is to protect the natural support network, that consists of relatives, family members, friends and neighbors or to restore it as swiftly as possible.

Acknowledgments. The study of Carlier et al. (1994, 1995) on the efficacy of debriefing was made possible by grants of the Prevention Fund, the Ministry of Home Affairs, the National Foundation for Mental Health, the Inspectorate for Mental Health Care, and the City of Amsterdam.

References

American Psychiatric Association. (1994). *Diagnostic and statistical manual of mental disorders*, 4th ed. Washington, DC: American Psychiatric Press.

Armstrong, K., O'Callahan, W., & Marmar, C. (1991). Debriefing Red Cross disaster personnel: The multiple stressor debriefing model. *Journal of Trauma and Stress*, 4, 581–594.

Auerbach, S. M., Kilmann, P. R. (1977). Crisis intervention: A review of outcome research. *Psychological Bulletin*, 84, 1189–1217.

Benyaker, M., Kutz, I., Dasberg, H., & Stern, M. J. (1989). The collapse of structure: A structural approach to trauma. *Journal of Trauma and Stress*, 2, 431–450.

Bisson, J. I. (1996). Critical incident stress debriefing: Does it work? Presented at the *Second World Conference of the International Society for Traumatic Stress Studies*, June 9–13, Jerusalem, Israel.

Bisson, J. I., Deahl, M. P. (1994). Psychological debriefing and prevention of posttraumatic stress. More research is needed. *British Journal of Psychiatry*, 165, 717–720.

Black, J. M. (1987). The libidinal cocoon: A nurturing retreat for families of plane crash victims. *Hospital and Community Psychiatry*, 38, 1322–1326.

Bloom, B. (1963). Definitional aspects of the crises concept. *Journal of Consulting Psychology*, 27 498–502.

Bohl, N. (1991). The effectiveness of brief psychological interventions in police officers after critical incidents. In T. T. Reese, J. M. Horn, C. Dunning (Eds.), *Critical incidents in policing*. pp. 31–37 Washington, DC: U.S. Department of Justice.

Bordow, S., & Porritt, D. (1979). An experimental evaluation of crisis intervention. *Social Science Medicine*, 13A,: 251–256.

Brom, D., Kleber, R. J., & Hofman, M. C. (1993). Victims of traffic accidents: Incidence and prevention of posttraumatic stress disorder. *Journal of Clinical Psychology*, 49, 131–140.

Bunn, T. A., & Clarke, A. M. (1979). Crisis intervention: An experimental study of the effects of a brief period of counseling on the anxiety of relatives of seriously injured or ill hospital patients. *British Journal of Medical Psychology, 52*, 191–195.

Butcher, J. N., & Maudal, G. R. (1976). *Crisis intervention*. In I. B. Weiner (Ed.), *Clinical Methods in Psychology*. New York: Wiley-Interscience.

Caplan, G. (1961). *An approach to community mental health*. New York: Grune & Stratton.

Caplan, G. (1964). *Principles of preventive psychiatry*. New York: Basic Books.

Carlier, I. V. E., & Gersons, B. P. R. (1992). Development of a scale for traumatic stress incidents in police work. *Psychiatrica Fennica Supplementum, 23*, 59–70.

Carlier, I. V. E., & Gersons, B. P. R. (1994). Trauma at work: Posttraumatic stress disorder; an occupational health hazard. *The Journal of Occupational Health and Safety—Australia and New Zealand, 19*, 254–266.

Carlier, I. V. E., & Gersons, B. P. R. (1995). Partial PTSD: The issue of psychological scars and the occurrence of PTSD symptoms. *Journal of Nervous and Mental Disorders, 183*, 107–109.

Carlier, I. V. E., Van Uchelen, J. J., Lamberts, R. D., & Gersons, B. P. R. (1994). Het effect van debriefen. Een onderzoek bij de Amsterdamse politie naar aanleiding van de Bijlmerramp (The effect of debriefing. A study at the Amsterdam police after the Bijlmer plane crash). Academic Medical Center at the University of Amsterdam, Department of Psychiatry (in Dutch only).

Carlier, I. V. E., Lamberts, R. D., Van Uchelen, J. J., & Gersons, B. P. R. (1995). Het lange-termijn effect van debriefen. Een vervolgonderzoek bij de Amsterdamse politie naar aanleiding van de Bijlmerramp (The long-term effect of debriefing. A continued study at the Amsterdam police after the Bijlmer plane crash). Academic Medical Center at the University of Amsterdam, Department of Psychiatry (in Dutch only).

Carlier, I. V. E., Fouwels, A. J., Lamberts, R. D., & Gersons, B. P. R. (1996). Posttraumatic stress disorder and dissociation in traumatized police officers. *American Journal of Psychiatry, 153*(10), 1325–1328.

Chemtob, C. M., Thomas, S., & Law, W. (1997). Post disaster intervention: A field study of the impact of debriefing on psychological distress. *American Journal of Psychiatry, 154*, 415–417.

Deahl, M. P., Gilham, A. B., Thomas, J., Searle, M. M., & Srinivasan, M. (1994). Psychological sequelae following the Gulf war. Factors associated with subsequent morbidity and the effectiveness of psychological debriefing. *British Journal of Psychiatry, 165*, 60–65.

Doctor, R. S., Curtis, D., & Isaacs, G. (1994). Psychiatric morbidity in policemen and the effect of brief psychotherapeutic intervention: A pilot study. *Stress and Medicine, 10*, 151–157.

Duckworth, D. H. (1986). Psychological problems arising from disaster work. *Stress and Medicine, 2*, 315–323.

Dyregrov, A. (1989). Caring for helpers in disaster situations: Psychological debriefing. *Disaster Management, 2*, 25–30.

Ellison, K. W., & Genz J. L. (1983). Stress and the police officers. Springfield, IL: C. C. Thomas.

Flannery, R. B., Fulton, P., Tausch, J., & Deloffi, A. Y. (1991). A program to help staff cope with psychological sequelae of assaults by patients. *Hospital and Community Psychiatry, 42*, 935–938.

Ford, J., Shaw, D., Sennhauser, S., Greaves, D., Thacker, B., Chandler, P., Schwartz, L., & McClain, V. (1993). Psychological debriefing after Operations Desert Storm: Marital and family assessment and intervention. *Journal of Social Issues, 49*, 73–102.

Foa, E. B., Hearst-Ikeda, D., & Perry, K. J. (1995). Evaluation of a brief cognitive-behavioral program for the prevention of chronic PTSD in recent assault victims. *Journal of Consulting and Clinical Psychology, 63*, 948–955.

Gersons, B. P. R., & Carlier, I. V. E. (1993). Plane crash crisis intervention: A preliminary report from Bijlmermeer Amsterdam. *The Journal of Crisis Intervention and Suicide Prevention, 14*, 109–116.

Griffith, J., & Watts, R. (1994). The Kensey and Grafton bus crashes: The aftermath. East Lismore: Instructional Design Solutions.

Hamada, R. S. (1995). School-based postdisaster interventions with children: Evaluation of outcomes. Presented at the *International Society of Traumatic Stress Study Annual Meeting*, November 2–6, Boston.

Hytten, K., & Hasle, A. (1989). Fire fighters: A study of stress and coping. *Acta Psychiatrica Scandinavia, 80*, 50–55.

Joseph, S., Andrews, B., Williams, R., & Yule, W. (1992). Crisis support and psychiatric symptomatology in adult survivors of the Jupiter cruise ship disaster. *British Journal of Clinical Psychology, 31*, 63–73.

Kazdin, A. E. (1992). Research design in clinical psychology. Boston: Allyn & Bacon.

Kenardy, J. A., Webster, R. A., Lewin, T. J., Carr, V. J., Hazel, P. L., & Carter, G. L. (1996). Stress debriefing and patterns of recovery following a natural disaster. *Journal of Trauma and Stress, 9*, 37–50.

Kilpatrick, D. G., & Veronen, L. J. (1984). Treatment for rape-related problems: Crisis intervention is not enough. In L. Cohen, W. Clairborn, & G. Specter (Eds.), *Crisis intervention* (2nd ed, pp. 165–185). New York: Human Sciences Press.

Lazarus, R. S., & Folkman, S. (1984). Cognitive appraisal processing. In R. S. Lazarus, & S. Folkman (Eds.), *Stress appraisal and coping* (pp. 22–52). New York: Springer.

Lee, C., Slade, P., & Lygo, V. (1996). The influence of psychological debriefing on emotional adaptation in women following early miscarriage: A preliminary study. *British Journal of Medical Psychology, 69*, 47–58.

McFarlane, A. C. (1988). The aetiology of post-traumatic stress disorders following a natural disaster. *British Journal of Psychiatry, 151*, 116–121.

McFarlane, A. C. (1993). Helping the victims of natural disasters. Unpublished manuscript. Dept. of Psychiatry, University of Adelaide. Adelaide.

Mitchell, T. J. (1983). When disaster strikes. *Journal of Emergency Medical Services, 8*, 36–39.

Mitchell, T. J., & Everly, G. S. (1995). Preventing work-related post-traumatic stress: The critical incident stress debriefing (CISD). In G. S. Everly, & J. M. Lating (Eds.), *Psychotraumatology: Key papers and core concepts in postraumatic stress*. New York: Plenum.

Orner, R. J. (1995). Intervention strategies for emergency response groups: A new conceptual framework. In S. E. Hobfoll, & M. W. de Vries (Eds.), *Extreme stress and communities. Impact and intervention.* Dordrecht: Kluwer Academic Publishers.

Raphael, B. (1977). Preventive intervention with recently bereaved. *Archives of General Psychiatry, 34*, 1450–1454.

Raphael, B., Meldrum, L., & McFarlane, A. C. (1995). Does debriefing after psychological trauma work? *British Medical Journal, 310*, 1479–1480.

Robinson, R. C., & Mitchell, J. T. (1993). Evaluation of psychological debriefings. *Journal of Trauma and Stress, 6*, 367–382.

Salmon, T. W. (1919). The war neuroses and their lesson. *New York State Journal of Medicine, 51*, 993–994.

Scott, R. T., & Jordan, M. (1993). The Los Angeles riots, April 1992. Presented at the *Second World Congress on Stress, Trauma and Coping in Emergency Service Professions*, Baltimore.

Searle, M. M., & Bisson, J. I. (1992). Psychological sequelae of friendly fire. *Proceedings of Military Psychiatric Conference Stress Psychiatry and War*, Paris.

Sloan, P. (1988). Post-traumatic stress in survivors of an airplane crash-landing: A clinical and exploratory research intervention. *Journal of Trauma and Stress, 1*, 211–229.

Solomon, Z., & Benbenishty, R. (1986). The role of proximity, immediacy and expectancy in frontline treatment of central stress reaction among Israelis in the Lebanon war. *American Journal of Psychiatry, 143*, 613–617.

Stallard, P., & Law, F. (1993). Screening and psychological debriefing of adolescent survivors of life-threatening events. *British Journal of Psychiatry, 163*, 660–665.

Steinmetz, C. H. D. (1990). Hulp aan slachtoffers van ernstige misdrijven (Helping victims of major crimes). (Dissertation, Arnhem: Gouda Quint (in Dutch only)).

Sutker, P. B., Uddo, M., Brailey, K., Vasterling, J. J., & Errera, P. (1994). Psychopathology in war-zone deployed and nondeployed Operation Desert Storm troops assigned graves registration units. *Journal of Abnormal Psychology, 103*, 383–390.

Turnbull, G. J. (1994), Debriefing of released British hostages from Lebanon. *Clinical Quarterly, 4*, 21–22.

Tyhurst, J. S. (1951). Individual reactions to community disaster: The natural history of psychiatric phenomena. *American Journal of Psychiatry, 107*, 23–27.

Vernberg, E. M. (1995). Helping children's adaptation following a natural disaster. Presented at the *International Society of Traumatic Stress Studies Annual Meeting*, November 2–6, Boston.

Yule, W. (1992). Post-traumatic stress disorder in child survivors of shipping disasters: The sinking of the "Jupiter." *Psychoter Psychosom, 57*, 200–205.

28

Coping and Community Resources in Children Facing Disaster

SHMUEL LAHAD, YEHUDA SHACHAM, AND SHULAMIT NIV

Background

This chapter describes an integrative model of coping with individual and community stress, developed by the Community Stress Prevention Center (CSPC) in Kiryat Shmona, a border town in the north of Israel. Two studies will illustrate the implementation of this working model. The first focuses on children evacuated from their homes during a military operation, and the second evaluates interventions in a school following two traumatic events involving children and teachers alike. The central theme across the studies is that of resiliency and the use of individual and community resources.

The CSPC was established in 1981, following a wave of attacks on border settlements. Since then it has served towns and villages in times of crisis and between them. Its aims are to prepare the civilian population for all too likely war events, to assist local authorities in organizing emergency responses, and to train professionals in intervention techniques. During crisis, the CSPC provides immediate help to individuals, families, and institutions.

The CPSC's working model draws on systematic observations of individuals, groups and communities under prolonged threat. It emphasizes resiliency and focuses on ways in which people survive and cope. This model is felt to be appropriate for both prevention and intervention following disaster. The model comprises six dimensions, or domains, related to coping with adversity (Lahad, 1997): Belief and values, Affect and emotion, Social interaction, Imagination, Cognition, and Physiological response (Alias: BASIC-Ph). It is believed that by using these dimensions, coping styles can be effectively identified in individuals and communities. Inappropriate use of such resources or mismatch between resources used and specific stressful situations may, subsequently, be mapped and become the object of corrective interventions. Following is a brief description of the model.

SHMUEL LAHAD, YEHUDA SHACHAM, AND SHULAMIT NIV • The Community Stress Prevention Center, Tel Hai Academic College, Kiryat Shmona, 11012, Israel.

International Handbook of Human Response to Trauma, edited by Shalev, Yehuda, and McFarlane. Kluwer Academic / Plenum Publishers, New York, 2000.

Belief and values are exemplified by Garborino et al.'s (1992) statement: "Ideology is a coping resource for adults, which may have important consequences for the treatment children receive, as well as for the interpretation offered for the children regarding stressful events ..." Affect is generally appraised as in Lazarus and Folkman (1984). Intense expression of affect characterizes a period of expectancy for a stressor; e.g., Gal et al. (1994) have noted that "In stressful events which are perceived as uncontrollable it is more efficient to use coping mechanisms focused on affect."

Several studies emphasize the importance of Social coping. For example, Dyregrov and Mitchell (1992) found that most emergency rescue teams used social support and contacts with other workers in coping with exposure to traumatized children. Solomon (1993) noted that families evacuated during the Gulf War were less distressed when they were together. Vogel and Vernberg (1993) similarly showed that the amount of social support given to children was a major predictor of subsequent problems.

The Imagination dimension is exemplified by Dyregrov and Mitchell's (1992) description of emergency teams being helped by trying to anticipate and imagine what their role would be on their way to assist survivors. Janis (1983) and Breznitz (1983) have argued that denial (e.g., of danger), as far as it does not distort reality, may enable better contact with it.

Many studies emphasize the role of logical or cognitive coping, which is expressed by seeking information, rationally organizing the situation, and behaving according to logical rules. With regard to children, Itzkowitz et al. (1994) suggested that "Information, together with the ability to process and organize it, gives children better understanding of the situation, and possibly better understanding of what might help them...."

Physical activity is expressed as preference for active participation in rescue effort, and as being comforted by having an active role (Dyregrov & Mitchell 1992). Gal and Lazarus (1975) report that physical activity provides a sense of control and lessens anxiety and helplessness in combat soldiers, regardless of their being directed toward the direct source of threat or elsewhere.

This model has been implemented in several incidents, such as the Gulf War, military operations, and suicide bomb attacks. The following studies exemplify its implementation in children.

Study I: Children Coping with Temporary Evacuation

In the summer of 1993, Israel decided to mount a military response in southern Lebanon. Over the period of a few days, large military forces were brought to the northern region, and no room was left for doubt regarding the impending operation, its dimensions, and its cost. As shelling of the Israeli side of the border commenced, civilian residents had mixed reactions. Some families had prepared themselves for eventual hostility before they began. Others had chosen to leave the town temporarily, and other families evacuated their children to a boarding school, in which summer activities were organized by the local authorities. Many families, however, remained at home throughout the entire operation. Following the operation's end, children were evaluated for stress responses and their use of coping resources.

An 80-item questionnaire asking about experiences during the military operation was administered at school by homeroom teachers to 797 school children, aged 9–15. In accordance with assumptions, it was found that the intensity of mobilizing coping resources was higher among children who stayed close to the border. Children evacuated to a summer camp showed higher mobilization of resources than those who left with their families. Differences were noted in global coping measure, as well as specific domains of affect, imagination, and physical activation. No differences were found in social interaction, belief, and cognition.

Expressions of anxiety, however, were higher in the group evacuated to the summer camp, compared with other children. When asked about the future, those evacuated to a summer camp said that they would prefer to stay with their families, even in a war zone. Levels of anxiety were higher in boys, both during evacuation and following the end of hostilities. However, the average rating by girls of their wish to leave the town in case of another incident was higher than that of boys. Younger children did not differ from adolescents in anxiety scores during the operation. Indeed, the average level of fear following the operation was higher among adolescents. Young children tended to mobilize more Affect, Imagination, and Cognition resources than older adolescents.

Contrasting with expectations, subjects who, prior to the incident, received "primary prevention" (i.e., whose families made explicit preparations for the event) exhibited higher levels of anxiety during the operation and thereafter. Subjects who were more prepared before the operation mobilized more resources during and after the operation.

Study II: Psychoeducational Prevention in Children Exposed to Recurrent Trauma

In January of 1994, an 8th-grade girl committed suicide by jumping from the fourth floor of a building next to her school. She was killed instantly. Students and the teachers were shocked. The dead girl was an ambitious, brilliant student, good-looking, and very popular among her peers. Many of her fellow students felt guilty for not noticing her desperate state. Psychologists from the CSPC were asked to help. An intervention based on Lahad's (1981, 1997), Ayalon's (1977, 1978), and Klingman's (1985, 1986; Klingman et al., 1991) models of stress reduction and prevention was planned with the following goals in mind:

- Help in "normalizing" teachers' reactions, such that individual responses, no matter how strong, would be perceived as "normal reactions to an abnormal situation."
- Encourage teachers to initiate open discussions with their students.
- Help students and teachers develop ways to address difficulties related to the girl's death and encourage discussions of similar problems in the future.
- Identify individuals who may be at risk, given how vulnerable some may become following such tragedy.

The intervention consisted of discussing the suicide with the staff, paying attention to prior signals, and recommending class activities for the days following the suicide. We stressed the importance for students of attending school the day after the suicide.

A few months later in April 1994, tragedy struck again . A terrorist exploded himself in a car near a bus by the same school's gate. Three girls (two from the 11th grade and one from 7th grade) and four adults (including two teachers) were killed. Eight students (seven of whom were in the 7th grade class) were injured, including two who were badly burned. Officials and psychologists from the area gathered together early the next day to discuss a plan to help children of all ages. In one way or another, the disaster involved everyone in the town. Most children knew the dead or injured students and teachers.

Because we had previous experience with this school, we were also assigned to help them this time. An element of research was included to study the effect of the previous intervention. Another junior high school in the same town provided a comparison group. The main dependent variable was the effect of the first intervention on current responses (prevention was not implemented in the other school). We expected that crisis intervention would also be helpful in reducing negative reactions in the future.

The current intervention consisted of debriefing sessions using the Mitchell & Everly (1996) model. The first stage involved reviewing the facts about the event. The second stage was to discuss the thoughts and decisions that students had made since the tragedy. The third stage required teachers to ask their students to recount their worst experiences during the tragic event. Finally, the fourth stage dealt with coping style and resources, following Lahad's (1997) integrative BASIC Ph model.

The research questionnaire was administered 6 weeks after the terrorist attack. It dealt with traumatic reactions and coping strategies utilized after the first and the second incidents. The independent variables were proximity to the incident, gender, age, and the amount of primary preventive activity the students had received. The dependent variables were levels of anxiety, emotional reactions, near-miss feelings, and coping skills. We gave the same questionnaire to the 8th- and 9th-grade students one year later.

We hypothesized that (1) there would be differences between children of the two schools and (2) there would be a correlation between the previous intervention and the children's personal coping, such that children from School "A" would cope better than students from School "B." We also hypothesized that the effectiveness of the previous intervention would be linked with children's preferred coping mode. Finally, we expected to find that proximity to the site of the explosion would be linked with more distress six weeks later. Six hundred and eighty-four students took part in the study (293 boys and 391 girls), including 240 from School "A" (the one that was hit but received prior intervention) and 292 Students from School "B."

At 6 weeks we found a significant correlation between intervention received before and students evaluation of their own coping with this disaster. As expected, students from School "A" which was hit harder, exhibited fewer post-traumatic reactions after the event. A significant correlation was also found between the effectiveness of the school activities following each of the traumatic events and the choice of coping resources. The more effective the activities (according to the students' reports), the more resources were activated after the suicide and in part after the explosion. The three major resources were Affect, Social integration, and Cognition. A year later, students from school "A" still felt that the more prevention activities they had, the more effective was the prevention.

With regard to proximity to the site of the event, we found a negative correlation between knowing the victims and their ways of coping. The better individuals knew those injured, the less well they coped with the disaster, and the less they thought that their lives had returned to normal. No significant correlation was found between knowing the victims and the intensity of post-traumatic reactions after 6 weeks.

Boys reported better coping with the explosion with less post-traumatic reactions at 6 weeks. More of them reported that "life had returned to normal." Girls frequently used Affect, Social interaction, and Activities as primary coping. One year later, boys still reported that they were coping significantly better with the explosion.

Discussion

In the first study we examined the effect of exposure to stressful events on emotions and mobilization of coping resources in children who live under continuous threat. Exposure to traumatic events is seen in the literature as related to fear and anxiety in a dose-response manner (e.g., Vogel & Vernberg, 1993; Pynoos et al. 1987). Pynoos (1993) and Klingman et al. (1991) further found that personal acquaintance with traumatized children was even more decisive than the physical proximity to the site of the trauma. Our findings confirm the above. They are in contrast, however, with previous findings in Israel by Ziv, Kruglanski & Shulman (1974) who reported a protective effect of local patriotism among children in settlements under bombardment. This may be explained by the different historical context: The nineteen years that have passed between the two studies have seen the Israeli society move from an uncompromising ethos of heroism and praise for staying put under attack into legitimizing evacuation of civilians in danger (Granot, 1994). Moreover, society may be more open to admit expressions of fear and anxiety, wereas the relationship of affective expression to poorer coping has not been established. Indeed, expressiveness may strengthen coping and resistance to threat (Lahad & Cohen, 1988).

The effect of age and gender on anxious responses to adversity in children are controversial (Klingman et al 1993 and Levinson et al 1994). Gender differences in expressiveness, greater willingness to report symptoms or different social expectations may mediate the higher responses reported in girls (e.g., Vogel and Vernberg, 1993).

This first study did not confirm the protective effect of preparation on levels of distress expressed during exposure (e.g., Ayalon, 1997; Lahad 1988). Quite the contrary, it was found that children in whose homes more prevention activities had taken place, were more anxious than those living in homes where fewer such activities took place. Possibly, preparations could have been laden by parental anxious expectation, which may have been communicated to the children (Diamants 1994; Gal, Or and Tennenbaum, 1994). Another explanation may be derived from Janis' (1971) construct of mental inoculation, according to which levels of anxiety should be raised to an "optimal" level for learning to take place. Accordingly, the study's results may be read as part of the "work of worry" suggested by Janis (1971).

Social and behavioral consequences of relocation have been studied extensively (e.g., Ressler, 1992), and it is generally shown that "When evacuation is necessary parents tend to leave together with their children in a desperate attempt to protect them." Such a trend, which is clearly prevalent (e.g., Zelinsky & Kisinski, 1991), is also considered to be appropriate for childrens' needs: "... if evacuation is deemed necessary, that children be evacuated as part of family unit, being kept with their primary care givers" (Ressler, 1992). In line with the above, this study shows that separating children from their families heightens anxiety even though it reduces exposure.

The second study found differences between gender similar to those found in the first one. Girls used more Social interactions and Affect in coping with disasters.

Younger children preferably used Belief, Social, and Cognitive coping, yet older children expressed more fear. Younger children also evaluated the prevention to be significantly more effective and made use of it more than the older ones. As in previous studies, we found that being an acquaintance of the victims had a negative effect on coping. Geographical proximity, on the other hand, did not seem to negatively affect coping. On the contrary, it probably made it possible for those exposed to receive help openly.

The two studies evaluated the integrative multimodal model intervention and its long-term preventive effect. They point out preferred modes of coping in children following extreme events and indicate that the active coping of families has major consequences on children. Last but not least, our observations support the long-standing knowledge that it is better to evacuate children with parents.

References

Ayalon, O. (1977). Preparing the education system for emergency. *Matters in Education*, 15.

Ayalon, O. (1978), *COPE, emergency kit for the education system.* Haifa University.

Breznitz, S. (1983). The seven kinds of denial. In S. Breznitz (Ed.), *The denial of stress* (pp. 257–286). New York: International Universities Press.

Diamant, M. (1994). The connection between anticipation and preparation, and perception of quality of functioning, different coping styles of men and women during the Gulf War. *Psychologia, D*, 1–2.

Dyregrov, A., & Mitchell T. (1992). Work with traumatised children, psychological effects and coping strategies. *Journal of Traumatic Stress, 5*, 1.

Erlich, C., Greenbaum, T., & Toubiana, Y. (1994). Prolonged exposure to stress–sex differences in children's reactions to the Gulf War. *Psychologia, D*, 1–2.

Folkman, S., & Lazarus, R. (1984). If it changes, it must be a process. *Journal of Personality and Social Psychology, 48*, 150–170.

Folkman, S., Lazarus, R., & Dunkel-Sheffer, C. (1986). Dynamics of a stressful encounter; cognitive appraisal, coping and encounter outcomes. *Journal of Personality and Social Psychology, 50*, 992–1003.

Freud, A., & Burlingham, D. (1943). *War and children.* New York: Ernest Willard.

Gal, R., & Lazarus, R. (1975). The role of activity in anticipation and confronting stressful situations. *Journal of Human Stress, 14*, 71–75.

Gal, R. (1994). People under scuds: Reactions of the Israeli population to the missile attacks during the Gulf War. *Psychologia, 4*(1–2), 182–192.

Gal-Or, Y., & Tannenbaum G. (1994). *Psychologia, 4*(1–2), 66–75..

Garborino, J., Dubow, N., Kostelny, K., & Pardo, C. (1992). *Children in danger–coping with the consequences of community violence.* San Francisco: Jossey Bass.

Granot, H. (1994). The golden hour: The individual and society in emergencies. Home Front Command: Dekel Academic Publications.

Itzkowitz R., Zeidner, M., & Klingman, A. (1994). Children's affective reactions to the Gulf war. *Psychologia, 4*(1–2), 170–181.

Janis, I. L. (1971). Stress and frustration: Personality variable in social behavior. New York: Harcourt, Brace, Jovanovich.

Janis, I. L. (1983). Preventing pathogenic denial by means of stress. In S. Breznitz (Ed.), *The denial of stress,* (pp. 35–76). New York: International Universities Press.

Klingman, A. (1985). Free writing: Evaluation of preventive program with elementary school children. *Journal of School Psychology, 23*, 167–175.

Klingman, A. (1986). Emotional first aid during the impact of a mass school disaster. *Emotional First Aid, 3*, 51–57.

Klingman, A., Koenigsfeld, E., & Markman, D. (1991). *Art activity with children following disaster; a preventive oriented crisis intervention modality. The art in psychotherapy,* Vol. 14, (pp. 153–166). Elmsford, NY: Pergamon.

Klingman, A., Sagi, A., & Raviv, A. (1993). The effect of war on Israeli children. In L. Leavitt & N. Fox (Eds.), *The psychological effects of stress and violence on children.* Hillsdale, NJ: Lawrence Erlbaum.

Lahad, M. (1981). Preparation of children and teachers to cope with stress: A multi-modal approach. Unpublished master's thesis, Hebrew University, Jerusalem.

Lahad, M. (1997). Basic Ph: The story of coping resources. In M. Lahad & A. Cohen (Eds.), Community Stress Prevention, Volumes 1 & 2 (pp. 117–143). Kiryst Shonona, Israel: Community Stres Prevention Centre.

Lahad, S., & Cohen, A. (1988), *Community stress prevention*, Vol. 1. Kiryat Shmona: CSPC.

Lahad, S. (1983). Evaluation of a multi-modal programme to strengthen the coping of children and teachers under stress of shelling. (Ph. D. Thesis, Columbia Pacific University).

Lazarus, R. S., & Folkman, S. (1980). *Stress appraisal and coping.* New York: Springer.

Levinson, S., Shulman, P., Frankov, S., & Erez, T. (1994). Emotional expressions of fear and personal and family support factors of children and adolescents from Tel Aviv after the Gulf War. *Psychologia, D,* 1–2.

Lonigan, C. (1991). Children exposed to disaster, risk factors for the development of post-traumatic symptomatology. *Journal of the American Academy of Child and Adolescent Psychiatry. 33,* (1).

Milgram, R., & Milgram N. (1976), the effect of the Yom Kippur War on the anxiety levels in Israeli children. *Journal of Psychology, 94,* 107–113.

Milne, G. (1977). Evacuation after Cyclone Tracy. *Australian Psychologist, 12.*

Mitchell, J. T., & Everly, G. (1996). Critical incident stress debriefing: An operations manual for the prevention of traumatic stress among emerging services and disaster workers. Ellicott City, MD: Chevron Publishing Corporation.

Pynoos, R. (1993). Traumatic stress and psychopathology in children and adolescents. In J. Oldson, M. Riba, & M. Tasman (Eds.), *American Psychiatric Press Review of Psychiatry* (pp. 205–238). Washington, DC: American Psychiatric Press.

Pynoos, R., Frederick, C., & Nader, K. (1987). Life threat and post-Traumatic stress in school age children. *Archives of General Psychiatry, 44,* 1057–1063.

Ressler, V. (1992). Evacuation of children from conflict area. Geneva: UNHCR & UNICEF.

Schwarzwald, J., Weisenberg, M., Waysman, M., Solomon, Z., & Klingman, A. (1993). Stress reactions of school age children to bombardment by Scud missiles. *Journal of Abnormal Psychology, 102,* 404–410.

Solomon, Z. (1993). *Combat stress reactions; the enduring toll of war.* New York: Plenum Press.

Vogel, M., & Vernberg E. (1993). Children's psychological responses to disaster (Task Force Report). *Journal of Clinical Child Psychology, 22* (4), 464–484.

Zeidner, M., Klingman, A., & Itskowitz, R. (1983), Children's affective reactions and coping under threat of missile attack. *Journal of Personality Assessment, 60,* 435–457.

Zelinski, W. I., & Kisinski A. (1991). Emergency Evacuation of Cities. Savage, MD: Bowman & Littlefield.

Ziv A., & Israeli, R. (1973). Effects of bombardment on the manifest anxiety of children living in Kibbutzim. *Journal of Consulting and Clinical Psychology, 40,* 287–291.

Ziv, A., Kruglanski, A., & Schulman, S. (1974). Children's psychological reactions to wartime stress. *Journal of Personality and Social Psychology, 30.*

VII

Healing Traumatized Societies and Preventing the Cycle of Violence

In the previous section, we discussed the treatment of individuals with post-traumatic disorders. In many areas of the world, however, exposure to traumatic stress occurs as a direct result of social conflict. Such conflicts, unfortunately, have the tendency to repeat themselves and create vicious cycles of hatred and vengeance that are perpetrated for generations. Ultimately, these toxic cycles result in environments which do not allow individuals to heal. The treatment of interpersonal violence requires more than attention to the individual and must extend to healing societies from the forces that give rise to, and perpetuate, individual victimization.

At first blush, it may appear unrealistic and overly ambitious even to contemplate how individuals may dare to begin healing societies. However, such efforts do exist and provide a worthy synthesis of humanitarian and therapeutic undertakings. Such efforts are of particular interest when they are directed toward ending racial conflicts. Merle Friedman has been involved in the "Truth and Reconciliation" committees in South Africa. These committees were formed as the rule in South Africa shifted to provide for more social justice. The new society allowed for reappraisal of previous practices of racial discrimination and violence that had been previously condoned. The question that is often raised when social paradigms shift in revolutionary ways is how to address acts that have now become unacceptable. The historical model has been to judge and if possible, punish previous perpetrators. However, ironically, such punishment may lead to further perpetuation of victimization. When large elements of societies have been involved as perpetrators or even bystanders, the implementation of retributive justice creates a new class of potential victims. Friedman's interpretation of the psychological underpinning of the South African model is that societies may heal through forgiving those who can clearly admit their wrongdoing. The implementation of such ideals is not without inherent conflicts that are clearly addressed.

Nancy Dubrow explores the Israeli-Palestinian conflict and makes the point that even during the stage of active conflict between two warring societies, mental health practitioners may be able to provide an initial step toward healing by transcending the social reality of actual violence and beginning a process of reconciliation. She describes a process through which mental health practitioners from Israel and Palestine have gone beyond the seemingly acceptable boundaries of their society to work together. We can only admire the courage of those mental health workers who, at substantial personal risk, have the vision to initiate constructive dialogue despite raging hostilities. Dubrow's chapter analyzes both the good that such acts can accomplish, as well as some of the difficulties that arise when mental health workers push beyond simple mental health practices.

One type of individual response to conflict within one's geographic boundaries is escape. Indeed, the last few decades have seen literally millions of people fleeing for their lives because of political turmoil and racial harassment. Hence, the traditional definition of refugees seeking asylum, which originally was meant to protect few individuals, has become insufficient to encompass the reality of the mass persecution and resultant displacement. Yet even those fortunate enough to be granted political asylum in a safe country are likely to face substantial difficulties, which often rival in intensity the original stressors that compelled them to seek asylum. Moreover, for societies who host such refugees, the problem of absorbing them as equals is formidable. Zachary Steel and Derrick Silove address the psychological aspects of seeking political asylum and underscore the dilemma presented to nations which despite their best intentions, often become a source of distress for those whom they wish to help.

This is the shortest section of this volume, and, in the best of circumstances, it would have been the longest. Ultimately, given the impact of traumatic stress on society, the role of the mental health professional will need to expand to affect individuals as well as societies.

29

The Truth and Reconciliation Commission in South Africa as an Attempt to Heal a Traumatized Society

MERLE FRIEDMAN

The Need to Address the Past

In April/May 1994 with the first ever democratic elections and the inauguration of President Mandela, the New South Africa officially came into being. It was a momentous occasion for the entire population and the world at large. An exceptional negotiated revolution and peaceful transition transformed South Africa from an internationally reviled oppressive regime to a beacon of hope for the possibilities of peaceful transformation. The present was indeed a miracle, but two serious and difficult questions remained: How does this new Rainbow Nation address the future, and how does it address the past?

The past is a very thorny issue for all South Africans regardless of the role they may have played in history. In fact, as we move into the future, we find, as the Himba people of Namibia describe, that the past is stretched out before us. The Himba see time as a river flowing past them. The future, which has yet to pass, is behind and invisible, whereas the past, which has already been experienced, is ahead and visible. Therefore, the Western idea of putting your past behind you and looking forward to the future is a senseless notion to the Himba (Jacobsohn et al., 1990).

What became clear during the negotiation process was that for most South Africans, and especially those historically disenfranchised, the past had to be addressed, and those parts of it that were invisible needed to be made visible. Thus, as part of the Interim Constitution, the Truth and Reconciliation Commission (TRC) was created. This was achieved with reference to and consultation with other truth commissions and

MERLE FRIEDMAN • Psych-Action, Sandton, 2046, South Africa.

International Handbook of Human Response to Trauma, edited by Shalev, Yehuda, and McFarlane. Kluwer Academic / Plenum Publishers, New York, 2000.

was based on the consensus that "the pursuit of national unity, the well-being of all South Africans and peace, require reconciliation between the people of South Africa and the reconstruction of society" (explanatory memorandum to the Parliamentary bill, 1994).

Essentially, the goals of the Commission were to establish the truth about the past, grant amnesty where appropriate, and establish measures for reparation, with the ultimate aim of rehabilitating and restoring the human dignity of victims of violations of human rights. The final clause of the Interim Constitution described the attitude under which the TRC was established: "A need for understanding but not for vengeance, a need for reparation but not for retaliation, a need for ubuntu* but not for victimisation." Consequently, a valiant attempt was made by the negotiating teams to address the needs and fears of all sectors of the diverse South African community. Yet, despite the consensus achieved among the negotiators, the TRC has remained one of the most hotly debated and conflict-ridden issues in the transition process. The major question is can the TRC meet the challenge to our society?

This chapter addresses, within a psychological framework, some of the major themes raised by this question. The primary theme to be addressed is how people exposed to unspeakable and protracted suffering may recover individually and collectively. The broader question posed is what kind of intervention will enhance the future functioning of this society. Additionally, the place of the TRC in the context of other attempts to redress evil acts of the past will be addressed. A model of healing and an evaluation of the TRC will be presented.

South Africa and the Legacy of Apartheid: South Africa's Willing Executioners

The history of racism in South Africa does not start with the birth of the apartheid regime in 1960 but was bequeathed by the colonial system established earlier in the history of the African continent. Lindqvist (1996) comments that European world expansion "… accompanied as it was by a shameless defence of extermination, created habits of thought and political precedents that made way for new outrages, finally culminating in the most horrendous of them all: the Holocaust."

The European tradition of racism goes back a long time. Hannah Arendt (1951) showed how imperialism necessitated racism as the only possible excuse for its deeds, a view exemplified in the words of the philosopher, Herbert Spencer (1850), that "imperialism has served civilization by clearing the inferior races off the earth." The history of Africa, and indeed the whole of the colonized world, is replete with gross human rights violations of the most heinous kinds—all supported by perspectives that dehumanized the native inhabitants, supported their utilization for economic gain, and excused their ultimate extinction as a Darwinistic evolutionary imperative.

With respect to South Africa itself, the approach was no different.

> No false philanthropy or racial theory can convince sensible people that the preservation of a tribe of South African kaffirs is more important to the future of mankind than the spread of the great European nations and the white race in general. Not until the native learns to produce anything of value in the service of the higher race, i.e., in the

*Ubuntu roughly translated means 'I am because we are'. This is an African concept implying the essence of a sense of community.

service of its and his own progress, does he gain any moral right to exist. (Paul Rorbach, 1912)

The context within which apartheid was conceived and developed was a fertile breeding ground for the institutionalization of racism within a statutory system. It is unsurprising then, that South Africa, situated within the context of European colonialism, and the Afrikaner nation in particular with its own history of oppression in the British concentration camps, should become South Africa's "willing executioners" (Goldhagen, 1966). The South African regime, epitomized in the apartheid system, treated the majority of the people of the country as inferior beings, based on theories and policies of unabashed racism. At the same time, it entrenched policies of privilege, also based on race, and produced, according to a 1989 survey, the world's most unequal society (Asmal et al.,1996).

Attempts to Address the Past

Attempts to deal with war crimes and human rights abuses have become of great national and international significance since the Nuremberg trials. It was here for the first time that individual responsibility for crimes against humanity during war was assumed (Buruma, 1995; Goldstone, 1997). The Nuremberg trials can be seen as an attempt to cleanse Germany of its Nazi past. They formed a ritualistic gesture that went beyond the national and the personal responsibility for such crimes. They were intended to be a symbolic punishment of the German people—"a moral history lesson cloaked in all the ceremonial trappings of due legal process" (Buruma, 1995 p. 145). Allied tribunals were also held in Japan and Southeast Asia. However, whereas Germany has accepted responsibility for atrocities committed during the war, Japan treated war crimes as military excesses that occur in any war—despite evidence to the contrary (Buruma, 1995).

Truth commissions have also been set up in Uruguay, Paraguay, El Salvador, Chile, and Argentina. The Latin American attempts, however, have been less than successful (Simpson, 1994). Argentina attempted to reconcile a limited prosecutorial process with the recovery of the truth but failed to sustain the punitive nature required because of political factors. The Chilean truth commission had inadequate investigative powers and so failed to uncover the details or to attribute individual responsibility for human rights violations. A more successful element of the Chilean process was the establishment of the "Corporation on Rehabilitation and Reconciliation" (Simpson, 1994). This body was set up to consider compensation for victims of human rights abuses and their families, to assist in searching for the remains of victims, and to formulate proposals for a culture respectful of human rights.

The South African Attempt

The period of negotiation that led up to the first democratic election in South Africa was complicated and volatile, and very strong motivations drove the different factions. In viewing the gross human rights violation of the past and the results of 40 years of oppression, the African National Congress (ANC) pressed for a judicial process where perpetrators of violations would be prosecuted and justice would run its course.

On the other hand, representatives of the apartheid regime wanted a blanket amnesty or indemnity from prosecution. This would have allowed all perpetrators of gross human rights violations to remain unanswerable for the actions they had taken during the apartheid era. Further pressures were represented by the threat of a South African Nuremberg type trial and by international human rights factions.

The contradictory nature of these positions resulted in ongoing conflict within the negotiating process, and the TRC was ultimately constituted as a strategic and political compromise between these opposing factions. Yet, even though it represented a compromise, the South African process of facing the past has a more ambitious scope than similar processes elsewhere. "Other efforts have sought to achieve an historically accurate picture of the past, or to confer amnesty, or to compensate victims. The South African Truth and Reconciliation Commission aims to achieve all of these together" (Asmal et al., 1996).

The Structure of the Truth and Reconciliation Commission (TRC)

The TRC comprises 17 members. The chair of the Commission is Archbishop Desmond Tutu, a Bishop of the Anglican Church and Nobel Peace Prize laureate. An Investigative Unit was set up to investigate anything pertaining to the Commission's powers, functions, and duties, including summoning people to give evidence under oath, where necessary. The Commission was planned to complete its work within 18 months after its constitution. The TRC comprises the three following elements:

The Committee on Human Rights Violations

The task of this Committee is to investigate gross violations of human rights in or outside South Africa and to record all allegations made by victims or others with personal knowledge or reliable information.

The Committee on Amnesty

The task of the Committee is to consider applications to grant amnesty. Persons who wish to apply for amnesty for any act, omission, or offence must satisfy the Committee that (a) The act, omission, or offence was associated with a political objective; (b) The act, omission, or offence took place between March 1, 1960 and the cutoff date, May 10, 1997; and (c) full disclosure has been made.

The Committee on Reparation and Rehabilitation

The task of this Committee is to deal with applications for reparation and rehabilitation by victims of gross violations of human rights.

Forgiveness

Although not overtly occurring in the wording or the structures of the TRC, the expectation and hope stated repeatedly in the media, especially by Bishop Tutu, is that forgiveness would be the outcome of this commission.

The Meaning of Reconciliation

The effects of exposure to gross human rights violations is devastating to individuals and society. More than 50 years after World War II, survivors of such abuses are still clamoring for the world to recognize and understand their continued pain and suffering and provide some form of relief. In turn, the effects produce an aftermath in the lives of the individuals, their families, and society as a whole. These consequences have been well documented in the broad literature on the Holocaust and are reinforced by complicated legal and moral problems that have emerged in relation to Japan, its role in the commission of atrocities during the war, and its refusal to assume moral responsibility for those acts.

By choosing the route of reconciliation, South Africa has rejected the legal solution to the problems of dealing with the past. The legal solution is a narrow, procedural conceptualization, assuming justice in the form of punishment, also termed retributive or punitive justice. It would have implied a Nuremberg type process, which was on the cards for South Africa, because apartheid had been declared a crime against humanity by the United Nations (Werle, 1996).

Reconciliation, a substantive, healing process, implies that all parties involved should come together and ultimately move forward in mutual understanding. As opposed to retributive justice, this has been termed restorative justice (Zehr, 1994; Bianchi, 1995).

To achieve this end, a clinically based intervention rooted in understanding traumatic stress provides the most encompassing approach. Such an approach must accommodate both individual and group processes. It should be context- and culture-sensitive and should deal not only with victims, but also with perpetrators and bystanders.

Adressing Individual and National Needs

If South Africa is perceived as a traumatized nation, it belies the resilience and health of individuals. Nevertheless, some people would in fact qualify for a diagnosis, and one that might be more applicable to those who have lived under oppression punctuated with multiple traumatic incidents may be within the realm of "complex post-traumatic stress disorder" (Herman, 1994). The most significant aspect that would qualify victims for such a diagnosis is the initial diagnostic element, "A history of subjection to totalitarian control over a prolonged period" (ibid, p.121).

A Psychological Framework: A Proposed Model for Understanding Healing The Effects Following Prolonged Traumatizations

The effects of extreme traumatic exposure are thoroughly addressed in the literature of the Holocaust, as well as in that of state sponsored terrorism. This literature addresses the moral, ethical, and psychological questions of how such acts of atrocity could be perpetrated and how to help victims to deal with their experiences and move beyond them. Bearing in mind that the South African situation was neither the Holocaust nor a genocide, lessons learned from those events are, nevertheless, relevant.

One such lesson is that it is important to address victims, perpetrators, and bystanders. In South Africa, people who belong to all three categories played some part in the past (Staub, 1989) and will be part of the future. Moreover, the public and statutory nature of some crimes calls for public attempts at recovery. Thus, the treatment for the nation, it is submitted, should involve both public and private interventions. Whereas private interventions may take the form of more traditional models of therapy for post-traumatic stress disorder, the public aspects need to be both reparative and symbolic in their aims and goals.

The legacy of the apartheid system is indeed complex. In considering its effects, it might be useful to remember that the violent abuses perpetrated by the system were in agreement with the more general goal of apartheid ("separateness"), i.e., to enhance division between groups of people. Impermeable boundaries were developed between racial groups, communication between them was practically severed. Even knowledge about each other was scant.

Metaphorically, one can extend to these group processes the fragmented structure of Dissociated Identity Disorder (DID), where a society, similarly to an individual, experiences having separate parts of the mind, divided from one another and partially autonomous. At the healing stage, however, past dividedness is exemplified by distress expressed at the atrocities and also at the lack of knowledge that they occurred. The words of Wynand Malan, Truth Commissioner (1997), accurately capture the feelings of a large sector of South African society today:

> We are horrified and feel betrayed. We feel done in. We feel our dignity impaired. That things like these were possible, right under our noses. How could this have happened? We are victims of the cruelest fraud committed against us! This is our experience of revelations made day after day—and the Lord knows—will still be revealed.

Consequently, the treatment for the nation should involve recovering memories of the past and making them accessible to the entire country, so that the truth will be known by all. As in DID, the ultimate healing will be in integrating the parts: "If we want to make a contribution to the future of a healthy South Africa, of a country where they can be us and we can be them, where we can all be us—then we will have to endure the larger pain of sharing their pain. Then we must get beyond the luxury of wallowing in our own pain" (Wynand Malan, 1997).

The following tripartite model, presents the author s formulation of the basic elements of group healing following violations of human rights. Its three parts are acknowledgment, apology, and reparation.

Acknowledgment

The question of memory is central both to victims and perpetrators. Oppressors and bystanders may need to forget and deny, as was the case during and after the Holocaust (Allen and Solkoff, 1988). Therefore, confessing to one's role is extremely difficult. "Many times people become so overwhelmed by the shame associated with admitting the role they have played in perpetrating destructive acts against others, that their rationalisation, denial, avoidance, and dissociation appear totally divorced from reality, psychotic, or just deceitful" (Bloom, 1997. p. 223.). On the part of the victims, in contrast, there is a need for remembrance. For example, Agger and Jensen (1996) emphasized the significance of testimony as a part of the therapy for victims of state terrorism in Chile.

For a healing process to take place, however, not only must the truth be told, it must also be heard. In fact, it is the combination of telling the story and the manner in which it is heard and understood that initiates healing. Herman (1992) describes how in therapy with individuals "this work of reconstruction actually transforms the traumatic memory so that it can be integrated into the survivor's life" (p. 174). By analogy, in the public forum, the telling of the stories and the acknowledgment of their veracity and effects transforms a private trauma into a public memory which can then be integrated into the historical memory of the nation. *Public* acknowledgment, therefore, is a significant element of the healing process, in which the victim bears witness and the nation hears and confirms the evil nature of deeds and the harm caused, thereby transforming and enabling transcendence of the trauma.

Apology

Apology is the next necessary step. Sincere apology on the part of the specific perpetrator to the victim would imply a process of having reflected in depth on violations committed, having some understanding of the resulting suffering, and expressing a genuine sense of remorse. Apology further confirms the traumatic experience of the victim and directly addresses the relationship between victim and perpetrator. Acknowledgment and apology together "rehumanize" the victims and allow them to reestablish an acceptable and accurate cognitive schema of self others. It is also the ultimate way in which suffering may be recognized. In some way the act of apology, following that of acknowledgment, validates the internal world of the victim. Furthermore, the victim is empowered by being able to accept or reject the apology, and the power balance is shifted, allowing individuals to emerge from victimhood.

For the apology to be acceptable, it needs to be sincere and remorseful and directed from the perpetrator to the victim. It is also important that apology occurs when the victim is ready and able to hear it and respond to it. The more severe the trauma, particularly when the trauma resulted in the death of a loved one, the more difficult it becomes to accept an apology. Justice implies that the system takes responsibility for inducing a similar level of suffering in both perpetrator and victim. Accepting an apology may signify that, to some degree, this need has been satisfied and that the remorse is perceived to be adequate.

Although one would hope that perpetrators would have remorse for their acts and seek pardon, it is not possible to legislate apology. The expression of true remorse requires a great deal of courage and support. "Such acts of contrition, however, require a social group that is willing to help the perpetrator tolerate the depth of self-annihilating shame that is the price to be paid for true remorse" (Bloom, 1997, p. 223). Finally, where apology is not made or is perceived to be inadequate, or when the victim is not ready to accept an apology, the seeking of retributive justice does appear to be a psychological impellent.

Reparation

The final stage, reparation, answers a call for leveling the playing fields. The victims need this repair to help them feel that oppression is over and that an equal chance of living a reasonable life exists. Reparation is different in each case and ideally should take the form that each individual determines.

Unless these three components are satisfied, the victim will continue to feel victimized and oppressed despite objective evidence to the contrary. Herman (1994, p.190) describes how a fantasy of compensation in survivors is fueled by "the desire for victory over the perpetrator that erases the humiliation of the trauma". Usually such fantasy includes more elements of psychological (or symbolic) "victory" than material gain. Acknowledgment of harm, apology, or public humiliation of the perpetrator represent such "symbolic" compensation.

Herman further suggests that, even though this compensation fantasy is about ideas of empowerment, it keeps the patient's fate tied to that of the perpetrator and holds the patient's recovery hostage to the perpetrator's whims. In societal circumstances, because of the social or public nature of prolonged trauma and the responsibility assumed by the state, the form of the TRC, for example, those aspects of the compensation fantasy, may operate as well.

Comments on, and Critiques of, the Proposed Model

Compared with a Nuremberg type trial or with a retributive justice system, the Truth Commission is a very generous solution for perpetrators. For victims, it carries a promise of repair, yet may also be perceived as, miscarriage of justice. For bystanders, the work of the TRC is often confusing and misunderstood, sometimes perceived as an unnecessary preoccupation with the past. Comparison with other models of dealing with human rights violation reveals the following differences and similarities:

Amnesty, Justice and Apology: Comparison of Different Models of Psychological Healing

Compared with the proposed components of *Acknowledgment, Apology*, and *Reparation*, the Chilean Truth commission's approach included seeking *Truth, Justice*, and *Compensation* (Agger & Jenson 1996). Reconciliation, according to the Chilean model, could take place only once these have been achieved. The Chilean model also included steps toward preventing further violations, such as by education regarding human rights (Figure 1).

The two models attempt to solve a similar question, yet, in different ways: Acknowledgment is also admitting to the truth. Yet, acknowledgment additionally includes the endorsement of personal responsibility for acts committed, whereas truth, as such, can be established whether or not the perpetrator takes such responsibility. Justice also differs from Apology in that it resolve pasts disputes by retribution and punishment

Proposed Model	Chilean Model
Acknowledgment	Truth
Apology	Justice
Reparation	Compensation

FIGURE 1. Proposed model for healing and the TRC in Chile.

(rather than by a deliberate gesture of the perpetrator toward the victim and the public). Reparation or compensation appear to be analogous and well agreed upon as a necessary and serious attempt to right the wrongs.

The South African TRC is dealing with perpetrators by a conflict- ridden procedure of granting amnesty (Asmal et al., 1996). Although such amnesty requires the full admission of having committed human rights violations, there is no mandatory requirement to acknowledge past acts as having been "bad" or "evil," nor is there a mandatory request for an expression of remorse. In that sense, amnesty has been perceived as too "painless" and not necessarily leading to genuine reconciliation. For genuine reconciliation to take place (Asmal et al., 1996), the perpetrator/s must effectively submit to (1) facing unwelcome truths and (2) taking responsibility for past activities (e.g., not claiming that they were innocent mistakes or they followed legal orders), and (3) Wedergutmaching—committment to making good again (Figure 2).

Upon examining of the models, it can be observed that the acknowledgment or the uncovering of truth is consistent in all models as is the aspect of compensation or reparation. The major discrepancy occurs in the second aspect. Where the model proposed by the author describes the apology as necessary, the Chilean Commission looked toward justice in the form of punishment. The TRC model replaces punishment by freedom from prosecutions via *Amnesty, granted* to perpetrators who acknowledge full liability (Figure 3). In that sense the models are in sharp contrast.

Therefore, a question must be asked whether the South African Truth and Reconciliation Commission can succeed in the aim of psychological healing. It may be said that the compromise made forced the negotiators "into a reconciliation whose terms were to be defined by those who would be forgiven" (Schmidt, 1987). Hans Habe (1976) has commented that amnesty granted to an unpunished murderer is a form of complicity in the crime. "It does not foster forgiveness, it precludes it." Eckhart (1988) comments, "When social outrage is absent, one should be concerned about the morality of the community" (p. 575)

Forgiveness and Repentance

In Bishop Tutu's explanatory memorandum to the Parliamentary bill (June 1994), one reads the following: "We will be engaging in what should be a corporate nation-wide process of healing through contrition, confession and forgiveness." From Bishop Tutu's speech it is evident that although forgiveness is not what is spelled out in the aims of the TRC, it is clearly an expectation. This position has and continues to evoke very strong feelings. Eckhart (1988), for example, argues that forgiveness is a complicated individual process that can neither be demanded nor expected other than in certain

Proposed Model	"Reconciliation Through Truth"
Acknowledgment	Facing Unwelcome Truth
Apology	Censoring of self
Reparation	Wedergutmaching

FIGURE 2. Proposed model for healing, compared with the requirements for Reconciliation Through Truth (Asmal et al., 1996).

Proposed Model	Chilean Model	South African Model
Acknowledgment	Truth	Truth
Apology	Justice	Amnesty
Reparation	Compensation	Reparation

FIGURE 3. Proposed model for healing, the Chilean model, and the South African Truth and Reconciliation Commission.

religious frameworks. She warns that too easy forgiving may perpetuate the very evil it wants to alleviate.

Conflicting Attitudes toward the TRC

In attempting to deal with trauma and reconciliation, the interwoven strands of victims, perpetrators and bystanders evoke contradictory positions. These different stake holders

> may have different and fluctuating assessments of both the reality of what has happened and of the extent of the victims suffering. As a result, victim and bystanders may have strongly conflicting agendas, such as to repair, forget or take revenge. These conflicts in assessment of the meaning of the trauma may set the stage for the trauma to be perpetuated in a larger social setting. Soon the allocation of blame and responsibility, not the trauma itself, may become the central issue." (van der Kolk et al., 1996, pp. 26–27)

Inadequate understanding of the psychological processes on which these responses are based may result in actions that deflect from the ultimate goal. At present, as various political parties are threatening and sometimes withdrawing from the TRC, the Minister of Justice threatens them with Nuremberg style trials if they do not cooperate. He likens the National Party that represents the former government to "a professional criminal pleading innocence in casting itself as a victim" (The Star, June 4, 1997).

On the other hand, attempts to bring the message of the TRC to the nation are proving successful. The media play a significant role in this process by bringing, nightly, extracts of the TRC's proceedings on the eight o'clock television news. The Sunday evening weekly summary of the TRC proceedings has been rated as the second most viewed television program. The written media, as well as radio, are also filled with reports and discussions of the process and outcomes of the TRC. Also as a result of the Amnesty clause and its promise of freedom from prosecution, there have been about 8,000 applications for amnesty (http://www.truth.org.za). Without the controversial feature of amnesty, it is highly questionable whether the truth would have been as forthcoming. Thus, the dissemination of information of the truth and its consequences is occurring.

African Cosmology

The extent to which ideas born in one society are applicable to others is another challenge to the process of reconciliation. The TRC is constituted in a Western framework, a context that may not be as sensitive to broader African cosmology as one would tend to assume. Africa is rich in cosmological ideas which, behind their diversity, are linked to a core of shared beliefs (Nyang, 1990). Traditional healing, which includes elaborate cleansing rituals, represents a strong and widely practiced approach to health and the prevention of disease. The sensitivity of the current process to the cultural needs of the majority of the victims and thereby its effectiveness as a work of healing is still unclear. A question that may be asked is whether a process that is more sensitive to the cultural needs of the majority of the victims would be more effective in the work of healing and thus reconciliation.

Inadequate Psychological Follow-Up of Testimonial Hearings

Witnesses who came before the TRC have had horrific traumatic experiences reevoked by testifying, with little, if any, follow-up, support, or therapy. There has been an implicit understanding that testimony is treatment and that the immediate relief expressed by victims in telling their story to the world would produce cures. For many, however, the opposite has been the case, with resulting disappointment, distress, and the replaying of traumatic memories. These were consonant with the lack of organized follow-up and with the fact that reparations have not yet been addressed.

Despite these critiques, there have been and continue to be many and varied very positive outcomes of the TRC. Many individuals, organizations, and churches have rallied to support victims. In the words of Bishop Tutu:

> The most heart-warming achievements, however, are the little-publicised acts of healing and reconciliation. It has been thrilling to hear of an individual in Kagiso, rejected by his community as an informer, now vindicated and rehabilitated; or to see the community of Phokeng, divided by the bantustan policy and a related killing, brought together again through the formalised mechanism of the amnesty process. One has similarly been overwhelmed by the qualities displayed by the daughter of an activist who says, 'I want to forgive, but I don't know whom to forgive' or by the Eastern Cape librarian, her body still full of shrapnel from a hand grenade, who says, extraordinarily, 'This experience has enriched my life.'

Bishop Tutu concludes that "The TRC is contributing to the healing and reconciliation process in our beautiful but wounded land" (*Sunday Times*, December 4, 1996).

Conclusion

The TRC as constituted can only partially meet its objectives, and is seriously hampered in its goal of reconciliation by the fact of Amnesty. The question of amnesty has already been the source of a great deal of distress and legal action, and its future implications remain to be seen. Moreover, on an individual level, the notion of "testimony as treatment" must be questioned. From the therapeutic perspective, the testimony as given in the TRC may be seen as an opening up of the therapeutic process, which needs to be continued. Interventions may include those who have given testimony, their families, and those whose trauma has been reevoked by exposure of the testimonies and the amnesty hearings. Such interventions should be culturally appropriate, and should also include mass ceremonies and rituals that have import for the entire nation (Agger & Jensen, 1996).

As the TRC grapples with the issues of reparation, other problems may surface. If the general aim is national reconciliation and healing, the attitudinal changes that are necessary and the required work for repair should be regarded as part of the TRC's mandate. For example, to soften the blow to the need for retributive justice on the part of some victims, an option of voluntary community work aimed at reconstruction and repair of both individual lives and communities could be offered to those applicants who are granted amnesty, as well as to bystanders, as a way for them to demonstrate remorse and work toward repairing the damage they have wreaked. Despite honorable intentions, forgiveness should be an outcome that is hoped for but not expected or requested. Hence, if the TRC is reconceptualized as, "beginning the process" of reconciliation, it may get closer to the stated objectives.

Finally, despite all the criticism that has and still will be leveled at the TRC as a model for reconciliation, it remains a valiant attempt and the best to date to move beyond the narrow notion of justice and toward a more inclusive and substantive aim of healing the nation in South Africa.

References

Agger, I., & Jensen, S. B. (1996). *Trauma and healing under state terrorism.* London & New Jersey: Zed Books.

Allen, W. S., & Solkoff, N. (1988). The role of psychological denial in the Holocaust. Presented at an International Scholars Conference. *Remembering for the Future* (pp. 1219–1225). Oxford: Pergamon Press.

Arendt, H. (1951). *The origins of totalitarianism.* Republished: Harcourt Brace (1973).

Asmal, K., Asman, L., & Roberts, R. S. (1996). Reconciliation through truth: A reckoning of apartheid's criminal governance. David Phillips Publishers Cape Town & Johannesburg in association with Mayibuye Books: University of the Western Cape.

Bianchi, H., (1995). Justice as sanctuary: Toward a new system of crime control. Bloomington: Indiana University Press.

Bloom, S. L. (1997). Creating sanctuary: Toward the evolution of sane societies. New York: Routledge.

Buruma, I. (1995). *Wages of guilt: Memories of war in Germany & Japan.* Reading, Berkshire, Great Britain: Cox & Wyman.

Eckhart, A. L. (1988). Forgiveness and repentance: Some contemporary considerations and questions. Paper presented at an International Scholars' Conference. *Remembering for the future* (pp. 571–583). Oxford: Pergamon Press.

Goldhagen, D. J. (1996). *Hitler's willing executioners: Ordinary Germans and the Holocaust.* New York: Random House.

Goldstone, R. (1997). Address on the 50th anniversary of the Nuremberg trials. Johannesburg, South Africa.

Habe, H. (1976). Quoted in Wiesenthal, S. (1976). *The sunflower* (p. 123). New York: Schocken Books.

Herman, J. L. (1992). *Trauma and recovery.* New York: Basic Books.

Jacobsohn, M., & Pickford, P. & Pickford, B. (1990). *Himba: Nomads of Namibia.* Cape Town: Struiks Publishers.

Lindqvist, S. (1996). *Exterminate all the brutes. One man's odyssey into the heart of darkness and the origins of European genocide.* New York: The New York Press.

Malan, W. (1997). Statement by Mr. Wynand Malan, Deputy Chair of the Human Rights Violations Committee of the Truth and Reconciliation Commission, (May 16).

Nyang, S. S. (1990). *Islam, Christianity and African identity.* Vermont: Amama Books.

Rorbach, P. (1912). *German thought in the world.* New York: The New York Press.

Quoted in Lindqvist, S. (1996). *Exterminate all the brutes. One man's odyssey into the heart of darkness and the origins of European genocide.* New York: The New York Press.

Schmidt, J. N. (1987). Those unfortunate Years. Nazism in the public debate of post war Germany. Lecture delivered at Indiana University, October 15, 1986 and published by the Jewish Studies Program, 1987, p. 10.

Simpson, G. (June 1994). Proposed Legislation on Amnesty/indemnity and the establishment of a Truth and Reconciliation Commission. Submission to the Minister of Justice, Mr. Dullah Omar.

Spencer, H. (1850). *Social statistics* (p. 416). Republished: Augustus M. Rielley Publishers (1970).

Staub, E. (1989). *The roots of evil: The origins of genocide and other group violence.* New York: Cambridge University Press.

Storm over Nuremburg trials for NP. (June 4, 1997). *The Star,* Johannesburg p. 1.

Tutu, D. Archbishop. Letter to the Sunday Times. *Sunday Times,* South Africa, December 4, 1996.

van der Kolk, B. A, McFarlane, A. S., & Weiseth, L. (1996). *Traumatic stress: The overwhelming experience on mind, body, and society.* New York: Guilford.

Werle, G. (1996). Confronting State Criminality: The German Experience. Conference: *Reporting the Truth Commission,* Johannesburg.

Zehr, H. (1994). Justice that heals. *The Vision Stimulus, 2*(3), 5–11.

30

The Role of Mental Health Professionals in Building Bridges of Peace

NANCY DUBROW

In the words of Maya Angelou, "I note the obvious differences in the human family ... but we are more alike, my friends, than we are unalike" (1994). Indeed, this is the fundamental principle upon which a symposium was built, associating Palestinian and Israeli colleagues in the hope for an imminent peace. June of 1996 appeared to be an appropriate time to articulate our work and the motivation for joint efforts. The political peace process was unfolding before us, and we had hoped that after so many years, all men, women and children would have an acknowledged nationality and enjoy all of their inalienable human rights and, thus real peace. However, between the time of the presentation in Jerusalem and the writing of this chapter, we have witnessed renewed conflict, and the resulting challenges to our professional work together are even greater.

Symposium members included professionals in the fields of medicine, history, and the behavioral sciences: Dr. Fathi Arafat, President of Palestine Red Crescent Society and the Higher Health Council of the Palestinian National Authority; Dr. Elia Awwad, Director of a Child and Family Consultation Center; Dr. Yair Hirschfeld, Professor at Haifa University and Economic Cooperation Foundation; Dr. Dan Bar-On, Professor at the Department of Behavioral Sciences and David Lopatie, Chair for Post-Holocaust Psychological Studies, Ben-Gurion University of the Negev; and Dr. Paul Hare, Professor, Department of Behavioral Sciences, Ben-Gurion University of the Negev.

We had come together on previous occasions to work on joint Palestinian-Israeli projects. For example, several members of the group have worked over the years to develop psychosocial responses to traumatized populations living in armed conflict (Dubrow et al., 1995; Halperin, 1997). Whether pursuing research, training, or public policy initiatives, each effort has been grounded in our collective belief in the value of shared knowledge, experience, and humanitarian goals. These "superordinate goals"

NANCY DUBROW • Taylor Institute, Chicago, Illinois 60622.

International Handbook of Human Response to Trauma, edited by Shalev, Yehuda, and McFarlane. Kluwer Academic / Plenum Publishers, New York, 2000.

or goals shared by individuals or groups, as described by Staub (1989), form the basis of our action. Although they often collided with reality, we understand that there is no other way to build a strong community of professionals and thereby contribute to peace.

The Challenge of Working in a Situation of Conflict

The conflict between Palestine and Israel presents unique physical and psychological barriers to joint efforts. The situation on the ground keeps changing. Israeli and Palestinian professionals who choose to work together must deal with flaring unrest, random incidents of violence, border closures, and revoked travel permits. For example, closure of checkpoints between cities often results in the cancellation of scheduled meetings between Israeli and Palestinian colleagues.

The psychological barriers have an even more pronounced effect on the work to be done. On an ongoing basis, we witness human rights violations, experience pressure from distrustful colleagues, and are humiliated by collective punishment resulting from the violent acts of others. All of these realities contribute to the stressfulness of working together for a common purpose and create challenges for professionals from both sides.

Dispelling the Myth of the Enemy

In an informal exchange with Joseph Sandler (1983), Anna Freud said "We know that with persecuted minorities, against whom atrocities are committed, the atrocities are preceded by a withdrawal of the feeling of sameness." She added that "without such preliminary withdrawal (or boundary setting) what happens afterwards cannot happen, because of the feeling of sympathy and empathy, of sameness, which has to be done away with."

Studies in human development reveal that children have empathy for others at a very early stage in their development. Before they have language, research demonstrates their responses to others in distress. Researchers in Norway (Raundalen, 1993) documented children as young as two years of age comforting crying adults with an empathetic touch of their hands. Based on these observations, the researchers postulated that loss of empathy for others during the formative years is a process of creating differences. This is in line with Staub (1989) who described how human beings devise "them" and "us" categories through a process of identifying group differences and thereby also create stereotypes and/or enemies.

Additionally, withdrawal of empathy from selected groups of people can occur if acting on behalf of others is not presented to children via adult behavior. Children seem to require familial and community models of humanitarian action to develop their own sense of shared humanity and empathy for others. Salient examples are those non-Jewish citizens of Europe who, during the Nazi Holocaust, risked their own lives to hide Jewish citizens in their homes. Research indicated that these individuals decided to provide safe havens for the Jews because they saw them as equal human beings and thereby could react to their need for protection.

In an effort to dispel the myth of the enemy, panel members have deliberately transcended their political, religious, ethnic, and cultural affiliations, committing themselves to continue their strong personal and professional relationships, trust, respect, and mutual understanding despite incidental violence and terror.

The Roots of Peace

Peace represents the highest achievement of civilization. It should begin within oneself, but this is not enough. Many people wish for peace for themselves, their families and communities. More rarely are such wishes extended to other groups or nations, particularly to enemies. As suggested by Dr. Arafat in the symposium, until one achieves peace outside of oneself, that is, desires peace for the other as well, one does not have real peace. Peace and war are often linked, one following the other, and one makes sense on the background of the other. Hence, negotiating peace always involved interaction between previous enemies and an extension of one's wish for peace to the other group. Such a process, however, must address the psychological sequelae of violence, the stress and the memory of humans harming other humans.

Supporters of peace have to contend with the simultaneous presence of supporters of war. The latter work to create an environment where no one feels safe; where the threat of violence must be considered daily; and where traditional safe havens, such as homes, schools, and hospitals, are disrupted or destroyed. These threats to safety, which are the essence of psychological trauma, affect one's fundamental trust in humanity and in the predictability and continuity of life itself (van der Kolk, 1987).

Building the Professional Community

An "architect" of the Oslo Accords, Dr. Yair Hirschfeld discussed the history of the current conflict and that of the Economic Cooperation Foundation (ECF), an organization established as an "incubator" for joint Israeli-Palestinian projects. The ECF brings together Israeli and Palestinian colleagues around issues of mutual interest and expertise, who need funding support.

Primary health care, the environment, peace education, and mental health are among the areas upon which the the ECF has focused. In the latter, for example,the ECF facilitated meetings between mental health specialists from both sides to develop a telephone "help line", an Israeli organization based in Tel Aviv and a Palestinian child and family consultation center serving the West Bank and Gaza. The Israeli organization had telephone hot lines working for several years. The ECF worked on developing funding support for a joint venture in which directors of both programs will work on implementing a culturally sensitive Palestinian telephone "help line" model.

Although funding for projects is essential, bringing Palestinian and Israeli professionals together is possibly more important. Professionals come to the table with shared interests and work on identifying commonalties rather than differences. By exchanging their experiences, knowledge, and time, they lay the foundations for peace between people. The ECF sees every such meeting as promoting positive and normalized experiences. As such experiences multiply, there is hope for better understanding and cooperation.

Understanding the "Other"

One of the most serious problems that children face when exposed to chronic violent trauma is a break of trust in human beings, in relationships, and in the future. This goes beyond the threat of physical injury to include psychological and moral injuries as well. Such danger stems from being put in situations that contradict previously internalized norms acquired from families and communities. Such norms may be the sanctity of life, yet children see people killed. They may have learned to define morality (right vs. wrong), yet they witness violations of human rights, humiliation, harassment, and disregard for justice (Dubrow, 1997).

One of the entry points to understanding and thus, restoring moral values is to study how each group perceives the "other." Palestinian and Israeli children have little or no opportunity to experience each other in schools, community centers, recreation, and sports activities. Therefore, their perception of each other is influenced by the media, by history lessons in school, and by parents and community discourse (Bar-On et al., 1997). Television images that conventionally portray Palestinian terrorist bombings and warring Israeli soldiers are extremely detrimental to children of both nations. As such expressions continue to be presented (e.g., Palestinian children to Israeli soldiers; Palestinian laborers to Israeli supervisors), it is not surprising that the myth of the bad "other" continues. The perceptions of the "other" was the focus of a study conducted by two psychologists, Drs. Elia Awwad and Dan Bar-On, who interviewed Israeli and Palestinian youth.

The following example illustrates problems in the perception of "others" (Awwad, 1996, 1997). Radwan is a 23-year-old male from the town of Beit Sahour whose father died when he was eight years old. At the age of 17 he was imprisoned for political reasons and held in Israeli prison for four years (1985–1989). He was then released, resumed his school, obtained the national certificate, and was arrested again for another year. His mother died of cancer while he was in prison for the second time. During his five years of imprisonment, Radwan was transferred to ten prisons and was subjected to interrogations, breakdown techniques, and what Hartman (1993) termed the "double bind" i.e., the need to choose between his physical integrity and his values, friends, or political organization. While in prison he describes feelings of confusion, disorientation, fear, anxiety, and distress. His mother's illness and subsequent death left him with guilt for not having assisted her and anger toward the authorities who prevented his assistance at his mother's funeral. Moreover, following his release from prison, he was abandoned by his political and social community as well, which further affected his self-esteem and identity. In other words, he became a "psychologically homeless" person (Awwad, 1996) or, as he says himself "I am a lost person with no direction."

In the light of these traumatic experiences, Radwan was asked about his perception of the Israelis. He said, "As a human being, I perceive the Israelis as human beings. Both of us need peace and security. This attitude will continue as long as the Israelis are ready to give me peace, security and allow me to live as an individual with all of my rights. In the past, I was a blind person. I learned to hate."

Palestinian and Israeli mental health professionals are responsible for assuring psychological well-being to individuals in their respective communities. In that context, helping resolve the trauma of fighting and violence is of central importance. Purely economic or political peace would remain unstable without concomitant psychological healing. A professional responsibility within a peace process is that of ensuring stable emotional recovery of those previously and presently traumatized.

This process of reestablishing psychological well-being is twofold: first, to identify the type of relationship that was developed throughout past years and second, to help heal resulting trauma experiences within the groups. Israelis and Palestinians have perceived one another and responded to each other in what is known as the "enemy image syndrome" (Spillman and Spillman, 1991). This syndrome comprises seven characteristics:

1. distrusting everything that originates from the enemy;
2. seeing the enemy as guilty and responsible for the underlying tensions;
3. assuming that everything the enemy does is intended to do harm;
4. identifying the enemy as the opposite of everything that one's own group is striving for and sensing that either the enemy or oneself can survive;
5. assuming that anything that benefits the enemy harms one's own group;
6. deindividuating the enemy, in which individuals' identities as "members of the other group" overshadow their personal character and action; and
7. refusing empathy by denying anything in common with the other group.

These characteristics are nonrational and subjective, and individuals should be helped out of this "enemy image syndrome" into a more rational and objective view. However, because this syndrome emanates from traumatic experiences, a second responsibility is to help resolve the trauma within societies. If left unattended, traumatic experiences may be turned inward in both. Hence, an unhealed trauma has the potential of being far more devastating than the violence that initially gave rise to it.

Conflict Resolution

Conflict resolution is an attempt to prevent further violence among individuals and populations. One example of a conflict resolution program is the "Seeds of Peace" nongovernmental organization, dedicated to bringing together youth from Israel, Palestine, Egypt, and Jordan. Seeds of Peace accomplishes this goal by hosting a camp in Androscoggin, Maine, United States, where youth have the opportunity to meet outside the situation of conflict in their respective countries. The youth are taught how to resolve conflicts peacefully by identifying problems, considering solutions, and coming to mutual agreement.

In some of the interviews with youth following their camp experience, they admitted that they had been extremely anxious before meeting the "other." Many had thought that they would fight and would not like the others. In fact, many of the youth entered the camp with the notion that the experience would be a failure. The results of the camp experience, however, were quite the opposite, and many emerged as strong advocates for peace, often more articulate than adults who did not have similar experiences. Moreover, upon return to their respective and segregated communites, relationships built during the camp appear to survive. The youth continue to communicate by the telephone, visit one another and stay overnight in each others' homes. Still, they lack a central meeting place to support continuation of their peace activities. A simple need, the difficulty of identifying such a neutral site, is reflective of the ongoing conflict.

The Children's Peace Museum

Throughout the world, increasing concern is being expressed for children's welfare during armed conflicts. As a result of a recommendation by the United Nations Committee on the Rights of the Child, the General Assembly asked the Secretary-

General to appoint an expert to study the impact of armed conflict on children. After two years of research, field visits, and consultations, Graca Machel, the Secretary-General's Expert on the subject and a former Minister for Education in Mozambique, submitted a report titled, The impact of armed conflict on children (1996), to the 1996 session of the General Assembly. The report addresses issues of rehabilitation of war-affected children. It points to the deterioration of moral values which have allowed children to be involved in war, which is defined as a violation of children's rights.

In the Middle East, the Taylor Institute is facilitating the development of an interactive Children's Peace Museum to encourage peace education activities for young children and youth. A team of Palestinian and Israeli artists, psychologists, and educators has been assembled to direct the implementation of this project. Interactive exhibits will encourage children and youth to explore ideas about our shared humanity and human rights issues. Children will be invited to explore the culture, ethnicity, and religions of other peoples. Additionally, children from different backgrounds will be invited to visit the museum simultaneously to encourage face-to-face interaction.

The rationale of an interactive Children's Peace Museum has at its core the idea that children and youth need to understand each other on a cognitive level, as well as through direct experience with each other. The Children's Peace Museum is foreseen as an international peace movement with plans to develop similar museums, for example, in Ireland and South Africa.

Conclusion

Working in the field of traumatic stress and particularly in areas of conflict requires professionals to be adept and to work not only with a theoretical base and experience, but also by improvisation. The joint efforts described in this chapter demand that professionals reexamine previously defined routines. They involve constant confrontation with unfamiliar and new situations. In *Composing a Life: Life as a Work in Progress*, Mary Catherine Bateson, daughter of Margaret Mead and Gregory Bateson, described the improvisatory art in life as the ability to combine the familiar with unfamiliar components in response to new situations, and to see in problem situations, solutions and opportunities for growth (1990). Symposium members work in this realm of uncertainty and with challenges to their creativity. Behind this work are the energy, the sincerity, and the commitment of Israeli and Palestinian professionals who embrace a vision of real peace and understanding of others (in the words of the Israeli writer Amos Oz (1994) "… to delve into the depths of the other's soul"). Work done by professionals on both sides gives rise to hopes that making peace and healing trauma may begin by building community among professionals.

References

Angelou, M., (1994). *The Human Family in the complete collected poems of Maya Angelou*. New York: Random House.
Arafat, F. (1996). Peace is the highest form of civilization. Presented at the *Second World Conference of the International Society for Traumatic Stress Studies*, Jerusalem.
Awwad, E. (1996). The effects of violence and trauma on the perception of the relevnt other: The Palestinian-Israeli experience during the peace process. Presented at the *Second World Conference of the International Society for Traumatic Stress Studies*, Jerusalem.

Awwad, E., (1997). Identity reconstruction of young Palestinians, Israeli Palestinians and Israeli Jews in the light of the Peace Process. In D. Halperin (Ed.), *To live together: Shaping new attitudes to peace through education*. Paris: United Nations Educational, Scientific and Cultural Organization (UNESCO).

Bar-On, D., Sagy, S., Awwad, E., & Zak, M. (1997). Recent research and intervention activities in the Palestinian-Israeli context: An overview. In D. Halperin (Ed.), *To live together: Shaping new attitudes to peace through education*. Paris: United Nations Educational, Scientific and Cultural Organization (UNESCO).

Bateson, M. C., (1990). *Composing a life: Life as a work in progress*. New York: Plume.

Dubrow, N., (1997). Children's human rights: The equation of justice and peace. *Palestine-Israel Journal*, *IV*(1), 6–11.

Dubrow, N., Liwski, N., Palacios, C., & Gardinier, M. (1995). Traumatized children: Helping child victims of violence: The contribution of non-governmental organizations. In Y. Danieli (Ed.), *International responses to traumatic stress: Humanitarian contributions, collaborative actions and future initiatives*. New York: published for and on behalf of the United Nations, Baywood Publishing.

Halperin, D.S. (Ed). (1997). *To live together: Shaping new attitudes to peace through education*. Paris: United Nations Educational, Scientific and Cultural Organization (UNESCO).

Hartman, L. (1993). Psychopathology of torture victims. *Torture*, *3*(2), 36–38.

Machel, G. (1996). Impact of armed conflict on children. United Nations document A/51/306 and Add.1.

Oz, A. (1994). *Israel, Palestine and peace essays*. San Diego: Harcourt Brace.

Raundalen, M. (1993). Empathy in young children. Presented to UNICEF Counsellor Training Program, Monrovia, Liberia.

Spillman, K. R., & Spillman, K. (1991). On enemy images and conflict escalation. *International Social Science Journal*, *43*(1), 57–76.

Staub, E. (1989). *Roots of evil*. Cambridge: Cambridge University Press.

van der Kolk, B. (1987). *Psychological trauma*. Washington, DC: American Psychiatric Press.

Volkan, V. (1988). *The need to have enemies and allies*. London: Jason Aronson.

31

The Psychosocial Cost of Seeking and Granting Asylum

ZACHARY STEEL AND DERRICK SILOVE

The Convention on Refugees adopted by the United Nations in 1951 represented a milestone in international initiatives to provide protection to displaced persons. Signatories to the Convention agreed to offer sanctuary to those persons fleeing state persecution who held a legitimate fear of returning to their homelands. The Convention and subsequent Protocol (1967) operated effectively over subsequent decades in an era when the number of refugees arriving in Western countries, mostly originating from the Eastern bloc, was relatively small and when the ideological climate was such that the newcomers were afforded high levels of public compassion and acceptance.

The mid-1970s marked a major change in patterns of refugee movement. With the ascendance to power of Communist governments in Vietnam, Cambodia, and Laos, an exodus began from Indochina which resulted in displacing millions of people during the following 20 years. United Nations agencies, such as the Office of the High Commissioner for Refugees, were ill-prepared and inadequately resourced to deal with this mass flow of people. As a consequence, the refugee camp, in which large numbers of stateless persons are held for protracted periods in countries of first asylum, has become established as a commonly used strategy to control the numbers seeking resettlement in Western countries (Mollica et al., 1993).

In the last 15 years, the problem of mass displacement of populations has grown in magnitude, and more than 100 regions around the globe are undergoing social upheaval as a consequence of war and other forms of political conflict (Kos et al., 1993; Vernez, 1991). The number of people fleeing war and other forms of social upheaval has reached more than 50 million, and approximately 20 million displaced people are seeking refuge in foreign countries. As a consequence, the numbers of people seeking political asylum in Western countries have increased significantly. In 1977, an estimated 30,000 persons sought asylum in Western Europe. This number increased to 186,000 by

---

ZACHARY STEEL and DERRICK SILOVE • Psychiatry Research and Teaching Unit, Liverpool Hospital, Liverpool, NSW 2170, Australia.

International Handbook of Human Response to Trauma, edited by Shalev, Yehuda, and McFarlane. Kluwer Academic / Plenum Publishers, New York, 2000.

1987 and to 543,000 in 1993 (European Consultation on Refugees and Exiles, 1994). In Australia, a corresponding increase in the number of asylum applicants has been observed, and more than 31,000 applications were lodged between 1989 and 1996.

During the same period, countries of Western Europe, North America, and Australia have faced increasing economic uncertainties, rising unemployment, and a resurfacing of ethnocentric tendencies—at least among a vocal minority group within society. From an administrative perspective, an increasingly sharp distinction has been made between "offshore" refugees whose applications have been lodged outside the country of intended resettlement, and "onshore" asylum seekers who cross borders illegally or are on temporary visas and then apply for asylum from within the country. It is argued that the numbers of new settlers arriving on the "offshore" refugee program can be closely monitored, whereas the influx of "spontaneous" asylum seekers is more difficult to control. As a consequence, most Western countries, including Australia, have responded to the increasing number of onshore asylum applicants by instituting stringent procedures to test claims for refugee status (Jupp, 1994; Silove et al., Becker, 1993; Summerfield et al., 1991). The problem of assessing such claims is made more complex by the escalating numbers of unauthorized immigrants entering Western countries for nonpolitical reasons, usually in search of work and better living conditions. A policy of so-called "humane deterrence," including detention in some instances and restrictions on those asylum seekers living in the community, has been applied to attempt to discourage all would-be settlers without established immigration rights from entering Western countries. Therefore, there is a danger that the restrictions aimed to deter unauthorized economic migration will be applied indiscriminately to asylum seekers who have genuine claims to refugee status. Thus, from a mental health perspective, there is a risk that the harsh conditions experienced in the postmigration environment may add to or complicate symptoms of PTSD, depression and anxiety in asylum seekers, particularly those who are survivors of torture and other forms of organized violence (Silove et al., 1993; Summerfield et al., 1991).

Trauma Exposure among Displaced Persons

During recent decades, several community studies focusing on displaced persons residing in Western countries have documented high levels of exposure to trauma among refugees. Few studies have focused on the issue of traumatic stress in asylum seekers per se, so that reference needs to be made to the literature on authorized refugees to assess the likely levels of trauma exposure and traumatic stress disorders experienced by the former group. Thus a brief overview will be undertaken of some key recent studies on the mental health of displaced persons.

Carlson and Rosser-Hogan (1991, 1993, 1994) found that more than 80% of Cambodian refugees in the United States reported the loss of a friend or a family member by political "disappearances" and approximately half had been personally assaulted (including rape) or had witnessed a family member being killed. Hinton et al. (1993) reported that approximately 20% of newly arrived Vietnamese refugees had been exposed to trauma and 5.5% reported imprisonment and torture. Mollica et al. (1992) found that more than 60% of 91 Indochinese refugees in the United States reported enforced isolation, being exposed to combat situations, or being close to death, and more than one-fourth tortured.

High levels of trauma exposure have also been documented among displaced persons in refugee camps. In a large random sample of Cambodian refugees living in Thailand-Cambodia border camps, Mollica and co-workers (1993) found that more than 85% reported that, before reaching the camp, they had been deprived of food, water, shelter, or medical care or had been subjected to forced labor. More than 50% had witnessed the murder of a friend or family member or had been close to death, and more than one-third reported past torture experiences.

As expected, such refugee populations generally manifest levels of post-traumatic stress disorder (PTSD) that may be as high as 86% (Carlson & Rosser-Hogan, 1991). Elevated rates of other psychiatric disorders such as depressive disorder have also been commonly observed. Hinton et al. (1993) found that 8.5% and 5.5% of 201 newly arrived Vietnamese refugees met DSM-III-R criteria for adjustment disorder and major depression, respectively. Westermeyer (1988) reported that 44% of 97 Hmong refugees met criteria for an Axis I disorder with adjustment reactions and that affective and paranoid disorders were most common.

Increasingly, it is recognized that the characteristics of the peri- and post-traumatic environments are important in determining the persistence and severity of ongoing PTSD symptoms (Hales & Zatzick, 1997; Yehuda & McFarlane, 1995). Emerging findings from refugee research tends to support such conclusions. For example, in a study of 223 Cambodian refugees resettled in New Zealand, Cheung (1994) found that an index of postmigration stress was as strong a predictor of PTSD status as the extent of exposure to premigration trauma. In a study of 308 Southeast Asian refugees, Abe et al. (1994) found that postmigration factors, such as the number of significant life changes experienced and the extent of the refugee's reliance on welfare support, were significant predictors of PTSD status. Similarly, Basoglu et al. (1994) found that the severity of psychosocial stressors in the peritraumatic environment influenced the expression of PTSD symptoms in a sample of 55 torture survivors.

In recognition of the psychiatric problems faced by refugees, services for survivors of torture and trauma have been developed in many countries (Cunningham & Silove, 1993; McGorry et al., 1995). Although, as noted before, severe stress may exacerbate symptoms of PTSD in some refugees, longitudinal research among resettled refugee populations has indicated that their psychiatric symptoms generally follow a favorable course, and symptom reduction and improvement in psychosocial well-being occur during the first three years of resettlement (Beiser, 1988; Beiser et al., 1989; Krupinski & Burrows, 1986; Rumbaut, 1989, 1991; Westermeyer et al., 1989).

In contrast to authorized refugees, many asylum seekers residing in Western countries live under conditions of deprivation and face the threat of forced repatriation during the prolonged period while they await the outcome of their refugee claims (Becker & Silove, 1993). Refugee applications may take years to process, and during the intervening period, asylum claimants may be denied ready access to work, education, social security, or health services (Cox & Amelsvoort, 1994). Aron (1992) expressed the concern that the complexities of the legal process involved in seeking asylum in the United States had the potential to retraumatize persons fleeing state terrorism. Making similar observations in relation to Europe, Baker (1992) concluded that the "... whole situation is fraught and weighted against the asylum seeker" (p. 93). For those asylum seekers held in detention while their refugee claims are being processed, the risk of "retraumatization" may be particularly high (Silove et al., 1993). In summarizing the experiences of mental health, legal, and welfare workers in Australia, Silove et al. (1993) concluded that there had been "... a marked increase in expressions of despair ... amongst asylum seekers prusuing claims for residency. Asylum seekers both in detention and living in the community show evidence of profound depression, helplessness, and hopelessness" (p. 607).

Research on Asylum Seekers

Few studies have focused exclusively on the mental health status of unauthorized asylum seekers in Western countries. Thonneau et al. (1990) reported that among 2099 asylum applicants in Quebec, 18% reported prior exposure to torture. Similarly, the Association pour les Victimes de la Repression en Exil found that 20% of people applying for asylum in France reported past torture experiences (Reid & Strong, 1987). Silove et al. (1993) estimated that approximately 26% of asylum seekers seeking assistance from a refugee legal aid service in Sydney, Australia, had suffered torture, and most of the remainder reported exposure to organized violence.

Hougen and Jacobsen (1988) reported that Lebanese asylum seekers ($N = 20$) who had been tortured displayed high rates of psychological distress compared to their non-tortured peers and to refugees participating in a previous study. Jensen et al. (1989) found that 70% of 49 "refugee" psychiatric patients (75% of whom were asylum seekers) suffered from PTSD, but refugees and asylum seekers were not compared directly. An unpublished report cited by the Inter-Church Committee for Refugees in Canada (Silove et al., 1993) found that 70% of asylum seekers surveyed reported high levels of tension, anxiety, and depression, but the method used to assess such psychological difficulties was not specified. More recently, Lavik et al. (1996) found a lower level of psychosocial functioning for the asylum seeker subgroup among a sample of 231 displaced persons referred to a psychiatric outpatient unit.

Silove et al. (1997) reported that, more than two-thirds of 40 asylum seekers attending a community assistance center in Sydney had experienced at least one traumatic event, such as witnessing killings, being assaulted, or suffering torture and captivity. Thirty-seven percent fulfilled DSM-IV criteria for PTSD. In addition to pre-migration trauma exposure, a number of postmigration stressors were associated with a current diagnosis of PTSD. Salient ongoing stressors included delays in processing refugee applications, being interviewed by or experiencing conflict with immigration officials, being denied a work permit, unemployment, and loneliness and boredom.

These studies suggest that asylum seekers, like other displaced persons, are at heightened risk of trauma-related psychiatric disorder. The research by Silove et al. (1997) also indicates that psychological distress among asylum seekers may be exacerbated or prolonged for those who encounter harsh conditions in the postmigration environment. The deprived and insecure nature of the circumstances in which many asylum seekers live provides an in vivo crucible, largely determined by administrative and political forces, that allows close examination of the effects of adverse post-traumatic environments on established traumatic symptoms. Furthermore, it has been postulated (Silove et al., 1993) that particular post-traumatic stressors, such as the threat of repatriation, may interact with experiences of past trauma to increase the severity of PTSD symptoms. As yet, such a postulate remains to be tested systematically.

Tamil Asylum Seekers Fleeing Sri Lanka

Asylum seekers in Western countries are diverse in their cultural and linguistic backgrounds, posing measurement difficulties in making accurate assessments across diverse cultural and language groups (Butcher, 1991; Garcia-Peltoniemi, 1991; Kinzie & Manson, 1987; Williams, 1987). For this reason, the present study focused on a single ethnic group, namely, Tamils, who comprise one of the largest populations of asylum seekers in Australia.

Since July, 1983 Sri Lanka has been in a state of civil war. The conflict between the larger Sinhalese and minority Tamil ethnic groups has involved civil violence, acts of terrorism, guerrilla attacks, reprisal actions, and conventional military warfare. Widespread allegations of torture and related human rights abuses have been made. Estimates suggest that 50,000 people drawn from the various ethnic groups have died during the years of conflict in Sri Lanka, more than a half million persons have been displaced internally, and more than 200,000 have fled overseas (Chandrakanthan, 1994). In 1995, the war escalated after sustained government operations were mounted against Tamil strongholds, and up to 400,000 Tamils were displaced from their homes in the Jaffna Peninsula.

In the only published study from the war zone, Somasundaram and Sivayokan (1994) examined 98 randomly selected adults living in a suburb of Jaffna, the largest Tamil city in northern Sri Lanka. Forty-nine percent of respondents had experienced the death of a relative due to war, 38% had experienced threat to life, 10% detention, 10% assault, 10% injury, and 1% torture. Twenty-seven percent suffered from PTSD, 26% from generalized anxiety disorder, and 35% from major depressive disorder. Because substantial numbers of the Tamil community have fled to Western countries where many have lived for prolonged periods as asylum seekers, they represent an appropriate group for investigating the premigration traumas and postmigration stresses that act on their own or in concert to increase symptoms of PTSD, anxiety, and depression.

Method

Sample

Tamils form a small and dispersed minority group in Sydney, making it impossible to apply strict epidemiological methods to sampling. In addition, asylum seekers are often mobile, do not have telephones, and may be suspicious of direct approaches made by strangers conducting research. Thus, a widespread publicity campaign was initiated to inform the Tamil community about the study. Information was provided through legal aid and resettlement services, ethnic radio stations, newspapers, newsletters, magazines, and community meetings. In advertising the study, it was emphasized that the research team was independent of government departments and that question-

ZACHARY STEEL AND DERRICK SILOVE

naires could be filled out anonymously. All adult Tamils were invited to participate, irrespective of their residency status, but the present report would focus on the asylum-seeker group alone. Legal agencies in contact with asylum seekers and the Ealam Tamil Association agreed to mail questionnaires to their clients or membership without revealing names to the researchers. The Ealam Tamil association provides a focus for information, cultural support, and social activities for the Tamil community in Sydney.

Measures

The questionnaire included a section on demographic information, as well as information about migration and residency status, the Hopkins Symptoms Checklist-25 (Parloff et al., 1954; Winokur et al., 1984), the Harvard Trauma Questionnaire (HTQ) (Mollica et al., 1992), and a postmigratory living problem checklist developed to assess typical ongoing stressors reported by asylum seekers.

The Hopkins Symptom Checklist-25 (HSCL-25)

The HSCL-25 has been validated on a community population (Winokur et al., 1984) and Indochinese versions have been translated and validated by Mollica et al. (1987). Several investigators have attested to the transcultural robustness of the measure (Butcher, 1991; Kinzie & Manson, 1987). The HSCL-25 includes 10 anxiety items and 15 depression items. A summary score is derived by adding all responses and dividing by the number of items answered.

The Harvard Trauma Questionnaire (HTQ)

The HTQ (Mollica et al., 1992) was specifically developed for use among refugee populations. The first section includes 17 items describing a range of traumatic and stressful experiences that displaced people commonly recall. For each item there are four categories of response: "experienced," "witnessed," "heard about," and "no" (exposure). Although not all categories conform strictly to the definition of trauma in DSM-IV, it was decided to retain the entire set to examine whether distinctions emerged across the categories in terms of their likelihood of predicting PTSD, depressive, and anxiety symptoms. The HTQ also includes 30 items that assess symptoms of PTSD using DSM-III-R criteria. The Indochinese versions of the HTQ have yielded close agreement between HTQ-derived PTSD diagnoses and those derived from a structured diagnostic interview administered by a clinician (Mollica et al., 1992).

Postmigration Living Difficulty Questions

A series of questions relating to postmigration living difficulties as developed following discussions with a wide range of legal workers, cultural advisers, and Tamil community leaders. The questions covered 19 common difficulties in the areas of employment, separation and isolation from family members, the procedures involved in applying for refugee status, access to health services, welfare support, poverty and work difficulties, acculturation difficulties, and boredom and isolation (see Table 2). Each item was rated on a 5-point scale ranging from "no problem" to "a very serious problem."

Translation and Analysis of Measures

All questionnaires were translated into Tamil by a bilingual worker with mental health experience and independently back-translated by a bilingual worker without such experience (Bontempo, 1993; Bracken & Barona, 1991). Both English and Tamil copies of the questionnaire were then sent to two bilingual experts (one medical practitioner, one psychiatrist) who had not been involved in the initial translation process (Bracken & Barona, 1991). Recommended revisions were incorporated into the final version of the Tamil questionnaire. Because the Tamil symptom measures have not been calibrated against structured interview diagnoses, no attempt was made to determine caseness (for example of PTSD, major depressive disorder). Instead, it seemed more conservative to analyze the data according to continuous symptom scores. For consistency of interpretation, Pearson's correlation coefficients will be presented as a measure of association for both numerical variables such as age, and discrete variables such as sex. The latter were coded using dummy variables (Cohen & Cohen, 1983).

Results

According to a conservative estimate provided by the Federal Department of Immigration, the number of asylum seekers (N = 62) who participated in the study represented approximately 60% of the Tamil asylum-seeking population in the Australian state of New South Wales (DIEA, 1993). Forty-eight (77%) of the asylum seekers were male and the mean age was 35 years (SD = 11). The average length of residency in Australia was 3.7 years (SD = 1.4). Forty-seven (82%) had completed secondary school and/or held higher qualifications. Before arriving in Australia, most were employed in full-time work (60%) or had been students (27%). Only a minority (42%) were working in Australia at the time of the study. Results from the larger pool of respondents (N = 196) which included Tamil immigrants and authorized refugees, have been reported elsewhere (Silove et al., 1998).

Trauma Exposure, PTSD, Depression and Anxiety

Asylum seekers' endorsement rates of trauma categories assessed by the HTQ are presented in Table 1. Forty-eight (77%) asylum seekers reported exposure to at least one traumatic event, and the mean HTQ categories endorsed was four (SD = 3.9). The most frequent trauma categories reported were the unnatural death of family or friends (47%), forced separation from family members (47%), murder of strangers (47%), being close to death (40%), and murder of family or friends (39%). Twenty-six percent reported exposure to torture. The mean score on the PTSD symptom measure of the HTQ was 1.73 (SD = .55), with a mean score of 1.9 (SD = .65) for the HSCL depression scale and 1.67 (SD = .63) for the HSCL anxiety scale.

Postmigratory Living Problems

As indicated earlier, participants were asked to respond to items on a checklist aimed at identifying problems they may have experienced in Australia during the past 12 months (Table 2). A substantial number of items were identified as "serious" or "very

TABLE 1. Frequency of Harvard Trauma Questionnaire Assessed Trauma Events Experienced by Asylum Seekers (N = 62)

	Experienced N (%)
Unnatural death of family or friends	29 (47)
Murder of stranger or strangers	29 (47)
Forced separation from family members	29 (47)
Ill health without access to medical care	25 (40)
Being close to death	25 (40)
Murder of family or friend	24 (39)
Lack of food or water	20 (32)
Lack of shelter	19 (31)
Forced isolation from others	17 (27)
Torture	16 (26)
Combat situation	14 (23)
Imprisonment	12 (19)
Serious injury	8 (13)
Lost or kidnapped	8 (13)
Brainwashing	7 (11)
Rape or sexual abuse	0 (0)
Mean number of trauma events experienced	3.9 (SD = 3.9)
Mean number of trauma events witnessed	2.8 (SD = 2.9)

TABLE 2. Frequency of Postmigration Stressors Causing Serious or Very Serious Problems for Asylum Seekers (N = 62)

	Rates as Serious/Very Serious Problem N (%)
Fear of being sent home	42 (68)
Delays in processing claims	34 (55)
Interviews by immigration officials	16 (26)
Conflict with immigration officials	20 (32)
Unable to return home in an emergency	52 (84)
Worries about family back home	44 (71)
Separation from family	39 (63)
No permission to work	28 (45)
Cannot find work	19 (31)
Bad job conditions	16 (26)
Difficult access to health care	38 (61)
Difficult access to dental care	39 (63)
Inadequate financial assistance from government	25 (40)
Inadequate financial assistance from charities	14 (23)
Poverty	11 (18)
Communication difficulties	10 (16)
Discrimination	10 (16)
Loneliness and boredom	23 (37)
Isolation	18 (29)

serious" problems by respondents, including issues such as anxieties about visiting family in an emergency (84%); fears of being sent home (68%); and obstacles in obtaining treatment for health (61%) and dental (63%) problems. Issues causing serious/very serious concerns in over one-third of respondents were delays in the processing of refugee claims (55%), not having permission to work (45%), lack of government financial assistance (40%), and loneliness and boredom (37%).

Predictors of Depression, Anxiety, and PTSD among Asylum Seekers

Demographic Characteristics and Premigration Trauma

Table 3 displays Pearson correlation coefficients for demographic and premigration variables with measures of anxiety, depression, and PTSD. Age, gender, and education showed no association with symptom scores. In contrast, the composite total of trauma categories endorsed by asylum seekers accounted for 23% of the variance ($r = .48$) of depressive symptoms. Analysis of individual postmigration items revealed that depression scores were higher for asylum seekers who had experienced forced separation from family members ($r = .44$), ill health without access to medical care ($r = .31$), the murder of family and friends ($r = .30$), lack of food, water ($r = .49$) and shelter ($r = .35$), being in a combat situation ($r = .42$), imprisonment ($r = .33$), kidnapping ($r = .31$), and torture ($r = .33$).

Thirty-one percent of the variance ($r = .56$) of anxiety symptoms was predicted by the composite score of trauma items. Anxiety was higher in those asylum seekers who

TABLE 3. Pearson's Correlation Coefficients for Demographic Variables and Premigration Predictors of Depression, Anxiety, and PTSD ($N = 62$)

Demographic and Premigration Trauma	HSCL Depression	HSCL Anxiety	HTQ PTSD
Age	.10	.16	.00
Gender	.08	.01	.10
Level of education (tertiary)	.19	.06	.08
Unnatural death of family or friend	.04	.33[b]	.08
Murder of stranger or strangers	.23	.40[b]	.22
Forced separation from family members	.44[b]	.44[b]	.54[b]
Ill health without access to medical care	.31[a]	.42	.38[b]
Being close to death	.23	.19	.21
Murder of family or friends	.30[a]	.39[b]	.20
Lack of food or water	.49[b]	.44[b]	.54[b]
Lack of shelter	.35[b]	.42[b]	.51[b]
Forced isolation from others	.11	.15	.33[b]
Torture	.32[a]	.26[a]	.37[b]
Combat situation	.42[b]	.59[b]	.40[b]
Imprisonment	.33[b]	.20	.34[b]
Serious injury	.24	.38[b]	.21
Lost or kidnapped	.31[a]	.18	.23
Brainwashing	.04	.22	.09
No. trauma events experienced	.48[b]	.56[b]	.57[b]
No. trauma events witnessed	.05	−.01	.22

[a] = $p < .05$.
[b] = $p < .01$.

reported the unnatural death ($r = .33$) or murder ($r = .33$) of family and friends, had witnessed the murder of strangers ($r = .40$), were forcibly separated from family members ($r = .44$), had been exposed to a combat situation ($r = .59$), or had been seriously injured ($r = .38$). Deprivations associated with living in a war-torn society, such as lack of food, water ($r = .44$), or shelter ($r = .42$), and not having access to health care when ill ($r = .42$) were also predictors of anxiety symptoms.

The total number of trauma categories endorsed predicted 33% ($r = .48$) of the variance in post-traumatic stress symptom scores. Individual traumas associated with such scores included forced family separations ($r = .54$), forced isolation ($r = .33$), combat exposure ($r = .40$), imprisonment ($r = .34$) and torture ($r = .37$), as well as war-related stressors such as a lack of food, water ($r = .54$), and shelter ($r = .51$), and not having access to health care when ill ($r = .38$).

Postmigratory Stressors

A substantial number of postmigration stressors emerged as significant predictors of symptoms of distress among Tamil asylum seekers (Table 4). Statistically significant predictors of depression scores included being separated from a spouse because of the asylum-seeking process ($r = .34$), family separations ($r = .29$), fears of being sent home

TABLE 4. Pearson's Correlation Coefficients for Postmigration Predictors of Symptoms of Depression, Anxiety, and PTSD among Asylum Seekers ($N = 62$)

	HSCL Depression	HSCL Anxiety	HTQ PTSD
Postmigratory stressors			
Time in Australia	.23	.22	.29[a]
Forced separation from spouse	.34[b]	.09	.32[a]
Level of contact with other Tamils	−.01	−.07	−.01
Problem checklist items			
Fears of being sent home	.41[b]	.35[b]	.34[b]
Delays in processing claims	.40[b]	.35[b]	.47[b]
Interviews by immigration officials	.25	.36[b]	.13
Conflict with immigration officials	.42[b]	.39[b]	.44[b]
Unable to return home in emergency	.21	.06	.10
Worries about family and home	.32[a]	.33[b]	.21
Separation from family	.29[a]	.11	.29[a]
No permit to work	.11	.12	.08
Cannot find work	.17	.22	.12
Bad job conditions	.16	.07	.14
Difficulty accessing treatment for health problems	.33[b]	.37[b]	.18
Difficulty accessing treatment for dental problems	.23	.27[a]	.20
Inadequate government assistance	.21	.32[a]	.23
Inadequate charity assistance	.11	.21	.17
Poverty	.33[b]	.39[b]	.31[a]
Communication difficulties	.09	.17	.21
Discrimination	.02	.24	.14
Loneliness and boredome	.53[b]	.27[a]	.54[b]
Isolation	.50[b]	.38[b]	.49[b]

[a] = $p < .05$.
[b] = $p < .01$.

($r = .41$), delays in processing refugee claims ($r = .40$), conflict with immigration officials ($r = .42$), difficulty in obtaining treatment for health problems ($r = .33$), poverty ($r = .33$), loneliness and boredom ($r = .53$), and isolation ($r = .50$).

Significant postmigratory predictors of anxiety scores included fears of being sent home ($r = .35$), delays in processing refugee claims interviews by and conflict with officials ($r = .35$ and $r = .39$, respectively), concerns about family not in Australia ($r = .33$), difficulties obtaining treatment for general health ($r = .37$) and dentistry needs ($r = .27$), lack of government financial assistance ($r = .32$), poverty ($r = .39$), loneliness and boredom ($r = .27$), and isolation ($r = .38$).

For symptoms of post-traumatic stress disorder, significant postmigratory predictors included length of time in Australia ($r = .29$), fears of being sent home ($r = .34$), delays in processing refugee claims ($r = .47$), conflict with immigration officials ($r = .44$), being separated from a spouse because of the asylum seeking process ($r = .34$), other family separations ($r = .29$), poverty ($r = .31$), loneliness and boredom ($r = .54$), and isolation ($r = .49$).

Moderating Effects of Premigration Trauma on Postmigration Stressors

Previous commentators (Aron, 1992; Baker, 1992; Silove et al., 1993) have raised the possibility that pressures associated with the process of applying for asylum, together with the multiple deprivations that asylum seekers experience, may compound the effects of prior trauma in generating distressing symptoms of PTSD, anxiety, and depression. In theory, pre- and postmigration stressors may be additive in their effects, or there may be specific interactions among them. A series of regression models was calculated for each postmigration stressor listed in Table 4. The regression models included the number of trauma categories endorsed, the postmigration stressor, and a term which reflected the interaction between the number of trauma events and the postmigration stressor. Evidence of a moderating effect as a consequence of prior trauma exposure on the impact of postmigratory stress is indicated by a significant interaction term over and above any main effects (Baron & Kenny, 1986). Table 5 displays the increments in variance (ΔR^2) associated with the introduction of a "number of trauma events $\times$ postmigration stressor" interaction term (only ΔR^2 that are statistically significant at the .05 level have been reported). Because zero-order correlations have been presented for the effects of trauma and postmigration stressors (see Tables 3 and 4), the main effects from the regression models are not presented.

The results provide evidence for selective interactive effects which can be grouped into two categories: interactive effects that augment a main effect between postmigration stressors and levels of psychiatric symptoms (signified by [a] in Table 5) and unique interactive effects of premigration trauma and a postmigration stressor where the latter form of stress alone does not predict symptom severity (signified by [b] in Table 5).

Asylum seekers with a history of exposure to trauma manifested heightened depression if exposed to either unemployment or "bad" job conditions ($\Delta R^2 = 9.1$ and 5.5, respectively) in combination. These postmigration stressors were associated with depression only in those asylum seekers with high levels of premigration trauma.

More extensive interactive effects were evident for anxiety symptoms. Asylum seekers with higher trauma exposure had higher anxiety scores associated with fears of being sent home ($\Delta R^2 = 4.6$) than was generally evident among asylum seekers reporting fears of being sent home. Other interactive effects for anxiety in addition to a

**TABLE 5. Change in R^2 Due to the Introduction
of a Trauma by Postmigration Stressor Interaction Term ($N = 62$)
(only Significant Interactions Are Presented)**

	Tamil Asylum Seekers $N = 62$		
Postmigratory Stressors	HSCL Depression	HSCL Anxiety	HTQ PTSD
Trauma × Forced separation from spouse		7.7[b]	
Trauma × Fears of being sent home		4.6[a]	4.5[a]
Trauma × Interviews by immigration officials		7.7[a]	
Trauma × Worries about family at home		6.0[a]	
Trauma × No permit to work			4.8[b]
Trauma × Cannot find work	9.1[b]		5.4[b]
Trauma × Bad job conditions	5.5[b]		
Trauma × Poverty		14.5[a]	
Trauma × Discrimination		4.5[b]	

[a]Significant interaction in addition to postmigration stressor main effect.
[b]Significant interaction with no evidence of postmigration stressor main effect.

significant main effect included interviews by immigration ($\Delta R^2 = 7.7$), poverty ($\Delta R^2 = 14.5$), and worry about family not in Australia ($\Delta R^2 = 6.0$). Important unique interactive effects also emerged. Anxiety symptoms were not generally higher for asylum seekers who had been separated from their spouses due to migration, but such separations were associated with anxiety in asylum seekers with a history of trauma. Similarly, problems associated with discrimination were associated with heightened anxiety symptoms only in those asylum seekers with exposure to past trauma.

Although the fear of being sent home in itself predicted levels of PTSD symptoms ($r = .34$), interactive effects of such fears with high levels of trauma exposure added to symptom severity ($\Delta R^2 = 4.5$). Furthermore, although there were no main effects evident for work-related stressors in relation to PTSD symptoms, not having a work permit and unemployment individually interacted with trauma to increase such symptoms ($\Delta R^2 = 4.8$ and 5.4, respectively).

Discussion

The findings reported in this chapter stand in stark contrast to the proposition that the majority of onshore asylum applicants are "economic migrants" or "queue jumpers" who are seeking to better their living standards rather than to escape from persecution (Silove et al., 1997). Consistent with research on other groups of displaced persons (Carlson & Rosser-Hogan, 1991; Hinton et al., 1993; Mollica et al., 1993), asylum seekers reported extensive exposure to premigration trauma and predictable levels of consequent psychological distress. In the present study, almost half the asylum seekers reported the unnatural death of family or friends, witnessing killings, and being forcibly separated from family members, and more than one-third reported suffering ill health without access to medical care, being close to death, and experiencing lack of food, water, or shelter. More than one-fourth reported torture or forced isolation from others.

One possible limitation to the extent to which these findings can be generalized is that the sample consisted of volunteers and therefore may not have been representative of the generality of Tamil asylum seekers in Australia. Based on government estimates, it was possible to calculate that the number participating in the study comprised approximately 60% of the Tamil asylum seekers in Sydney at the time of the study. Thus, the extent of trauma exposure in the whole Tamil asylum-seeking population in Sydney would still be substantial even if the 40% of those who were not assessed suffered substantially lower levels of such experiences. The findings also contribute to a growing consistency across studies that asylum applicants in Western countries are a high-risk group in terms of prior trauma exposure. Such consistent findings are particularly significant considering that the studies have employed a variety of sampling methodologies, have been conducted in different countries, and have examined asylum applicants from diverse regions and cultural backgrounds. For example, in another Australian-based study, Silove et al. (1997) reported levels of trauma exposure similar to the present sample among 40 asylum seekers originating from 21 different countries in Asia, Latin America, the Middle East, Europe, and Africa. Thonneau et al. (1990) found that 18% of asylum seekers reported prior exposure to torture in a survey of all new applicants to Quebec, and the Association pour les Victimes de la Repression en Exil found that 20% of people applying for asylum in France reported past torture experiences. Such prevalence rates of torture are broadly similar to the 26% rate reported in the present study.

Although one study has been undertaken in the war zone in Jaffna (Somasundaram & Sivayokan, 1994), no psychiatric data have been available on Tamils displaced to Western countries by the long-standing conflict in Sri Lanka. Assessment of psychiatric symptoms in this study was undertaken by using the Hopkins Symptom Checklist-25 and the Harvard Trauma Questionnaire. These measures have been shown to yield valid and reliable data when applied in cross-cultural settings and have been widely used in previous refugee research (Mollica et al., 1992). However, it must be acknowledged that, although appropriately translated and back-translated, these measures have not been calibrated to assess caseness for the Tamil population. Therefore, it seemed more conservative in this study to focus on symptom scores as dimensional variables rather than to determine caseness (for example, of PTSD) by imposing threshold criteria derived from studies of other cultural groups (Beiser et al., 1994). Further limitations of the study include its cross-sectional design and the associated risk of recall bias in reporting trauma exposure. Caution is also necessary in drawing causal inferences because it is possible that ongoing affective symptoms might have colored the perspective of respondents in reporting postmigration living difficulties. Such distortions could have been increased in a group such as asylum seekers, who have a vested interest in drawing public attention to their plight. However, in a separate analysis of this data, Silove et al. (1998) found that the sample of asylum seekers did not report levels of trauma or psychiatric symptoms higher than authorized refugees, suggesting that there was no general tendency for the latter group to exaggerate their difficulties.

Notwithstanding the foregoing caveats, premigration trauma appeared to be a powerful predictor of psychological symptoms. Such events accounted for 33% of the variance in post-traumatic stress symptom scores. Specific trauma categories displaying significant correlations with post-traumatic stress symptoms included forced family separation, forced isolation, torture, combat exposure, imprisonment, and war-related stressors. It is interesting to note that although a number of these war-related stressors, such as a lack of food, water, or shelter and not having access to health care, do not conform strictly to the definition of trauma in DSM-IV, nevertheless, they emerged as highly salient predictors of post-traumatic stress symptoms. One possible explanation is that in extreme war-related situations, such experiences can be life-threatening. On the other hand, in interpreting such findings, it should be noted that only zero-order associations were presented. It is possible, for example, that the association between a variable, such as lack of food and water, and post-traumatic symptoms may be due to a second-order association, such as being in a combat situation where food or water were inaccessible. More complex analyses requiring a larger sample size would be necessary to elucidate such possible relationships.

Higher levels of trauma exposure were also related to depressive and anxiety symptoms in asylum seekers, a finding which is consistent with the observation that post-traumatic stress symptoms constitute only one pathogenic outcome associated with trauma (Yehuda & McFarlane, 1995). The total number of trauma categories endorsed by Tamil asylum seekers accounted for 23% of depressive symptoms, and individual trauma events found to predict high depression scores included forced separation from family members; ill health without access to medical care; the murder of family and friends; lack of food, water, or shelter; being in a combat situation; imprisonment; kidnapping; and torture. Thirty-one percent of the variance in anxiety scores was predicted by the composite index of trauma experienced. More specifically, anxiety scores were higher for those asylum seekers who had been exposed to unnatural death or murder, enforced separation from family, or to combat situations and personal injury. Deprivations associated with living in a war-torn society such as a lack of food, water, and shelter and lack of access to health care when ill, were also predictors of anxiety symptoms.

The pattern of responses to the postmigration stress questions testifies to the high levels of living difficulties experienced by asylum seekers residing in Australia. More than 50% of asylum seekers rated as serious or very serious such difficulties as accessing emergency and long-term medical or dental care, separation from family, worry over family not in Australia, being unable to return home in an emergency, fears about being sent home, and delays in the processing of their refugee applications. These high endorsement rates provide systematic evidence to support the concerns raised by previous observers that asylum seekers face high levels of stress while awaiting the outcome of their refugee applications (Cox & Amelsvoort, 1994; Moss, 1993; Silove et al., 1993).

Two general hypotheses were investigated concerning the impact of postmigration stress on asylum seekers. In the first instance, it was postulated that exposure to high levels of stressful events in the postmigration environment would be directly linked to levels of depression, anxiety, and post-traumatic stress. Secondly, to test the assertion of previous commentators (Aron, 1992; Baker, 1992; Silove et al., 1993), it was hypothesized that the stringent procedures for processing asylum applicants and the associated deprivations experienced in the postmigration environment would compound the risk of psychological symptoms in those asylum seekers with a history of premigration trauma exposure. Such a trauma-induced sensitivity model was tested by regression equations that included both indexes of trauma exposure and postmigration stressors as interaction terms.

Evidence for both direct effects of postmigration stress and trauma-induced sensitivity effects were found. Postmigration stressors which emerged as significant predictors of depression scores fell into three general categories: problems associated with the asylum seeker process, such as being separated from a spouse or other family members; challenges intrinsic to making refugee claims, such as fears of being sent home, delays in processing refugee applications, and conflict with immigration officials; and difficulties arising from exclusion from services, such as health care. Other predictors of depression scores, such as loneliness and boredom and social isolation, may have reflected general adaptational difficulties associated with migration or may have been an outcome rather than a cause of the emotional disturbance. Evidence of trauma-induced sensitivity effects were not strong for depression, except in relation to unemployment and poor job conditions.

Postmigratory predictors of higher anxiety scores fell into three domains: those specifically associated with the asylum-seeking process, such as fears of being forcibly repatriated, delays in processing claims, and interviews by, as well as conflict with immigration officers; deprivations associated with administration restrictions, such as difficulties accessing health and dentistry care, lack of financial assistance and associated poverty; and personal factors, such as threat to family, boredom, and isolation. Anxiety responses to postmigration stresses showed particular evidence of trauma-induced sensitivity effects. For example, although asylum seekers who reported fears of being sent home were generally more likely to be anxious, those with higher levels of trauma exposure experienced even greater levels of anxiety symptoms as a consequence of such fears. Interviews by immigration, poverty, and worry about family not in Australia also showed significant interactive effects with past trauma exposure. In addition, there were some unique interactive effects, and separation from spouse and exposure to discrimination led only to significant increases in levels of anxiety in those asylum seekers with higher levels of trauma exposure.

Finally, the current research provided further evidence to verify the importance of the post-traumatic environment in determining the severity of ongoing PTSD symptoms (Hales & Zatzick, 1997; Yehuda & McFarlane, 1995). Significant postmigratory predictors of PTSD symptoms included length of time in Australia, stressors associated with the asylum seeking process including fears of being sent home, delays in processing refugee claims, and conflict with the department of immigration, as well as other factors, such as poverty, boredom, isolation, and family separation. Those asylum seekers with the highest levels of trauma exposure displayed an additional sensitization effect to fears associated with forced repatriation and stressors due to unemployment or not having a work permit.

Concluding Comments

Controversy continues in Western countries about whether most asylum claimants are bona fide refugees or illegal migrants seeking to better their economic circumstances (Silove et al., 1993). The findings reported in this chapter, when considered in concert with other international research, present a consistent picture of asylum seekers as a highly traumatized population at risk of persisting emotional disturbance. The results of this study suggest that the postmigration environment for asylum seekers may be characterized by high levels of stress, often directly related to the conditions of uncertainty and fear created by stringent refugee determination procedures. In addition, asylum seekers often live under conditions that deprive them of basic services such as access to medical care (Sinnerbrink et al., 1996). Many of those stressors appear to be associated with symptoms of depression, anxiety, and PTSD. Additionally, as anticipated by previous commentators (Aron, 1992; Baker, 1992; Silove et al., 1993), particular postmigration stressors, such as the threat of repatriation, appear to interact with experiences of past trauma to increase the severity of anxiety and post-traumatic stress symptoms experienced by asylum seekers. Regardless of whether the majority of asylum applicants in a country are ultimately recognized as bona fide refugees, it seems important for public policy to be formulated to take into account the levels of stress faced by this population. It is an unfortunate irony that, at a time when many Western countries are promoting public health strategies aimed at preventing mental ill health, other policies may be pursued that are demonstratively destructive to the psychological well-being of certain vulnerable minorities such as traumatized asylum seekers.

References

Abe, J., Zane, N., & Chun, K. (1994). Differential responses to trauma: Migration-relation discriminants of post-traumatic stress disorder among southeast Asian refugees. *Journal of Community Psychology, 22*, 121–135.

Aron, A. (1992). Applications of psychology to the assessment of refugees seeking political asylum. *Applied Psychology: An International Review, 41*, 77–91.

Association pour les Victimes de la Repression en Exil (no date). *Proposal by the AVRE to Establish a centre for the care of victims of torture and cruel, inhuman or degrading treatment.* Paris: Association pour les Victimes de la Repression en Exil.

Baker, R. (1992). Psychosocial consequences for tortured refugees seeking asylum and refugee status in Europe. In M. Basoglu (Ed.), *Torture and its Consequences* (pp. 83–106). Cambridge: Cambridge University Press.

Baron, R., & Kenny, D. A. (1986). The moderator-mediator variable distinction in social psychological research: Conceptual, strategic, and statistical considerations. *Journal of Personality and Social Psychology, 51*, 1173–1182.

Basoglu, M., Paker, M., Ozmen, E., Tasdemir, O., & Sahin, D. (1994). Factors related to long-term traumatic stress responses in survivors of torture in Turkey. *Journal of the American Medical Association, 272*, 357–363.

Becker, R., & Silove, D. (1993). Psychological and psychosocial effects of prolonged detention on asylum-seekers. In M. Crock (Ed.), *Protection or Punishment: The detention of asylum seekers in Australia* (pp. 81–90). Sydney: The Federation Press.

Beiser, M. (1988). Influences of time, ethnicity, and attachment on depression in Southeast Asian refugees. *American Journal of Psychiatry, 145*, 46–51.

Beiser, M., Turner, R. J. & Ganesan, S. (1989). Catastrophic stress and factors affecting its consequences among Southeast Asian refugees. *Social Science and Medicine, 28*, 183–195.

Beiser, M., Cargo, M. & Woodbury, M. A. (1994). A comparison of psychiatric disorder in different cultures: Depressive typologies in southeast Asian refugees and resident Canadians. *International Journal of Methods in Psychiatric Research, 4*, 157–172.

Bontempo, R. (1993). Translation fidelity of psychological scales: An item response theory analysis of an individualism-collectivism scale. *Journal of Cross-Cultural Psychology, 24*, 149–166.

Bracken, B. A., & Barona, A. (1991). State of the art procedures for translating, validating and using psychoeducational tests in cross-cultural assessment. *School Psychology International, 12*, 119–132.

Butcher, J. N. (1991). Psychological evaluation. In J. Westermeyer, C. L. Williams, & A. N. Nguyen (Eds.), *Mental Health Services for Refugees* (pp. 111–122). Washington, DC: U.S. Government Printing Office.

Carlson, E. B., & Rosser-Hogan, R. (1991). Trauma experiences, posttraumatic stress, dissociation, and depression in Cambodian refugees. *American Journal of Psychiatry, 148*, 1548–1551.

Carlson, E. B. &, Rosser-Hogan, R. (1993). Mental health status of Cambodian refugees ten years after leaving their homes. *American Journal of Orthopsychiatry, 63*, 223–231.

Carlson, E. B., & Rosser-Hogan, R. (1994). Cross-cultural response to trauma: A study of traumatic experiences and posttraumatic symptoms in Cambodian refugees. *Journal of Traumatic Stress, 7*, 43–58.

Chandrakanthan, A. J. V. (1994). An exodous sans destination: Refugees and the internally displaced in Sri Lanka. Presented at the *4th International Research and Advisory Panel Conference*, University of Oxford.

Cheung, P. (1994). Posttraumatic stress disorder among Cambodian refugees in New Zealand. *International Journal of Social Psychiatry, 40*, 17–26.

Cohen, J., & Cohen, P. (1983). *Applied Multiple Regression/Correlation Analysis for the Behavioural Sciences*. Hillsdale, NJ: Lawrence Erlbaum.

Cox, D. R., & Amelsvoort, A. V. (1994). *The well-being of asylum seekers in Australia: A study of policies and practice with identification and discussion of the key issues*. Victoria: Centre for Regional Social Development, La Trobe University.

Cunningham, M., & Silove, D. (1993). Principles of treatment and service development for refugee survivors of torture and trauma. In J. Wilson & B. Raphael (Eds.), *International handbook of traumatic stress syndromes* (pp. 751–762). New York: Plenum Press.

DIEA. (1993). Statistics request: Sri Lankan refugee applicants. Canberra: Australian Department of Immigration and Ethnic Affairs.

European Consultation on Refugees and Exiles (1993). *Asylum in Europe: An introduction*, 4th ed. London.

Garcia-Peltoniemi, R. E. (1991). Epidemiological Perspectives. In Westermeyer, J. Williams, C. L. & Nguyen, A. N. (Eds.), *Mental health services for refugees*. Washington, DC: U.S. Government Printing Office.

Hales, R. E., & Zatzick, D. F. (1997). What is PTSD? (editorial). *American Journal of Psychiatry, 154*, 143–145.

Hinton, W. L., Yung-Cheng, J. C., Nang, D., Tran, C. G., Lu, F., Miranda, J., & Faust, S. (1993). DSM-III-R Disorders in Vietnamese refugees: prevalence and correlates. *Journal of Nervous and Mental Disease, 181*, 113–122.

Hougen, H. P., & Jacobsen, P. (1988). Physical and psychological sequelae to torture: a controlled clinical study of exiled asylum applicants. *Forensic Science International, 39*, 5–11.

Jensen, S. B., Schaumburg, E., Leroy, B., Larsen, B. O., & Thorup, M. (1989). Psychiatric care of refugees exposed to organised violence. *Acta Psychiatrica Scandinavica, 80*, 125–131.

Jupp, J. (1994). Australian immigration and settlement: history and current trends. In I. H. Minas, & C. L. Hayes (Eds.), *Migration and mental health. Responsibilities and opportunities* (pp. 3–11). Melbourne: Victorian Transcultural Psychiatry Unit.

Kinzie, D. J., & Manson, S. M. (1987). The use of self-rating scales in cross-cultural psychiatry. *Hospital and Community Psychiatry, 38*, 190–196.

Kos, A., Perren-Klinger, G., Groenenberg, M., Mollica, R., De Martino, R., & Petevi, M. (1993). Draft guidelines on the evaluation and care of victims of trauma and violence. Geneva: United Nations High Commissioner for Refugees.

Krupinski, J., & Burrows, G. (1986). *The Price of freedom: Young Indochinese refugees in Australia*. New York: Pergamon Press.

Lavik, N. J., Hauff, E., Skrondal, A., & Solberg, O. (1996). Mental disorder among refugees and the impact of persecution and exile: Some findings from an outpatient population. *British Journal of Psychiatry, 169*(6), 726–732.

McGorry, P. (1995). Working with survivors of torture and trauma: The Victorian Foundation for Survivors of Torture in perspective. *Australian & New Zealand Journal of Psychiatry, 29*, 463–472.

Mollica, R. F., Wyshak, G., de-Marneffe, D., Khuon, F., & Lavelle, J. (1987). Indochinese versions of the Hopkins Symptom Checklist-25: A screening instrument for the psychiatric care of refugees. *American Journal of Psychiatry, 144*, 497–500.

Mollica, R. F., Caspi-Yavin, Y., Bollini, P., Truong, T., Tor, S., & Lavelle, J. (1992). The Harvard Trauma Questionnaire: Validating a cross-cultural instrument for measuring torture, trauma, and posttraumatic stress disorder in Indochinese refugees. *Journal of Nervous and Mental Disease, 180*, 111–116.

Mollica, R. F., Donelan, K., Tor, S., Lavelle, J., Elias, C., Frankel, M., & Blendon, R.J. (1993). The effect of trauma and confinement on functional health and mental health status of Cambodians living in Thailand-Cambodia Border Camps. *Journal of the American Medical Association, 270*, 581–586.

Moss, I. (1993). Refugees and asylum seekers. In I. Moss (Ed.), State of the Nation: A report on people of non-English speaking background. Australia: Human Rights and Equal Opportunity Commission.

Parloff, M. B., Kelman, H. C., & Frank, J. D. (1954). Comfort, effectiveness, and self-awareness as criteria of improvement in psychotherapy. *American Journal of Psychiatry, 3*, 343–351.

Reid, J., & Strong, T. (1987). *Torture and trauma: The health care needs of refugee victims in New South Wales*. Sydney: Cumberland College of Health Sciences.

Rumbaut, R. D. (1989). Portraits, patterns and predictors of the refugee adaptation experience. In T. C. Owan (Ed.), *Southeast Asian mental health: Treatment, prevention, services, training, and research* (pp. 433–486). Rockville, MD: National Institute of Mental Health.

Rumbaut, R. D. (1991). The agony of exile: a study of the migration and adaptation of Indochinese refugee adults and children. In F. L. Ahearn. & J. L. Athey (Eds.), *Refugee children: Theory, research, and services* (pp. 53–91). Baltimore: Johns Hopkins University Press.

Silove, D., McIntosh, P., & Becker, R. (1993). Risk of retraumatisation of asylum-seekers in Australia. *Australian and New Zealand Journal of Psychiatry, 27*, 606–612.

Silove, D., Sinnerbrink, I., Field, A., Manicavasagar, V., & Steel, Z. (1997). Anxiety, depression and PTSD in asylum seekers: Associations with pre-migration trauma and post-migration stressors. *British Journal of Psychiatry, 170*, 351–357.

Silove, D., Steel, Z., McGorry, P., & Mohan, P. (1998). Trauma exposure, post-migration stressors, and symptoms of anxiety, depression and posttraumatic stress in Tamil asylum seekers: comparisons with refugees and immigrants. *Acta Psychiatrica Scandinavica, 97*, 175–181.

Sinnerbrink, I., Silove, D., Manicavasagar, V., Steel, Z., & Field, A. (1996). Asylum seekers: general health status and problems with access to health care. *Medical Journal of Australia, 165*, 634–637.

Somasundaram, D. J., & Sivayokan, S. (1994). War trauma in a civilian population. *British Journal of Psychiatry, 165*, 524–527.

Summerfield, D., Gorst-Unsworth, C., Bracken, P., Tonge, V., Forrest, D., & Hinshelwood, G. (1991). Detention in the UK of tortured refugees (letter). *Lancet, 338*, 58.

Thonneau, P., Gratton, J., & Desrosiers, G. (1990). Health profile of applicants for refugee status (admitted into Quebec between August 1985 and April 1986). *Canadian Journal of Public Health, 81*, 182–186.

United Nations convention relating to the status of refugees (1951). New York: United Nations Publications.

Vernez, G. (1991). Current global refugee situation and international public policy. *American Psychologist, 46*, 627–631.

Westermeyer, J. (1988). DSM-III psychiatric disorders among the Hmong refugees in the United States: a point prevalence study. *American Journal of Psychiatry, 145*, 197–202.

Westermeyer, J., Neider, J., & Callies, A. (1989). Psychosocial adjustment of Hmong refugees during their first decade in the United States: A longitudinal study. *Journal of Nervous and Mental Disease, 177*, 132–139.

Williams, C. L. (1987). Issues surrounding psychological testing of minority patients. *Hospital and Community Psychiatry, 38*, 184–189.

Winokur, A., Winokur, D. F., & Rickels, K. (1984). Symptoms of emotional distress in a family planning service: stability over a four-week period. *British Journal of Psychiatry, 144*, 395–399.

Yehuda, R. & McFarlane, A. C. (1995). Conflict between current knowledge about posttraumatic stress disorder and its original conceptual basis. *American Journal of Psychiatry, 152*, 1705–1713.

Afterword

Future Perspectives

Trauma never happens in a social and cultural vacuum, nor can the effects of trauma be relegated to the psychology or biology of an individual. Therefore, it is imperative to avoid reductionist discussions of the impact of traumatic stress. It is not easy for professionals to negotiate the multifactorial causation of traumatic stress responses and the varying dimensions of human tragedy. This book has attempted to lay out some of the factors that are currently pertinent to the field of traumatic stress. Indeed, in uncovering the extent of human traumatization by describing its consequences in an official nomenclature of diseases, the ancestors of the International Society for Traumatic Stress Studies may have opened a Pandora's box, the depth of which is still unknown. Those currently involved in the field—whether as therapists, neurobiologists, or anthropologists—may not realize the full extent of this relatively new discourse.

Preventing society from using its usual denial of human traumatization may have a profound effect. More than eighty years ago, 60,000 casualties taken in a single day of the Battle of the Somme could have been absorbed without shock or protest in their societies. Indeed, the casualties sustained actually perpetuated more violence because each society became even more willing to continue with the hostilities, which lasted three more years and resulted in millions of deaths and even more in permanent psychological scars. Ultimately, the test of the traumatic stress paradigm will be in whether providing information as to how high the social costs are and how malevolent and long-lasting the effects of traumatization can be, can result in minimizing future interpersonal trauma or at least recognizing its true effects.

Many nations are engaged in war now, and others may be perpetually violating human rights, particularly those of individuals such as women and children. Very few of these victims are even likely to have the opportunity to receive any sympathetic support, let alone receive systematic treatment. The second challenge of the traumatic stress paradigm is to expand its scope to reach a larger proportion of those in need. While doing so, we cannot ignore the cultural boundaries that might render some of the traumatic stress propositions alien and therefore ultimately useless. However, at the same time, we cannot use cultural differences as an excuse for not actively offering education and assistance.

Possibly the most salient discovery in the area is that the human brain and body can suffer only so much without severely reorganizing one's internal capacity for adaptation. The biological sensitization that has been recently described in many trauma survivors provides a cogent metaphor for the injurious effects of trauma and at the same time offers an explanation for the way exposure to a single trauma will ultimately magnify all subsequent reactions to future adversities. A tendency to become permanently frightened and terrorized may be deeply embedded in our genes. Traumatic stressors may cause such trends to be expressed, in which case it may be very difficult to achieve a new equilibrium.

Reversing such effects requires medical and psychological treatment but may not be complete until family and community environments are challenged. Therefore, community among professionals should not be limited to those few who—by virtue of personal courage—transcend social and political boundaries. It is imperative that those who cling to narrow paradigms be ready to apprehend their own limitations and share the task with others, whose language and concept may seem foreign and often threatening. Editing this volume, among three professionals from three continents, has been a stimulating and edifying experience.

Appendix

The International Society for Traumatic Stress Studies: Childhood Trauma Remembered

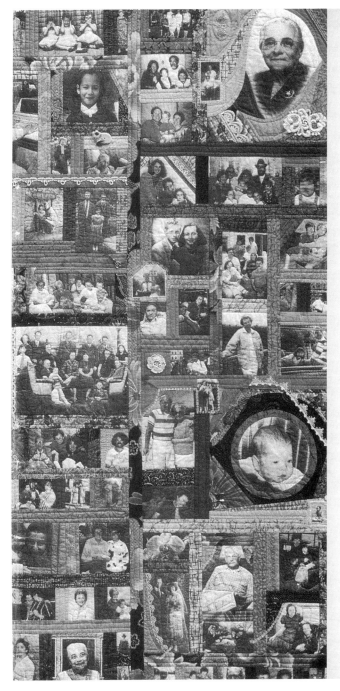

Childhood Trauma Remembered

A Report on the Current Scientific
Knowledge Base and its Applications

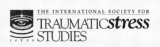

THE INTERNATIONAL SOCIETY FOR
TRAUMATIC*stress*
STUDIES

443

INTRODUCTION

O ver the past several years, the topic of memories of childhood trauma, particularly childhood abuse, has led to considerable debate among professionals and nonprofessionals alike. The debate has attracted the attention of the popular media, which has both reflected and created a wide-ranging interest in questions relating to the memory, in adulthood, of traumatic experiences in childhood.

The degree of popular and professional interest in questions about the validity of memories of childhood abuse has helped to establish a cultural backdrop against which personal, clinical and legal issues for survivors of childhood abuse are considered. On the one hand, a considerable amount of attention has been drawn to the prevalence and enduring effects of the abuse of children by adults who control their access to nurturance, love and material resources. On the other hand, an air of suspicion often surrounds accounts of recovered memories of childhood trauma, whether they occur in response to cues or triggers in the popular media, in psychotherapy, in the courtroom or in response to family life. For the most part, what has been missing in the public eye is a balanced report on the current scientific knowledge base relating to memories of childhood trauma, and the implications of this knowledge base for clinical and forensic practice. The purpose of this report is to provide that information in a readily accessible way.

The initiative for this report comes from the leadership of the International Society for Traumatic Stress Studies, with strong support from its membership. The Society (ISTSS) is perhaps uniquely prepared to take on the task of gathering the expertise necessary to present the state of the art in scientific understanding about memories of childhood trauma. ISTSS is a professional organization of worldwide influence which is dedicated to the discovery and dissemination of knowledge and to the stimulation of policy, program and service initiatives that relate to the occurrence and consequences of traumatic stress. For the present document, we have received input from some of the most distinguished clinical researchers and scholars on traumatic memory in order to provide you with the best available knowledge and its most thoughtful practical application.

1

The International Society for Traumatic Stress Studies

**Additional Reading for
Introduction**

*Below are reports of professional
organizations on the topic of
memories of childhood abuse:*

Alpert, J., Brown, L., Ceci, S.,
Courtois, C., Loftus, E., &
Ornstein, P. (1996). *Working group
on the investigation of memories of
childhood abuse: Final report.*
Washington, DC: American
Psychological Association.

American Medical Association.
*Memories of Childhood Abuse
Report of the Council on Scientific
Affairs* (CSA Report 5-A-94).

American Psychiatric
Association. Statement on
Memories of Sexual Abuse
approved by the Board of
Trustees of the American
Psychiatric Association on
December 12, 1993.

Hammond, D.C. et al. (1994).
*Clinical hypnosis and memory:
Guidelines for clinicians and for
forensic hypnosis.* American
Society of Clinical Hypnosis Press.

Recovered memories. The
Report of the Working Party of
the British Psychological Society
(1996). In Pezdek, K. & Banks,
W. (Eds.), *The recovered memo-
ry/false memory debate.* New
York: The Academic Press.

This report is organized into five short sections. In the **first section**, accumulated scientific findings about the prevalence of childhood trauma and
its psychological consequences are discussed, and the relationship of these
findings to the traditions of trauma-focused psychotherapy and assessment
is explained. In the **second section**, the scientific evidence for the forgetting
of childhood traumatic events, for the delayed recall of traumatic events
after a period of forgetting, and for "false memories" of childhood trauma is
presented. This section is the center of our report, and the remaining three
sections provide the elaboration and application of the information presented here. In the **third section**, what cognitive psychologists and neurobiologists understand about human memory is outlined, based on recent scientific discoveries, and then the implications of this research for an understanding of traumatic memories in general, and forgetting and delayed
recall of traumatic events in particular are described. Finally, in the **fourth
and fifth sections**, the focus is on how to best apply this current knowledge
in clinical and forensic practice with trauma survivors. Gaps in the knowledge base are also identified.

This report represents and incorporates the work of a diverse group of
scholars with expertise in a variety of different topic areas and professional
contexts. It is a statement of the state-of-the-science that is expected to
evolve as new information becomes available. Finally, this effort is in keeping with what has been produced by other professional organizations (see
reports at left), and is in the spirit of finding middle ground and a convergence of various points of view and areas of expertise.

This report is not meant to be a comprehensive research review, but rather
an overall summary of the major issues involved in the recall of childhood
trauma. Therefore, instead of the usual format of citing specific references
for each issue, representative references and suggested readings are listed as
a sidebar for each section.

Childhood Trauma Remembered

SECTION I

PREVALENCE AND CONSEQUENCES OF CHILDHOOD TRAUMA

Altogether too many children experience serious traumas in childhood. Major accidents from cars or fire, involving broken bones or concussions, are common. Children also unfortunately experience life-threatening diseases such as cancers, leukemia and systemic infections. Some children get caught up in natural and human-made disasters like earthquakes, floods, wars or ethnic persecution. Children experience violence in their communities; they get kidnapped, raped or watch assaults on others. And although much of this was once hidden from public view, we know today that children are too often the victims of battery or sexual abuse by those taking care of them, or are witnesses to episodes of abusive violence between parents.

We do not know the exact number of children who experience serious trauma, but given the variety of forms it can take, the number is not small. In recent years, many efforts have been made to estimate the occurrence of particular kinds of childhood trauma. Sexual abuse is the type of trauma that has received the greatest amount of study. The estimate that 20% of girls and 5-10% of boys experience such unwanted sexual contact and molestation while growing up is based on a large number of community epidemiological studies that have interviewed adults about their childhoods. It appears that only a fraction of these cases get disclosed to authorities while they are occurring, which accounts in part for why only approximately 300,000 cases get reported to U.S. child welfare authorities each year.

Both science and personal experience tell us that these childhood events sometimes leave scars that last until adulthood and interfere with healthy adult functioning. It is one of the most consistent scientific research findings that traumas and adversities in childhood tend to put an individual at risk for a large variety of later difficulties. This is true for all kinds of early traumas, including accidents, disasters and the observation of violence. But we know it to be especially true for victims of child abuse and neglect, who have been the subject of a particularly large amount of research. Those who were severely abused as children are two to five times more likely to experience a mental illness as an adult than those who were not. They are more likely to suffer from low self-esteem and difficulties in social, academic and occupational performance. Children who were abused or neglected are also more likely to get caught up in patterns of later delinquent and criminal behavior, violence, alcohol and drug abuse.

The International Society for Traumatic Stress Studies

Additional Reading for Section I

Briere, J. & Elliott, D. (1994). Immediate and long-term impacts of child sexual abuse. *The Future of Children*, 4 (2), pp. 54-69.

This article reviews evidence about the long-term impact of early traumatic sexual abuse.

Finkelhor, D. (1994). Current information on the scope and nature of child sexual abuse. *The Future of Children*, 4 (2), pp. 31-35.

This article reviews evidence on the prevalence of childhood sexual abuse in the general population.

U.S. Department of Health and Human Services. (1997). *Child maltreatment 1995. Reports from the states to the National Child Abuse and Neglect Data System, Contract no. ACF-105-95-1849.* Washington, DC: U.S. Government Printing Office.

This publication provides the most recent information on the large numbers of child abuse cases currently being reported and investigated by state agencies.

Of course, the relationship between childhood traumas and later difficulties is not a simple or inevitable one. Not all traumatized or maltreated children by any means suffer from later problems. Many recover, sometimes very quickly, and have successful lives. And some traumatized children suffer later problems not directly due to their trauma, but due to other factors such as poverty or genetic vulnerabilities that put them at risk for trauma in the first place. But overall, the weight of research evidence points very strongly toward childhood trauma as one important causative factor in later adult maladaptive functioning.

Given that childhood trauma can play such an important role in adult problems, most psychotherapeutic approaches currently in practice carry the assumption that it is important and even essential to gather a comprehensive trauma history in order to plan treatment. The details surrounding traumatic experiences can provide clues to the depth and seriousness of a person's difficulties. Knowledge about these traumas and some of their possible effects can also help therapists in formulating the kinds of corrective experiences that might alleviate current distress and maladaptive patterns of functioning. While it is not certain that trauma-focused treatments are necessarily better than other kinds of treatment for trauma survivors, and while controlled studies are just now being done with many trauma populations for the first time, research has nevertheless shown trauma-focused treatments to be effective. Patients report relief from anxiety and depression, and resolution of intrusive thoughts and feelings about traumatic childhood events. The practices of trauma-focused assessment and psychotherapy have grown in popularity in recent years for these reasons, and we will return to this topic in Section IV.

SECTION II

DELAYED RECALL OF TRAUMATIC EVENTS
AFTER A PERIOD OF FORGETTING

A t the root of the debate about memories of childhood trauma is the question of how common it is for adults to fail to recall traumas that occurred in childhood. People forget myriad ordinary experiences, but do people forget childhood *trauma*? While there is a period in infancy and early childhood during which scientists don't expect memory for any life events, the debate about recovered memory centers on traumas that occurred after this period of approximately the first two or three years of life.

Evidence for the forgetting of childhood trauma

Evidence that people forget childhood traumas comes from clinical and nonclinical studies, and encompasses a range of traumas. The evidence is not limited to people in treatment or to people whose trauma is sexual abuse. Clinical reports of trauma-related forgetting in individual patients can be found in psychiatric literature spanning the last hundred years. In the last 10 years, scholarship on this topic has included research with larger clinical samples of women and men in treatment for the consequences of sexual abuse. This research reveals that many adults who recall childhood sexual abuse report prior periods during which they did not remember the abuse. Recent scholarship has also included nonclinical samples of adults who report a broader range of traumas, and here, too, there are reports of high rates of prior periods of forgetting. One difficulty with these studies is that reports of prior forgetting are also subject to memory problems. We cannot assume that individuals' assessments of their prior forgetting are necessarily accurate. *Prospective* studies of documented abuse that evaluate current forgetting suggest, however, that a significant proportion of women and men with documented cases of sexual abuse *in childhood* do not appear to recall the documented incident when reinterviewed as young adults. Some of the research findings from retrospective and prospective studies are summarized below and on the next page.

Evidence for Forgetting Childhood Traumas
- Herman & Schatzow (1987) found that 28% of their clinical sample of women in group therapy for incest reported "severe memory deficits" for their abuse.
- Briere & Conte (1993) found that 59% of 450 women and men in treatment for sexual abuse reported that, at some time prior to age 18, they had forgotten the sexual abuse they suffered during childhood.

The International Society for Traumatic Stress Studies

448

Additional Reading for Section II

Hyman, I., Husband, T. H., & Billings, F. J. (1995). False memories of childhood experiences. *Applied Cognitive Psychology*, **9**, pp. 181-197.

This paper provides evidence that individuals can be made to believe that they had unusual childhood experiences that did not actually occur. After a third suggestive interview, 25% of the subjects claimed to recall events that had not occurred.

Hyman, L. E. & Pentland, J. (1996). The role of mental imagery in the creation of false childhood memories. *Journal of Memory and Language*, **35**, pp. 101-117.

This article provides evidence that individuals who are asked to form a mental image of an event and to describe it to an interviewer were more likely to create a false event. They were also more likely to recover memories of a previously unavailable true event.

6

■ Loftus, Polonsky & Fullilove (1994) reported that 31% of their sample of sexually abused women in treatment for substance abuse reported at least partial forgetting or incomplete memory for their abuse. 19% reported prior periods of total lack of recall of the abuse.

■ Elliot (1997), in a national, stratified, random sample of 505 women and men, found that 20% of the 116 people in the sample who reported a history of childhood sexual abuse said that there was a period of time when they had no memory of the event. Complete to partial forgetting was reported after every form of traumatic experience, with child sexual abuse, witnessing a murder of a family member and combat exposure yielding the highest rates.

■ Williams (1994), and Williams & Banyard (1997) followed up women and men who, in the early 1970s, were seen in a hospital emergency room for child sexual abuse. They found that at the time of their study, which was 17 years later, 38% of the women and 55% of the men did not recall the documented abuse. Of the women who did recall the abuse, 16% stated that there was a time in the past when they did not remember that it had happened to them.

■ Widom & Morris (1997) found that 32% to 60% of women and 58% to 100% of men with court-substantiated reports of child sexual victimization did not report such abuse on reinterview some 20 years later.

It should be noted that the above findings have been challenged in a number of critiques that address methodological concerns with the retrospective studies as well as with the Williams study (see Pope & Hudson, 1995).

Sources: Herman, J. L., & Schatzow, E. (1987). Recovery and verification of memories of childhood sexual trauma. *Psychoanalytic Psychology*, **4**, pp. 1-14; Briere, J. & Conte, J. (1993). Self-reported amnesia for abuse in adults molested as children. *Journal of Traumatic Stress*, **6**, pp. 21-31; Loftus, E., Polonsky, S. & Fullilove, M. T. (1994). Memories of childhood sexual abuse: Remembering and repressing. *Psychology of Women Quarterly*, **18**, pp. 67-84; Elliot, D. M. (1997). Traumatic events: Prevalence and delayed recall in the general population. *Journal of Consulting and Clinical Psychology*, **65**, pp. 811-820; Williams, L. M. (1994). Recall of childhood trauma: A prospective study of women's memories of child sexual abuse. *Journal of Consulting and Clinical Psychology*, **62**, pp. 1167-1176; Williams, L. M. (1995). Recovered memories of abuse in women with documented child sexual victimization histories. *Journal of Traumatic Stress*, **8**, pp. 649-675; Williams, L. M. & Banyard, V. L. (1997). Gender and recall of child sexual abuse: A prospective study. In Read, J. D. & Lindsay, D. S. (Eds.), *Recollections of trauma: Scientific evidence and clinical practice*, pp. 371-377. New York: Plenum Press; Widom, C. S., & Morris, S. (1997). Accuracy of adult recollections of childhood victimization: Part 2: Childhood sexual abuse. *Psychological Assessment*, **9**, pp. 34-36.

Childhood Trauma Remembered

Evidence for delayed recall of trauma after a period of forgetting

If we accept the evidence that a significant minority of people do in fact forget childhood trauma, at least for some period of time, then other interesting questions arise. When people report that they recall instances of childhood trauma that they had previously forgotten, clinicians and researchers have been interested in the factors relating to this "delayed recall," and in the accuracy of these "recovered memories." Research findings suggest that age at the time of the childhood trauma is associated with forgetting, and that those who were younger are more likely to have forgotten and to report recovered memories. A wide variety of triggers seem to be associated with the recovery of memory for childhood trauma, including watching a television program or reading some materials about trauma, undergoing a similar experience at a later time, and discussions with family and friends. It is likely that situations that have some characteristics that are similar to the original event are associated with recovered memories. Interestingly, a majority of recovered memories are reported to occur outside of therapy.

Regarding the accuracy of recovered memories, several cases in the public record of reported delayed recall of childhood abuse that were corroborated provide evidence for accuracy, as do preliminary studies of recovered memories of documented traumatic events that occurred in childhood. In the research project mentioned above, for example, Williams was able to compare women's current accounts of their abuse with the details of the abuse that had been recorded in the 1970s. She found that the women who reported prior periods of forgetting and the experience of having recovered memories, and those who had always remembered had the same number of discrepancies when their accounts of the abuse were compared to the reports from 17 years earlier. This evidence suggests that memories of childhood trauma can become accessible after periods of forgetting. A summary and synthesis of more than two dozen studies on trauma-related forgetting is described in Scheflin and Brown.

Additional Reading for Section II

Loftus, E. F. & Pickrell, J. E. (1995). The formation of false memories. *Psychiatric Annals*, 25(12), pp. 720-725.

This paper relies on the "lost in shopping mall" paradigm to show that adults could lead a child to believe that he or she had been lost in a shopping mall, suggesting that memories of at least one mildly traumatic event can be implanted.

Pope, H. G. & Hudson, J. I. (1995). Can memories of childhood sexual abuse be repressed? *Psychological Medicine*, 25, pp. 121-126.

This article provides a thoughtful methodological analysis of the limitations of studies concerning forgetting of childhood sexual abuse and constructive suggestions for the design of future studies.

Scheflin, A. W. & Brown, D. (1996). Repressed memory of dissociative amnesia: What the science says. *Journal of Psychiatry and Law*, 24 (2), pp. 143-188.

This paper presents a summary and synthesis of more than two dozen studies on trauma-related forgetting.

7

Additional Reading for Section II
Schooler, J. W. Bendiksen. M. &
Ambadar, Z. (1997) Taking the
middle line: Can we accommodate both fabricated and recovered memories of sexual abuse?
In M. Conway (Ed.), *False and
recovered memories*, pp. 251-292.
Oxford: Oxford University Press.

*This paper provides evidence of
recovered memories and also
reports that some individuals may
exaggerate their prior forgetting,
believing they had forgotten about
their abuse during periods in
which they are known to have
talked about it.*

Williams, L. M. & Banyard, V. L.
(1997). Perspectives on adult
memories of childhood sexual
abuse: A research review. In
Spiegel, D. (Ed.). Section II
*American Psychiatric Review of
Psychiatry*, **16**, Chapter 9, pp. II-
123 to II-151.

*This chapter provides a review of
empirical evidence that supports
the likelihood that child sexual
abuse can be forgotten, that memories of abuse can be implanted
and that memories of abuse once
forgotten can be recovered.*

There is no scientific evidence that adults are likely to intentionally fabricate allegations of abuse in childhood when surveyed using standard victimization screening techniques, or when reporting abuse histories to friends, family or therapists. However, a critical question is whether some proportion of report-ed accounts of recovered memories of childhood trauma, although sincere, are inaccurate (i.e., what have been called "false memories").

Evidence that memories can be implanted

A large body of laboratory research on memory and suggestibility supports the position that memory is reconstructive and imperfect, that memory can be influenced and distorted, that confabulation can occur to fill in memory gaps, and that subjects can be persuaded to believe they heard, saw or expe-rienced events which they did not. Evidence has accumulated that inaccurate memories can be strongly believed and convincingly described. Much of the laboratory research on suggestibility of memory has involved paradigms in which subjects view an event in which they are not a participant, are later provided incorrect information about the event and, finally, are asked about what they saw. Incorrect information is likely to be incorporated in the later reports of memories of the event. This is termed the "misinformation effect," and it is argued that this effect applies as well to memories for experiences of childhood trauma or child sexual abuse. It is asserted that similar processes may lead to a client's false belief that he or she was sexually abused or other-wise traumatized if such a history is suggested by a therapist.

Criticisms of the application of laboratory research to questions of memory of childhood trauma in general, and to child sexual abuse specifically, have focused on the ecological validity of the studies (i.e., their applicability to the real world experience of trauma experienced in childhood, and child molestation and its aftermath). Changing or adding a feature to an event, as is the procedure in much of the laboratory research, is not the same as caus-ing someone to believe that an entire new event occurred. Critics have argued that implanting memories for traumatic events, and generally for events in which one is a participant, may be a very different matter. Of course, research ethics preclude any experiment that would attempt to implant memories of something as serious as sexual abuse.

Recently, a number of studies have been conducted to directly assess the implantation of memories for events that would be mildly traumatic had they occurred, to examine types of events that are more likely to be successfully implanted, and to study the factors associated with successful implantation of memories for events which did not occur. Several designs or paradigms have been used in these studies, but all have in common an attempt to get younger family members of the researchers' collaborators to "remember" events that did not occur. In these studies, researchers were usually able (sometimes after several attempts) to get between 20% and 40% of participants, depending on the strength of the experimental manipulation, to believe that experiences that did not occur actually did happen to them. There is some literature to suggest that those who "remember" events that did not occur may score higher on measures of dissociation and creative imagination. Interestingly, when individuals were asked to form a mental image of an event and to describe it to an interviewer, they were not only more likely to create a false event but they were also more likely to recover memories of a previously unavailable true event. Although these studies all rely on fairly small samples, and although the majority of participants in these studies resisted implanted memory, the findings suggest that certain situational and personal characteristics may maximize suggestibility and that some individuals will report a false or substantially inaccurate memory of childhood trauma. While much needs to be learned about the factors that may contribute to inaccurate recovered memories of childhood trauma and about factors associated with such memories, the provocative laboratory findings on suggestibility and memory point to the value to trauma clinicians and researchers of having a firm grounding in knowledge of human memory processes.

9

SECTION III
HUMAN MEMORY PROCESSES, TRAUMATIC MEMORY AND DELAYED RECALL OF TRAUMATIC EVENTS

1. Memory is not a simple unitary process.
2. Memories are not stored as complete and separate "packets" of information.
3. Memory is not a perfect representation like a photograph.
4. There are two basic forms of memory: explicit and implicit memory.
5. Traumatic memories may be different than ordinary memories.
6. There are a number of as yet unproven mechanisms that might explain how traumatic memories are "forgotten."
7. There is currently no scientific consensus regarding the question of how a "forgotten" memory can be later "recovered."

Until recently, it was generally believed that memories for specific events were stored as discrete bits of information. The Greek philosopher, Plato, likened the memory process to an aviary in which each bird represented a different memory. Remembering, according to Plato, was the process by which the mind attempted to capture the correct bird so that the full memory of a specific event could be viewed by the conscious mind. This concept of memory persisted in various forms for 2000 years. Memory, from this perspective, was simply identifying a single complete representation of a past event in the mind's collection of memories.

Based on recent scientific discoveries, such models of the memory process are no longer accepted. In this section, we will outline some of the most important scientific findings of cognitive psychologists and neurobiologists pertaining to human memory processes. It must be emphasized at the outset, however, that the scientific questions in this field are very complicated. Thus, the following is only a simplified summary of our current state of knowledge:

1. Memory is not a simple unitary process.
Memory involves three complicated processes that depend on multiple brain regions and connections:
- Encoding is the creation of the memory.
- Consolidation is an intermediate step whereby the memory is constructed so that it can be stored over time.
- Retrieval is the process by which the memory is removed from storage and made available to consciousness.

2. Memories are not stored as complete and separate "packets" of information.
Recent research in cognitive psychology suggests that the memory of a specific event is not processed or stored in any one location within the brain but is distributed, instead, across a network. That is, different dimensions of the memory such as visual quality and spatial location are stored in separate areas. It is believed that consolidation of such a memory involves the linking of separate brain regions that together store the memory of the entire event. In order to recall an event it appears that the brain must somehow reconstruct the memory.

10

Childhood Trauma Remembered

Contemporary cognitive psychologists have rejected Plato's birds in favor of a model of memory storage that is more like a spider web in which specific memories are represented by the pattern of connections among fibers in the entire network. Memory is not a process of locating intact bits of information but rather involves partially recreating a pattern of associated threads of information across an entire network. Attempts to retrieve a certain memory might be associated with a particular pattern of vibration throughout the network. Sometimes the retrieval process might actually activate a close approximation of the original memory, one that is similar but not exactly the same as the original memory. This *Connectionist Model of Memory* explains, for example, how memories of similar events can influence one another, and how people often remember some but not all aspects of a past event. It generally helps us understand common errors in remembering.

3. Memory is not a perfect representation like a photograph.

The human capacity to remember and retrieve past events is largely accurate, but it is not perfect. Memory is a selective process which prioritizes information thought to be most important at the time it first occurred. Although most errors in retrieved memory will be small, sometimes they can be quite large. Some common errors in remembering that people make are:

- People sometimes are unable to recall vast portions of their past experiences.
- People sometimes fail to accurately identify the source of their memories.
- People may mistake memories of imagined events for memories of real events.
- People are suggestible; social influence may generally affect the memory retrieval process, and recall of an event may be influenced by misinformation.

4. There are two basic forms of memory: explicit and implicit memory.

Explicit memory, also referred to as the *declarative memory system*, records consciously available information about past experiences. *Implicit memory*, also referred to as the *nondeclarative memory system*, is information that is not consciously available. Skills or attitudes that are "second nature" and relatively automatic are examples of implicit memories. Implicit memory may also contribute to strong emotional memories. Currently available information about these two basic forms of memory is useful for an understanding of traumatic memories:

Additional Reading for Section III
Davis, S. (Ed.). (1992). *Connectionism: Theory and practice*. New York: Oxford University Press.

This book presents an excellent collection of chapters on the connectionist model of memory.

Roediger, H. L. (1980). Memory metaphors in cognitive psychology. *Memory & Cognition, 8*, pp. 231-246.

This paper provides a thoughtful review of the evolution of models of memory processes from ancient times to the present.

Schacter, D. L. (1996). *Searching for memory: The brain, the mind and the past*. New York: Basic Books.

This is the authoritative book on brain mechanisms and memory.

Shobe, K. K. & Kihlstrom, J. F. (1997). Is traumatic memory special? *Current Directions in Psychological Science, 6*, pp. 70-74.

This article provides a thoughtful critique of claims that traumatic memory is special, and a careful analysis of data on which those claims are based.

11

Additional Reading for Section III
van der Kolk, B. A. (1996).
Trauma and memory. In van der
Kolk, B. A., McFarlane, A. C. &
Weisaeth, L. (Eds.). *Traumatic
stress: The effects of overwhelming experience on mind, body
and society.* New York: Guilford
Press.

*This chapter provides a compre-
hensive review of data suggesting
that the processing of traumatic
memories is different than for
other memories.*

*Also suggested are four chapters
from:* Yehuda, R. & McFarlane,
A.C. (Eds.). (1997). Psychobiology
of posttraumatic stress disorder.
*Annals of the New York Academy
of Sciences,* **821.** New York:
Academy of Sciences:
    van der Kolk, B. A.,
Burbridge, J. A. & Suzuki, J. The
psychobiology of traumatic
memory: Clinical implications
of neuroimaging studies, pp. 99-
113.
    Cahill, L. The neurobiology of
emotionally influenced memory:
Implications for understanding
traumatic memory, pp. 238-246.
    Roozendaal, B., Quirarte, G.
& McGaugh, J. L. Stress-activat-
ed hormonal systems and the
regulation of memory storage,
pp. 247-258.
    Armony, J. L. & LeDoux, J. E.
How the brain processes emotional information, pp. 259-270.

12

- Different brain structures serve explicit vs. implicit memory.
- Implicit memory may play a role in the processing of events associated with fear, anxiety and other strong emotions. It may also be involved in creating memories concerning nonemotional information such as skill acquisition and priming.
- Different drugs may affect the two systems differently.
- Implicit memory mechanisms appear to play a key role in the processing of some traumatic memories, although explicit mechanisms are also important.

5. Traumatic memories may be different than ordinary memories.

There are a variety of points of view or emphasis among researchers and scholars with regard to the memory of traumatic vs. nontraumatic events. Some researchers believe that the same basic memory processes can account for the forgetting of both traumatic and nontraumatic memories. Others, however, believe that while traumatic and nontraumatic memories may share many similarities, there may also be important differences between these two types of memories in certain aspects of encoding, con-solidation and retrieval. Some researchers propose that memories of trau-matic events are less distorted, longer-lasting and less susceptible to inaccu-rate recall, suggestibility or social influence. This is because traumatic stress activates both explicit and implicit memory to a much greater extent than is the case for nontraumatic events. Emotional arousal associated with trau-matic events may also be accompanied by elevations in stress hormones and neuromodulators that facilitate memory formation. The amount of arousal that occurs during a traumatic event, however, may influence the quality of memory formation. Some researchers argue that moderate levels of arousal will lead to more reliable memories, but that extreme levels of arousal may limit attention so much that little memory of the event will be retained. Still others propose that highly charged traumatic memories may sometimes mobilize active efforts to forget a memory. One such theoretical mechanism (among others) that has been widely discussed is called "repression," which prevents conscious recall of such memories. Repression is a concept, originally postulated in psychoanalytic theory, that has not been empirically demonstrated in the laboratory.

These different views about memory for traumatic vs. nontraumatic events continue to stimulate a great deal of exciting research. In spite of our gaps in knowledge and differences in opinion, it is generally accepted that the memory of both childhood and adult traumatic events may sometimes become irretrievable ("forgotten") after exposure. There has also been a great deal of speculation about the mechanisms that might explain the forgetting of childhood trauma.

6. There are a number of as yet unproven mechanisms that might explain how traumatic memories are "forgotten."

It is not currently known how traumatic memories are forgotten, and different mechanisms may operate under different circumstances. These questions are of great interest to researchers, and we can expect a rapid growth in information in this area over the next decade. Among explanatory mechanisms that have been proposed to account for "forgetting" are the following:

- **Failure to encode:** a failure to create a memory at the time of the event.
- **Dissociation:** an altered cognitive state which sometimes occurs during a traumatic event and which may interfere with the normal processes for remembering (encoding, consolidation or retrieval) of such events.
- **Simple forgetting:** the fading of a memory over time (a normal phenomenon with non-traumatic memories).
- **Repression:** a theoretical psychological process hypothesized to actively prevent conscious retrieval of memories.
- **Conditioned extinction:** a laboratory phenomenon by which certain conditions can activate inhibition (or reduce the availability) of previously learned behavior.
- **State dependent learning:** a mechanism that would explain why traumatic memories can be retrieved only when the individual is in the same emotional, environmental and neurobiological state that was present during the original traumatic event.
- **Long-term depression:** a cellular mechanism which suppresses the transmission of data from certain nerve cells to others; this could theoretically impair the retrieval of previously accessible information.

7. There is currently no scientific consensus regarding the question of how a "forgotten" memory can be later "recovered."

Since there is evidence that "forgotten" memories of traumatic events are sometimes "recovered," it is necessary to understand how this might occur. The key to answering this question is first to understand how the initial memories became inaccessible in the first place. It is expected that once we have a better understanding of the mechanism(s) of "forgetting," we will be able to address the question of memory "recovery" in a systematic manner. It is, of course, equally important to understand how inaccurate memories that appear to have been "recovered" can be so compelling as to make some individuals believe that such events really happened. The challenges presented by the "recovered" memory debate have stimulated a burst of creative research activity that will undoubtedly enhance understanding of the complex cognitive psychology and neurobiology of human memory processes.

The International Society for Traumatic Stress Studies

13

SECTION IV
APPLICATION OF THE CURRENT SCIENTIFIC KNOWLEDGE
BASE TO CLINICAL PRACTICE

Trauma, like other aversive life events, is associated with a range of negative psychological consequences. Reviewing these past experiences is considered an important component of many treatment approaches. Key tasks in such therapies involve understanding the impact of traumatic events on current functioning and addressing unresolved consequences of such experiences. Memory for trauma is relevant when individuals seek treatment for the specific problems that may be related to traumatic experiences, disclose trauma histories in the course of therapy, or recall previously forgotten experiences while in treatment. Therapy does not always or exclusively focus on trauma memories, but therapy must focus on aspects of the trauma such as emotions and cognitions when they are a source of distress.

Many posttraumatic symptoms are related to traumatic memories and include intrusive thoughts, intensification of emotional and physiologic reactions at recall, flashbacks and nightmares. Specific memories of traumatic events are especially likely to be disturbing and, because of this, become a focus of trauma-specific treatment. Along with such memory-related symptoms, there may be alterations in assumptions about self that derive from actions taken and not taken during and after traumatic events. Cognitive and emotional processing are effective treatments for Posttraumatic Stress Disorder (PTSD) that involve talking specifically and in detail about the experience. Pharmacological interventions can reduce stressful and uncomfortable symptoms associated with traumatic memories, thereby improving the functional capabilities of patients.

Memory for trauma, like all memory, is reconstructive; it may be essentially true, contain significant inaccuracies or, in some cases, be illusory. Competent therapists recognize that memory is fallible and that certain therapeutic approaches may increase the likelihood of distortion or confabulation. In therapeutic situations, when clients have experienced traumatic events, the literal accuracy of the memory may be less relevant than perceptions and meaning. On the other hand, it is harmful for patients to believe they have had traumatic experiences when they have not. Therapy that creates or reinforces false beliefs of trauma may have negative consequences for clients and for third parties.

14

Childhood Trauma Remembered

Current controversies about recovered memory have led professional societies in North America, Europe, Australia and New Zealand to produce position papers on the topic. Although there are certain differences in content and emphasis among them, there is agreement on several points: (1) traumatic events are usually remembered in part or in whole; (2) traumatic memories may be forgotten, then remembered at some later time; (3) illusory memories can also occur. A general consensus is that at present unresolved scientific questions about the mechanisms of remembering and forgetting exist. Finally, professionals agree that there is no standard procedure for establishing the veracity or accuracy of memories in individual cases without evidence or corroboration; therefore, differences of opinion may result among therapists when evaluating the validity of individual reports. While a therapist in an individual clinical situation may develop a hypothesis about the validity of the report, it is ultimately up to the patient, not the therapist, to come to a conclusion about what happened in the past.

Clinicians are advised to be cognizant of these issues and to adhere to recognized principles of therapy. Some specific practices or procedures are outside the standard of care or are potentially risky. For example, one should never assume that certain symptoms or symptom clusters in and of themselves indicate a trauma or abuse history. The diagnoses of Posttraumatic Stress Disorder and Acute Stress Disorder are only given when the patient reports a history of a traumatic stressor as well as the requisite number of trauma-related symptoms. All other psychological symptoms, even those commonly noted in trauma survivors, may have a variety of etiologies. Suggesting to clients that they must have had traumatic experiences, or encouraging clients to imagine that they were traumatized without a reported history are not only contraindicated, but may promote the development of illusory memories. Hypnosis or amytal interviews that are conducted for the purpose of uncovering past experiences and that contain suggestions regarding possible trauma may also produce false memories. Thus neither procedure, when used, should contain suggestions that affect post hypnotic or post amytal memories. Furthermore, clinicians should be aware that when a client is hypnotized or given amytal, they may not thereafter, in some U.S. states, be allowed to testify in any kind of civil or criminal legal proceeding.

Additional Reading for Section IV

Berliner, L. & Briere, J. (in press). Trauma, memory, and clinical practice. In L. Williams (Ed.). *Trauma and memory.* Thousand Oaks, CA: Sage.

This chapter reviews relevant literature on the impact of trauma on memory, the fallibility of memory and therapy practices with regard to memories. Implications for practice are discussed.

Briere, J. (1996). *Therapy with adults molested as children.* New York: Springer.

This is a revised edition of an earlier, seminal book on treatment with adults who have been severely abused. There are updated sections on treatment with specific reference to the handling of memory issues.

Courtois, C. A. (1997). Guidelines for the treatment of adults abused or possibly abused. *American Journal of Psychotherapy,* 51, pp. 497-510.

A set of guidelines for therapy practice where recovered memory is at issue.

15

The International Society for Traumatic Stress Studies

Additional Reading for Section IV

Courtois, C. A. (1997). Informed clinical practice and the standard of care: Proposed guidelines for the treatment of adults who report delayed memories of childhood trauma. In J. D. Read and D. S. Lindsay (Eds.). *Recollections of trauma: Scientific research and clinical practice*, pp. 337-361. New York: Plenum.

This chapter identifies key issues in the treatment of adult survivors who report childhood abuse or recall abuse in therapy. It provides specific guidelines for therapy practice.

Dalenberg, C. & Carlson, E. (in press). Ethical issues in the treatment of the recovered memory trauma victims and patients with false memories of trauma. In S. Buckey (Ed.). *The comprehensive textbook of ethics and law in the practice of psychology*. New York: Plenum.

This chapter describes the various clinical situations where memory or lack of memory for trauma becomes an issue. It identifies the various and complex dilemmas that clinicians face, and suggests therapeutic approaches in light of these dilemmas.

16

Individuals sometimes have vague or incomplete memories about childhood abuse, or become concerned about a possible abuse history based on related childhood memories, information from others or current symptoms. Understandably, in many cases, they want clarification about whether they were abused, and if so the nature and extent of the experience. When clients raise these concerns in psychotherapy, they are an appropriate therapeutic focus. Therapists can provide an opportunity for patients to examine the basis for their suspicions, consider alternative explanations, learn about the various abuse and nonabuse related origins of psychological distress, and become informed about the ways that memory works and can be altered or distorted. Patients who wish to explore their past may choose to talk with family members or others, and obtain school, medical and counseling records. They may want to record their relevant thoughts or feelings over this period. This information may become part of the therapeutic process. Therapists should refrain from confirming or disconfirming the validity of memories and instead assist patients in arriving at their own conclusions.

Clients sometimes consider taking certain actions with accused offenders and/or family members during the course of therapy for childhood abuse. These actions may include confronting offenders, informing others about the abuse, restricting, and in some cases severing family relationships, or taking legal action against an alleged perpetrator. It is appropriate for therapists to explore with clients the potential positive and negative impacts that different choices may have on psychological and social functioning. It is not appropriate for therapists to instruct or pressure clients to take a particular course of action.

Therapists treating clients who have suffered trauma or report a trauma history have a duty to promote a therapeutic environment that is supportive regarding the trauma, but acknowledges that memory is imperfect. Clients must not be discouraged from revealing and talking about traumatic experiences because of therapist discomfort with the traumatic material or because of undue skepticism about client reports. However, it may be advisable, especially with delayed recall of memories for events that occurred in the remote past, that therapists convey information about the reconstructive nature of memory.

Therapists and patients need not be deterred from exploring trauma histories; however remembering for its own sake should not be a goal of therapy. Effective therapy for trauma helps patients resolve trauma-specific symptoms, leads to an accurate and meaningful interpretation of the traumatic event and allows the experience to be put in perspective.

While reviewing past traumatic experiences is often an important component of the preferred treatment approach, this does not preclude a correspondent treatment emphasis on the present. In treating adult survivors of childhood trauma, the ultimate goal is to address the enduring impact of childhood trauma so that patients can improve their current and future lives. Whether or not there is traumatic material under discussion, improving current functioning is ultimately the major goal of treatment. While childhood traumatic experiences may always remain an important part of a survivor's identity, after successful treatment survivors are likely to be facing forward rather than looking back.

Additional Reading for Section IV

Knapp, S. & VandeCreek, L. (1996). Risk management for psychologists: Treating patients who recover lost memories of childhood abuse. *Professional Psychology: Research and Practice*, 27, pp. 452-459.

This paper recommends a series of basic precautions that practitioners can take to reduce legal risks with clients including maintaining boundaries, obtaining informed consent, seeking consultation, and maintaining careful documentation.

Knapp, S. & VandeCreek, L. (1997). *Treating patients with memories of abuse: Legal risk management.* Washington, DC: American Psychological Association Press.

A volume devoted to treatment issues that therapists should attend to as legal risk management.

Read, J. D. & Lindsay, D. S. (Eds). (1997). *Recollections of trauma: Scientific evidence and clinical practice.* New York: Plenum.

An edited book of papers and commentaries from the 1996 NATO conference of the same title.

17

SECTION V
APPLICATION OF THE CURRENT SCIENTIFIC KNOWLEDGE
BASE TO FORENSIC PRACTICE

T he topic of recovered memories of childhood abuse is one that often arouses a strong emotional response. For one thing, it is very difficult to accept the fact that adults sometimes fail to protect or actually inflict harm on children, especially if those adults are family members. It goes against our moral grain and our need for a sense of security and comfort with the social order. Also, the whole issue of child abuse is very difficult to discuss. In fact, until very recently, there hasn't been a public forum in which this topic could receive full public discussion and consideration.

Another related way to understand the strong emotional response to the topic of recovered memories of childhood trauma is to realize that because of society's persistent commitment to justice, there is a strong universal commitment to identify perpetrators of child abuse accurately. It is as important to ensure that innocent people not be accused of such reprehensible behavior as it is that victims see their perpetrators held responsible. This concern for justice is complicated by ambiguities inherent in situations in which the validity of the memory of abuse might be called into question. Thus the emotional outrage about childhood abuse must be tempered when there is concern that a recovered memory of childhood trauma might be false and might result in someone being falsely accused. Perhaps nowhere is the strong emotional response to the topic of recovered memories of childhood abuse so apparent as in the legal arena. In the effort of our legal and judicial systems to balance both the rights of alleged victims as well as the rights of alleged perpetrators, the current scientific controversy concerning recovered memory has received considerable forensic attention. This concern has led to legal initiatives that have been designed to broaden both the protections available to alleged victims who have recovered memories of prior abuse as well as protections for alleged perpetrators who have been falsely accused.

The laws against child abuse have the purpose of providing legal mechanisms for protecting children from harm within their families, protecting the community from convicted criminals, exacting retribution for violation of the law or obtaining monetary compensation for intentional harmful or negligent acts. Different countries have different types of legal systems that are governed by legal principles, rules and precedents. Under the adversarial legal system that exists in the common law countries of England, Scotland, Ireland, Canada, Australia and the United States, the government or private party bringing the lawsuit must prove the allegations before individuals lose custody or access to their children, their liberty or their assets.

Mental health practitioners may become involved in legal actions in a variety of ways. One circumstance involves reporting suspected child abuse to government entities. In the United States, Canada and some Australian states, mental health providers are legally required to report suspected child abuse to the child protection or criminal justice authorities. In many other common law countries, suspected child abuse may be reported to government agencies which are empowered to conduct investigations and intervene. Other countries have nongovernment agencies or designated individuals who receive reports and carry out interventions. In those countries with formal child protection laws or systems, practitioners are generally granted some degree of immunity for making good faith reports. Practitioners should be familiar with their specific obligations and protections. In the United States, although mandated reporters such as psychiatrists or psychologists have legal immunity, there have recently been cases in which mandated reporters have been civilly sued or reported to licensing boards by alleged perpetrators.

Most jurisdictions that mandate child abuse reporting do not require reports about childhood abuse revealed by adult patients. However, there may be an obligation where the practitioner has knowledge that another child is currently at risk. In countries or jurisdictions with agencies that receive reports, practitioners may choose to make a report because they believe that official inquiry is necessary for the protection of a child. Familiarity with the relevant statutes and implications of reporting is a professional responsibility.

Additional Reading for Section V

Bowman, C. G. & Mertz. (1996). A dangerous direction: Legal intervention in sexual abuse survivor therapy. *Harvard Law Review*, **109**, pp. 551-563.

This is a summary article of legal issues surrounding memory recovery and therapy.

Brown D., Scheflin A. W. & Hammond, D. C. (1998). *Memory, trauma treatment, and the law.* New York: W. W. Norton.

This book was written for clinicians, researchers, attorneys and judges to provide a critical review of memory research, trauma treatment and relevant legal cases.

Knapp, S. & VandeCreek, L. (1996). Risk management for psychologists: Treating patients who recover lost memories of childhood abuse. *Professional Psychology: Research and Practice*, **27**, pp. 452-459.

This paper recommends a series of basic precautions that practitioners can take to reduce legal risks with clients including maintaining boundaries, obtaining informed consent, seeking consultation and maintaining careful documentation.

19

Additional Reading for Section V
Pope, K. S. & Brown, L. S.
(1996). *Recovered memories of
abuse: Assessment, therapy,
forensics.* Washington, DC:
American Psychological
Association.

*This book was written for clini-
cians and expert witnesses working with clients who report recovered memories of childhood
abuse. Forensic issues for therapists providing treatment and for
forensic expert witnesses are
addressed.*

Practitioners may also become witnesses in criminal or civil legal actions.
They may be fact witnesses because they have information that is relevant
and admissible. In such cases their testimony may be compelled by subpoe-
na and the patient-practitioner privilege may be abrogated. Or, practitioners may be involved as expert witnesses. Experts for plaintiffs or defendants
may be called to testify about a particular patient because they have conducted a forensic evaluation or reviewed case materials. They may be asked
to give opinions about whether the traumatic event occurred and about the
psychological damage that has resulted from the traumatic event(s). They
may also testify as to whether a practitioner met the standard of care in situations where professionals are sued for malpractice or are reported to
licensing or professional bodies. Sometimes experts testify about relevant
scientific and clinical knowledge without specific reference to a particular
individual.

Several new areas of law have emerged in recent years that directly relate to
questions of memory and may involve practitioners as fact or expert witnesses. For example, many jurisdictions through legislation or case law have
extended the statutes of limitations (the period of time by which a legal
action must commence) for child abuse criminal prosecutions or civil damage suits. This has occurred in response to increased awareness that some
victims remember their experiences long after the fact, or only belatedly
recognize the link between current dysfunction and past victimization.
Statutes of limitations exist in recognition that over time memory fades,
evidence may be lost, witnesses may disappear or die and as a result, a
defendant's right to an adequate defense and a fair trial may be compro-
mised. These limits on the time elapsed between the perpetration of a damaging act and the filing of a suit by an alleged victim to claim damages for
such an act may be extended by legal interpretation or by new legislation
based on the "delayed discovery rule." This legal principle recognizes that
there are circumstances where it is not possible for a victim to know about
a crime or a negligent act and its harmful effects until the statute of limitations has expired. In these cases, the statute of limitations does not start to
run until the time that a victim remembers or recognizes the harm.

Another relevant legal development in the United States has been malpractice suits against therapists initiated by third parties who are not clients or otherwise participants in their therapeutic relationship, but claim to have been harmed by the therapists' actions. Under traditional malpractice law, therapists can be sued for malpractice *only* by their clients. For example, some legal actions have been brought by clients who claim that their therapist exerted undo pressure on them to recall previous trauma or who initially accused a family member of childhood abuse, later retracted such accusations, and currently hold the therapist responsible for promoting the initial accusations. Recently, however, some courts have allowed cases to proceed in which "third parties" — usually a member of the client's family — claim that the therapist has committed malpractice by engaging in activities that may have led clients to develop false memories about the third party. These cases have proceeded even when the adult client does not wish to bring an action against the therapist and has not taken any legal action against the alleged perpetrator. In addition to law suits, third parties have also been successful in making complaints to disciplinary boards that have resulted in restrictions on practice or the loss of license to practice. In many of these cases, the patients themselves have not supported the actions and have not believed they were harmed by the therapy. One result of these developments is that some therapists have become increasingly reluctant to address their patients' traumatic memories, even when such therapeutic attention seems necessary.

Practitioners who conduct forensic evaluations or serve as expert witnesses must adhere to the professional standards of practice in their respective disciplines. For example, forensic practice differs from clinical practice in terms of the role of the practitioner, the purpose of the professional activity and the generally accepted methods and approaches. Forensic evaluations are intended for use in legal decision-making, although the evaluator does not always testify in court. Such evaluations are ordinarily requested by lawyers or courts. Patients are informed of the nature of the evaluation and agree to the release of information to designated parties. Practitioners generally assume a neutral stance and rely on a variety of sources of information in addition to patient report. In addition, experts must be familiar with the current scientific and clinical knowledge about trauma and memory.

Additional Reading for Section V

Tracy, C. E., Morrison, J. C., McLaughlin, M. A., Bratspies, R. M., & Ford, D. W. (1996). Brief of the International Society for Traumatic Stress Studies and the Family Violence & Sexual Assault Institute as *Amici Curiae* in support of the state. No. 95-429; State of New Hampshire v. Joel Hungerford; State of New Hampshire v. John Morahan; Appeal of an Order of the Hillsborough County Superior Court, Northern District, Pursuant to RSA 606:10; In the State of New Hampshire Supreme Court, 1996 term, July session.

This "friend of the court" legal document is concerned with the admissibility of testimony concerning recovered memories about childhood sexual abuse, and more specifically, with the court's recognition of traumatic amnesia as a well-documented symptom that may result from severe trauma.

21

The International Society for Traumatic Stress Studies

This is a field that is rapidly expanding and new research findings are regularly reported in peer-reviewed journals and at professional meetings. Although there is no requirement that experts be academic researchers, since expertise can be a function of extensive experience, clinical experts would do well to be aware of the general principles and facts that are accepted by the relevant scientific community.

It is important for practitioners to understand that laws and legislation related to statute of limitations, the application of delayed discovery and third party law suits are state specific and may change frequently. It is recommended that practitioners consult their malpractice carriers for information regarding the laws in their states.

Childhood Trauma Remembered

SUMMARY AND CONCLUSIONS

Childhood trauma involving interpersonal violence occurs frequently and plays an important role in later adult maladaptive functioning. Correspondent with a general increase in trauma-focused scholarship has been an increase in knowledge about delayed recall of traumatic events and about memory processes relevant to an understanding of traumatic memories. We know that people forget childhood traumas and that this is not limited to people in treatment or to people whose trauma is sexual abuse. We also know that people can accurately recall memories of documented childhood trauma that they report having previously forgotten, and that a wide range of triggers seem to be associated with these memories. Most memory recovery appears to be precipitated in situations that include cues that are similar to the original trauma and does not occur as a direct result of psychotherapy. However, it is possible, and indeed many would argue likely, that therapists who fail to conform to accepted standards of practice may promote a "recovered memory" of an event that never occurred.

23

While there is some evidence that recovered memories of childhood abuse can be as accurate as never-forgotten memories of childhood abuse, there is also evidence that memory is reconstructive and imperfect, that people can make very glaring errors in memory, that people are suggestible under some circumstances to social influence or persuasion when reporting memories for past events and that at least under some circumstances inaccurate memories can be strongly believed and convincingly described. While traumatic memories may be different than ordinary memories, we currently do not have conclusive scientific consensus on this issue. Likewise, it is not currently known how traumatic memories are forgotten or later recovered. These are all fundamental questions that have stimulated a great deal of important research on the memory process in general and on traumatic memories in particular.

Trauma-focused approaches to assessment and treatment have also promoted a sophisticated articulation of the purpose, process and standards of care. While competent therapists must provide a therapeutic environment in which recovered memories of childhood trauma can be addressed, they must also recognize that memory is fallible and that certain therapeutic approaches may increase the likelihood of distortion or confabulation. Professionals agree that there is no standard procedure for establishing the accuracy of recovered memories in individual cases and that in clinical practice, it is up to the patient to come to his or her own conclusions about whether or not he or she was previously traumatized and about the specific details of such events. Professionals also agree that it is not the role of therapists to instruct or pressure patients to take a particular course of action with accused offenders and/or family members during the course of therapy for childhood abuse.

There is a strong commitment in contemporary society to accurately identify perpetrators of child abuse, and it is as important that innocent people not be accused of such a crime as it is that victims see their perpetrators held responsible. In the efforts of our legal and judicial systems to balance the rights and protections of both alleged victims and alleged perpetrators, the current scientific controversy concerning recovered memory has received considerable forensic attention and has led to a number of legal initiatives. Both alleged perpetrators and those held responsible for alleged false accusations, including therapists, have been targets of legal action. While there is currently not a standard protocol for the determination of the validity of individual reports of recovered memories of childhood trauma, our current scientific knowledge base provides consensual and balanced information that can be essential in forensic practice.

This pamphlet was developed by the International Society for Traumatic Stress Studies to inform the general public about the complex and important issues that are involved in the current controversy about memories of childhood sexual abuse. We address the questions of childhood trauma, traumatic memory, the memory process, clinical issues and forensic implications pertaining to this controversy. We have tried to present a balanced review of these issues. As an international organization dedicated to promoting the best research and education in this field, we believe it essential that people who grapple with this controversial topic be equipped with the most accurate and comprehensive information possible. We hope that this pamphlet has served this purpose.

Childhood Trauma Remembered

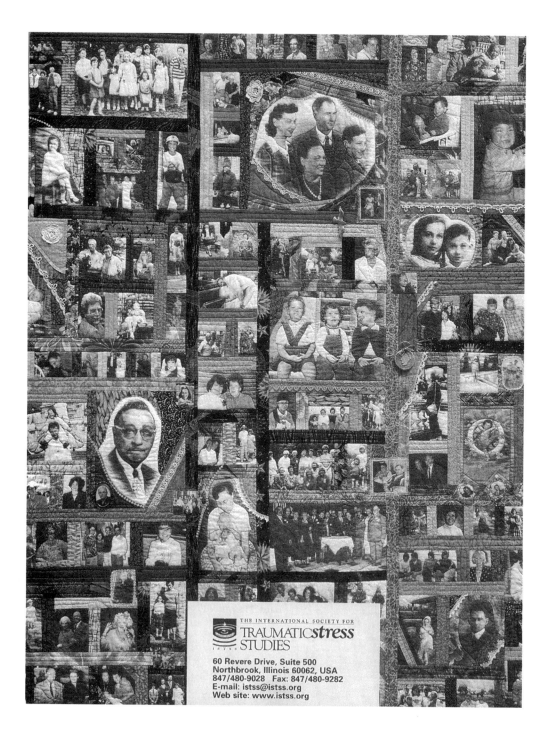

THE INTERNATIONAL SOCIETY FOR
TRAUMATIC**stress**
STUDIES

60 Revere Drive, Suite 500
Northbrook, Illinois 60062, USA
847/480-9028 Fax: 847/480-9282
E-mail: istss@istss.org
Web site: www.istss.org

Index